Coronary Thermodilution

Pitt O. Lim

Coronary Thermodilution

Unravelling Angina with Invasive Cardiology

Springer

Pitt O. Lim
Department of Cardiology
St George's Hospital
London, UK

ISBN 978-3-032-10733-6 ISBN 978-3-032-10734-3 (eBook)
https://doi.org/10.1007/978-3-032-10734-3

This Springer imprint is published by the registered company Springer Nature Switzerland AG
The registered company address is: Gewerbestrasse 11, 6330 Cham, Switzerland

Dedicated to my parents, Margaret
and Joseph,
and my family, Doreen and Serena Leigh

Materiam Superabat Opus

Preface

Imagine that it's possible to know,
The actual coronary blood flow.
Would this not remove all doubt,
If chest pain is the heart's shout?
(British Journal of Cardiology 2022;29:67-72)

August 31, 2024, was a momentous day. The 47th European Society of Cardiology (ESC) Congress returned to London after a 9-year hiatus and was in full swing at ExCel Conference Centre, which is in the Royal Docks of East London, next to the Custom House Station, this time easily accessible by the new Elizabeth Line that was unveiled by the 96-year-old Queen Elizabeth II, 837 days before. In the main auditorium at 2.00 pm in the afternoon, Vijay Kunadian on behalf of the ESC upgraded to *Recommendation Class I Level B Evidence* invasive cardiology management in its guidelines for angina with non-obstructive coronary arteries (ANOCA) [1], formerly known as cardiac syndrome X, from IIa/b C in 2013 [2]. ESC recognises the complexity of angina, with threefold characterisation of *coronary vasodilatory capacity*, *vasoreactivity* and *resistance* with the aid of acetylcholine (ACh) [3]. In addition, ESC admits, as do researchers, that this is a fast-moving field with new indices and techniques around the corner [4]. However, in laypersons' term, cardiac catheter-based investigation of ANOCA has just become standard of care (SOC) in those with persistent symptoms. This is following the footsteps of radial access, aspirin and statin use, coronary angioplasty for myocardial infarction, coronary artery bypass grafting (CABG), etc.; most ideas from seeding to fruition take on a journey of 25 years. Thus, by 2034, coronary physiology study will undoubtedly be mainstream.

Why is this book written by someone from St George's Hospital? Brand St George's, in its long history since 1733, initially sited at Hyde Park Corner, before moving to Tooting in 1980, is an early adopter of new ideas and technologies. In cardiology, angina pectoris was first described by William Heberden the Elder (1710–1801) from there in 1768, its link to coronary artery disease was also first postulated by Edward Jenner (1749–1823) there, and extensive research on ANOCA was undertaken there, including the collaborative formulation of the ACh bolus dosing now adopted by ESC. The ENCORE-Stuttgart-London Sequence was introduced by Juan Carlos Kaski to me, which I adopted for use at St George's with Peter Ong on March 12, 2013 [5]. Ong was Kaski's visiting fellow from Stuttgart, and Kaski was trained by Attilio Maseri (1935–2021). Maseri was a giant in ANOCA and had used ACh to elicit coronary artery spasm both at the epicardial and microvascular levels. Most of today's leaders in coronary pathophysiology can be traced back to him. Maseri was puzzled by ANOCA without provocable spasm, and without flow reduction demonstrable by coronary flow reserve, i.e. the flow more than doubling to meet demand (CFR $\geq$ 2.0—K. Lance Gould 1974). This book hopefully will provide some pointers to the readers in untangling this *Gouldian knot* of ANOCA with the emerging technique of continuous thermodilution.

I had the good fortune of meeting Hein J. J. Wellens (1935–2020) in Stockholm at the 62nd (old count from 1952) ESC Congress on August 30, 2010—his description in 1982 of an ischaemic electrocardiographic pattern signifying high risk acute coronary syndrome, that involving the left anterior descending artery, the Wellens' pattern, gives a sense of urgency for action, its recognition continues to save lives, and it is an easy attributory eponymous code to use [6]. In my 20-year career in invasive cardiology at St George's, I have dealt with countless patients with Wellens' syndrome. I have undertaken over 10,000 procedures to date, which means that I am an expert by Malcolm Gladwell's standard, and my observations in measuring the absolute coronary flow in selected cases had readily been accepted by reputable peer-reviewed journals, suggesting that there is an interest and a knowledge gap in this topic.

This project started with the first email to Hexacath (Rueil-Malmaison, France) dated July 27, 2021, enquiring about the RayFlow infusion microcatheter, which is required for continuous thermodilution to allow absolute volumetric coronary flow to be estimated. I am thankful to Yannick Giraud who was ever so helpful, culminating with my first case on September 8, 2021.

This was 61-year-old woman with ANOCA and hypertension, who developed severe and diffuse coronary artery spasm with ACh 100 ug, but surprisingly, her flow increased by 90% from baseline, and she had a CFR of 2.6, which was 1.8 with the established technique of bolus thermodilution. Endothelial dysfunction turns out to be far more complicated than is generally thought and taught. It is not just about nitric oxide which has dominated and slanted the field. This book traces the folk etymology and history of ACh and looks under the bonnet of bolus thermodilution to understand its strengths and weaknesses. Based on current methodology this patient would be told that she has spasm in her artery, started on a calcium channel blocker, and the cardiologist moves on to the next patient. Yet, patients such as her will keep coming back again and again with angina. Are we missing something?

Coronary physiology in the individual setting is still at the early phase; principally there is a need to address *three philosophical questions*. **First**, a diagnostic test based on a ratio captures all, that is, sensitive but lacks specificity, used because it is convenient, expedient, and due to a lack of precise methodology, for instance, the left ventricular ejection fraction (EF). Many patients with a low EF, including athletes, live a normal life. The brain natriuretic peptide (BNP), the absolute value of which is both sensitive and specific, has led to a proliferation of acronyms; heart failure (HF) with reduced, moderate, preserved and supranormal EF (HFrEF,

HFmrEF, HFpEF and HFsnEF). Heart failure physiologically is difficult to pin down unless an invasive pressure-volume loop is constructed for each patient, which is not feasible when dealing with a large population.

This applies too to one cause of ANOCA, the coronary microvascular dysfunction (CMD), defined by coronary flow reserve (Gouldian CFR < 2, failure of the coronary circulation to double its flow to keep up with demand), which is a ratio between maximal hyperaemic and basal flows. There lies the problem: what is basal flow? A naturally low one that is due to a disease process in the microvasculature, or an adaptively high one when there is diffuse small vessel epicardial coronary artery disease, or simply due to procedural stress, or drug treatment? CFR works in epidemiological studies because it is inclusive. But when applied to the individual patient at hand, it can be imprecise, as noted by Bernard de Bruyne [7], one half of a duet of pioneers, with Nico H. J. Pijls, defined modern coronary physiology, which included the introduction of coronary continuous thermodilution, the subject of this book. They showcased this technique in their 19th Aalst-Einthoven Coronary Physiology Course in Belgium on November 19–20, 2015, which I had the honour to attend. Compared with CFR, the fractional flow reserve (FFR) which was also introduced to the world by de Bruyne and Pijls, used to assess a *fixed stricture* in the coronary artery, is incredibly reproducible in practice. The question is, does ANOCA's flow restriction behave like a static "stricture", or is it a different beast altogether?

Second, ANOCA is a broad term, akin to anaemia; it has multiple aetiologies. Is it due to a structural state which is persistent, or a functional phase that is subject to change? My practice by default is set out to prove conclusively that an ANOCA patient has a normal heart with the protocol described in these pages, and reassure. Unfortunately, nearly all of those with persistent symptoms have demonstrable pathology. Much of what is written here is conjectural, as assessing the absolute coronary flow is like charting a new continent. There is also the dilemma of *symptomatology-pathology disconnect* which is still poorly understood. A well-conducted trial of an endothelin-A antagonist, Zibotentan 10mg daily in patients with CMD and genetic predisposition for excess endothelin did not alter symptoms, despite objective measures in increased blood flow on cardiac imaging [8]. Perhaps this is related to the fallacy that *association* does not equate *causation* as per Koch's threefold postulates.

Third, coronary haemodynamics are subject to beat-to-beat change in values, not unlike the definition of what is hypertension. The same ESC Congress updated the level by which blood pressure should be lowered (< 130 mmHg), and its treatment threshold is reduced too in the presence of comorbidities [9]. Interestingly, outcome is known to be "U-shaped"; this risk does not *plateau* until a systolic blood pressure of about 100 mmHg, as observed in people who lived up in the mountains on a subsistence diet, where their blood pressure does not rise with age [10]. Thus, the coronary circulation, though unique in some ways, is not disconnected from the systemic circulation; hence the definition of what constitutes abnormality is equally uncertain. The heart muscle contracts during systole and myocardial perfusion mostly occur during diastole, but the driving pressure is not at the diastolic "trough" pressure as it is measured, but nearer to the mean systemic blood pressure by convention. Although coronary flow starts immediately after closure of the aortic valve, corresponding to the second heart sound, and the arterial dicrotic notch. Continuing throughout diastole, well until the mitral valve closes and before the aortic valve reopens, when the heart starts to contract - the isovolumetric contraction phase. To the purist, this whole-diastole integrated coronary perfusion pressure (CPP) which requires simultaneous aortic and left ventricular pressure monitoring, is the area bounded by the 2 pressure-time curves, is the genuine gradient that drives coronary perfusion. This is used as a research tool to calculate the "diastolic" FFR to assess the myocardial bridge, a *dynamic* coronary constriction, where the traditional FFR fails. However, all these complexities of *pressure-derived flow surrogates* can be bypassed, in one fell swoop, by measuring *actual* coronary flow. On the other hand, the systolic blood pressure is more prognostic than the diastolic blood pressure; it is what other organs see, and when this is partially transmitted to the coronary circulation, it causes coronary hypertension which increases microvascular resistance.

This book is not a compendium of published works; neither does it contain an exhaustive review of the topic at hand. Books are usually outdated by the time they are printed on paper. Instead, it reflects my personal considered opinion reading much of the materials which are hard to digest; nobody can be an expert all the way from biochemistry to experimental physiology, least a clinician at heart. What I can make sense of is written for a wide audience, from the expert patient to the diehard coronary physiologist, readers can be selective in choosing pages that interest them.

The three overarching principles followed in this tome are: (1) image focus. A picture is worth a thousand words; (2) succinct and simple English with present-is-pleasant tense framing where natural, while treading a fine line between clarity and pedantry. To quote Woodrow Wilson (1856–1924), "If I am to speak for ten minutes, I need a week for preparation; if fifteen minutes, three days; if half an hour, two days; if an hour, I am ready now"; and (3) historical context, as much as possible, tracing the origin of ideas and how they come about. This immeasurably aided the understanding of why things are done in certain ways, and if there are better ways to do them. I have incorporated within these pages tips and tricks I have acquired over the years which are helpful to me, and safe for the patients, especially the distal radial and slender techniques, the latter using the smallest of catheters possible, as many ANOCA patients have challenging and vasoreactive vascular access.

This book has 11 chapters; the first describes an abridged history of cardiology relevant to coronary physiology, its assessment, and principle and practice of continuous thermodilution. Each of the next nine chapters has a theme. I have included myocardial infarction patients whom I had treated with the stent-free approach of drug-coated balloon, my third area of interest. The last chapter synthesises the overall thrust of this book. A total of 42 cases are described in detail. The chapters were sequentially written over the course of a year; inevitably there will be repetitions, but this will only serve to reinforce recurrent encounters and to familiarise with new concepts. In some cases, the interpretation may have shifted. One clear example is the reason why flow falls with low-dose ACh in the absence of epicardial vasospasm, only to rise again with high-dose ACh—the biphasic ACh response. Is this microvascular spasm that can be overcome by ACh, or something else?

I owe a debt of gratitude to all the patients I had the privilege to care for, who ever so kindly allowed their case histories to be described in these pages. Also, I am thankful for the support from my colleagues, who are too numerous to list here, but as a shorthand, all the staff in the Department of Cardiology, who made this book a possibility. Last but not least, I would like to thank Enhui Yong, my assistant for the last four years, who was instrumental in the success of the continuous thermodilution programme at St George's Hospital.

London, UK
28 August 2025

Pitt O. Lim

References

1. Vrints C, Andreotti F, Koskinas KC, Rossello X, Adamo M, Ainslie J, et al. 2024 ESC Guidelines for the management of chronic coronary syndromes. Eur Heart J. 2024. https://doi.org/10.1093/eurheartj/ehae177.
2. Task Force M, Montalescot G, Sechtem U, Achenbach S, Andreotti F, Arden C, et al. 2013 ESC guidelines on the management of stable coronary artery disease: the Task Force on the management of stable coronary artery disease of the European Society of Cardiology. Eur Heart J. 2013;34(38):2949–3003. https://doi.org/10.1093/eurheartj/eht296.
3. Lim PO. Angina: The Ischemic Triad. Am J Cardiol. 2024;223:118–9. https://doi.org/10.1016/j.amjcard.2024.05.023.
4. Sinha A, Rahman H, Demir OM, De Silva K, Morgan HP, LiKamWa ME, et al. Microvascular resistance reserve predicts myocardial ischemia and response to therapy in patients with Angina and nonobstructive coronary arteries. Circulation: Cardiovasc Interv.0(0):e014477. https://doi.org/10.1161/CIRCINTERVENTIONS.124.014477.
5. Ong P, Athanasiadis A, Borgulya G, Vokshi I, Bastiaenen R, Kubik S, et al. Clinical usefulness, angiographic characteristics, and safety evaluation of intracoronary acetylcholine provocation testing among 921 consecutive white patients with unobstructed coronary arteries. Circulation. 2014;129(17):1723–30. https://doi.org/10.1161/CIRCULATIONAHA.113.004096.
6. de Zwaan C, Bar FW, Wellens HJ. Characteristic electrocardiographic pattern indicating a critical stenosis high in left anterior descending coronary artery in patients admitted because of impending myocardial infarction. Am Heart J. 1982;103(4 Pt 2):730–6. https://doi.org/10.1016/0002-8703(82)90480-x.
7. Mahendiran T, Wilgenhof A, De Bruyne B. The Elusiveness of "Rest": The Challenges of Assessing Resting Coronary Physiology. Circulation. 2025;152(3):147–9. https://doi.org/10.1161/CIRCULATIONAHA.125.074343.
8. Morrow A, Young R, Abraham GR, Hoole S, Greenwood JP, Arnold JR, et al. Zibotentan in Microvascular Angina: A Randomized, Placebo-Controlled, Crossover Trial. Circulation.0(0). https://doi.org/10.1161/CIRCULATIONAHA.124.069901.
9. McEvoy JW, McCarthy CP, Bruno RM, Brouwers S, Canavan MD, Ceconi C, et al. 2024 ESC Guidelines for the management of elevated blood pressure and hypertension: Developed by the task force on the management of elevated blood pressure and hypertension of the European Society of Cardiology (ESC) and endorsed by the European Society of Endocrinology (ESE) and the European Stroke Organisation (ESO). European Heart Journal. 2024. https://doi.org/10.1093/eurheartj/ehae178.
10. He J, Tell GS, Tang YC, Mo PS, He GQ. Effect of migration on blood pressure: the Yi People Study. Epidemiology. 1991;2(2):88–97. https://doi.org/10.1097/00001648-199103000-00002.

Contents

Part II

Part I

Chapter 1
Crowned Heart

Abstract The heart wears its blood vessels like a crown; hence the term "coronary", first used in Renaissance Padua 500 years ago. Angina from obstructive coronary artery disease was described 250 years later in Enlightenment London. Yet the era of coronary physiology is quite recent, dating back only 50 years to the mid-1970s. The key insight was that, when an obstructive coronary artery is unable to double its blood flow to the subtended myocardium during stress, the coronary stenosis is physiologically significant and likely to cause ischaemia. Because direct coronary flow measurement was impossible in humans, clinicians instead relied on a pressure surrogate, the fractional flow reserve, to assess the severity of coronary lesions during hyperaemia, a state when flow and pressure are proportional. However, it is now clear that, even in the absence of blocked coronary arteries, cardiac ischaemia can still occur, purportedly due to coronary microvascular dysfunction, a condition that affects the small vessels of the heart. This realisation, which marks the next phase of coronary physiology, has been facilitated by the advent of bolus thermodilution, while continuous thermodilution offers a highly reliable absolute coronary flow measurement, crucial for unravelling the diverse mechanisms of angina with non-obstructive coronary arteries.

1.1 Historical Background

The naming of the arteries that supply the heart is somewhat incongruous. The artery serving the brain is termed cerebral, that of the spleen splenic, and that of the liver hepatic; by this convention, the heart's artery should be cardiac, but it is not. This divergence traces back to Andreas Vesalius (1514–1564), who was a Flemish doctor born in Brussels on December 31, 1514, at that time part of the Habsburg Netherlands [1]. He began his medical education at the University of Leuven in 1530, 15 miles east of Brussels, where human dissection was not permitted. In 1533, he left for Paris, studying under Jacques Dubois (Jacobus Sylvius, 1478–1555) and Jean Fernel (1497–1558), where limited human dissections took place, typically once a year and usually performed by barber surgeons and assistants. Dubois was a Galenic scholar whose Latinised surname *forest* has a namesake in Leiden

P. O. Lim, *Coronary Thermodilution*,
https://doi.org/10.1007/978-3-032-10734-3_1

who gave the brain its Sylvian fissure, which is just above the temporal lobe, but he named many blood vessels, including the femoral or thigh artery which became the preferred vascular access to the heart. Fernel coined the word, *physiologia*; it is a combination of physis (nature, φύσις) and logos (study, λόγος): the study of nature or normal functioning of the body. Fernel systematised physiology within his medical triad that included pathology and therapy, a framework that became standard in medical teaching [2]. Thus, Vesalius' two teachers provided terms used in this book, but one would severely condemn him later.

Due to religious fervour and political unrest in France in 1537, Vesalius returned to Leuven where he reworked with Galenic lens, the Latin translation of Ninth Book of Rhazes (Persian physician, Abu Bakr Muhammad Ibn Zakariya Al-Rāzī, 865–925) as his first published work in February 1537, printed locally [3, 4], before he relocated to Padua, which was part of the Republic of Venice, to continue his medical studies. He qualified shortly thereafter, and within the same year in December, at age 23, he was appointed Professor of Surgery and Anatomy at the University of Padua [1, 5]. Altogether, he studied medicine for 7 years across three domains at a time when the concept of a "country" as a centralised nation-state did not exist.

Vesalius's later more sympathetic reading of Al-Rāzī's medical compendium critical of Galen inevitably shaped his worldview, emboldening him to challenge convention where he saw inconsistencies [6]. Al-Rāzī was a vocal critic of the Galenic cornerstone of bloodletting and noted that when applied to patients with chest pain, those with weak pulses, or having vomited blood, death came soon after the treatment. Bloodletting persisted in Europe until late nineteenth century; notable deaths included those of John Keats (1795–1821) at 25 in Italy, as treatment for tuberculosis, and Lord Byron (1788–1824) at 36 to treat his probable malarial fever in Greece. Six years after beginning his lectureship, in 1543, Vesalius published his magnum opus, *De Humani Corporis Fabrica* (On the Fabric of the Human Body) [7]. In Book III of VII, page 299, he wrote:

> But from the same trunk, from which the great artery ascending from the heart is sent out, another artery arises, which, although it should be counted among the lesser arteries, brings the greatest benefit to the heart itself.
>
> This artery itself, as soon as it arises, gives off two slender branches, which, *in the manner of a crown, encircle the base of the heart* together with the *coronary* vein, and send little branches along the length of the heart, so that the whole heart is, as it were, made reticulated by these twigs.

Thus, that was how the heart got its "crown", a term likely imbued with religious connotation and allegory. Vesalius referred to the coronary artery in Latin as "coronalis arteria" and was notably struck by the ring these vessels form as they encircle the base of the heart. In his anatomical description, Vesalius observed how the main arteries, arising from the aorta, send out branches (surculi) in the manner of a crown (coronae prorsus modo), together with the coronary vein, thus surrounding the base of the heart and distributing smaller branches throughout its length. While Vesalius did not use the names like "circumflex", "right coronary", "obtuse marginal", "posterolateral", "posterior descending", "left anterior descending", or "diagonal" arteries, his account clearly anticipates the pattern; arteries fan out from the base and supply the entire heart to its apex, forming a vascular crown that gives the coronary arteries their name.

Fabrica was updated and revised 12 years later as second edition in 1555, printed by the same publisher in Basel, the Swiss printer Johannes Oporinus (Johann Herbst, 1507–1568), famed for his high quality illustrations and scholarly printings. Mass printing was relatively new in Europe, having begun with Johannes Gutenberg's (c. 1400–1468) reinvention of movable type. The Chinese had pioneered woodblock printing as early as the seventh century and developed movable type by the eleventh century, following their invention of paper, which Cài Lún (c. 50–121 CE) in 105 CE presented to Emperor Liú Zhào (79–105 CE) of Eastern Han Dynasty (25–220 CE, capital in Luòyáng, Hénán) [8]. Papermaking technology reached Europe much later, with the first paper mills appearing in the Islamic Iberian peninsula in Spain (Al-Andalus), nearly a thousand years after its invention in China, arriving via Silk Road interactions between East and West. Gutenberg conducted his first printing runs in the 1440s in Mainz, in what is now Germany. The spread of printed words would go on to ignite Europe's Renaissance [9].

Pope Boniface VIII (1294–1303; Benedetto Caetani, of Italy, c. 1235–1303) issued the 1299 decree *De Sepulturis* (On Burials), which forbade the transport of crusaders' body parts for burial. Ever resourceful, Italian scholars during the Renaissance interpreted the decree for what it did not say. Namely, that it did not forbid human dissections for scientific and educational purposes. The University of Bologna was first to conduct such dissections, in January 1315, mostly on executed criminals, followed by other institutions, including Padua, which subsequently became famous for its regular public dissections in the anatomical theatre it built in 1594 [5].

Vesalius was at Padua between 1537 and 1543. After he printed his book in Basel, he returned to Brussels and became imperial physician to Charles V (1500–1558), the Holy Roman Emperor and King of Spain, who ruled over a vast territory encompassing much of Western and Central Europe, including parts of Italy. In the final chapter of his life, Vesalius took a leave of absence from the royal court and undertook a pious journey to the Holy Land, which was then under Ottoman rule (1299–1922). The Sultan was Suleiman I the Magnificent (1494–1566), who, as the tenth ruler of the Ottoman Dynasty, reigned from 1520 and expanded his empire across Southeastern Europe, from Greece to Hungary and Crimea. Vesalius died on October 15, 1564, aged 49 years and 9.5 months following a short illness on the Greek island of Zakynthos, in Ionian Sea, in the return leg of his journey for which his ship was diverted to. His Santa Maria della Grazie church grave was lost to earthquakes in 1893 and 1953, but a marble bust of him bearing his name in Greek (ΑΝΔΡΕΑΣ ΒΕΖΑΛ) was erected on the 400th anniversary of his death in 1965, behind the OTE (Hellenic Telecommunications) building in Zakynthos town centre, in the Andreas Vesalius Square section, close to Dionysios Solomos Square; a bronze statue based on Vesalius's anatomical drawings was placed in the latter area in front of the Municipal Library to mark the quincentenary celebration of his birth in 2014 [1, 10].

On the other hand, in 1958, Charles V had his triumphant marble statue with an unsheathed sword and a vanquished foe under his right foot erected within Puerta Nueva de Bisagra (from Al-Andalus Arabic, Bab al-Saqra or "Gate of Falcon"—10th century), a reconstruction which he commissioned 10 years before and which was completed posthumously in 1559, the northern monumental city gate of Toledo (etymologically—city on a hill, Roman *Toletum*), a medieval Castilian capital, embraced on three sides by the River Tagus, on the 400th anniversary of his death. After 374 years of Islamic rule, the Christians retook Toledo in 1085; it became a city of learning, the confluence of Arabic, Hebrew and Latin scholarship led to translation of ancient Greek manuscripts expanded with Arabic annotations, adaptations and innovations into Latin, which seeded Europe with medicine and science within the next hundred years. The pre-eminent Spanish literature, Don Quixote (part 1—1605 and part 2—1615), written by Miguel de Cervantes (1547–1616), was based on a fictional manuscript attributed to a Moorish chronicler mocking Spanish society found in Toledo. Cervantes's 400th birth anniversary plaque dated 1947 is next to the right-sided archway wall in the quadrangle, right to Charles V's statue, well within his stony gaze. Thus, sword and pen confined together in the same space.

The celebrated Castilian knight, Rodrigo Díaz de Vivar (c. 1043–1099) "El Cid" (from Arabic al-Sayyid, "the Lord") who recaptured and ruled Valencia (Christian-held 1094–1102), fought alongside Alfonso VI of León and Castile (c. 1040–1109) against Islamic attempts to retake Toledo in the Battle of Consuegra, 40 miles south of the city in 1097. In that battle, he lost his only son, Diego Rodríguez (c. 1078–1097). However, one of his daughters, María (c.1080–1105), became progenitor of the Kings of Aragon. In 1492, her progeny, Ferdinand of Aragon (1452–1516) and his wife, Isabella I of Castile (1451–1504) through their Alhambra decree, expelled from Spain all non-Christians who refused to convert, followed by Portugal in 1496, where their daughter, Isabella of Aragon (1470–1498) was married into the Portuguese royal household. The Sephardic Jews and the Muslim Arabs took their fortune; papermaking, printing and publishing skills; commercial, scientific and medical know-how elsewhere, contributing to European revival. These people indirectly educated Vesalius and printed his books.

New Spain gained an empire, which it could not administer because of brain drain. Other rising European powers rapidly overshadowed it, beginning with the defeat of the Spanish Armada in 1588 by England's Elizabeth I (b. 1533, r. 1558–1603). Her royal chief physician from 1581, Rodrigo López (c. 1525–1594), whom she reluctantly executed for treason after a court intrigue, was a Sephardic Jewish converso. Benjamin Disraeli (1804–1881), Conservative Victorian British Prime Minister (1868, 1874–1880), was also a Sephardic Jewish descendant. One of his many memorable paraphrased quotes that can serve as a theme for this book is "*Change is inevitable. Change is constant*" [11]. John R. R. Tolkien (1892–1973), an Oxford don who was familiar with El Cid's epic poem, *Cantar de mio Cid* (The Song of my Cid), and medieval Iberian saga, might have subtly drawn inspirations for his *Lord of the Rings* trilogy: a returning knight redeemed his crown and unified a nation; light and shadow struggle; and House of Aragorn [12].

Vesalius studied the Toledan Galenic translation as part of his medical education since the Arabic-Latin texts were standard curriculum. When he started human dissections, he initially wondered whether Galen was lost in translation. He was able to obtain the Byzantine Greek to Latin five-volume translation of Galen while in Padua (a time when fleeing Greek scholars, scribes and intellectuals took their prized and precious manuscripts to Venice, Florence and Rome following the fall of Constantinople in 1453 to the Ottoman Turks) and he also learned enough Greek to read the originals. It was then he conclusively proved to himself that Galen was indeed wrong when it came to human anatomy and cleared up the translational confusion between vein and artery [1]. As Galen was embedded into Christian Orthodoxy, a contrarian view was regarded as heretical, and this exacted a price for Vesalius subsequently.

Both Vesalius's grandfather and father were in aristocratic medical services. It was only natural that he would receive a job offer from Emperor Charles V which he could not refuse, based on his royal connection, exalted academic status in Padua and *Fabrica*. Thus, reaching the pinnacle of his medical career at 28 as a court physician in Brussels, which unfortunately curtailed his scientific enquiry. He was denounced by his former teacher in Paris, Dubois [10], openly mocked by many, including his 1543 replacement in Padua, Renaldo Colombo (1516–1559), who listed errors in his book, who in fact correctly deduced pulmonary circulation instead of Galenic ventricular septal pores between right-to-left heart which he retained, even in his more refined second edition in 1555. Although he conceded that they must be too small to be seen by naked eyes. His second successor in 1551 was Gabriele Falloppio (1523–1562), who was more respectful in his analysis of *Fabrica*, which he published in 1561. Vesalius saw this and responded line-by-line Falloppio's critiques that he printed on May 24, 1564, in Venice, shortly before he embarked on his ill-fated trip from there; this included his defence of his version of autonomic nervous ganglia and plexuses around the pericardium [1, 13].

Charles V grief-strickenly abandoned Toledo following the death of his wife Isabella of Portugal (1503–1539), aged 35, during her sixth childbirth in the city. He was 39, wore black and mourned her for the rest of his life, while keeping close by a life-sized portrait of her, painted by Tiziano Vecellio (Titian c. 1488–1576) now in Madrid's Museo del Prado. Then they had three surviving children, Philip, Maria and Joanna, aged 11, 10 and 3 respectively. The eldest became Philip II (1527–1598), who inherited Spain and a vast empire at 28, when Charles V abdicated in 1555 through ill health and gout and retired to a monastery. Philip II united Portugal in an Iberian union which expanded his empire to the largest the world had ever seen till then, and Philippines was named in his honour. As for Vesalius, losing his more receptive patron of 13 years at 41, then moving to Madrid to serve the deeply religious Phillip II who disapproved of his dissections and anti-Galenic views, resulted in court politics, culminating with his fateful pilgrimage [1]. Vesalius's tale exemplified the interconnectedness of a globe where acceptance of human diversity and open-mindedness are more receptive to change for the better, as pithily verbalised by Disraeli; yet, going against the grain requires hindsight, insight and foresight—this also demands considerable courage to face objection, rejection and dejection;

thus, it is not for the faint-hearted. In Vesalius's case, his life was cut short, but he was the man who crowned the heart.

William Harvey (1578–1657) was taught by Vesalius's 19-year-removed third successor at Padua, the Italian Girolamo Fabricius ab Acquapendente (1533–1619) appointed in 1565, who inaugurated the anatomical theatre in January 1595. Fabricius was the world's first embryologist studying chick embryos and described the venous valves, works which later inspired and facilitated Harvey in his research. Harvey obtained his Doctorate in Medicine after 3 years in 1602. He was the first to put forth the notion of a closed-loop circulatory system. Laid out in his publication, *Exercitatio Anatomica de Motu Cordis et Sanguinis in Animalibus* (An Anatomical Disquisition on the Motion of the Heart and Blood in Animals) in 1628 [14].

Harvey defined cardiac output as the product of stroke volume and heart rate ($CO = SV \cdot HR$) and estimated this to be roughly 4.2 L/min in an adult man. In so doing, he directly rebutted the ideas of Galen (129–216 CE), a Greek doctor who served as personal physician to Emperor Marcus Aurelius (121–180 CE) in Rome. Galen's understanding of the heart was based on animal dissections, as human dissection was strictly forbidden at the time. Nevertheless, he described the heart as *enwreathed* by a couple of veins that sprang forth from within its cavity and that the heart nourished itself directly via them [15]. While working in Pergamon in modern-day Turkey, Galen also gained experience by treating gladiators' wounds, which provided rare insights into human anatomy. Despite the limitations of his methods, Galen's views on the heart and circulation dominated Western medicine for 1400 years.

Harvey reasoned that if blood was made in the liver and consumed by various organs, as was proposed by Galen, the whole body blood volume would be depleted within 30 min. Hence, blood must be recycled by the heart straddling the systemic and pulmonary circulations. He observed blood flow in chick embryos studying the genesis of the heart. He further demonstrated the directionality of veinous flow through their one-way valves in the arm and hypothesised the presence of connecting vessels (capillaries) between the artery and vein, rather than through pores between the right and left hearts as taught by Galen. He was proven correct when the Italian physician Marcello Malphigi (1628–1694) saw these under microscope 33 years later in 1661 [16].

1.2 Estimating Cardiac Output

The Reverend Stephen Hales (1677–1761) is an English Anglican Parish Priest and experimental scientist who intubated the left femoral artery, not the carotid artery as is popularly illustrated, of animals and measured the "force of the blood" with an open-ended glass tube in Teddington, ten miles west of St George's Hospital in Tooting. His publication in 1727, *Vegetable Staticks*, which primarily dealt with plant sap pressure and physiology, in it he described 2 horses, the blood column went up eight feet three inches for one and eight feet nine inches for another, it was five feet six inches for a small dog, seven feet for a large spaniel (dog) and five feet seven inches in a fallow doe (deer) [17]. These would be equivalent to 197, 209, 131, 167 and 133 mmHg.

In Hale's second volume, *Haemastaticks*, printed in 1733, he calculated cardiac output using Harvey's equation by making wax heart casts of oxen and horses, demonstrated microvascular resistance, showed that the microvasculature in the gut is capable of vasodilatation with "warm water hyperaemia", and interstitial hydrostatic filtration in lungs and guts [18]. By modern standards this was unusual; he was elected Fellow of the Royal Society in 1718 at 41, well before his publications, via his sheer reputation as an experimenter and through his network within the scientific community.

It became possible to calculate cardiac output using Adolf E. Fick's (1829–1901) method. He was a German doctor who did his earlier research in the University of Zürich, Switzerland. He proposed that a substance taken up by an organ per unit time equals to its concentration difference in the artery and vein that perfuse the organ under study. By measuring oxygen uptake, VO_2 from room air minus that in exhaled air, dividing this by the arteriovenous oxygen content difference, cardiac output (CO) can be calculated:

$$CO = \frac{\dot{V}O_2}{C_aO_2 - C_vO_2}$$

For example, 250 mL O_2 per minute divided by 20–15 mL O_2 per dL of blood = 50 dL/min or 5 L/min. By convention, basal VO_2 uptake is defined as 3.5 mL/Kg/min or 1 metabolic equivalent (MET), and *VO_2 maximum* is used to judge fitness, as a surrogate for cardiac output. Based on this, a world class athlete could achieve an eight times increase in cardiac output in terms of exercise intensity.

The Fick principle was adapted in 1970 by Harold J. C. Swan (1922–2005) and William Ganz (1919–2009) in the pulmonary circulation to measure absolute right heart cardiac output with their balloon-tipped flow-directed pulmonary artery (PA) catheter which also transduces pressure. This Swan-Ganz PA catheter has 3 ports; distal pulmonary artery lumen to collect mixed venous blood, proximal right atrial lumen to deliver drugs or inject a saline bolus, and an air-port to inflate the 1 mL flotation balloon. By inputting 3 variables, oxygen uptake, VO_2 from the bedside ventilatory metabolic cart, oxygen content from radial or femoral artery blood sample, and pulmonary artery mixed venous blood sample, cardiac output could be precisely calculated.

A thermistor-tipped version of the PA catheter was introduced shortly, allowing Swan and Ganz to utilise the thermodilution approach first described in man in 1968 which simplified cardiac output measurement [19]. They published their results in 1972 [20, 21]. It boils down to a single action, a 10 mL of saline at 0–4 (iced) or 21 (room) °C temperature is injected into the right atrium, the exact temperature of this injection is detected by an in-line miniature *proximal thermistor* at Y-connector and the instantaneous change in blood temperature against time is detected by the *distal thermistor* in the pulmonary artery, creating a cooling-time plot, the *first-pass area under the curve* (AUC, °C·s) is the **zeroth moment**; it represents the total "temperature change" signal over time as the indicator passes. In other words, this denominator contains the information of how low the temperature falls in the blood and for what duration is inversely proportional to cardiac output as per the Stewart–Hamilton equation [22–24], Flow (Q):

$$Q = \frac{T}{\int_0^{\infty} \Delta T(t)dt}$$

The numerator is the product T, which is 10 mL · (Baseline pulmonary artery temperature—Injectant temperature °C) ·1.08·60. The composite constant 1.08 is the density and heat transfer property of either isotonic saline or dextrose in relation to blood (k_1), and instrument calibration and heat exchange factors specific to equipment (k_2), and 60 is the conversion from second to minute, and denominator, the *zeroth-moment* AUC—summation of ΔT(t), which is change of temperature over time, using integrative algebraic calculus, ∫dt. For example, 10 mL·(37–4 °C)·1.0 8·60/4.5 °C·s = 4752 mL/min or 4.75 L/min.

Despite the user-friendliness of the Swan-Ganz PA catheter, it's general use to monitor intensive care patients was curtailed 30 years later due to non-supportive randomised controlled trials (RCT) data. Nevertheless, compared with the gold-standard of Fick's method, thermodilution has an intra-subject coefficient of variation of < 5% and a mean difference of < 10% between measures, making it highly precise and reliable in measuring cardiac output, and by extension, blood flow [19, 20]. And 5% of the cardiac output goes to the coronary arteries; this proportion, interestingly, does not appear to change with stress or exercise intensity [25].

1.3 Estimating Coronary Flow

George N. Stewart (1860–1930) was a Scottish doctor who settled in Cleveland, Ohio. He conducted a series of canine experiments, in which he injected 1.6% hypertonic (normal 0.9%) saline into the left ventricle (LV) via the left carotid artery and placed a pair of hook-shaped platinum electrodes on the right femoral artery. Since saline is a conductor that lowers blood's electrical resistance, he used this property to measure the peak transit time of the saline, used it to divide the saline-diluted blood volume, giving the cardiac output and extrapolating this to 5.8 L/min for humans in 1897 [24].

Replacing saline with a non-diffusible brilliant bright red synthetic dye, given intravenously from the antecubital fossa and femoral artery blood samplings every second for up to 15 s in humans, William F. Hamilton (1893–1964), a physiologist from Louisville, Kentucky, was able to construct a time-concentration plot to calculate the AUC for a more precise mathematical estimation of cardiac output, christened the *Stewart-Hamilton equation* in 1931. Although in practice his estimation of cardiac output was x1.75 magnitude higher, which could be an inherent systematic methodological overestimate, having the indicator cross over from pulmonary to systemic circulation is the inflationary tendency with the bolus dilution technique. However, as discussed in the previous section on *estimating cardiac output*, using the same methodology, but confined just to the right heart and the pulmonary artery, the Swan-Ganz PA catheter is able to produce more accurate results.

William Ganz (1919–2009) was 20 years old when the Nazis occupied Czechoslovakia and shut down Charles University School of Medicine in Prague, his medical school, after 1 year of study in 1939. And being a Slovakian Jew, he was drafted into Hungarian forced labour battalions which were formed in 1940, Hungary having annexed Košice, his city of birth in 1938. He was back in Košice after two and half years' hard labour and managed to acquire false papers given to him by Oliver Rácz Sr. (1918–1997), whose fiancée, Katalina Nyiszli (1919–1996) was Jewish whom he also helped escape to the Hungarian city of Budapest. Rácz Sr. was working as a clerk in the Košice camp, with ready access to documents and official stamps. Ganz's forged labour camp release identified him as a Hungarian Christian soldier. Rácz Sr also gave him a matching uniform, which allowed him an escorted travel by train to Budapest, where Ganz went into hiding with the Jewish resistance network and met his future wife, Magda Weisz (1920–2005), whom he married after Soviet liberation of Budapest in 1945. Thus, avoiding the May–July 1944 Košice deportations to Auschwitz-Birkenau, Poland, when Germany occupied Hungary in March 1944. He almost certainly would have perished as a Holocaust victim, as fewer than 10% of deportees survived, with most being sent directly to the gas chambers upon arrival [26].

He resumed his medical studies qualifying top of his class in 1947 after the war. A year later there was a Communist coup in 1948, despite which he undertook post-graduate research into the complex mathematics of thermodilution and applied it in animal experiments and human studies, including the effects of nitroglycerine on coronary flow at the Cardiovascular Research Institute in Prague with a colleague, Arnost Fronek (1923–2020) [27, 28]. Fronek proposed a flow-directed balloon flotation in the pulmonary circulation, although it was not his original idea [29, 30], which Swan independently took up in the US and perfected it into the Swan-Ganz PA catheter in collaboration with Edwards Laboratories (now Lifesciences, Irvine), Santa Ana, California [31]. Fronek first immigrated to the US in 1962. Ganz, at 47 in 1966 followed his footsteps and defected via Vienna to the US with his wife and 2 sons, later settling as a staff physician at Cedars-Sinai Medical Center in Los Angeles, California, where he continued his pivotal trials in cardiovascular physiology [32, 33].

Between 1968 and 1970, in parallel with testing the Swan-Ganz PA catheter, Ganz himself primarily experimented on his *coronary sinus continuous thermodilution flow catheter*, which he designed with Wilton Webster Manufacturing Company in Altadena, California [34]. This is a bespoke 7 French 100 cm of Dacron polymeric tubing with 2.3 mm outer diameter and a pre-formed 45–60° distal bend moulded into the distal 45–50 mm to allow "self-seating" in the coronary sinus under fluoroscopy. It has an 0.75 mm internal diameter nylon inner tube running down the shaft and ends in a single 0.4–0.5 mm side-hole that is 20 mm proximal to the closed tip. There are two tiny thermistors encased in biocompatible epoxy within the wall. One internal at the side-hole to record injectate temperature, the other external 10–15 mm upstream to sample mixed blood temperature. There are lead bands marking the thermistor locations for fluoroscopic positioning.

This catheter was designed to be manoeuvred via the antecubital fossa as per Werner Forssmann's (1904–1979) technique described in 1929, for which Forssmann was awarded the Nobel Prize for Medicine or Physiology in 1956, and it sits well within the coronary sinus by design. Isotonic 5% dextrose is delivered through the catheter using a Harvard model 921 infusion pump which has a reservoir of 200 mL, to ensure a constant infusion rate of 35–40 mL/min for 20 s (12 mL) at room temperature (20–25 °C). The coronary sinus flow could be calculated with only 3 temperature variables, resting blood (T_b), infusate (T_i) and mixed blood (T_m) temperatures; T_i is measured in the distal luminal thermistor and T_i and T_m by the proximal external thermistor. The numerator, T_b-T_i represents the initial thermal driving force, or how cold the injectate is, and denominator T_b-T_m, how much of the heat is dissipated by the flow, when this ratio is multiplied to the injectate flow rate, it estimates the blood flow. The heat exchange constant of 1.08 is not added for dextrose 5% as it has the same property as blood. It has an exceptional Bland-Altman coefficient of variation of 2.4% and a mean difference of 4% with estimates of coronary sinus flow of 83–167 mL/min in both normal subjects as well as those with coronary artery disease in his published series [34].

Although coronary sinus flow is of limited clinical utility, it only captures about 1/3–2/3 of coronary flow since the rest is drained directly into cardiac chambers via anterior cardiac, thebesian and sinusoidal veins/shunts. Further, later studies found that the catheter is prone to respiratory displacement of 0.5–2.0 cm making sequential measurements highly variable, with 10% variation during quiet respiration [35], and up to 10% cases of coronary sinus dissection albeit usually subclinical [36]. This latter report in 2003 appears to be the last publication on the use of the 7 French retrograde *coronary sinus continuous thermodilution flow catheter* (CCS-7 U-90B, Webster Laboratories, Altadena, California). The catheter was phased out from production when the company merged into Biosense Webster (Irvine, California), a subsidiary of Johnson and Johnson Medtech which shifted its focus to electrophysiological products in 1998.

1.4 Coronary Thermodilution

1.4.1 Coronary Pressure Wire

It is inevitable that the technology and knowhow brought by Ganz from Prague, which he perfected in the US in the 1970s, would be miniaturised and applied to the coronary artery. This involved pioneers from the three kingdoms of Sweden,

Netherlands and Belgium working collaboratively to define clinical coronary physiology. The pressure wire was introduced in 1991 by a Swedish company, the Radi Medical System, Inc., Uppsala, Sweden, co-founded by Lars Tenerz in 1988. Tenerz tested his **fibreoptic pressure sensor** with a diameter of 0.45 mm mounted on a standard 0.018″ angioplasty guidewire at Sahlgrenska Hospital, Göteborg, Sweden a couple of years later, and found that it was small enough not to influence post-coronary angioplasty pressure increase, unlike the deflated bulky balloon introduced by Andreas R. Grüentzig (1939–1985) in 1977 [37].

Meanwhile, around the same time, Nico H. J. Pijls in the Netherlands applied to the coronary artery the indicator-dilution methodology based on the *Stewart-Hamilton equation*, adapted by Paul Meier (1924–2011) and Kenneth L. Zierler (1917–2009) in 1954 into the *central volume principle*; $V = Q \cdot Tmn$ [38, 39], i.e. which applies to an indicator that dissipates within the microvascular bed, as a marker of *tissue* penetration or opacification, and not just confined to the vascular compartment as it was originally envisaged. This equation underpins quantitative perfusion in positron emission tomography (PET), cardiac magnetic resonance (CMR) and CT coronary angiogram (CTCA).

When applied to coronary physiology, V which is the *volume of distribution* of contrast passing within the myocardium, but when contrast is injected under *maximal hyperaemia*, it becomes a constant, and could be conveniently dropped out of the equation, or ignored; then flow, $Q \propto 1/Tmn$, Tmn is the *first-moment* mean transit time of the contrast bolus, or the average dwell time of a contrast within the zone of interest [40]. This contrasts with zeroth-moment AUC of the original Stewart-Hamilton equation which reflects total contrast mass within a **closed** vascular compartment as opposed to an **open** volume that disperses into the tissues. Since only a region of interest is examined, and not the whole circulation, AUC cannot be used without knowing total volume and injectant dose. To account for this, Tmn is used instead, which relates to AUC via V, and q, the amount of contrast or indicator injected; $Tmn = (V/q) \cdot AUC$ [38]. It is important to note that when Tmn is used in a Swan-Ganz model, and Tmn is plotted against AUC, it systematically overestimates flow.

Pijls used 6 mL of contrast, injected at 4 mL/s down the coronary artery, the "dilution" of which was calculated at a region of interest within the heart subtended by the coronary artery in which the contrast was injected, using cine-angiographic videodensitometry [41]. The change in grayscale level plotted a dilution curve. He pursued one key concept pioneered by K. Lance Gould [40], instead of relying on contrast-induced hyperaemia; he induced maximal hyperaemia, with dipyridamole in his canine experiments and intracoronary papaverine in humans, and demonstrated that 1/Tmn is a better index than peak time and density in correlating with flow against a ring-mounted Doppler probe around the circumflex artery. In humans, it was reproducible with 5% of variation and allowed post-coronary angioplasty maximal flow ratio (*MFR*) to be calculated to judge procedural success [42–45]. In 40 subjects, an MPR > 1.6 or 60% increase in post-procedural coronary flow had a positive predictive value of 96% for reversal of ischaemic exercise testing in 7–10 days following treatment. This work was the precursor to the next phase.

1.4.2 Fractional Flow Reserve

In 1990, Pijls met Bernard De Bruyne, a Belgian Cardiologist at the 9th Annual Scientific Meeting of the American College of Cardiology (ACC) at New Orleans, Louisiana in March 18–22, [46] and then set out to concept proof his idea of using coronary pressure as a surrogate for flow, to simplify and consolidate the research he had done in the Netherlands [47]. Pijls and de Bruyne from then on forged an unrivalled collaboration that introduced a new field of invasive coronary physiology, published as joint authors between 1993 and 2025, at least 150 research articles, averaging 4–5 papers per annum, and co-authored a book on coronary pressure 7 years later from their meeting [48].

In 1974, Gould conducted a series of canine experiments which were similar to what Pijls had done in the Netherlands a decade and a half later, measuring absolute volumetric coronary flow in the circumflex (Cx) artery, but with electromagnetic flowmeter which was surgically implanted. He found that contrast hyperaemia could increase coronary flow fourfold, from 6 s, lasting as long as 3 min. Complete occlusion of the artery for 10 s could also produce a hyperaemic response 3–7 times above resting levels. He noted that when the Cx was increasingly constricted with the implanted micrometer, the rest flow was not affected even when the lesion was very severe, but hyperaemic flow started to fall with a stenosis between 30 and 45%, and disappeared with a stenosis approaching 88−93%, akin to Starling's curves in 1915 [40]. He used radionuclide imaging to prove Cx territory myocardial ischaemia with hyperaemic stress when the Cx lesion became severe. Based on the experimental data, Gould proposed a *hyperaemic-to-rest ratio* of < 1.5 as being a significant stenosis, but 2.0 corresponded with an 80% stenosis. This ratio become known as the *coronary flow reserve* (CFR); further canine experiments and positron emission tomography (PET) studies in humans correspond a CFR < 2 with coronary ischaemia and stenoses > 80–90% [49]. When CFR is mapped to absolute stress perfusion in mL/min/g, it produces a chart with colour codes; low values on both ↓CFR and ↓maximal flow predict the worse prognosis; this at any region of the heart carries a mortality of 14% over 4 years. This does make sense. CFR is a unitless ratio; it can be low because of increased baseline flow, giving a low CFR or a type I error; this can be overcome when paired with regional or absolute stress flow [50, 51].

Pijls was familiar with Gould's work undertaken 15 years earlier and he had learnt three of things from his own research and others', Gould's in particular:

1. Coronary cine-angiographical assessment of a coronary stenosis is anatomical; it correlates poorly with angina, especially with *moderate lesions*.
2. Physiological evaluation of a coronary stenosis involves a *flow gradient*. From his stint working on MFR which is a ratio, 60% improvement in flow post-coronary angioplasty predicts a good result, i.e., resolution of exercise ECG ischaemia. But these are all patients with obviously severe angiographic coronary disease. There are many patients who have exercise ECG ischaemia with what appears to be a moderate lesion. His method is too elaborate, cumbersome and laborious. Further, MPR is a post-procedural index; what he needs is a pre-

procedural index. Gould's CFR is exactly the ratio he needs to replicate, but how could he adapt it without measuring actual flow; this could be down with Ganz's coronary sinus continuous thermodilution flow catheter, but it is for the whole heart, not for a selective coronary artery, and the catheter is too bulky.

3. Anything that moves is governed by three factors. The electrical analogue Ohm's law can be applied to the circulatory system as utilised by Swan and Ganz, $\Delta P = Q \cdot R$; ΔP for pressure gradient, Q for flow and R, resistance. In other words, like water flowing from high to low ground, a principle used by the Romans to construct their aqueducts, pressure is generated to push flow forward against resistance within an artery. The coronary stenosis is a *localised, fixed and static resistance* to flow. The question is how to quantify this in a clinically expedient way. From Pijls' previous experience where he freezes out V from $V = Q \cdot Tmn$, of the central volume principle to derive $Q = 1/Tmn$ during maximal hyperaemia, V becomes a constant, he reasons that the same can be applied to Ohm's Law. Under maximal hyperaemia, R too becomes a constant, then $P \propto Q$; any fall in P beyond a lesion reflects a fall in Q too, without *actually* measuring the absolute flow, which at the time cannot be achieved in small arteries. Plus, he needs to work out how to make sense of and tame the various pressure values in different parts of the pressure gradient impacting the coronary circulation.

During his postdoctoral time in Huston, Texas, Pijls performed further canine experiments, continuously measuring absolute coronary flow in the Cx with a calibrated perivascular ring-mounted Doppler probe, which he had used before, but this time with an ultrathin 0.015″ × 15 cm fluid-filled pressure-monitoring guidewire (Advanced Cardiovascular System, Santa Clara, California) [47]. This allowed a non-intrusive measurement of Pd, the pressure beyond the coronary lesion; other pressure indices he obtained were: Pa, proximal or aortic pressure, Pw, coronary wedge pressure, obtained with the artery occluded that reflects collateral supply pressure (added, which reduces effective Pa) from the microvascular bed in question and finally Pv, central venous pressure in the right atrium (right atrial pressure, RAP) as a surrogate for LVEDP.

In this model, the coronary perfusion pressure (CPP) is Pa − Pv, but he was interested in the actual flow from the S*upplying* epicardial coronary artery under study (Qs), across the microvasculature (Q), that is independent of pre-existing C*ollateral* circulatory supply (Qc):

$$Q = Qs + Qc$$

$$Pa \rightarrow (\text{lesion}) \rightarrow Pd \rightarrow (-)Pw \rightarrow (\text{microvasculature}) \rightarrow Pv$$

Hypothetically, during *maximal vasodilatation with hyperaemia*, the **proportion** of blood received by the microvasculature from the supplying epicardial coronary artery, Qs and via the collaterals, Qc **becomes a constant** with **or** without a coronary artery lesion, as do their respective resistances, hence, $Q \propto P$, **only P matters.**

Therefore, effective pressure after and before the coronary lesion, the ratio of which is the *pressure-derived* fractional flow reserve (FFR):

$$\mathrm{FFR}_{\mathrm{cor}} = \frac{\mathrm{Pd} - \mathrm{Pw}}{\mathrm{Pa} - \mathrm{Pw}}$$

→Fractional flow across the *coronary lesion*, corrected for competing collateral flow.

$$\mathrm{FFR}_{\mathrm{myo}} = \frac{\mathrm{Pd} - \mathrm{Pv}}{\mathrm{Pa} - \mathrm{Pv}}$$

→ fractional flow across the *myocardium or microvasculature*; this correction is important when LVEDP is raised as in heart failure.

$$\text{Fractional collateral flow} = \mathrm{FFR}_{\mathrm{myo}} - \mathrm{FFR}_{\mathrm{cor}}, \text{or}$$

$$\mathrm{Q_c} = \left(\mathrm{FFR}_{\mathrm{myo}} - \mathrm{FFR}_{\mathrm{cor}}\right) \cdot \mathrm{Q}$$

→ Post-coronary angioplasty, Pd rises, $FFR_{myo} \approx FFR_{cor}$, which causes the collateral supply to fall dramatically despite the same Pw.

Finally, assuming that there are **no collaterals**, and the **cardiac function is normal**; Pw and Pv are "0", therefore they are omitted, then:

$$\mathbf{FFR} = \frac{\mathbf{Pd}}{\mathbf{Pa}}$$

To rehash, the key assumption is that flow, Q, through the microvasculature is the same, with or without an epicardial lesion under *maximal vasodilation during hyperaemia*, with minimised resistance becoming a constant, but the driving pressures to achieve this in the two scenarios are different, their pressure ratio is a measure of the physiological severity of the obstruction, the FFR.

Pijls experimented on 5 dogs, aside from the Doppler probe; he added a circular ballon occluder to create 12 graded stenoses from mild to severe. Maximal hyperaemia was induced with intracoronary 8 mg papaverine bolus (verified against hyperaemia provoked by 20 s of coronary occlusion, as an opportunity to obtain Pw too) before each stenosis, and varying aortic BP provoked with phlebotomy, vasodilator such as nitroprusside or nitroglycerine for hypotension, and phenylephrine was used to create hypertension. With these haemodynamic upheavals, during maximal hyperaemia as he theorised, FFR_{myo} matched coronary blood flow Doppler velocities obtained, before and after stenoses were created and for FFR_{myo}, after stenoses were created; there are near perfect linear relationships in all five dogs between FFR_{myo} and doppler velocities. However, when FFR_{myo} is plotted on Y-axis against CFR on X-axis, they are *not mirror image*; the slope is shallow < 1, suggesting that FFR_{myo} is systematically lower than CFR. This is thought to be due to increasing flow inertia and turbulence it generates, as the stenosis gets tighter, pressure drops faster than flow as per Young-Tsai fluid dynamic equation [52, 53] for transstenotic pressure drop, adapted from the works of Gotthilf H. L. Hagen (1797–1884), Jean L. M. Poiseuille (1797–1869) and Daniel Bernoulli (1700–1782) [52, 54, 55].

$$\Delta P = \frac{8\pi \mu L}{An^2} \cdot Q + \frac{\rho}{2}\left(\frac{1}{As} - \frac{1}{An}\right) \cdot Q^2$$

Where ΔP is the transstenotic pressure drop (mmHg), μ is blood viscosity (0.03 g/cm/s), L is the stenosis length (mm), A_s is the stenotic cross-sectional area (mm^2), A_n is the "normal" reference area (mm^2), ρ is blood density (1 g/cm) and Q is mean flow (mL/s). When flow is *strictly laminar in the absence of a stenosis*, the **quadratic inertia term** becomes negligible, and the equation reduces to the **laminar viscous term**; Hagen-Poiseuille's law:

$$\Delta P = \frac{8\pi \mu L}{An^2} \cdot Q$$

$$\Delta P = \frac{8 \mu L}{\pi r^4} \cdot Q$$

$$\Delta P = R \cdot Q$$

→ R is the hydraulic resistance; note that π and μ, blood viscosity, are constants, changes in vessel radius have a dramatic geometric effect on resistance; doubling the radius reduces resistance 16-fold.

The equation was popularly christened as *hydraulic equivalent of Ohm's law* in 1956 by Arthur C. Guyton (1919–2003) from the first of his eight single-authored editions, a work that grew into the eponymous 14th revision (2020) of his physiology book, now the standard text for medical students. However, this electrical analogy was in fact first invoked by Otto Frank (1865–1944) in 1899, in his paper on the Windkessel model, which he wrote in German; *Nach dem Ohmschen Gesetze gilt für den Kreislauf Δp = Q · w; Δp—druckdifferenz and Latin pressura, Q—fluss but Latin Quantitas, w—widerstand* (According to Ohm's law, the pressure difference equals flow times resistance in the circulation) [56, 57].

Windkessel is a German firefighters' term for a metal vessel with an air cushion inside; when water is pumped in, albeit intermittently, the flow emerging at the other end remains almost constant. The trapped air stores energy and then releases it smoothly. In the vascular analogy, that "air cushion" is the arterial diastolic compliance or recoil, which damps the heart's pulsatile output so flow entering the microvasculature stays steady. Frank showed that once the aortic valve closes and no new blood enters, arterial pressure decays exponentially.

$$P(t) = P_0 e^{-t/\tau}$$

→ R is systemic vascular resistance or $\Delta P/Q$, C is total arterial compliance, and τ, tau, is time-constant of the pressure fall by 1/e, measured from the diastolic pressure curve; $\tau = R \cdot C$, thus, $C = \tau/R$, in mL/mmHg, normal range is 1.5–2.0 for artery and 3.0–6.0 for LV, although the latter is calculated differently, from LV pressure-volume (PV) loop's slope of the diastolic limb, $\Delta V/\Delta P$, measured at mid to late filling, slope of the end-diastolic PV relationship or curve (EDPVR)—*passive stiffness* or how stretchy the LV is. Whereas the τ of the LV is measured during isovolumic relaxation, similarly how quickly LV pressure falls by 1/e, this is *active relaxation* or lusitropy of the LV. Thus, in the LV, there is no relationship between τ and C, or LV compliance, although both would be abnormal in diastolic heart failure.

The $\Delta P = Q \cdot R$ equation itself was originally derived by Poiseuille in his capillary-tube experiments in 1835–1846, with fixed *resistance* [58]. On the other hand, Ernest H. Starling (1866–1927), who was fluent in German, was familiar with Frank's research, also used the electrical parallel, and modelled variable *resistance* in 1912 with his Starling resistor [59]—a collapsible elastic tube from altering external chamber pressure to simulate systemic vascular tone.

Starling connected this resistor to isolated feline and canine hearts, feeding it via the right innominate artery (upstream) and exiting it through the superior vena cava (downstream). He reported two key findings, 1. Within 30–40 °C, heart rate fell with temperature, between 23 and 26 °C, the heart dilated and then fibrillated, and between 45 and 46 °C, the heart became irregular and then stopped, and 2. He injected air inside the chamber in which the rubber tubing was and read the pressure within this chamber in mmHg (jacket pressure). At low jacket pressure, the flow increased with pressure—*ascending limb*, between 20 and 40 mmHg, reaching a plateau at 70–90 mmHg; the heart's generated pressure matched the jacket pressure between 80 and 150 mmHg—the *autoregulatory range*, i.e. the heart worked harder in response to increasing pressure to maintain the same flow rate. Beyond this upper limit, flow rapidly fell when the heart was overloaded—*descending limb*. This observation illustrated the idea that within the autoregulatory range, with constant flow, *resistance becomes and equals pressure*. Which implies that treating hypertension and heart failure by lowering resistance do not reduce cardiac output but instead reduces cardiac work and improves prognosis. This is a very important therapeutic principle in cardiology.

Others extended Starling's finding of falling flow, when the resistance overcomes the heart's capacity to generate pressure to the keep the microvasculature open. This is the controversial "waterfall effect", when neither reducing the downstream or venous pressure would augment flow as is expected [60–62]. In other words, this breaks Ohm's law, which applies to *rigid tubes*, where widening ΔP by either increasing upstream arterial perfusion pressure or lowering downstream venous pressure would increase flow. However, in *collapsible microvasculature*, a minimal opening "zero-flow" pressure, Pf_0 is needed to avoid the vessels collapsing, and when the vessels are shut, widening the pressure gradient, ΔP by reducing venous pressure do not augment flow, thus the dissociation between pressure, ΔP and flow, Q. However, and paradoxically, increasing the venous pressure with coronary sinus reducer (CSR) appears to significantly relieve angina by redistribution of adenosine-induced hyperaemic flow to the subendocardium [63].

These fluid dynamic equations are elegant and beautiful, yet unintelligible to the uninitiated, but knowing them at least nominally help make sense of much of coronary pathophysiology in daily clinical practice. Blood circulation fundamentally is about the *physical movement of particles within a closed system.* Thus, Isaac Newton's (1643–1642) three laws of motion are applicable. In other words, blood flow down the coronary artery is a tug of war between *inertia* and *viscosity.* Inertia is derived from Latin, *iners* which means lazy, and was first used as an astronomical term, formalised by **Newton into his first law of motion**—an object when sets in motion will continue in the same trajectory, resisting external influences on its course. When the heart contracts, a "stroke" volume of blood is ejected. This cardiac work or power (P, joules) overcomes systemic vascular resistance and generates an accelerating *inertial force*, **Newton' second law motion**, F = m (kg)·a (m/s^2) or *Newton* as the unit of measure, that maintains a *momentum* (p, mass · velocity, kg·m/s) of the blood circulating with its *inertia* (mass, kg). So that blood flow is continuous, even in diastole, and it does not stop to wait for the next cardiac contraction. Inertia relates to blood *density* (ρ, g/cm^3) which basically is mass concentration and *volume* (cm^3). Therefore, *inertia is weight*, a weighty ball rolled on the ground keeps on rolling, resisting change in its course, unlike a light ball that bounces off its path when it hits an obstacle.

On the other hand, *viscosity* is the physical property of a collection of particles within the ball interacting with each other; when this is fluid, in the case of blood, it acts as an internal brake to inertia. Viscosity (μ, Pascal x second, Pa·s) is how thick or sticky the fluid is, e.g., honey and water have the same density, but honey being more viscous flows slower. *Dynamic viscosity* is the internal friction between fluid layers when it is flowing. In orderly laminar flow in a straight vessel, it appears as parabolic, generating gradual velocity gradients between layers, dragging on the vessel wall surface as *shear stress,* translating into a tangential force per unit area acting *parallel* to the surface. A pulsatile shear stress is necessary to maintain normal endothelial function and keeps the artery semi-dilated and compliant.

In fluid dynamics, when inertia overcomes viscosity, turbulence occurs, resulting in increased shear stress, endothelial dysfunction and inflammation; leading to the atherosclerotic process, which begets further atherogenesis, culminating with the vulnerable plaque which ruptures, causing a thrombotic occlusion. Analogous to a gentle brush on the vessel wall with low shear stress and a sandpaper rubbing with high shear stress. With each heartbeat, the pulse wave generated stretches the vessel wall, and its recoil through the Windkessel effect propels the blood forward, adding to the inertia; it dissipates peripherally but bounces back to the heart as a reflected wave, akin to a kickback from shooting the pistol. When this is well timed, it closes the aortic valve, creating the dicrotic notch and facilitates coronary flow; the pressure that drives coronary flow is not the diastolic or trough BP, but throughout the diastole—from the dicrotic notch to the diastolic BP—**Newton's third law of motion**, to every action is a reaction.

To succinctly summarise the complex fluid dynamics as applied to the coronary atherogenesis, Ohm's law describes how a fluid is ejected from the heart and courses down a circulation, determined by the force by which it is expelled and resistance by which it must overcome in order to flow, facilitated by a pressure gradient in the process. Weak heart, low flow; and low resistance, high flow; and vice versa. The flow itself is conditional of two properties: viscosity and inertia. Viscosity is the **internal friction** to flow; the more viscous a fluid is, the more orderly and laminar its flow is, albeit slow. Inertia is **external friction** to flow; the higher inertia a fluid has, the more it resists a change in its course once it is flowing. When a fluid trips over itself, so to speak, or inertia overcomes viscosity, it is when turbulence occurs and disorderly non-laminar flow exerts non-uniform wall stress, resulting in either too much or too little friction on the vascular wall; the former in a straight vessel causes increased stress, and the latter in a bifurcation reduced stress. Both induce endothelial dysfunction and inflammation with plaque formation; high flow with high wall stress provokes plaque rupture, and low flow with low stress, stasis and thrombosis. That is why the site of myocardial infarction (MI) nearly always, is at a coronary bifurcation. Finally, for a fluid in flow, viscosity is a fluid's inert and intrinsic property that only comes into being with movement, hence the prefix, "dynamic". When it is multiplied by its velocity gradient, i.e. in a vessel, change of velocity from mid lumen to vessel wall, this exerts a horizontal shear stress along the wall. As for inertia, its weight, the heavier the fluid, the higher the wall shear stress when the flow is turbulent, with a disproportional drop in pressure in relation to flow rate beyond a stenosis. *Hence the shallower slope or gradient when pressure in y-axis is plotted against flow in x-axis in Pijls'canine experiments, as the stenosis gets tighter*. These insights explain why long stents, and stents at bifurcation in the coronary artery often fail in time by promoting the double drawback of endothelial dysfunction and flow turbulence.

Further, with regards to Pijls' FFR_{myo}-CFR plot described earlier, there is a consistent positive intercept on Y-axis at 0.2–0.4, at zero flow on Doppler, implying that collateral flow could be *dynamically recruited*, but this is partly correctable with FFR_{cor}, when Pw is deducted from Pa and Pd. Although, there is also the "waterfall" phenomenon of very low perfusion pressure causing collapse of the microvasculature, the postcapillary venules are more susceptible, raising the resistance disproportionately, as observed with Starling's resistor [64, 65]. Later studies suggest that pre-existing collateral flow limits infarct size and is associated with 80% reduction in mortality over 16 years in a large cohort study [66]. It can be assessed with pressure-derived collateral flow index (CFI) or collateral FFR as proposed by Pijls. CFI $\geq$ 2.5 carries survival advantage. But it could also be an adverse reflection of microvascular obstruction in acute myocardial infarction, where Pw no longer reflects collateral supply [67].

$$\mathrm{CFI} = \frac{\mathrm{Pw} - \mathrm{Pv}}{\mathrm{Pa} - \mathrm{Pv}}$$

As with FFR, Pv can be dropped and Pw is easily obtained during a routine FFR-guided coronary intervention, and it still is a hyperaemic index, by virtue of balloon-induced ischaemic reactive hyperaemia, 20 s of coronary occlusion increases flow by 4–5 times above the basal flow, an effect that lasts for 30 s as demonstrated by Pijls in his canine experiments [47]. But to obtain CFI, a steady state is required for a stable Pw, and 60 s occlusion is recommended. When this is done without provoking chest pain or ST elevation, it is a sign of adequate collateral recruitment or supply [66, 68].

In lockstep, de Bruyne [54] used the same fluid-filled pressure-monitoring guidewire in 37 patients undergoing a single vessel coronary angioplasty to measure pressure fall across coronary stenoses. Tested in vitro first, it underestimated true pressure by ≤ 5%, and showed predictable overestimation of gradients in very tight lesions, while in vivo it safely crossed 97% of stenoses and accurately tracked pre- and post-coronary angioplasty mean gradients (falling from 30 to 3 mmHg). However, it was not suitable for use in small vessels with tight lesions, which resulted in dampened pulsatile signals, limiting its further development as a high fidelity tool for FFR in the clinical setting.

Pijls came upon Tenerz's publication in the niche *Catheterization and Cardiovascular Diagnosis* (1975–1998) journal in 1991 about a first-in-man trial of a fibreoptic pressure wire in Sweden. The journal was mid-rank in impactfulness, but was widely read within the interventional cardiology community. Therefore, it was not easy for Pijls to miss the article. From Tenerz's point of view, his use of a fibreoptic pressure wire was a proof of principle of his PhD project. Its development stalled, for lack of an obvious clinical indication, until Pijls reached out to him in 1992. The standard practice at the time was angiographic visual assessment of a coronary lesion and balloon pullback gradient post-angioplasty, a methodology that had remained unchanged since Grüntzig introduced it in 1977, and the coronary angioplasty doctors were comfortable with this time and tested approach, which had been around for over 15 years.

The collaboration that was to come between Pijls, de Bruyne and Tenerz with the latter's company, Radi Medical Systems, Ltd., Uppsala, Sweden, culminated with the birth of FFR in 1996, and a value of < 0.75 has 93% accuracy in predicting cardiac ischaemia on non-invasive tests [69]. Through subsequent large RCTs with long-term data, FFR is firmly established in routine clinical practice and a prognostic threshold of ≤ 0.80 is established. However, the rationale, theoretical underpinning and methodology advanced by Pijls, de Bruyne and Gould, in the coming era of advanced computer digitisation and modelling of fluid and flow dynamics with artificial intelligence (AI), being applied in the cardiac catheterisation laboratory and high-resolution CT coronary angiogram, will usher in *wire-free* FFR or flow-derived surrogate of CFR for coronary lesion assessment and microvascular function testing [70].

1.4.3 Bolus Thermodilution

The miniaturisation of pressure sensing using fibreoptic microscopic reflective diaphragm allows continuous pressure transducing, as alternative to the traditional fluid-filled manometry, plus it could be fitted on a coronary 0.014″ guidewire, upgraded from an earlier 0.018″ prototypic Pressure Guide [37, 69], marketed by

Radi Medical Systems, Uppsala, Sweden, introduced as PressureWire® in 1993. A *thermistor* was added in 2007 as the Certus model. Radi was acquired by St Jude Medical, St. Paul, Minnesota, in 2008, which innovated it into the PressureWire™ X Guidewire with wireless connectivity, launched in 2016. The following year, St Jude was integrated into Abbott's Cardiovascular Division, Plymouth, Minnesota. The pressure wire has, in effect, turned into a shrunken Swan-Ganz PA catheter in concept, but with methodological differences in its use, adapted to the coronary artery.

There are often situations whereby the FFR is non-significant, but the patient has a positive ischaemic non-invasive test and continuing angina, grouped as angina with non-obstructive coronary arteries (ANOCA). In general, one third of patients with chest pain undergoing a diagnostic coronary angiogram have significant epicardial coronary artery disease. These are treated with coronary angioplasty, coronary artery bypass grafting (CABG) or escalating anti-anginals. The other two-thirds, most are labelled as having non-cardiac chest pain, reassured and discharged from specialist care. But a significant number continued to have chest pain; many repeatedly presented themselves to the emergency department, underwent multiple invasive coronary procedures, and were treated with empirical polypharmacy, often with multiple drug intolerance [71–73].

In the absence of epicardial coronary stenosis, if the angina is convincing, and chronically experienced, then by virtue of Ockham's razor, it must be the microvasculature that is at fault. This is when Ohm's law as described earlier comes into play, $\Delta P = Q \cdot R$. Here is where it gets a bit confusing with many assumptions and trade-offs. The pressure that drives flow across the myocardium, ΔP, is the pressure gradient with an *upstream* driving pressure and a *downstream* minimal pressure (LVEDP)—the coronary perfusion pressure (CPP). For convenience and expediency, the right atrial pressure (RAP) or the central venous pressure (CVP) is used for accessibility, as was used by Ernest H. Starling (1866–1927) and others in their animal experiments as a surrogate for LVEDP. RAP is subject to loading status, right heart function and lung condition, therefore it is not an accurate reflection of the LVEDP. Next, the left atrium is not accessible but the Swan-Ganz PA catheter when wedged (pulmonary capillary wedge pressure, PCWP) offers a reasonable estimate of the LVEDP, but on the proviso that there is no mitral valvular dysfunction. Fundamentally, when it comes to the whole heart, the driving pressure across the organ is aortic pressure minus right atrial or central venous pressure (Pa-Pv), but in the context of a single coronary artery perfusing a segment of myocardium, the pressure across the microvasculature is Pd-(Pw)-LVEDP. But even this is an over-simplification, it gets more complicated.

As for the actual aortic pressure when the coronary artery starts to flow is after the closure of aortic valve, corresponding to the aortic *dicrotic notch* when the aortic pressure equalises, then exceeds the LV pressure, i.e. the LV end-systolic pressure (ESP) which is the start of isovolumic relaxation with flow entering the LV subepicardium, and from mid-diastole with opening of the mitral valve the LV rapidly fills, when peak flow occurs with subendocardial perfusion. Intra-aortic balloon pump

(IABP) is timed and triggered at the dicrotic notch to augment diastolic coronary flow [74].

Since the peak aortic systolic BP is easier to pinpoint under any circumstances, a commonly used rule-of-thumb is that dicrotic notch ESP is at 90%, but this is true in normotensives under resting condition, it becomes unreliable under stress [75, 76]. Alternatively, the mean BP can also be accurately determined, this is used in FFR. Mean BP is roughly diastolic BP plus a third of pulse pressure (systolic BP—diastolic BP). This aligns with mid diastole but changes according to heart rate, with bradycardia it shifts to late diastole, and in critical care, a mean BP of > 65 mmHg is recommended [77]. Mean BP is used to calculate the workload of the heart: (Mean BP—LVEDP) ·Stroke volume, mmHg·mL or Joules—similar to the area within an LV pressure-volume loop. On the other hand, in classic open-chested canine *beating* heart experiments, the CPP was defined as diastolic BP (trough) minus RAP < 50 mmHg, when autoregulation failed, cardiac ischaemia ensued with ventricular fibrillation [78]. But the tradition of using the diastolic BP as the upstream pressure for CPP does not make logical sense but is used conceptually more for teaching than for practice. At that stage, just prior to the aortic valve opening, the myocardial perfusion would have completed anyway. Which potentially means that in humans and through the research of Pijls on coronary collaterals, the failure of autoregulation might be even lower at 25–30 mmHg.

Indeed, when a semi-compliant balloon was gradually inflated within a stent in the proximal left anterior descending (LAD) artery of a 63-year-oldman, as the distal LAD pressure fell to 13 mmHg, the coronary flow down the LAD remained unperturbed at rest [79]. During hyperaemia, CFR < 2.0 corresponded with an FFR of < 0.20, suggesting an even more potent microvascular adaptation in humans. Conversely, as Pijls and de Bruyne demonstrated in their canine experiments in 1993, that during hyperaemia there was a linear relationship between pressure and flow [47], in this detailed and precise report, an *FFR of 0.80 which is the current standard for coronary intervention*, paralleled a CFR of about 3.5, albeit in this single case study. This highlights a mismatch between physiology and trial data with an FFR ≤ 0.80. With this enforced FFR threshold, coronary angioplasty reduced angina by a third at 30 days in the milestone FAME 2 trial reported in 2014 [80]. This finding has been confirmed by a sham-controlled ORBITA 1 trial in 2018 [81]. Important to note that elective coronary angioplasty for stable angina does not alter prognosis, neither short-term, nor long-term. In other words, procedural complications such as MI and stent failures including stent thrombosis, usually balance out natural history events of patients treated medically, in equal measure. Pedantically, since 70% of patients responded well to medical therapy, at least in the first month, if these patients were granulatedly analysed and stratified according to FFR all the way down to 0.20, it is like that CFR < 2.0 remains the physiological threshold for angina, as per Gould's adopted definition of functional ischaemia he established in 1974 [40, 82]. He also noted this was associated with a stenosis of > 85%, and CFR started to fall with > 50% stenosis during hyperaemia in his canine experiments. But in reality CFR falls linearly without a stenotic threshold [79].

There is evidence that CFR is measured concurrently, resulting in a discordance, i.e., FFR ≤ 0.8 and CFR ≥ 2.0, coronary intervention appears not to be beneficial according to data from the ILIAS Registry, reported in 2022 [83, 84], that was added on top of an earlier long-term follow-up study [85]. Although the CFR in this registry was obtained with different techniques with significant technical limitations, with regard to reliability of signals from Doppler wire and repeatability of bolus thermodilution, including CFR being sensitive to high baseline flow, making it prone to type I error or false positive results, the findings are still relevant for further investigations [83]. In contrast, FFR is incredibly reproducible.

In the unpublished dataset from DEFINE-FLOW study presented at TCT on October 16, 2020, delivered online because of the COVID-19 pandemic, originally scheduled for Miami Beach Convention Center, Florida, FFR ≤ 0.80 had double composite event rates, comparing CFR < 2.0 and ≥ 2.0 (5.8% vs 10.8%), with CFR measured using the Doppler wire, over 2 years—but the primary endpoint was driven by coronary revascularisation, rather than by either death or MI. Data from this study looking at 133 lesions, which also included the IDEAL registry dataset [86], when CFR was interpreted with maximal hyperaemic flow as coronary flow capacity (CFC) mapping, this outperformed FFR ≤ 0.80 in predicting $\geq 50\%$ post-PCI hyperaemic flow gain [87]. This philosophy boils down to the fact that FFR is discrete lesion specific, while CFR is a global index that includes both epicardial disease and microvascular function. *High CFR suggests that the microvasculature is capable of diastolic filling by active suction despite low FFR*, as foreseen by Francisco Torrent-Guasp with his helical ventricular myocardial band (HVMB) model of the heart [88–90].

A recent take on CPP is the *diastolic pressure-time index* (DPTI, mmHg·s) which is the area of the aortic pressure during diastole that exceeds the LV pressure [91, 92]. It is a measure of myocardial perfusion or blood supply during diastole, the bigger the area the more blood the heart gets. The Buckberg index is obtained as a ratio between DPTI with systolic pressure-time index (SPTI), the area under systolic LV pressure curve, as a maker of myocardial oxygen demand, a value < 0.7 suggests a mismatch between supply and demand, and it is believed to be a marker for subendocardial ischaemia.

Pijls applied his videodensitometry contrast-dilution method to the new pressure wire with temperature sensing, a miniature Swan-Ganz PA catheter. He and de Bruyne described the first coronary artery *thermodilution* with a 3 mL saline bolus-injectate at room temperature, delivered at the guide catheter tip, placed in the ostium of a coronary artery. This approach of estimating coronary flow, which then allowed Ohm's law to estimate microvascular resistance with mean coronary perfusion pressure would be applied to ANOCA. First, to demonstrate the gold standard of reduced vasodilatory capacity in ANOCA, i.e. CFR < 2, and second, to calculate the hyperaemic microvascular resistance.

While Swan and Ganz applied the Stewart–Hamilton equation in full, Q is proportional to inverse of cooling-time integral $\int_0^\infty \Delta T(t)\mathrm{dt}$ of the **first-past of all-of-the saline bolus at zeroth moment** within a well-defined, confined space and closed system, Pijls applied his earlier work with the mean transit time, Tmn, which was adapted for an undefined contrast volume (V) of distribution, but focusing on one particular area of interest, using Meier-Zierler's *central volume principle*; V = Q · Tmn. And his work with FFR using intravenous adenosine for inducing hyperaemia. In this context, Tmn is a measure of the "average" time it takes for the saline bolus to cross a segment of an artery, rather than an indicator's average appearance time on a defined piece of organ. Mathematically, this is calculated as the **first moment** an indicator appears, its concentration (C) or signal intensity per unit time (C·t).

$$\text{Tmn} = \frac{\text{First moment curve}}{\text{Zeroth moment curve}}$$

$$\text{Tmn} = \frac{\int_0^\infty \text{t}\cdot\Delta T(\text{t})\text{dt}}{\int_0^\infty \Delta T(\text{t})\text{dt}}$$

→ In practice, Tmn is calculated by computer with a sampling rate of 100 Hz or 0.01 s, using the Trapezoid rule, ΔT_i = temperature change from baseline at time t_i, and Δt = interval width.

$$\text{Tmn} = \frac{\sum_{i=1}^{n} t_i \cdot |\Delta T_i| \cdot \Delta t}{\sum_{i=1}^{n} |\Delta T_i| \cdot \Delta t}$$

For example, using a sampling at of 0.1 s (Δt):

Time (s)	ΔT (°C)
0.0	0.00
0.1	0.10
0.2	0.50
0.3	0.80
0.4	0.60
0.5	0.30
0.6	0.10
0.7	0.00

Numerator:

(0.0 × 0.00) + (0.1 × 0.10) + (0.2 × 0.50) + (0.3 × 0.80) + (0.4 × 0.60) + (0.5 × 0.30) + (0.6 × 0.10) + (0.7 × 0.00) = 0 + 0.01 + 0.10 + 0.24 + 0.24 + 0.15 + 0.06 + 0 = **0.8 °C·s**

Denominator (AUC):

0.00 + 0.10 + 0.50 + 0.80 + 0.60 + 0.30 + 0.10 + 0.00 = **2.4 °C**

$$\text{Tmn} = \frac{0.8°\text{C} \cdot \text{s}}{2.4°\text{C}}$$

$$= 0.33\text{s}$$

This mix and match of three methodologies allowed him to calculate the *flow-derived* CFR. These are the five reasons why the highly precise Swan-Ganz methodology could not be adopted.

1. The 3-mL saline bolus does not all travel down the coronary artery where the wire-tip thermistor is in the mid-to-distal vessel; it dissipates down the aorta and down other main branches. If the wire is in LAD, saline volume is lost in the Cx; therefore the volume of distribution (V) is unpredictable and is unknowable. But doing this under resting conditions and during hyperaemia, the numerator V could be cancelled out.
2. The travel time of the saline bolus is under 1 s, making Tmn less variable, a full cooling-time AUC integral would square the error.
3. The high flow in coronary artery recirculates the saline bolus instantly with heat lost to the vessel wall, adding to a long tail, which would overestimate the cooling-time AUC integral.
4. Instead of volume of distribution (V), the numerator of the Stewart–Hamilton equation includes an injectate-specific heat/density constant (k_1) and an equipment calibration constant (k_2) which include catheter dead space and heat exchange characteristics. These constants are challenging to standardise and tend to amplify measurement errors.
5. Bolus thermodilution measures heat dilution of a saline bolus along a short distance of an artery and uses Tmn from the central volume principle, which is designed to evaluate tissue perfusion. While Pijls's initial work in the 1990s with fluoroscopic videodensitometry to assess myocardial contrast blushing following direct coronary injection is a valid use of the methodology, this is *adapted or misapplied*, since heat changes within the myocardium are not measured, nor are they measurable. In other words, the derived indices of bolus thermodilution reflect flow over an artery segment, not tissue perfusion.

Bolus thermodilution is elegant in its simplicity, despite the considerable theoretical workarounds and assumptions underlying its use [93]. With the pressure-thermistor sensors ≥ 6 cm from the guide catheter tip, Tmn is obtained in triplicates, these should be within 20% in variation, otherwise repeated measures are undertaken until this is achieved. The average of three Tmn at rest and during hyperaemia; CFR = $\text{Tmn}_{\text{rest}}/\text{Tmn}_{\text{hyperaemia}}$. When FFR and Pa (mean aortic pressure) are taken into account to address the epicardial flow resistance and aortic driving pressure; microvascular resistance reserve (MRR) could be derived [94–96]:

$$\text{MRR} = \frac{\text{CFR}}{\text{FFR}} \cdot \frac{\text{Pa}(\text{rest})}{\text{Pa}(\text{hyperamia})}$$

Since some ANOCA patients have coronary microvascular dysfunction (CMD), aside for vasodilatory incompetence with reduced CFR or MRR, and a normal FFR confirming non-obstructive epicardial coronary arteries, a complementary microvascular index is necessary. This came in the form of index of microvascular index (IMR) obtained during hyperaemia, adapted from Ohm's law of $R = \Delta P{\cdot}Q$; $\Delta P = Pd - LVEDP$ and $Q \propto 1/Tmn$, assuming $LVEDP = 0$, thus:

$$IMR = Pd \cdot Tmn_{hyperaemia}$$

The corrected IMR which takes into account driving aortic pressure, epicardial coronary artery disease and collaterals:

$$IMR_{Corr} = Pa{\cdot}Tmn_{hyperaemia}{\cdot}\frac{Pd - Pw}{Pa - Pw}$$

IMR underwent, as with other coronary physiology indices, vigorous validation against other techniques, in vitro, and in vivo, both in animal experiments and in human studies, in particular with epicardial coronary artery disease and following MI for the latter [97–101]. Equipped with bolus thermodilution-derived CFR and IMR, which are ideally suited for the diagnosis of ANOCA, the Coronary Microvascular Angina (CorMicA) study reported in 2018 a cohort of 391 patients undergoing an elective coronary angiogram for angina [102]. Of these, 151 had non-obstructive coronary arteries and they all had invasive coronary function test with bolus thermodilution defining CMD as a cause of microvascular angina using $CFR < 2$ and/or $IMR \geq 25$, with acetylcholine spasm testing—3/145 (3%) had brady-arrhythmia.

The ANOCA patients were randomised in 1:1 to a usual care group, and an intervention group ($n = 75$, women 71% and median age 62, interquartile range 54–69 years) was divided into a grid of 4; 1. Normal 6 (8%), 2. CMD 43 (57%), 3. VSA or vasospastic angina 12(16%), and 4. Mixed CMD/VSA 14 (18.7%). The intervention group was managed according to their coronary physiology, CMD treated with beta blockade, e.g. nebivolol, risk factor management, reducing unnecessary drugs, weight lost and cardiac rehabilitation. The VSA group was treated with calcium channel blockade, long-acting nitrates and smoking cessation; endothelial dysfunction (epicardial vasoconstriction to acetylcholine < 90%) was treated with ACE inhibitors and statins. By 6 months, the physiology-guided group achieved a mean 11.7-point greater improvement in angina severity (Seattle Angina Questionnaire summary score) with parallel gains in quality of life and treatment satisfaction, compared to the usual-care group. This was a breakthrough trial which highlighted that ANOCA could be rationally managed with an outcome that was sustained for 1 year [103, 104].

A larger study by the same group, this time with patients pre-identified with CT coronary angiogram (CTCA) from the outpatient setting, and following $FFR > 0.80$ also underwent the same coronary physiology study followed by CorMicA treatment algorithm in 115/231 patients, but this did not yield a positive result with an up to 2 years' follow-up [105, 106]. The utility of bolus thermodilution in these studies was not specifically looked at. Nevertheless, with its increasing adoption, and with further clinically based studies, CFR and IMR have not been found to be as reproducible as originally thought [107, 108]. They are subject to multiple confounders, making their reliability on a personalised care level unacceptable for a positive result because of type I error. However, bolus thermodilution is a useful test for ruling out CMD, with CFR $\geq$ 2.5 and IMR $<$ 25, and if undertaken with intracoronary adenosine, this allows for repeated studies at the same sitting with incremental escalating 200 μg doses up to 1000 μg for the LAD, when hyperaemia is not in doubt [108, 109]. A lower starting adenosine dose for the right coronary artery can be used, from 100 to 200 μg.

1.4.4 Continuous Thermodilution

Pijls and de Bruyne demonstrated a prototypic continuous thermodilution in their 19th Aalst-Einthoven Coronary Physiology Course in Belgium on 19–20 November 2015 [25]. Using a St Jude PressureWire™ Certus™ Guidewire which was inserted down the 25 mm monorail segment of a RayFlow® infusion microcatheter, manufactured by Hexacath In., Rueil-Malmaison, Paris, France. They advanced by 6 cm the 0.014″ combined pressure-thermistor tipped wire to the mid LAD of a study volunteer. The RayFlow stayed in the proximal vessel. It has four laser-cut 100 μm infusion holes, two at 7 mm and another two at 8 mm from the tip, radially oriented at 0°, 180°, 90° and 270° in pairs, respectively. Saline exits through these side holes as four evenly spaced radial jets, coalescing into a uniform cylindrical sheath of fluid for rapid, homogeneous mixing with blood. At 9 mm from the tip, there are 2 further side holes to house the wire sensors [110].

Saline was infused at a flow-controlled mode of the injector; the pump pressure was set at an upper safety limit of 500 pounds per square inch (PSI), more than enough to deliver 20 mL/min [111, 112]; a higher rate at 25 or 30 mL/min may be necessary to induce maximal hyperaemia that will require a pump pressure increase [113], but rarely the rate is reduced to 15 mL/min if there is bradycardia and dropped heartbeats with 20 mL/min. In this case, the saline infusion caused hyperaemia within 20 s, the mixed temperature noticeably fell on the Abbott Coroventis CoroFlow™ software interface, stabilising into T_m. The wire was then pulled back into the RayFlow with the opaque segment just outside the microcatheter, and temperature curve plunged, to a steady infusate temperature (T_i), almost instantly but a stable line was allowed to run for 20 s. In general, the two key temperature measurements together could be obtained within 30–45 s, making repeat studies feasibly easy. Absolute volumetric coronary blood flow (Q) is calculated with the following equation:

$$Q = 1.08 \cdot \frac{T_i}{T_m} \cdot Q_i$$

This set-up reproduced Ganz's coronary sinus continuous thermodilution flow catheter "lock, stock and barrel" in concept and theory, but with major adaptations made as described above. Ganz's version has two thermistors: working with one thermistor makes moving the wire up and down the artery necessary for repeated measures. Another novel adaptation is the introduction of saline hyperaemia.

Stephen Hales (1677–1761) first noted intestinal microvascular resistance to warm water injected down the descending aorta in his canine experiments. He injected 542 cubic inch (8.9 L) of water, that was equivalent to 13 pounds (5.6 L) of blood; seeped out in 400 s through a whole-length cut gut, whereas it took 140 s through the mesenteric arteries, and 30 s to pass through the aorta—he concluded that the mesh of small blood vessels in the gut "retarded" blood flow by threefold. Further, despite driving the water in at a normal arterial pressure, the blood vessels did not rupture, implying that they had capacity to dilate and accommodate the increased volume. Hale therefore was the first person to describe microvascular resistance, and compliance or vasodilatation, and by a tenuous implication, hyperaemia [18]. Earlier, he calculated cardiac output of a dog by directly funnelling blood from the ascending aortic and calculated the cardiac output to be about 1.9 L/min, which is within range for a medium-sized dog.

In slow flow or no reflow following coronary angioplasty in acute MI, a forceful 10 mL saline flush through the thrombectomy catheter, which could be repeated two or three times, improves flow, demonstrable with angiography and pressure transducing through the thrombectomy catheter [114]. This flushes out the microvascular plugs, causes microvascular dilatation and reduces ST elevation. Saline infusion at 20 mL/min causes red cell haemolysis, releasing adenosine triphosphate (ATP) that acts on the vascular smooth muscle cell (VSMC) through multiple endothelial pathways to promote hyperaemia [115]. In theory, caffeine which blocks A_2 adenosine receptor, its abstinence, as is required prior to many tests including FFR, where adenosine is used to induce hyperaemia, is not necessary. But, in the presence of microvascular endothelial dysfunction, saline hyperaemia could be blunted. Which means diabetics with low CFR with saline hyperaemia perhaps should be retested with intravenous adenosine at the same sitting, or assess for acetylcholine responsiveness [116]. Potentially, ionic shifts could also contribute to the saline phenomenon. Myron Prinzmetal (1908–1987) in 1959 found that when he soaked 1% hypertonic saline over the ischaemic myocardium where the coronary artery was ligated in dogs, the ST elevation settled. Increasing extracellular sodium through the Na^+/Ca^{2+} exchanger causes cytosolic sodium influx and calcium efflux in VSMC, delaying ischaemic repolarization and causing vasodilatation; thereby leading to reduction in ST elevation and vasodilatation [117].

This first iteration of the Pijls-de Bruyne's coronary continuous thermodilution technique was submitted 1 month after the demonstration in the course, and published 7 months later on 7 July 2016 [110]. In Vitro, with simulated LV and coronary artery, flow rates of 50–300 mL/min were tested with RayFlow infusion rates of 15, 25 and 30 mL/min; they found strong correlation between actual and estimated flow, with a Spearman's rank coefficient, $\rho = 0.976$ ($p < 0.0001$). Over the three infusion rates, the mean biases were −12, −5.4 and −1.1 mL/min, at higher 30 mL/min infusion rate, it tracked the actual flow within 1 mL/min. When repeated under the same condition, the Bland-Altman repeatability coefficient of variation was 8% [110].

In humans, an infusion rate of 15 and 20 mL/min down the LAD matched intravenous adenosine given at the rate of 140 μg/kg/min. Combining adenosine and saline infusion did not generate more hyperaemic flow [112]. In order to calculate the CFR, *basal flow* is needed, and a lower rate of infusion at 10 mL/min was used against the Doppler wire. In this follow-up human study in which 27 coronary arteries were tested, this was verified by Pijls and de Bruyne. CFR obtained with continuous thermodilution and Doppler wire were similar; 2.78 ± 0.91 versus 2.76 ± 1.06, with a mean bias of −0.02 (limits of agreement −0.95 to +0.91; $p = 0.935$), Pearson $r = 0.90$ (95% CI 0.78–0.95, $p < 0.001$), and Passing–Bablok regression intercept = 0.03 (95% CI −0.61 to 0.55), slope = 1.01 (95% CI 0.79–1.30), indicating no systematic or proportional bias. Nevertheless, if the two methods were treated as repeat measures, the CFR has a Bland-Altman coefficient of variation (CoV) of 17 (0.47/2.77) %. Still a CoV of < 20%, to suggest a clinically meaningful equivalence between the two techniques. Therefore, saline infusion at 10 mL/min is reliable in estimating the rest or basal flow, and it could be used as the denominator to calculate CFR with the flow rate obtained at hyperaemic flow using a saline infusion rate of 20 mL/min. However, for smaller codominant circumflex and right coronary arteries, it can cause partial hyperaemia, noticeable with a drifting Pd/Pa. In which case, a lower 8 mL/min saline infusion can be used instead to estimate the basal flow [118]. But in practice, the focus is on the LAD; discordant results between different coronary territories in the absence of structural cardiac abnormalities; the so-called half-hearted CMD phenomenon, although it has been reported, should be regarded as biologically implausible [119].

The next task was to compare it with bolus thermodilution and apply it in patients with ANOCA. Haemodynamic indices of CFR and MRR obtained with bolus thermodilution were found to be systematically overestimated by at least 1 unit on average, with significant albeit modest correlation with Pearson $r = 0.26/0.28$ [95, 96, 120]. And, with regards to repeatability, the bolus thermodilution indices were three times more variable, Bland-Altman coefficients of correlation for CFR and MRR compared with continuous thermodilution were 13% versus 31%, and 12% versus 33%.

In ANOCA, the MRR is an obvious index to pursue. After all, given that in these patients the epicardial coronary arteries are non-obstructive, the reasoning goes: it must be that the microvasculature is dysfunctional, hence the terminology of CMD. The question is whether CFR < 2 is a robust measure for cardiac ischaemia due to coronary artery disease. How is MRR any different? it is an index with added variables derived from Ohm's law, which would add to its inaccuracy and variation. From studies using continuous thermodilution, MRR ≥ 2.7 is normal and < 2.1 is diagnostic of CMD [94, 121, 122]. In a cohort of 305 patients with chest pain and unobstructed coronary arteries, 184 had an MRR ≥ 2.7 on the LAD; mean age 58 ± 9 years, 83% female, stratified to three mean age groups of 47, 59 and 69. The rest and hyperaemic flow were 74 and 224, 74 and 228, and 69 and 211 mL/min, while rest and hyperaemic resistance were 1374 and 412, 1381 and 418, and 1483 and 462 Wood units—MRR of 3.9, 3.7 and 3.5 [123]. These changes were not significant across age groups, but there was a trend for increased resistance and reduced vasodilatory reserve with age.

This is the controversial part. It is time to pay less attention to microvascular resistance for these following three reasons:

1. Flow is autoregulated; by definition, flow is kept constant for any given BP. It is the resistance that changes beat-to-beat as is the BP. Resistance is like a sluice gate in a dam; it opens and it shuts to keep the flow steady [124]. *Logically, resistance tracks BP and as per the hyperaemic theory, when resistance is minimised, and becomes a constant, $P \propto Q$* [125], now that flow is measurable, its absolute value should be interpreted on its own merit. Indeed, Gould knows this and his coronary flow capacity (CFC) mapping is purely based on flow indices [50, 126]. Why measure an everchanging index (R), when a stable and regulated index (Q) is measurable?
2. Absolute microvascular resistance (Rμ) is not knowable. Ohm's law of ΔP = Q x R, therefore R = ΔP/Q; while absolute flow (Q) can be measured with continuous thermodilution precisely, ΔP is elusive, The Pa is at the aorta nominally taken as mean BP, the Pd is 6 cm in mid vessel, but beyond Pd, the pressure could be significantly lower, FFR should be undertaken with the pressure wire in distal vessel and a pullback gradient is recorded, in many patients with diffuse distal vessel disease, Pd/Pa is significantly lower in distal vessel compared to mid vessel. This is one reason why IMR is significantly higher in distal LAD compared with mid LAD [127]. Pw (coronary wedge pressure for collaterals) is not measured, and Pv (downstream right atrial pressure, RAP, which also measures extracardiac constraint) or left ventricular end-diastolic pressure (LVEDP, a marker of intracardiac compression and left ventricular stretch) is not factored in, further, the microvasculature includes basal and mid left ventricle, but the focus is at the LV apex. Thus ΔP is not definable, nor measurable—it is fuzzy.
3. Hypertension management is never based on a single measure, but on multiple readings, better taken at home. A 24-hr blood pressure monitoring (ABPM) is a superior test for sustained hypertension and its response to drug treatment. Since coronary flow is kept constant, blood pressure tracks resistance—that is the implication of the Ohm's law, if you know the absolute coronary flow, and the aortic pressure, then there is no need to know what the microvascular resistance is. If the BP is high, the coronary microvascular resistance will be high too. Nevertheless, there can be a simple rule of the thumb, hyperaemic Rμ ≥ 500 Wood units, divided by 20, is roughly equivalent to an IMR ≥ 25 which suggests a clearly elevated microvascular resistance, notwithstanding the above reservations, but in practice, when it is < 400 Wood units, it is barn door normal [128, 129]. Although Ohm's law cannot be precisely applied to a single coronary artery, it can in fact be applied to the *whole heart.* In a back of envelope calculation—total myocardial blood flood via the coronary arteries, 250 mL/min or 5% of cardiac output, ΔP = aortic BP 135/85 mmHg – Pv 5 mmHg, right atrial pressure or central venous pressure: total heart myocardial resistance is 387 Wood units, with higher systemic BP; BP 180/100 → 466 Wood units, and 220/120 mmHg → 593 Wood units, although the real value at any given coronary territory is 3 times higher. And interestingly, an explanted rabbit's heart has 10–20% higher resistance during arrest while maximally adenosine-vasodilated compared with when it is beating—which defies physics and logic to

suggest that precise measurement of resistance is methodologically challenging [130]. As mentioned earlier, Ohm's law holds true for a steady-state laminar and hyperaemic flow in a controlled vascular experiment, resistance, R, is held as a constant value, that is when pressure, P, linearly tracks flow, Q, or $P \propto Q$. When turbulence, pulsatility, vasoreactivity and myocardial compression are factored in, vis-à-vis the coronary flow being kept steady over a range of perfusion pressures—the autoregulatory curve, and at low, as well as supranormal flow, Ohm's law is no longer linear or valid [131–133]. In reality, microvascular resistance is somewhere between $\Delta P/Q$ and $\Delta P/Q^2$. And it changes beat-to-beat autoregulating flow irrespectively of the driving pressure, perhaps is should be depicted as a probability range and not a single figure.

The microvascular resistance that is calculated with Ohm's law is a combination of epicardial and microvascular resistance; Poiseuille's hydraulic resistance (R_h) and microvascular resistance, the former is normally ignored, if the artery is smooth and disease-free. In contrast, take for example a 10 cm LAD with diffuse disease, and calculate R_h using Poiseuille's inverse power equation against diameter:

5 mm → 2.8 Wood units
4 mm → 7.6 Wood units
3 mm → 22 Wood units
2 mm → 105 Wood units
1 mm → 1778 Wood units

Since a diseased vessel does not vasodilate significantly during hyperaemia, small vessel disease contributes significantly to coronary flow resistance—the microvasculature vasodilates using part of its vasodilatory capacity to compensate for this, thus giving a low CFR. This is usually described as functional CMD, when the microvascular resistance reserve becomes depleted. And Gould's report in 1974 the notion that cardiac ischaemia occurs when the heart is unable to double its flow under stress, CFR < 2 remains a powerful prognostic factor [124, 134]. It is the gold standard for cardiac ischaemic testing in invasive or non-invasive functional testing modalities, in particular the PET scan and now perfusion CMR.

FFR is highly reproducible and is well established in assessing epicardial coronary artery disease but in the presence of high microvascular resistance which raises Pd, it may be underestimating the epicardial coronary artery disease. However, this discordance between FFR and epicardial coronary artery disease can be associated with normal or high CFR. That is, high hyperaemic microvascular resistance does not preclude normal diastolic suction of blood into the microvasculature, even when it impedes pressure-driven forward flow [89]. Further, hyperaemic microvascular resistance is subject to multiple confounders; it might stay high because of ineffective hyperaemia from caffeine intake, inadequate intravenous adenosine dosing, polycythaemia [135], or reactive hypertension from anxiety [108]. Therefore, defining CMD based on IMR, or hyperaemic minimal resistance is biologically discordant and implausible in its utility. That is why there is an appeal to redefine CMD without the resistance component [89, 136].

Hyperaemic pressure-derived flow surrogates in the form of FFR and CFR are meaningful clinical tools as outcome measures for both prognosis and guidance for revascularisation [137, 138]. Attention could be redirected to absolute volumetric flow that is measured with precision and certainty using the continuous thermodilution methodology, its utility should be for tracking "instantaneous" flow changes in response to vasoactive agents. Also, less weight should be placed on the question, has maximal hyperaemia been achieved, or is this flow truly maximal? For example, pushing RayFlow saline infusion rate $\geq$ 30 mL/min to achieve this is associated with bradycardia, heart block and cardiac ischaemia in many patients [113]. Maximal stress is the province of athletes, but for most, a dose-response changes in flow under submaximal stress could be more informative; for example, submaximal exercise BP predicts future hypertension and it relates LVH [139].

1.5 Three Rules of Uncertainty

1.5.1 The Principle of Emergence

Tobias Mayer (1723–1762), a German astronomer, observed the Moon from Göttingen Observatory and charted the Moon's course by tracking the Manilius Crater as his primary reference point into highly accurate lunar tables for cross-referencing with Greenwich Mean Time (GMT). He used his "method of averages"—by dividing his consecutive 27 nightly observations (one observation per night at the same time) into three groups of 9 days in 1750 and solving in turn the astronomical equations devised by Newton in 1702 [140] with their averages, deriving three coefficients that denoted β (baseline longitude), α (wobble amplitude), and θ (phase shift) that characterise the Moon's main oscillation amplitude and the phasic timing of that oscillation to precisely predict the Moon's position and motion. Mayer submitted his findings to the British Board of Longitude in 1755. Although he died aged 39 in 1762 after a short febrile illness, his posthumous prize of £3000 was awarded to his widow, Maria V. Mayer, in 1765 [141].

Longitude is measured along meridians (great circle lines running from the North to the South Pole), with the prime meridian at Greenwich defined as 0°. By convention, longitudes West of Greenwich run from 0° to −180°, and East from 0° to +180°. Mayer's tables present a simple lookup—no further calculations are required. For example, imagine a man in 1780 shipwrecked in the middle of the Atlantic Ocean who drifted in a small boat to Liberty Island. Using a horizontal sundial at twilight, he determines his local solar time (LST) to be 18:00. He then measures the lunar distance from the Sun with a nautical sextant, getting 55° 30′, then consults Mayer's tables, finding that this separation occurs at 22:56 GMT. The time difference is 4 h 56 min (GMT is later, so he is West), and at 15° per hour the earth rotates, that corresponds to 4.933 h × 15°/h ≈ 74° West.

When Mayer's lunar tables were incorporated into the British Nautical Almanac in 1767, they made possible calculation of longitude at sea accurate to about ½°, comparing local time and GMT. This allowed Great Britain to assert maritime supremacy in traversing oceans, chart new territories and project power between 1780 and 1840 [142]. On the other hand, Pierre-Simon Laplace (1749–1827) applied Mayer's work to derive a series of mathematical equations to accurately predict solar and planetary orbits—thus, solving the Jupiter-Saturn's orbital wobbling due to interplanetary pull as they come close to each other in their respective courses, as per Newton's gravitational inverse square law [143]. Therein lies two key concepts: *first*, multiple measures reduce errors and *second*, accurate data is necessary to interpret meaningfully any subject under study.

Multiple measurements in physical systems such as the Moon allow *regression to the mean*, or the real value, cancelling out the measurement errors. This is also applicable in biology and that is why large epidemiological studies conducted using less accurate methods could inform on a net treatment effect—the law of large numbers. But when applied to the *individual patient*, it becomes problematic since errors cannot be easily accounted for, so-called ecological fallacy.

This can be illustrated by a hypothetical blood assay with moderate accuracy for haemoglobin, with a 20% measurement error and this is applied to a large population. Test it in a randomised controlled trial (RCT) to assess the treatment effect of iron supplementation. Undoubtedly, the broad conclusion will be that anaemia as diagnosed with this blood test will response to iron treatment. However, when applied to the individual patient, 20% or more patients are misdiagnosed with anaemia, and those with genuine anaemia, a significant proportion due to other causes such as folate or B12 deficiency, will not responsd to oral iron intake. This is the same issue faced with bolus thermodilution in diagnosing CMD, with its over 20% coefficients of variation for CFR and IMR, and an overly inclusive criteria [95, 96, 120].

1.5.2 The Principle of Convergence

The discovery of the structure of deoxyribonucleic acid (DNA) as complementary, anti-parallel, right-handed double helix genetic code of life by James D. Watson (1928–2025) and Francis H. C. Crick (1916–2004) on 25 April 1953 epitomises the idiom, "the time is ripe". That is, accumulating strands of evidence coalesce into a recognisable pattern, which then requires sufficiently accurate data obtained with a new tool or technique to finally pin down the insight. Different people or groups might come up with the same idea or solution to a problem. One analogy is the invention of the telescope, suddenly all newly visible planets and stars are discovered by different people.

Watson and Crick were neither formally tasked nor employed to work on DNA. Nevertheless, their research interest was to explore the theoretical basis and application of *X-ray crystallography*, which had been around for 40 years, to large proteins in the emerging field of molecular biology. Watson was a postdoctoral fellow, supported by the National Foundation for Infantile Paralysis; he obtained his PhD on bacteriophage genetics from Indiana University, Bloomington in 1950. Crick started his PhD at University College of London in 1937 which he had to abandon because of the second world war, and he enlisted for another PhD in Cambridge in 1950. They were theorists rather than trialists while at Cambridge. The weight of emerging data they were party to at the time was such that DNA's conclusive structure would be elucidated at some stage; if not by them, it would be by someone else, but this is not, in any shape or form, belittle the immensity of their achievement [144].

With Linus C. Pauling (1901–1994), a future double Nobel Laureate (Chemistry 1954 and Peace 1962) close at the heel, his son, Peter J. Pauling (1931–2003), who was pursuing a PhD on the structure of protein, announced to Watson and Crick that his father had solved the riddle of DNA 1 week before Christmas in December 1952. On 28 January 1953, he gave them as proof his father's soon-to-be-published article on triple helix DNA, a permutation that, seemingly they themselves had constructed with cardboard and wire, and discarded following a review visit by the King's College Group, 1 year earlier [145, 146]. The three of them, and Jerry Donohue (1920–1985), Pauling's former student, all shared a small room as an office on ground floor of the Austin Wing in Cambridge's Cavendish Laboratory. Studying the draft and finding flaws in Pauling's paper, Watson and Crick were duly relieved and revisited their DNA modelling. Incidentally, model building was pioneered by Pauling at the California Institute of Technology, where he conceived the α-helical protein fold in 1948, and published the idea 3 years later, which precedented Cambridge's own pursuit of the same structure [147]. Watson and Crick communicated their critiques directly to Pauling on 21 March 1953, and also attached him, their draft letter to *Nature* [148]. This was rapidly published a month later as a concise, 889-word Letter to the Editor, that included an *acknowledgement to King's College team for their unpublished DNA data.*

Watson visited Maurice Wilkins (1916–2004) at King's College with Pauling's preprint on 30 January 1953, intimating to him the urgency of solving DNA's structure. That was when he saw a print copy of **Photo 51** in Wilkins' office, which was developed over 2–6 May 1952 [144]. Watson at the time was novice at interpreting X-ray crystallography, but Crick likely to have discussed with him the theoretical helical features of diffraction patterns [149–151]. Watson was struck by the clarity of the 10 × 3.4 Ångström (Å, 0.1 nanometre) meridional stacked-and-layered "X" on photo 51. Hence, his eureka moment as he described in his book, "The Double Helix" published in 1968 [144]. But this momentary intellectual flash alone in no way solved DNA's structure. Its helical nature had long been suspected, including Pauling's DNA with triple helix, although photo 51 was first to show the helical signature on a 92% hydrated B-form DNA sample, close to its natural, cell state, purified from calf thymus glands by Swiss biochemist Rudolf Signer (1903–1990) [152].

Wilkins was a fortunate recipient of a bottle of this highly purified, fibrous A-form DNA from Signer, when Signer attended the Faraday Society meeting in

Cambridge on 12 May 1950 to discuss his method of DNA preparation [153, 154]. Wilkins initially worked on this 0.1 mm fibrous DNA sample with his PhD student, Raymond G. Gosling (1926–2015). He confirmed the 3.4 Ångström base pair axial rise (with hindsight), known since 1947 [155]. They found that semi-crystalline DNA with *50% humidity* which was a *mixture of A-form and B-form DNA*, on the basis of perpendicular light reflection, and infrared and ultraviolet light adsorption, pointed towards a *helix*. When rehydrated, it became elongated, as more DNA strands converted to the B-form, from the highly packed and stacked dehydrated A-form. This insight of the effect of hydration on DNA was the key that unlocked the DNA structure [156].

Against Wilkins' will, his departmental head, John T. Randall (1905–1984) redirected the bulk of DNA research, as well as reassigning his PhD student, Gosling to a newcomer with expertise in X-ray crystallography he had recruited, who started work on 5 January 1951. Nevertheless, Wilkin presented his DNA results at *Symposium on Submicroscopical Structure of Protoplasm* which took place at The Zoological Station in Naples, Italy on 22–25 May 1951, coincidentally attended by Watson which inspired him, when he was a postdoctoral fellow in Copenhagen (September 1950–September 1951) [157, 158]. There was to be a tug-of-war within King's College's Biophysics Department, whether DNA was really a helix as Wilkins believed, and tragically, two camps arose that worked in silos [156].

DNA is made up of nucleotides, like Lego pieces. Each nucleotide has three components: external phosphate-and-sugar backbone (ribbon) and an internal nitrogenous (pairing) base; consisting of two purines, adenine and guanine, and two pyrimidines, thymine and cytosine. Adenine can only pair with thymine and guanine with cytosine to form the complementary double helix DNA; this was inferred by Erwin Chargaff (1905–2002) in 1950 [159].

Soon after Watson's sight of Photo 51, on 9 February 1953, Max F. Perutz (1914–2002), a member of the Medical Research Council (MRC) Biophysics Research Committee under whom Watson and Crick worked, handed them the MRC progress report containing unpublished DNA experimental results which was handed out during a site visit to King's College on 15 December 1952 [160]. These DNA data belonged to Rosalind E. Franklin (1920–1958), who had expected that the Cambridge team would see them. In any case, there had been earlier collaborative discourses and mutual site visits between them. Although these were mostly on the dry A-form DNA. But perhaps, not on Photo 51, the data of which were included in the report too. Wilkins was keen to have Franklin working *under him* for his DNA project but not as an equal partner she was led to believe by Randall when she took up the job. She was initially recruited *to lead* her own project on protein work, since she was uniquely qualified in X-ray crystallography.

The resulting clashes of personality made her leave her job 6 months earlier, her three-year Turner & Newall postdoctoral fellowship at King's College's Biophysics Unit. She moved to Birkbeck College, University of London, where she began work on 16 March 1953, on the Tobacco Mosaic Virus funded by the Agricultural Research Council (ARC), which was modest in stipend. She took with her all her notes, her prototypic micro-focus (spot 4.0×40 μm, a single DNA fibre 30–40 μm), high-intensity X-ray tube with electrostatic lens system that could be mounted on a Phillip 2-inch micro-camera for DNA work which was on loan from Birkbeck College, built by Werner Ehrenberg (1901–1975) and Walter Spear (1921–2008) [160], and her photographs (including Photo 51), but left behind the original glass-plate negatives [161]. The Ehrenberg-Spear sealed tube X-ray was later patented, commercialised and it became standard for crystallography. Pauling was not privy to Franklin's data; in his reply to Watson and Crick 1 week later, he wrote that the jury was still out and reaffirmed his confidence in his triple helix hypothesis. But conceded when he visited Cambridge in late April 1953, when he saw the DNA model and read the *Nature* articles.

This *Nature* letter [162] has been cited over 20,000 times to date, far exceeding the accompanying article by Franklin on *B-form DNA* that was cited just over 2000 times, which contained three key pieces of information that helped clinched DNA's structure:

1. DNA is a helix.
2. It consists of two chains with ten nucleotides per turn (34 Å).
3. The paired nucleotides face inward, with the negatively charged phosphate groups on the exterior.

Extraordinarily, Franklin appeared to give precedence to Watson and Crick, by adding in her article, "Thus, our general ideas are not inconsistent with the model proposed by Watson and Crick in the preceding communication" [152]. She died 6 years later, aged 37 from metastatic right ovarian cancer on 16 April 1958. She had not regarded solving the DNA structure was a race. She had become friends with Watson and Crick after she left King's College. Following the International Union of Crystallography symposium in Madrid on 2 April 1956, she spent 1 week with the Cricks exploring Toledo, Seville and Córdoba in the South of Spain [163]. She was to be diagnosed with cancer in 5 months and died exactly 2 years later.

Not without a sense of irony, Franklin investigated the DNA, and she succumbed to a potentially heritable illness, although she had no public record of a family history of cancer [163]. Being of Ashkenazi Jewish heritage, her incidence of BRCA gene mutation would have been 1-in-40 [164], about five times higher than that of the general population. There is also speculation that her hours of exposure to ionising radiation, some DNA plates required over one hundred hours to develop, Photo 51 needed 62 hours [165], could have compounded her risk of developing a cancer. Radiation protection was proposed in 1928, but the guidelines were not followed consistently in the 1950s [166]. Equipment shielding was standard then, but lead thyroid shields and aprons, though available, were not mandatorily enforced that they were worn. Franklin was banned for about 6 weeks (February–March 1948) from the X-ray laboratory in Paris when her dosimeter registered a quarterly high radiation exposure. She was a postdoctoral fellow with Jacques Méring (1904–1973) in Laboratoire Central des Services Chimiques de l'Etat (LCSCE, Central Laboratory of State Chemical Services) (February 1947–June 1950) [167]. In her cooling off period, she wrote up a few papers on coal crystallography, and thought about an ideal micro-focus X-ray tube for her future research [168]. In London, her cumulative radiation exposure would have been minimal, despite the long hours she worked, because of her use of the novel Ehrenberg-Spear sealed tube X-ray she specified and worked with. Of note, her contemporaries, who might be similarly exposed, many lived to their 80 s; Gosling 89, Wilkins 88, Perutz 88, Randall 79, Chargaff 97, Watson 97, and Crick 88.

With the benefits of hindsight, Watson and Crick's solution to the DNA structure was crucially dependent on Franklin's unpublished DNA data [169]. They were awarded the Nobel Prize for Medicine or Physiology 9 years later in 1962, and both continued to help crack the complex genetic code, work that ultimately contributed to the completion of the human genome in 2003 [162]. Fascinatingly, comparative analyses reveal that roughly half of human genes have homologues in fungi, underscoring the deep evolutionary relationship between animals and mushrooms [170].

Franklin's role in the discovery of DNA's structure has been re-evaluated from a sidelined scientist who did not understand her findings, to a highly capable and meticulous female researcher, and a stage play, "Photograph 51" chronicling this episode of her life premiered in Los Angeles in 2009, leading to a cheeky Twitter (now, X) quip, "What did Watson and Crick discovered in 1953? Franklin's data" [163, 169, 171, 172]. Franklin not recognising what photo 51 entailed, back on 6 May 1952, turned out to be a myth [163, 173].

Franklin had actually submitted on **6 March 1953** two papers to *Acta Crystallography*, on A-form DNA which were published 6 months later, including a third in the series submitted on 29 October 1955 [174–176]. A third paper on B-form DNA with the Photo 51 was finalised in typescript on **17 March 1953** [173]. Whereas Watson and Crick completed their second attempt DNA model on **7 March 1953** [160], *26 days* after they had use of *Franklin's submitted but unpublished data*, in particular the A-form DNA part II paper she sent to *Acta Crystallography*, 1 day before the DNA model was completed. Watson and Crick circulated their *draft letter* to *Nature* to Wilkins and Pauling, on 17 [145] and 21 March 1953 respectively, but the actual submission date was **2 April 1953**, coordinated with two accompanying articles, Franklins' pre-prepared third paper with Photo 51, and another from Wilkins.

A critical re-appraisal of this letter with modern eyes reveals the impossibility of the DNA model without Franklin's data [173, 177], but it had upended her seminal contribution as secondarily important, denying her due credit. In other words, it sounded like, Franklin's *subsequent* data were consistent with *prior* predictions from Watson and Crick's hypothetical DNA model. Instead of, Watson and Crick's DNA model was based in large part on Franklin's published results, if it was unveiled after 10 September 1953, following publication of Franklin's *Acta Crystallography* papers. The second scenario would put primacy on Franklin's research. As it turned out, they barely made a "*splash*" with 673, 159, 31 citations to date respectively, for her trilogy of A-form DNA papers. The *Nature* letter acknowledged thus:

> We have also been stimulated by a knowledge of the *general nature* of the unpublished experimental results of Dr. M. H. F. Wilkins, Dr. R. E. Franklin and their co-workers at King's College

A later paper submitted on 24 August 1953 to Proceedings of the Royal Society of London [178], footnote on page 82:

> It is observed* that DNA can exist in two different forms, a crystalline form structure A, and a paracrystalline form structure B.
>
> *The information reported in this section was very kindly reported to us prior to its publication by Drs Wilkins and Franklin. *We are most heavily indebted in this respect to the King's College Group, and we wish to point out that without this data the formulation of our structure would have been most unlikely, if not impossible*. We should at the same time mention that the details of their X-ray photographs were not known to us, and that the formulation of the structure was largely the result of extensive model building in which the main effort was to find any structure which was stereochemically feasible.

Franklin could adjust her humidity chamber such that conversion to B-form DNA was complete by raising the relative humidity (RH) to ≥ 75% (often carried out at 80–92%), yielding 30 weight % water (~ 20 H_2O/nucleotide). This pure form gave the high quality DNA diffraction, resulting in the Photo 51. Conversely, she drove the humidity below 40% RH to fully convert to A-form, with only 6 H_2O/nucleotide, at which point the fibres became crystalline enough to demonstrate molecular packing of a face-centred *monoclinic C2 cell* (a = 22.0 Å, b = 39.8 Å, c = 28.1 Å; β = 96.5°) and revealed a 2_1 screw axis. From the repeat of 28.1 Å and 11 phosphates/turn, she deduced an axial rise of ≃ 2.55 Å per base in A-form DNA. Following rehydration the helix "stretched" by ≃ 30% (28 → 34 Å) as 11 bases/turn → 10 bases/turn; this phenomenon of 180° rotation + ½-turn translation of the 2_1 screw axis leaves only an **anti-parallel double helix** [175]. She first laid out these A-form DNA dimensions in her departmental colloquium on 21 November 1951, which Watson attended but did not grasp the full extent of data [179]. Nevertheless, Watson and Crick had their first attempt at DNA modelling, resulting in a triple helix DNA model, and invited Franklin to view it, which she did 8 days later in Cambridge [163].

Watson's 1968 book, it was candid about colleagues, it caricatured Franklin, and conflated photo 51. Chargaff, whose review of the book appeared on 29 March 1968 issue of *Science*, was incisive and highlighted Wilkins' showing of Photo 51 and Perutz' sharing of the MRC report [180]. Perutz replied 15 months later on 27 June 1969, attaching the *full MRC report* in question [179]. He reflected that he should have sought permission from the King's College Group before giving the MRC report to Watson and Crick but pointed out that none of the data in the report had not been shared between units, in one form or another. Crick's *final piece* for the DNA puzzle was the A-form DNA results, which Watson failed to recognise in November 1951—at Franklin's seminar after 10.5 months into her job, and she had submitted the same data to *Acta Crystallography*, 1 day before Watson and Crick announced that they had completed their DNA model, 26 days after they had the MRC report.

Wilkins and Perutz were sufficiently embarrassed and both sought amends through their later actions about attribution and transparency in research conduct [181, 182]. Wilkins expressed regrets about sharing photo 51, and his poor working relationship with Franklin, and Perutz, being a world-class crystallographer would have known instantly Franklin's MRC data would help solve the DNA structure, yet he gave them to Watson and Crick as an unspoken gesture of interdepartmental research collaboration, but later expressed deep remorse that Franklin was not credited. Franklin's name was not mentioned during the Nobel ceremony in 1962, neither after [183].

Photo 51 had already been meticulously measured by Franklin, the data of which were among other data in the December 1952 MRC report, and they subsequently appeared in *Nature* as the short article in support of Watson and Crick's letter [152]. Watson's sight of Photo 51 on 30 January 1953 excited him, but a helical DNA was not a novel idea. Franklin herself jotted down in her notes dated 24 February 1953 that DNA could be helical based on her experimental data [173]. In the end, it was down to one man, Perutz [163]. Had he not shared the MRC report with Watson and Click, the world would have to wait for Franklin's twin papers on 10 September 1953 in *Acta Crystallography*. Crick had since admitted through interviews [163], and in his book published in 1988 [184] that without Franklin's data, it would be like *building the DNA model in the dark*.

Data sharing was communal and MRC funded both units; directly or indirectly for Crick, Watson and Wilkins, but not Franklin. She never thanked the MRC in any of her publications, yet she submitted a page [179] describing her work which was included in the December 1952 MRC site visit progress report [152, 162, 174–176, 185]. *Franklin's page is reproduced in full in Perutz's response to Chargaff in 1969*. There is an indirect quote from Franklin that she was relaxed about her unpublished data being shared [169], that was departmental policy, to facilitate interdepartmental discourse. Further, on 29 November 1951 when she visited Cambridge to see Watson and Crick's first triple helix model, it was figuratively demolished when she asked, "*But where are the water molecules?*" [163]. The negatively charged phosphate-and-sugar backbone squeezed tightly inside a dehydrated core with the hydrophobic nucleotides facing out; this configuration is as volatile as a powder keg—this was one of the critiques for Pauling's model. The derivatives of nucleotides are ubiquitous; they are involved extensively in cell signalling and energy regulation—as fuel, when the phosphate bond is hydrolysed, this releases energy.

Emil Fischer (1852–1919), a German chemist who won the Nobel Prize in Chemistry in 1902, coined the term purine in 1898 from *purum uricum* (pure uric acid) which he degraded to the parent bicyclic base of a pyrimidine (6 carbons—hexagon) and imidazole (5 carbons—pentagon) fused side-by-side at C4 and C5, making a flat bicyclic double-ring nitrogen base ($C_5H_5N_5$) [186]. When an amino (-NH_2) group is added to C6, it becomes adenine. It got its name from bovine pancreas where it was first isolated in 1885 by Albrecht Kossel (1853–1927)—Greek word ἀδήν (adēn, "gland") [187]. Further, Kossel, a German biochemist and geneticist was awarded the Nobel Prize in Medicine or Physiology in 1910 for his work on genetic materials, he found and named all the DNA.

The adenine nucleotide of DNA in full nomenclature is 2′-deoxyadenosine 5′-monophosphate (dAMP)—adenine base +2′-deoxyribose +5′-phosphate; this is the residue actually present in DNA strands, where the 5′-phosphate of one nucleotide links with the ribose 3′-carbon of the adjacent nucleotide, forming the phosphodiester chain (phosphate-and-sugar backbone).

It becomes *adenosine* when adenine instead bears the naturally occurring D-ribose (right-handed enantiomer), which carries a hydroxyl (-OH) group at the 2′-carbon of the 5-carbon pentose sugar (i.e. the DNA form has only -H there, hence the prefix "deoxy-", or missing an oxygen ion), attached to (cis) β-N9 position of the adenine. It is classed as a *nucleoside* (nucleo + oside), a cellular **nucleu**s-derived material, adenine and glyco**side**, a ribose sugar, hence, adenosine. Adenosine in its pure form was first isolated from a yeast nucleic acid in 1909 by Phoebus A. T. Levene (1869–1940) and Walter A. Jacobs (1883–1967) at the Rockefeller Institute [188].

If one phosphate (PO_4^{3-}, fully deprotonated) group is ester-bonded to the 5′-carbon position of the ribose, it becomes a nucleotide for ribonucleic acid, adenosine 5′-monophosphate (AMP); during RNA synthesis this residue is incorporated from ATP by RNA polymerase after pyrophosphate release. If it has two intramolecular ester bonds (an internal phosphodiester link) with ribose at the 3′-OH and 5′-OH, it becomes the ring-shaped nucleotide cyclic adenosine 3′,5′-monophosphate (cAMP), an important second messenger that transduces signals. In vascular smooth muscle cells (VSMC), β_2-adrenoceptor activation by catecholamines stimulates adenylyl cyclase, converting ATP to cAMP; the rise in cAMP activates protein kinase A (PKA) and promotes vasodilatation. If two or three phosphate groups are strung along the first phosphate of adenosine, it becomes adenosine 5′-diphosphate (ADP) or adenosine 5′-triphosphate (ATP), respectively, whose high-energy phosphoanhydride bonds serve as cellular fuel. Thus, adding and subtracting the phosphate group regulate cellular energy. In the context of the DNA, as Franklin pointed out, the phosphate groups outside the DNA attract, and soak up water, encasing the molecule in a shield, stabilising it.

Relevant to coronary physiology, interstitial adenosine was noted to be increased in the ischaemic myocardium and its exogenous administration causes microvascular vasodilation. Adenosine has 4 types of receptors, two of them, A2A and at higher concentrations, A2B, in the endothelium and VSMC stimulate adenyl cyclase, open KATP (potassium) channels and produce profound microvascular dilatation through cAMP and PKA. The A1 receptor predominates in the atrioventricular node; that is why bolus intracoronary adenosine down the RCA, which perfuses the node, is associated with transient high-grade heart block, albeit lasting seconds; the pause is brief because the nucleoside's intravascular half-life is < 10 s. In contrast, A2A and at higher concentrations, A3 receptors are also involved in ischaemic preconditioning and inflammatory modulation with the potential of limiting infarct size [189].

The hyperaemic property of intravenous adenosine has been utilised for ischaemic testing. At a dose of 140 μg/kg/min, it has been shown to elicit near-maximal coronary hyperaemia (about 4.4-fold resting flow) at steady state, matching the effect of intracoronary papaverine in 84% of patients, while causing only modest systemic changes (mean arterial pressure −6 mmHg, heart rate +24 bpm) in 1990 [190]. A higher dose of 180 μg/kg/min may sometimes be required [191]. However, the systemic effects of adenosine might not be tolerable in a small but a significant proportion of patients, and using an intravenous (IV) cannula with a running infusion can be clumsy (the line may tissue or the pump may malfunction). Activation of A1 receptors in the lungs stimulates pulmonary vagal nerves and causes the sudden sensation of breathlessness, while stimulation of these receptors on cardiac afferent nerves triggers characteristic angina-like chest discomfort [25].

Alternatively, adenosine could be given via the intracoronary (IC) route. Diluting a 30 mg in 10 mL (3 mg/mL) ampoule in a 50 mL syringe with 20 mL of saline added results in 1000 μg/mL. A repeat dilution of a 1 mL aliquot with 9 mL of saline in a 10 mL syringe produces a convenient 100 μg/mL concentration. Using this, 80 μg in the LAD and 40 μg in the RCA yield FFR values nearly identical to standard IV infusion [191, 192]. Bolus thermodilution can also be performed with IC adenosine; escalating doses up to 100–200 μg in the RCA and 200–1000 μg in the LAD allow repeated studies in quick successions [193–195]. However, while a concordantly normal result (high CFR and low IMR) on bolus thermodilution is reassuring, when CFR is low, it can be difficult to determine whether this reflects true CMD (by definition CMD is a failure to induce hyperaemia despite adequate adenosine dosing) or other factors such as adenosine underdosing (especially via the IV route) or caffeine intake, among many other reasons [25]. Thus, with a low CFR with bolus thermodilution, the aetiology for this finding needs to be teased out, ideally with an ad hoc continuous thermodilution. This allows high baseline flow to be excluded as a reason for the low CFR (see Fig. 1.2 below).

Coming back to Watson and Crick's triple helix, it was the first and last attempt at DNA modelling in Cambridge until February 1953. Franklin was a methodical experimentalist who was data driven and was sceptical about molecular modelling. Since there was no active collaboration and she was unaware that DNA modelling had resumed, she would not have thought her unpublished data would be of any use to anyone. However, if there had been no confusion about roles and responsibilities, the discovery of DNA could have been 1 year earlier; leveraging one unit's practice, with another unit's theory. In the end, decoding the DNA was not even a race, it would only become one *when anyone could have come up with the same solution given the evidence*, in this case, if Franklin's data were published first.

Despite the evasive acknowledgement for the use of Franklin's unpublished data, the Nobel Prize website on the 1962 Nobel Prize in Physiology or Medicine has recently been updated with a *Speed read*, "Deciphering life's enigma code", explicitly states that Wilkins and his colleague, Franklin provided the key X-ray diffraction patterns that Watson and Crick used in building the double helix model of DNA [196]. The Eagle Pub in Cambridge near the old Cavendish Laboratory where Watson and Crick purportedly announced that DNA was solved on "28 February 1953", Watson returned and unveiled a Blue Plaque with this date crediting himself and Crick on 25 April 2003 (50th anniversary). Crick did not attend as he was nearly 87 and battling colonic cancer, and he died just over one year later in San Diego, while Watson then was 75, and died on 6 November 2025 in New York, aged 97 as this book was being proofread. Over the next two decades, the Blue Plaque degraded and was repeatedly graffitied with "+ Franklin". It was replaced on 30 August 2023 adding the names of Franklin and Wilkins, but the folklorian date of 28 February 1953 remained. The DNA model was actually completed one week later and Crick wrote to his 12-year-old son, Michael, who was at a boarding school in Hampshire, describing the DNA structure to him on 19 March 1953. Franklin had an effusive obituary in *The Times*, Saturday 19 April 1958, written by John D. Bernal (1901–1971), Franklin's mentor and departmental head at Birkbeck, who also penned the *in memoriam* piece published in *Nature* on 19 July 1958, despite the admiration, unfortunately framed her as an exceptional technician [197].

Franklin's final resting place is in the Willesden Jewish Cemetery, Brent, London, which is 7 miles by road Northwest of St George's Hospital in Tooting, London. With an epitaph, *Scientist. Her research and discoveries on the viruses remain of lasting benefit to mankind.* Her pivotal role in the discovery of DNA would have been lost to history if it was not for Aaron Klug (1926–2018), her collegiate collaborator at Birkbeck who safeguarded her notes. He won a Nobel Prize in Chemistry in 1982 for his application of crystallographic diffraction analysis, a technique that Franklin excelled in, to electron microscopy. In his Nobel lecture on 8 December 1982, he publicly credited Franklin as the person who mentored him and set him on his career path. In 1986, he became the second successor to Perutz (who retired in 1979) as Director of the MRC Laboratory of Molecular Biology in Cambridge.

Watson's book in 1968 inadvertently thrust to the limelight Franklin's name. Chargaff, who knew Franklin personally, was annoyed by her *persiflage* portrayal [180], and Perutz's response to it highlighted the centrality of Franklin's data in Watson and Crick's DNA model [179], followed by Klug's detailed study of Franklin's notes were published on 24 August 1968 in *Nature* [198]. Klug followed up with another article in *Nature* in 1974 [199], and a final comprehensive review published 8 years post-retirement in 2004 [173]. A Lancet piece on *Nobel Chronicles* in 1999 firmly placed Franklin's name among the Nobel Laureates [157]. These secured Franklin's scientific legacy—a molecular biology topic that is overwhelmingly complex and thus impenetrable to the casual reader.

Advancement in science is tool-driven, although little credit was extended to Birkbeck's Ehrenberg and Spear, whose development of a prototype micro-focus, high-intensity sealed tube X-ray source enabled the creation of Photo 51—the image that made the double helix DNA conceivable [200]. In this regard, continuous thermodilution with its high level of reliability in measuring coronary flow tracks the true haemodynamic changes. It is likely that this technique will open up a new direction in coronary physiology. Also, Franklin's mastery of altering DNA's *water* content solved DNA's structure. Could changing *water* quantity within the microvasculature resolve the puzzle of angina that persists long after a trigger has ceased?

1.5.3 The Principle of Inference

Reverend Thomas Bayes (c. 1701–1761) was an English Presbyterian minister at Little Mount Sion chapel, Tunbridge Wells, Kent, who was interred at Bunhill Fields, close to Old Street tube station and about 8 miles by road north of St George's Hospital in Tooting, London. Owing to his non-conformist family background, he had to be educated in Edinburgh, Scotland, as Dissenters were barred from English universities [201]. He was also an amateur mathematician. Bayes was elected Fellow of the Royal Society in 1742, aged 41, purportedly for his work defending Isaac Newton's (1643–1727) calculus in 1736. This involved demystifying the notion of infinitesimals of the derivative dY/dX is not obtained by "making something vanish" but by taking the ratio ΔY/ΔX over ever-smaller intervals until it converges to a single, well-defined limit, i.e. the slope of the curve at that point as X → 0. To illustrate this, imagine a cyclist and graphing the journey. Y-axis is the distance in miles, and X-axis is the time of the day in minutes, between 12:00 and 13:00; then at 12:30, the slope at that time point is the velocity travelled, the derivative of *instantaneous change*, or a movement captured in a moment, in this case in miles/min [202]. Using this technique, the velocity of the cyclist can be determined at any time point, and so the *minimum* or *maximum* speed could be precisely measured. Another example is the LV relaxation time constant τ, measured during LV isovolumic relaxation phase, immediately after closure of aortic valve and before opening of mitral valve, at any instant in that interval, change of pressure, ΔP, against time, Δt:

$$\frac{dP}{dt} = \lim_{\Delta t \to 0} \frac{\Delta P}{\Delta t}$$

→ so dP/dt is simply the slope of the pressure curve, not a "*ghostly disappearance*" of t. Using mono-exponential analogue of Otto Frank's Windkessel model, "Weiss" τ [203] is the time for LV pressure to fall to 1/e (about 37%) of its value at t = 0. In other words, this zero time is traced backwards to the moment the aortic valve closes, where peak negative dP/dt is (minimum, P_0), and duration of decay to P_0/e is the τ, or time between pressure at aortic valve closure and fall of this pressure by 1/e. A smaller τ therefore means faster active relaxation, normally 30–40 ms, > 48 ms suggests slower active relaxation, seen in diastolic heart failure or HFpEF, but it is influenced by age, bradycardia, and hypertension. The coronary pressure wire can be advanced into the LV, and the Coroventis CoroFlow™ software will report the τ, plus the LVEDP [204, 205]. However, τ is of limited value in its clinical utility, because it is invasively obtained with a catheter in the LV. But a modest echocardiographic surrogate, *average* E/e′—the ratio between transmitral early-diastolic flow velocity (E) and mean of septal and lateral mitral annular early tissue velocities (e′), could be used, < 8 is normal and > 14 suggests abnormal LV diastolic function [206].

In addition, Bayes was able to calculate, using binomial distribution, the limits of the *Doctrine of the Mean* in astronomical measurements (see Tobia Mayers above); the range of error reduction is modest with a small numbers of observations [207]. However, he was best known for his posthumous paper, "*An Essay towards solving a Problem in the Doctrine of Chances*", which appeared in the Philosophical Transactions in 1763 [208].

The mathematical foundation of relating *a priori and a posteriori* probabilities was formalised by Laplace, who had independently formulated and published his method in his mémoire in 1774. Upon learning that Bayes had previously published a similar idea, albeit in a more conceptual format, Laplace graciously referred to his result as the *théorème de Bayes* (Bayes' theorem) in his updated mémoire of 1814

[209]. This is also convergence. Other convergent discoveries include the fluid dynamic analogue of Ohm's law by Gotthilf H. L. Hagen (1797–1884) and Jean L. M. Poiseuille (1797–1869); and derivative and integral mathematics of change described earlier, used in calculating LV relaxation, cardiac output and coronary flow. Isaac Newton (1643–1727) called his version *fluxions*, which he kept private until 1693, and Gottfried W. Leibniz (1646–1716) named his version, *calculus*, which he published in 1684 with "∫ and d" symbols that have become standard. Moreover, Leibniz was sent in 1701 from France, a woodblock sheet of 64 hexagrams from Shào Yōng's (1011–1077) Yìjīng by Joachim Bouvet (1656–1730), a Jesuit priest while on furlough from Emperor Kāng Xī's (1654–1722) Court in Běijīng, during the Qīng Dynasty (1644–1911) China. Leibniz annotated the print and recognised the symbolic duality, which reminded him of a numeral system he had devised in 1679. The synchronicity he thought was divinity, and he published his binary arithmetic in 1703, which led to modern computing [210].

These mathematical innovations provided the basis for today's machine learning and artificial intelligence (AI). In particular, Bayesian inference provides a framework whereby a prior probability influences the outcome. For example, the likelihood of finding the Pope anywhere in the world is one in 8 billion; the chances of bumping into him in Vatican City on an ordinary day are one in 10,000; and seeing him on the balcony of St Peter's Basilica on an Easter Sunday is essentially 100%. In other words, foreknowledge reduces the uncertainty of a future event [201].

Take a frequentist solution to a problem: a pot containing 20 red balls and 80 black balls, representing a 20:80 ratio, or 20% red balls. If one ball is drawn, its colour noted, and then replaced before drawing again, this process must be repeated approximately *246 times* to estimate the true red ball proportion within a ± 5% margin of error at 95% confidence. However, if multiple balls are drawn per trial, still with replacement, the number of trials required *decreases accordingly*. For example, drawing 5 balls per trial requires only *49 trials*; 10 balls, *25 trials*; 20 balls, *13 trials*; 50 balls, *5 trials*; and 100 balls, just *1 trial*, since the entire population has effectively been observed. This illustrates how sampling efficiency improves with larger batch sizes and how statistical confidence can be maintained with fewer repetitions when more information is gathered per trial. This principle reflects the *law of large numbers*, which states that estimates become more accurate as sample size increases.

To restate this puzzle in Bayesian terms, suppose a *prior belief* is assumed, that the pot contains a 50:50 ratio of red to black balls. Drawing one ball at a time with replacement, suppose *20 trials* are done, and 4 red and 16 black balls are observed. Applying Bayes' theorem with a uniform prior Beta (1, 1), the posterior distribution becomes Beta (5, 17), reflecting the updated belief about the red ball proportion. The mean of this posterior is approximately 0.227 [5/(5 + 17)], which closely aligns with the true underlying proportion of 20%. This Bayesian approach not only incorporates prior beliefs but also quantifies uncertainty through a posterior probability distribution rather than relying solely on point estimates or confidence intervals. It also deals with measurement errors by modelling the uncertainty in observed data and integrating over the possible true values to produce corrected, probabilistic estimates, thus providing a shortcut in estimating the true treatment effect.

The frequentists' RCT has co-opted the evidence base in medicine for good reasons, but comparing two drugs or devices when the outcome measure is small and infrequent, leads to use of composite endpoints potentially distorting priorities. One example is the systematic use of coronary stent in MI, a previous trial conducted over 20 years ago using the "eye-balling" angiographic coronary restenosis at follow-up after 6 months, despite no significant differences in death and MI, as a composite endpoint, drove the positive outcome [211–214]. Also, use of broad entry criteria and adjudication of, or selective use of outcome measures, with cherry-picking time points for follow-up studies, create controversies [215–217]. Many of these very expensive RCTs sponsored by key opinion leaders provide guidelines for the practising clinicians [218, 219].

The Bayesian method is more organic in learning and updating information. It is designed to answer the question, how much better is A than B, and what is trend, than the all-or-nothing set with a p-value of < 0.05 [220]. Yet, its adoption in evidence gathering in medicine is lagging. Only about 1.8% of articles in leading medical journals even mention Bayesian techniques, versus about 30% in top statistics journals [221]. One recent application in cardiology is to find out whether a 60 μm thin-strut stent is better than the conventional stent with thicker 80 μm strut in MI [222]. By using data from a previous study, the follow-up trial only needed to recruit about 1300 new patients, or 1700 in total recruits, instead of the conventional RCT that needs 4400 patients for stent failure of 6% vs 4%, at $\alpha = 0.05$ and 80% power; thus, a 60–70% reduction in patient numbers, while giving the same result, but stated in posterior probability of 0.986 [223, 224]. The superiority of thin-strut stents have since been validated in multiple conventional trials [225]. Regardless of statistical methods, it is the replication of the result that eventually matters the most, either in follow-up studies, or post-marketing surveillance whether rare events are observed. On a separate note, if thinner strut is good, what about no-strut coronary angioplasty with the drug-coated balloon (DCB, Chap. 5) [212–214]?

Relevant to CMD, before embarking on an invasive coronary physiology study, the symptom of angina has to be typical and exertional, rest or night pain suggests a vasospastic aetiology. William Heberden's (1710–1801) definitive 250 year-old description of angina pectoris as a pressure-like central or left sided chest pain, with a gradual onset and radiation up the jaw or down the left arm is important to elicit [226]. Stabbing, paraesthetic, spasmodic and sudden onset are non-typical features.

Structural cardiac abnormalities should be excluded on imaging studies, such as an echocardiogram or a cardiovascular magnetic resonance (CMR) scan. Echocardiographic wall motion abnormalities and ST depression on a 12-lead 24-hour Holter or on functional testings are pointers for an irrefutable ischaemic cause [227]. However, failure to demonstrate cardiac ischaemia does not rule out angina [227–232]. It might be that the symptom occurs at a lower threshold compared to an objective or visible ischaemia on cardiac imaging or ECG. Furthermore, coronary vasoreactivity can only be tested invasively with acetylcholine, but the clinical value of spasm-positivity remains mixed, especially in stable patients and in women [233–235]. One view is that coronary vasoreactivity is just an expression of vascular endothelial dysfunction and caused by any atherosclerotic plaque disruption. As was originally described by Myron Prinzmetal, a series of young men who smoked had intermittent coronary vasospasm with transient hyperacute ST elevation [236]. The coronary vasoreactivity usually resolves in time following healing of the disrupted plaque but could carry an adverse prognosis in men [235, 237].

The traditional coronary risk factors especially smoking, diabetes, hyperlipidaemia and hypertension are all associated with endothelial dysfunction, including menopause status in women, demonstrable with acetylcholine testing to elicit vasoreactivity. In the absence of these, as per Bayes' theorem, coronary artery disease is highly unlikely. There are only three ways cardiac ischaemia can occur; epicardial coronary artery disease, vasoreactivity and vasodilatory incompetence [238]. But in practice, they collectively contribute to angina, and it may not be possible to apportion each one's relative contribution, in a patient who has multiple coronary risk factors. Thus, these risk factors frontload the a priori probability for an abnormal coronary physiology study outcome.

1.6 Three Physio-anatomical Factors

1.6.1 LVEDP

From 1844, and over the next two decades, Parisians; Claude Bernard (1813–1878), Étienne-Jules Marey (1830–1904) and Jean-Baptiste A. Chauveau (1827–1917) through their experiments on dogs and horses, definitively consolidated percutaneous right and left heart catheterisations, proved what causes the precordial pulsation and charted simultaneous aortic and LV pressures to define the cardiac cycle [239–241]. When the same techniques were applied to humans, the Nobel committee in 1946 awarded the Medicine or Physiology prize to Werner Forssmann (1904–1979), André F. Cournand (1895–1988) and Dickinson W. Richards Jr. (1895–1973).

However, modern day left heart physiology was comprehensively studied and clarified by Otto Frank (1865–1944) and Carl J. Wiggers (1883–1963). Frank working with isolated frogs' hearts reported in 1895 the connection between LV filling and contractility, i.e. increased preload leading to filling and stretching of the LV increases BP when the afterload is constant [242]. On the other hand, Wiggers studied intact dogs' hearts with a multimodality approach, measuring with high fidelity pressure probes in left atrium (LA), LV, aorta, and concurrently recording ECG and heart sounds.

Wiggers divided the cardiac cycle into seven phases in 1921, later simplified by Thomas Lewis (1881–1945) [243]; **1. Atrial contraction** or systole (generating a fourth heart sound if LV is stiff and a-wave in LV, or *LVEDP which is after atrial kick* approximately corresponding to ECG R-wave, or a rough pressure estimate at the Z-point between v-wave and a-wave on *left atrial pressure tracing* indicating mitral valve opening when LA and LV pressures equilibrate, before atrial kick, measurable as wedge nadir with Swan-Ganz PA catheter (PCWP)—in a normal heart, 2–4 mmHg lower than LVEDP, in AF PCWP z-point = LVEDP), **2. Isovolumetric contraction** (begins with mitral valve closure against a closed aortic valve → first heart sound and a sharp LV pressure rise), **3. Rapid ejection** (aortic valve opens as systemic arterial elastance is overcome and blood ejected, marked by an *LV incisura, a left-sided LV dicrotic notch or impulse gradient*), **4. Reduced ejection** (LV pressure peaks and domes), **5. Isovolumetric relaxation** (begins when aortic valve closes → *aortic dicrotic notch, second heart sound and coronary filling, which roughly corresponds with mean BP or at a third of pulse pressure added to diastolic BP*), **6. Rapid filling** (mitral valve opens with *diastolic LV suction* and a third heart sound in an overloaded LV), and **7. Diastasis** (passive filling before atrial kick). Wiggers' description, and that modified by Lewis in 1921 of left heart cardiac cycle with multiple pressure tracings still stands for over 100 years and is adapted and adopted for today's physiological textbooks [244, 245].

Contemporaneously, at University College London, Ernest H. Starling (1866–1927) extended Frank's stretch-tension strip experiments in isolated canine heart-lung preparations (1914) and presented his results in his 1915 Linacre Lecture, "Law of the Heart" in Cambridge [246, 247]. Starling openly acknowledged Frank's earlier frog-heart work. He plotted right atrial pressure (RAP) against cardiac output, surmising and formulating the resulting curve into the *preload-dependent autoregulation of stroke volume,* which was henceforth christened the Frank-Starling Law.

Underpinned by the viscoelastic theory of the muscle in general, complete with a *descending limb*, when the fibres are stretched beyond its elastic recoil leading to contractile failure. Starling's close collaborator, Archibald V. Hill (1886–1977), whom he recruited to University College London in 1923, who had just won a Nobel Prize in 1922 for measuring heat release during muscle contraction, was a proponent of the viscoelastic theory. This turned out to be imprecise because muscle contraction with shortening requires additional energy compared to isometric contraction, disproving the pure elastic recoil hypothesis [248, 249].

Further, increasing preload via fluid loading thus elevating the RAP does not necessarily increase the end-diastolic volume (EDV), which is a better marker of LV stretch in an intact rather than an isolated heart-lung preparation of an animal. Current studies in humans correlating EDV with cardiac output show an ascending limb which then plateaus excessive LV filling just increases the LVEDP and precipitates pulmonary oedema without boosting further cardiac output [250, 251].

Thus, the descending limb of Frank-Starling's law has disappeared from textbooks, but in its modified form, it still holds true and is utilised daily in intensive care practice. The ascending limb is the pre-load sensitive zone, whereas the preload independent state is the plateau, *LVEDP* $\geq$ *15 mmHg*. Importantly, the molecular basis of the Frank-Starling's law is calcium sensitization from titin stretch within the myocardial sarcomere—this cannot be blocked by calcium channel blockers, which would otherwise impair preload sensitivity in raising cardiac output [252]. These calcium ions are cytosolic, cycling from the sarcoplasmic reticulum, via Ryanodine receptors (RyR), distinct from L-type calcium channels which are antagonised by drugs such as diltiazem or verapamil.

On the other hand, increased *afterload* through reduced forward flow, thus increasing end-systolic LV volume (ESV) and by extension end-diastolic LV volume (EDV), recruiting the same fibre-stretch reserve, sometimes termed the *Anrep effect*, could also increase cardiac output. This is why pure α-adrenergic vasopressors such as metaraminol elevate BP and, why sympathetic surges (e.g. procedural anxiety) transiently increase BP and where there is LV diastolic dysfunction, raise the LVEDP too [253]. When utilised in critical care, the Anrep effect is most effective at LVEDP 4–8 mmHg [254]. Thus, not so useful in patients with cardiogenic shock and high LVEDP.

A raised LVEDP is the hallmark of heart failure and it correlates with NT-ProBNP. In systolic heart failure, the increased ESV is an adaptive mechanism to utilise the fibre-stretch reserve. But when the "efficiency range" is depleted, this process becomes energy inefficient, and the heart failure process spirals. Most prognostic heart failure drugs counterintuitively *reduce cardiac output and BP* via blunting of heart rate, offloading preload and dispersing afterload (BP↓ = CO↓ x SVR↓, CO↓ = SV↓ x HR↓). These actions, via reduced EDV, reset myocardial fibre at a more energy efficient contraction-relaxation range.

The LVEDP is measured at end-expiration at the downslope of a-wave, which indicates the start of LV isovolumic contraction; this usually coincides with the R-wave of the ECG. Under normal circumstances, it should be < 12 mmHg. Raised LVEDP ≥13 mmHg carries adverse prognosis and even poorer outcome if it is ≥ 25 mmHg in the setting of stable and unstable coronary artery disease, in spite of coronary revascularisation [255, 256]. Notably, many patients with ANOCA as will be seen throughout this book have this level of LVEDP, in the absence of systolic dysfunction, neither overt diastolic dysfunction. Why?

1.6.2 VAC

The next phase of mechanistic study into the cardiac cycle was pioneered by Japanese researchers. In 1974, Hiroyuki Suga and Kiichi Sagawa reported the first pressure-volume (PV) loop from an isolated canine heart [257]. The experimental works were carried out in 1973 by Suga while he was a postdoctoral fellow working under Sagawa at John Hopkins University Medical School, in Baltimore, Maryland, US. The PV loop is a chart of LV pressure against LV volume; this creates a medieval church door shape in a counterclockwise closed-circuit that divides the cardiac cycle into 4 phases; (1) starting from LV diastolic filling between mitral valve opening and closing, the latter defines the end-diastolic PV relationship (**EDPVR**)—*LVEDP plotted against end-diastolic volume (EDV) in response to changing preload*, a right-ward, relatively low pressure shallow-angled ascending limb close to the X-axis (volume, Y-axis is pressure), (2) a right-sided upstroke of rapid LV pressure rise, the isovolumic contraction after closure of mitral valve to aortic valve opening, with rising LV pressure without volumetric change, (3) when aortic valve opens, there is an anticlockwise dome-shaped swoop of ejection systolic pressure driving the volume out of the heart, culminating with the pressure at aortic valve closure that defines the end-systolic PV relationship (**ESPVR**) or *LV pressure* *charted against end-systolic volume (ESV) with varying loading conditions*—important to note that this is not peak LV pressure, it corresponds to the beginning of *aortic dicrotic notch*, therefore not brachial systolic BP either, and (4) finally, a left-sided vertical descend of rapid fall in LV pressure between aortic valve closure and mitral valve opening, the isovolumic relaxation, for a single beat, and the cycle repeats. The enclosed area is the stroke work in mmHg·mL (1 mmHg·mL ≈ 0.000133 Joules); the stroke volume (SV) is between isovolumic contraction and relaxation, and ESPVR is diametrically opposite to EDPVR.

ESPVR and EDPVR are obtained by changing preload, usually with impeding venous return using balloon occlusion in the inferior vena cava (IVC) for 5–10 s. The resulting 8–15 heartbeats with changes in end-systolic LV pressure (ESP) at end-systolic volume (ESV) plots an ascending limb, the gradient of this line extrapolated to X-intercept defines the load-independent intrinsic contractility or **end-systolic elastance** (Ees); a strong heart is one that generates high pressure with less volume, i.e. steeper ascending line → ESP/ESV. A flatter line implies systolic impairment—low ESP and high "residual" ESV, which is synonymous to the Frank-Starling curve despite the different theoretical underpinning. This is also the reasoning behind ESV obtained with non-invasive imaging being a powerful prognostic factor [258].

In contrast, end-diastolic LV pressure (LVEDP) at end-diastolic volume (EDV) plots a non-linear gentle upward slope; this represents LV compliance, i.e. the ability of the LV to accommodate volume with minimal pressure rise. EDPVR that shifts left and up is seen in pericardial constraint, diastolic heart failure or HFpEF. In LBBB, the PV loop is narrow with reduced stroke volume and shifted right and up, the dyssynchronous septum causes a notched and prolonged isovolumic contraction instead of a vertical upstroke, right-ward shift of ESP at higher ESV and ultimately a smaller area suggesting cardiac inefficiency. When tested with multisite pacing, both right ventricular septum and apex pacing do not alter the PV loop, but lateral free wall pacing appears to normalise the PV loop; this is the basis for cardiac resynchronisation therapy (CRT) [259].

In 1983, Kenji Sunagawa and his colleagues at John Hopkins University Medical School, in Baltimore, Maryland, US, followed up with the concept of **effective arterial elastance** (Ea), which is a *composite* index of total arterial load encompassing systemic vascular resistance, arterial compliance (including wave reflection, which rises with heart-rate) and aortic stiffness in order to eject blood. This is simply calculated as Ea = ESP/SV, mmHg/mL [260]. When the heart's work, Ees is matched to the arterial load, Ea, then the system is most efficient, ventriculo-arterial coupling, VAC = 1. VAC is derived as Ea/Ees = ESP/SV ÷ ESP/ESV, simplified as *VAC = ESV/SV*, by cancelling out ESP, and this is a dimensionless ratio. Since ESV and SV can be easily obtained by echocardiography or cardiovascular magnetic resonance (CMR) scan, this volume-derived VAC is readily captured in clinical practice [261]. VAC ranges 0.6–1.0, > 1.0 suggests LV systolic dysfunction and < 0.6 is commonly seen in pericardial constraint, hyperdynamic circulation and HFpEF [262]. In other words, VAC is how many stroke volume multiples are left in the heart after contraction. Under normal circumstances, this should be one,

VAC = 1. VAC can also be further simplified to 1/EF − 1, e.g. EF 65%, VAC (1/0.65) − 1 = 0.54, which is the definition for heart failure with supranormal election fraction (HFsnEF) [263], and an EF under 50% gives a VAC of > 1.0, consistent with the standard definition of LV systolic dysfunction.

Non-invasive Ea could also be calculated with the *single-beat method*, 0.9 · cuff systolic BP ÷ SV, SV is measured either with echocardiography or CMR, with a normal range of 1.5–2.5 mmHg/mL; < 1.5 mmHg/mL → low afterload, sepsis and in athletes, and > 2.5 mmHg/mL → high afterload in hypertension, elderly with stiff artery and aortic stenosis. Working backwards, Ees = Ea/VAC, ranges from 1.5 to 3.5 mmHg/mL; < 1.5 mmHg/mL → systolic dysfunction and > 3.5 mmHg/mL → stiff LV with diastolic dysfunction [75]. Thus, with non-invasive BP and any imaging modality, PV loop indices can be estimated from three simple equations. Although their accuracy and utility are yet to be defined for routine clinical practice, especially that the derived measurements are not simultaneously or instantaneously obtained, which would the case with a high fidelity PV loop catheter in the LV [264]:

$$\mathrm{Ea} = \frac{0.9 \cdot \mathrm{SystolicBP}}{\mathrm{SV}}$$

$$\mathrm{VAC} = \frac{1}{\mathrm{EF}} - 1$$

$$\mathrm{Ees} = \frac{\mathrm{Ea}}{\mathrm{VAC}}$$

1.6.3 SEI

All cellular tissues start as a string, tube or sheet. Similarly, a muscle band requires two fixed points to contract from or pull against. The heart is a muscular Gordian knot in its complexity and many anatomists after Wiliam Harvey (1578–1657) had tried to unravel it for over three hundred and fifty years [265]. But who could have thought that the ventricles are actually made up of a *single muscular band, origamically folded into a helical figure-of-eight with three turns*? Francisco Torrent-Guasp (1931–2005), while a fourth year medical student at the University of Salamanca, he peeled apart with his fingers a human heart and could not match what he saw with diagrams in his anatomy text. Encouraged by Gómez Oliveros, his anatomy and physiology supervisor, he self-published his student research into a booklet before he even graduated in 1954 as a 129-page monograph, *El ciclo cardíaco* (The Cardiac Cycle), which raised doubts about cardiac muscle arrangement, including his hypothesis that blood enters the ventricles through active suction, an idea first expounded up by Erasistratus of Chios (304–250 BC) that was overturned by Harvey [266, 267].

These questions he carried with him to Dénia, Alicante, a port city on the Mediterranean coast of eastern Spain, where he practiced long-term as a family doctor from 1959 for over 30 years. There, he had a makeshift laboratory behind his clinic, where he boiled animal hearts to soften the connective tissue, then used blunt-finger dissection to follow the natural fibre direction. He noted that when he removed the thin layer of aberrant muscle fibres crossing the anterior interventricular sulcus from left to right ventricle, he could open the heart like woman's purse by detaching the RV from LV as the first step (see Chap. 6 on myocardial bridging). In his out-of-hours self-sponsored research, he dissected over one thousand hearts of different species, including worms, fish, reptiles, mammals and humans [268]. Based on what he saw, he did elaborate sketches of cardiac evolution across the species [269]. Thirteen years later, he presented his discovery at the Sixth European Congress of Cardiology, held in Madrid on 23–30 September 1972, organised at the behest of the Spanish Society of Cardiology [270]. The following year he was invited by Donald N. Ross (1922–2014) to demonstrate his helical ventricular muscle band (HVMB) at the National Heart Hospital in London. His revolutionary idea was met with admiration, scepticism and ridicule in equal measure [271]. Tried as he might, his submission to reputable international journals was flatly rejected and he settled for a Spanish journal 7 years later in1980 [272]. As he gained wider recognition within the international scientific community, he reduced his general medical commitments in his sixties to focus on invited lectures and collaborative research. As fate would have it, with a twist of irony and doing what delighted him, at 73, on 23 February 2005, after delivering his Pedro Zarco Lecture, entitled, "Ventricular filling is the consequence of an active muscular contraction: effect of CRT" scheduled at 7.05 pm to a group of prominent cardiac electrophysiologists at the 16th Madrid Arrhythmia and Myocardium 2005 — "Atrial fibrillation, sudden death and heart failure", he left to get ready for the gala dinner, but collapsed on the hotel corridors and suffered a fatal cardiac arrest, despite attempts by some meeting delegates to resuscitate him [273]. This hotel was just across the road within the vicinity of Palacio Municipal de Congresos (Campo de las Naciones, now renamed in 2019 to IFEMA (Institución Ferial de Madrid), accessible via Feria de Madrid Metro Line 8) where the meeting was held [270]. His death certificate was signed by one of the organisers of the conference, Jerónimo Farré.

The HVMB starts from pulmonary trunk and right ventricular outflow tract (RVOT), then becomes **right segment**, which is the right ventricular free wall band. Transitioning beyond the posterior interventricular sulcus, it continues as **left segment**, wrapping the basal portion of posterolateral and lateral LV free wall, followed by **descending segment** of the LV apical loop that courses *subendocardially*, covering the inner anterior and septal walls of the LV. At the apex, like a Möbius strip, the band loops back and ascends along the LV free wall, then crosses the outer anterior and anteroseptal wall as the *subepicardial* **ascending segment**, and finally becomes the LV outflow tract (LVOT) and aortic root [274]. This creates a continuous loop, with the two ends of the muscle band "glued" together into the cardiac fulcrum [275].

Torrent-Guasp followed up in 1998, 44 years from his initial spark of curiosity, formalising his idea that sequential peristaltic contraction along the muscle band is responsible for blood ejection and suction [276]. The way that the muscle band courses, the heart is functionally an inverted piston, analogous to the car engine. The piston is the cardiac apex, which appears fixed, when it is infarcted or stunned as in Takotsubo cardiomyopathy, with loss of the ventricular diastolic suction, the heart is filled via Harveian positive forward pressure. The left atrial (LA) systole contribution rises from 15% to 20% to over 40%, which drives up the LVEDP and causes both LA and LV dilatations [271].

Nature has its own experiment too; over the last 20 years, there are nearly 40 reported cases of patients with isolated left ventricular apical hypoplasia (ILVAH). They usually present after their twenties with fatigue, chest pain or heart failure with a spherically dilated LV and raised LVEDP [277–280]. The converse is congenital LV aneurysm (CLVA), a third is the apical variant, altogether, heart failure occurs and accounts for half of the 13% mortality below the age of 18 with a mean 5-year follow-up [281–283]. There is also a subset with LV diverticulum which causes no heart failure, nevertheless associated with LV rupture in infancy or childhood, and rarely trigger ventricular arrhythmias in later years but does carry a relatively benign prognosis.

There are *four clinical implications* predicable from the HVMB concept, First, as described above, what happens when the LV apex loses its crucial diastolic function. Second, the anatomical overlap of descending and ascending segments creates a double-layered reinforcement, which is demonstrable microscopically by the differing orientation of muscle fibres in the subendocardium and subepicardium. This insight helps explain where the subendocardial layer exists without a protective outer subepicardial wrap, such as the LV apex, anteroseptum and apical to mid anterior wall are particularly vulnerable to rupture after myocardial infarction. In other words, the absence of an outer buttressing layer renders the LV structurally weaker in the non-overlap areas [284].

Third, where the descending and ascending segments overlap, the inner layer or the subendocardium receives blood last. Since the coronary arteries are epicardial, through arterioles and capillaries they provide a meshwork of transmural perfusion. Further, the subendocardial descending segment and epicardial ascending segment contract sequentially by a 60 ms delay [285]. Put another way, the diastolic perfusion of the descending segment could be impacted by systolic compression of the ascending segment where they overlap. In the presence of high LV wall stress, the subendocardium is squeezed by the outer layer, exacerbated by hypertension coupled with LV hypertrophy (LVH) and raised LVEDP. In canine experiments, ligating the LAD is associated with earlier ECG ST elevation followed by hypocontractility in the subendocardium. Outer or epicardial layer ischaemia becomes prominent only at more advanced stages of ischaemia or near-total coronary occlusion [286].

Fourth, while the LV apex is essential for normal LV diastolic function, the base excels in LV systolic function, contributing to 70–90% of the stroke volume ejection in human and animal studies [287]. The sequence of contraction has been elucidated by up-to-date imaging and electrophysiological studies as envisioned by Torrent-Guasp. However, there is electromechanical disparity. The right segment is activated via the right bundle and descending segment is activated by the left septal Purkinje fibres concurrently; this leads in the LV, early right basal circumferential contraction and a flicker in the septum respectively, followed 10 ms later via the left posterior hemifascicle the Purkinje system, which causes left segment contraction of the left basal hoop. This completes the circular "belt-tightening" of the LV base. The descending segment continues its right-handed helical counterclockwise contraction in tandem pulling the base to the apex, reducing the mitral annular diameter, closing the mitral valve, ejecting the blood and completing the systole. The ascending segment with its left-handed helical configuration, contracts 60 ms later, further pull the base towards the apex, paradoxically lengthening the LV, akin to pulling a bow. It relaxes and releases the stored twist with rapid clock-wise "snap-back", creating an immediate 2–4 mmHg pressure fall, widening the mitral annulus by as much as 25%, facilitating mitral valve opening and creating a rapid LV filling by suction from left atrium [267, 285]. Therefore, the net mechanical effect, the base contracts first, followed by the apex. When there is a high afterload, such as uncontrolled hypertension or aortic stenosis, this sequential contraction could cause the base to work against the apex, producing an LV mid-cavity gradient leading to LV mid-cavity obstruction (MCO), increasing apical wall stress, and reducing perfusion to the LV apex, even in the absence of epicardial coronary artery disease, causing subendocardial ischaemia (SEI). Figure 1.1 shows an example of MCO related to uncontrolled hypertension.

To recap, on the basis of the HVMB model, the way that the LV is configured, the following could be predicted and concluded: (1). The LV apex is instrumental in maintaining diastolic LV filling and keeping the LVEDP low, (2). Non-overlapped myocardial segments are predisposed to rupture following myocardial infarction, (3). Overlapped myocardium is subject to SEI with high LV wall stress and raised LVEDP, and (4). Differential LV basal and apical contractility where there is high afterload causes varying degrees of LV mid-cavity gradient with increased apical wall stress culminating with MCO and mid-to-apical ring-like SEI. Gould, who originally proposed CFR < 2 as an ischaemic threshold [40], analysed 14,008 stress PET scans performed at his Houston centre in Texas between 2007 and 2024. After excluding caffeine-positive tests and any scan with a ≥ 5% relative perfusion defect which suggests regional ischaemia or infarction, 7416 studies (53% of the total cohort) remained [126]. Of these, 51% exhibited SEI despite intact global flow. Another 388 scans (5% of the 7416 defect-free studies; 2.8% of the total cohort) showed *reduced transmural hyperaemic perfusion while preserving the endocardial-to-epicardial ratio*, but only 11 of these (0.07% of all scans) provoked angina or ST depression during stress, thereby defining CMD. Gould regards SEI as due to diffuse small vessel disease, high wall stress and raised LVEDP. Thus, his very strict criteria in diagnosing CMD [107, 288–290].

In contrast to the US which is PET focussed, Europe is more adenosine-perfusion CMR-orientated. CMR has a higher spatial resolution of 2–4 mm compared to PET's 5–7 mm; hence, it could detect circumferential SEI as a marker of reduced subepicardial-to-subendocardial flow gradient, even in the absence of reduced global blood flow. First described in 2002 by Dudley J. Pennell's group at Royal Brompton Hospital, London [291]. SEI is well described in hypertrophic cardiomyopathy [292] and has been reported in hypertensive heart disease, especially with LVH, but its prevalence in hypertension is not well defined [293]. Large cohort

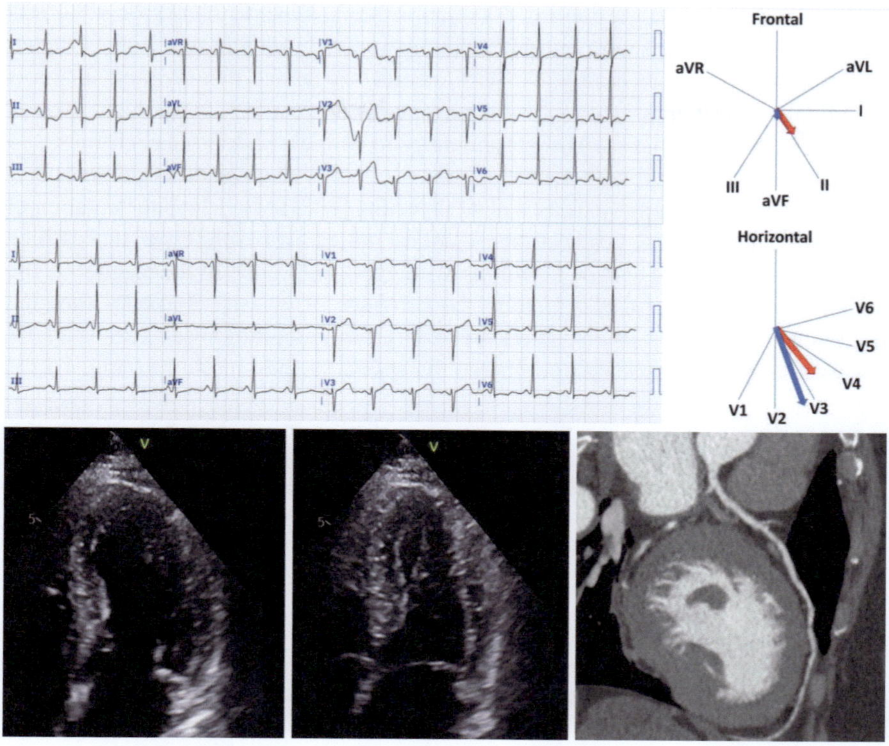

Fig. 1.1 Mid-cavity obstruction of the hypertensive left ventricle A 68-year-old Black woman with a BMI of 38.6 kg/m^2, who has hypertension presented with chest pain while watching television. Her BP fell from 147/84 mmHg to 101/62 mmHg after sublingual nitroglycerine. (**Top and middle panels**) Her initial ECG with a heart rate of 106 bpm showed widespread ST depression, with ST elevation in right-sided precordial leads and aVR. If there were ST elevation in I and aVL this would indicate left main coronary artery ischaemia. Her bedside echocardiogram found LVH and significant LV mid-cavity obstruction (MCO) with a gradient of 50 mmHg. When her ECG was repeated 45 minutes later, the ischaemic changes resolved, now with a heart rate of 97 bpm, but with ECG criteria of LVH plus a strain pattern. The *ST vector* on the frontal plane, *red arrow* is that of the first ECG—1.8 mm, 54°, second ECG with *blue arrow*—0.5 ($\leq$ 1.5) mm, 90°; corresponding horizontal place: 3.7 mm, 53°, and 5.3 mm, 70°. Taken together, at baseline, with LVH there was resting repolarisation abnormalities or *septal subendocardial ischaemia*, and when the MCO caused apical left ventricular ischaemia, the ST vector swung left toward the left ventricular apex. (**Bottom, left to right**) Her departmental echocardiogram done the following day, with a heart rate of 70 bpm showed concentric LVH (septal 1.4 cm and posterior 1.2 cm, < 1.1 cm) with MCO, EF 60–65% and average E/e' 9 (< 8). Apical 4-chamber long-axis views—in diastole (opened mitral valvular leaflets) and in systole showing MCO (closed mitral valvular leaflets). Her troponin T was not elevated and CT coronary angiogram confirmed unobstructed coronary arteries, therefore the chest pain in this woman was due to subendocardial ischaemia from LV MCO with a characteristic ECG pattern. Important to note that BP in these patients can be deceptively low to the extent causing syncope or collapse, because of the of the MCO. The mainstay treatment is beta blockade to reduce hypercontractility of the LV basal segments

studies have yet robustly established a relationship between either Myocardial perfusion reserve (MPR) [294], or SEI [295] and angina burden in ANOCA. Whether these CMR indices are modifiable with medical or device therapy, and if this is accompanied by symptomatic alleviation remains unclear [63, 296]. Also, there is no clear consensus what the MPR(I) should be to define CMD; it ranges from <1.84 to 2.19 [294, 297–299], with a dose of controversy where research fraud was committed [300, 301], but more trials will be reporting [302]. Also, the interpretation of *any ratio* such as MPR taken at face value is subject to baseline variation which creates a false positive or type I error in overdiagnosing CMD. In the meantime, the definitive diagnosis of CMD remains the province of invasive coronary function testing [303]. Although as discussed above, bolus thermodilution can also be overly generous in diagnosing CMD, compared to continuous thermodilution (Fig. 1.2).

1.7 Three Practical Steps for Continuous Thermodilution

1.7.1 Vascular Access

The Mayo Clinic which has extensive experience in coronary physiology study in ANOCA recommends 6 French femoral access because many of these patients are highly vasoreactive. They develop radial artery spasm, especially that radial cocktail that includes verapamil should be avoided as it could alter the vascular haemodynamics [304]. However, this would deny these patient of post-procedural comfort of radial access. Interestingly, despite the reticent that verapamil given intra-arterially through the radial sheath would interfere with acetylcholine spasm testing, this turns out not to be the case [305]. Intra-arterial verapamil is mostly locally active, and the small spillover amount is degraded via first past metabolism within the pulmonary circulation. Therefore verapamil is devoid of systemic effects when given intra-arterially.

The challenges of radial access can be minimised with the slender technique. Radial artery spasm even after upfront 5 mg of verapamil is dependent on sheath size, as is radial artery occlusion, and forearm haematoma. Patent haemostasis post-procedure reduces radial artery occlusion, but this is difficult to implement in a busy cardiac unit as it requires heavy nursing input. Nevertheless, the drawbacks of the radial approach could be significantly mitigated by doing the puncture more distally in the snuffbox, beyond the deep palmar arch. Post-procedure compression at this site will not interrupt continuing radial artery flow through the superficial palmar arch—this is akin to a natural patent haemostasis. That is why the rate of radial artery occlusion is well under 1% compared with 5% for standard radial access. Further, within the confined space of the snuffbox, if there is bleeding, the pressure from the localised haematoma automatically "tamponades off" the puncture wound, making haematoma extension to the forearm leading to a compartmental syndrome

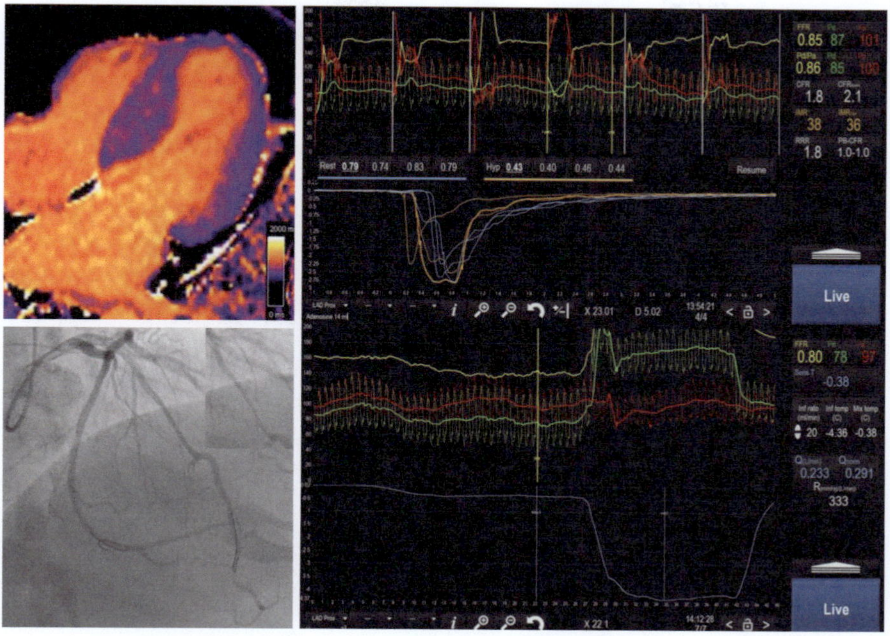

Fig. 1.2 Hypertrophic obstructive cardiomyopathy—discrepancy between bolus and continuous thermodilution A 55-year-old man with 6 years' history of angina was admitted for a one-stop coronary physiology study. His chest pain was exertional and with radiation down his left arm. His ECG showed tall QRS amplitude with "benign early repolarisation" and peaked T-wave in anteroseptal leads, and echocardiogram found asymmetric septal hypertrophy measuring 1.9 (< 1.1) mm, EF 70%, dilated left atrium (LA) at 4.4 (< 4.0) mm, ESVI 12 ml/m^2, SVI 37 ml/m^2, VAC 0.32, and left ventricular outflow obstruction (LVOTO) of 20 mmHg at rest, rising to 60 mmHg with squats and valsalva manoeuver resulting in complete systolic anterior motion (SAM) of the anterior mitral leaflet. These investigations were consistent with a diagnosis of hypertrophic obstructive cardiomyopathy (HOCM) (**Left, top and bottom panels**) Cardiovascular magnetic resonance (CMR) scan shows an EF of 72% with thickened left ventricle and mid-cavity obliteration; the anteroseptum measures 2.6 mm with a moderately dilated LA 36 (< 20) cm^2, ESVI 13 (15–37) ml/m^2, SVI 34 (41–65) ml/m^2 and VAC 0.38. There is widespread scattered increase in T1 signals (orange) indicating fibrosis. The coronary angiogram reveals unobstructed coronary artery, but there is a long segment of *systolic* myocardial bridging (MB) in mid left anterior descending (LAD) artery (*right upper corner inset*). With the pressure wire down the LAD, the Pd/Pa and RFR are 0.89 and 0.78 (> 0.89). (**Right, top and bottom panels**) Bolus thermodilution (BTD) using systemic adenosine infusion at 140 μg/min/kg over 1 minute derived the following indices—FFR 0.85, CFR 1.8, IMR 38 and MRR 2.1. With continuous thermodilution (CTD), the basal and hyperaemic values are—flow 121 and 233 mL/min, and resistance 819 and 333 Wood units—FFR 0.80, CFR 1.9, IMR_{CTD} 17 and MRR 2.5. **Interpretation**. BTD suggests CMD, but looking at the absolute values obtained with CTD, a different picture emerges; he in fact has low baseline coronary resistance and high basal flow, which means that his vasodilatory range is recruited, and neither is his MB obstructive. His heart rate during the procedure was 95 bpm on bisoprolol 5 mg od; this was increased, and he was started on a cardiac myosin inhibitor.

very unlikely [306]. Indeed, this has yet been reported. As with the radial approach, rarely pseudo-aneurysm can occur, particularly in the elderly on anticoagulation [307]. Another rare complication is a distal radial arteriovenous fistula, albeit iatrogenic [308]. On the other hand, deliberate distal radial arteriovenous fistula performed under local anaesthesia is commonly undertaken for renal replacement therapy [309].

The first distal radial access (dRA) for coronary intervention was described by Avtandil Babunashvili, a Russian Cardiologist in 2011 when he recanalised an occluded radial artery of a couple of patients within 6 days after a previous access, for a follow-up coronary procedure [310]. Ferdinand Kiemeneij, a Dutch Cardiologist, who is a credited pioneer of radial access coronary angioplasty, who introduced the technique in 1992 [311], took to the social media Twitter (now X) a campaign promoting dRA on February 14, 2014, which generated a lot of interest. He published his series of left dRA in 70 patients with 88.6% success in 2017 [312].

Kiemeneij is a promoter of slender techniques, i.e., using small sheaths and catheters, ideally suited for ANOCA patients. However, dRA access has a steeper learning curve, a report suggests it takes 200 cases to master the technique, in contrast to 50 for standard radial approach [313]. The challenges faced with dRA are not dissimilar to that of standard radial access [314, 315].

Diagnostic coronary angiogram can be undertaken without heparin via dRA with 4 French sheaths and catheters, post-procedure, the puncture site is manually pressed for 10 min achieving haemostasis in most cases [316]. For ad hoc progress to coronary intervention, the 4 French sheath can be replaced with any standard 5 French guide catheters, introduced sheathlessly with a 260 cm exchange length 0.035″ guidewire and a 4Fr MPA2 125 cm diagnostic catheter as an introducer (Fig. 1.3). A 5 French guide catheter has an external lumen of 1.67 mm, which is about the same size as a 4 French sheath, with an internal lumen of 1.47 mm, that is big enough to house the pressure wire with RayFlow, plus an additional guidewire. This is invaluable in stabilising the guide catheter when a patient has a short left main coronary artery, or separate origins for LAD and Cx. One caveat is there is a need for frequent flushing of the system to prevent pressure-damping during a coronary physiology study. This set-up is generally well tolerated, with rare incidences of radial artery spasm or access site bleeding. For older patients aged ≥ 70, left dRA is advisable to avoid the task of overcoming the calcified right subclavian artery tortuosity and grip [317]. The same can be done for femoral access, using a sheathless 5 French system that makes a 4 French puncture. At completion of the procedure, a 4 French femoral sheath can be inserted. When the activated clotting time (ACT) is under 150 s, the sheath can be pulled with a 10 min compression time to achieve complete haemostasis. Access site bleeding complications are rare with slender equipment.

The cannulation of dRA requires familiarity with anatomical landmarks. It is important to clearly identify the snuffbox, viewing the hand half-pronated dorsally,

Fig. 1.3 (continued) recanalised, she had procedural hypertension with a raised LVEDP implying LV diastolic dysfunction and ACh provoked microvascular spasm that was ameriolated by verapamil pre-treatment, but the flow did not rise by 50% suggesting intrinsic endothelial dysfunction. The notion of early flow reduction with low-dose ACh, only to rise with higher-dose ACh with or without verapamil pre-treatment—the biphasic ACh response is discussed elsewhere (Chap. 7)

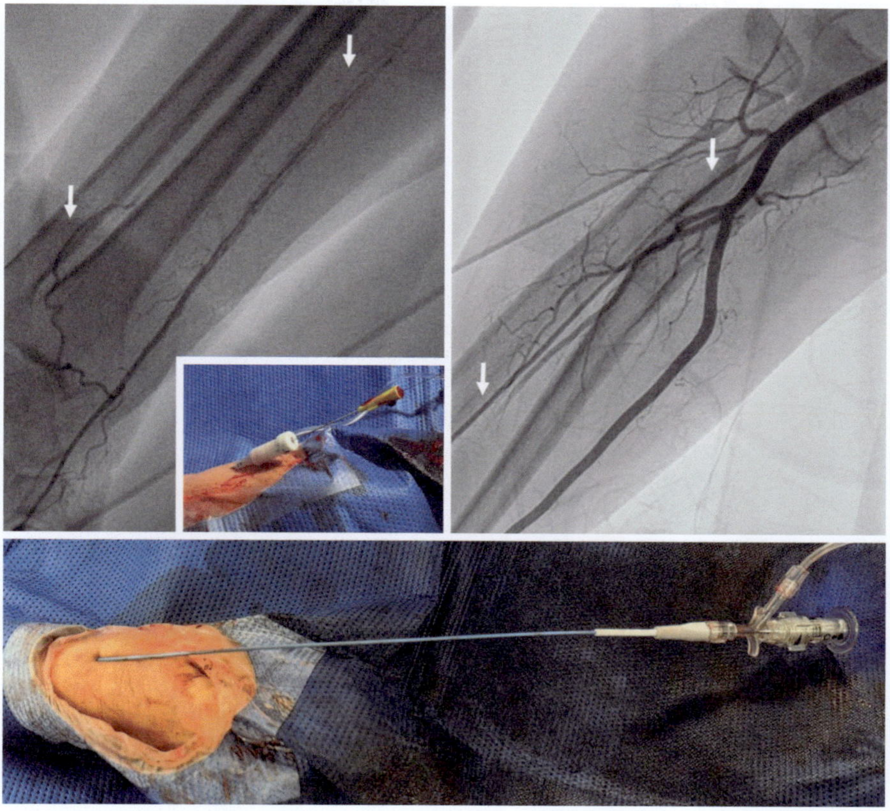

Fig. 1.3 Reaccessing the subtotally occluded radial artery via the distal radial approach A 60-year-old woman has excertional angina. She had a prior 4 French right radial approach diagnostic coronary angiogram that revealed non-obstructive coronary arteries over 8 years previously; her LVEDP was 12 mmHg then. She was a smoker of 20/day for 20 years but stopped smoking in her forties. Her heart was structurally normal on CMR and on echocardiogram that found an average E/e' of 12 (< 8) suggestive of LV diastolic dysfunction. When her distal right radial (dRA) artery was punctured, the guidewire could not be passed beyond the previous radial puncture site. A Cook® microcatheter was inserted and a radial angiogram was taken (**Left top panel**), this shows a subtotally occluded radial artery (*top arrow*) and a collateral vessel from the interrosseous branch (*bottom arrow*). The *inset* shows the microcatheter in situ. The radial artery was traversed with a coronary guidewire, followed by placement of a 4 French sheath. A 4 French pigtail was inserted into the LV, her LVEDP measured 25 mmHg, with a corresponding central aortic BP of 160/70 mmHg, which gradually settled to about 140 mmHg systolic during the rest of her procedure. This response was likely to be related to procedural stress, but the high LVEDP suggested a non-compliant LV. A sheathless Cordis 5 Fr XB 3.5 guide catheter was used to engage her left coronary artery to carry out her coronary physiology study (**Bottom panel**). Her basal and hyperaemic flow and resistance were repeated twice with continuous thermodilution: Q 75, **75**, 233 and **201** mL/min, and Rμ 1477, **1465**, 453 and **478** Wood units: picking the repeated pairs gave a CFR of 2.7 and MRR of 3.1. Acetylcholine (ACh) challenge with 2, 20 and 100 μg were associated with reduced fractional flow from baseline of 0.89, 0.83 and 0.95—associated with inferolateral ST depression without epicardial vasospasm—suggesting "isolated microvascular spasm". Verapamil 1 mg increased the flow x1.75 and rechallenge with ACh 100 and 200 μg were associated with no symptoms and fractional flow of 1.2 and 1.37, respectively. Repeat radial angiogram revealed a patent artery (**Top right panel**, *arrrows*). In summary, this lady had her right radial artery

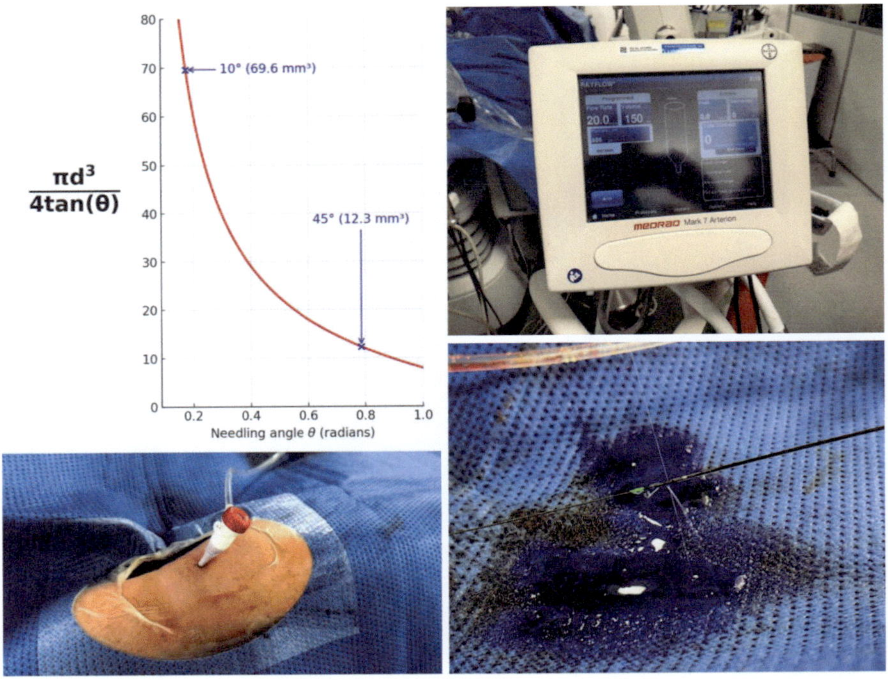

Fig. 1.4 Tangent rule and distal radial access (**Left, top and bottom panels**) The tangent rule suggests that a shallow needling angle increases the likelihood of puncturing the artery at first pass (see text for explanation). A distal right radial artery with a 4 French sheath in situ. (**Right, top and bottom panels**) The automated pump used to infuse saline, and note the four jets of saline coming off the RayFlow microcatheter

gently medial-flexed and standing on the right side of the patient, it is an elongated triangle bounded distal laterally by extensor pollicis longus, beyond which is the web between the thumb and the index finger, medially by twin tendons of extensor pollicis brevis and abductor pollicis longus, and proximally by the scaphoid bony floor. The crease of the wrist joint, if followed volar-palmarly into the snuffbox, points exactly at the puncture site for the right dRA. The dRA should be accessed on anatomical landmarks alone. Feeling the pulse and attempt to puncture under the palpating finger often results in a more distal puncture, beyond the extensor pollicis longus resulting in hand haematoma due to retrograde bleeding from the uncompressible deep palmar arch. It is a general principle in interventional artery access that there should be a bone under which the artery can be compressed against to achieve post-procedural haemostasis. Finally, after a generous 5 mL of 1% lidocaine infiltration around the snuffbox, which is rubbed in, the angle of needle approach determines success of cannulation if this not done with ultrasound guidance.

$$\theta \to \frac{\pi d^3}{4\tan(\theta)}$$

There is a mathematical relationship between the angle with which the needle pierces the skin and the potential volume of the artery which is available for cannulation. The needle tip with bevel facing up sees a cylindrical volume as per the tangent rule above, *d* is the diameter of the artery and θ in radians, the angle between the needle and the skin surface (Fig. 1.4). Hence, assuming an artery diameter of 2.5 mm, a needle inserted at 45° potentially sees an arterial volume of 12.3 mm^3, whereas a needle that is inserted at 10° would see a larger arterial volume of 69.6 mm^3, increasing by 5.7-fold the volume of artery available for cannulation. Hence a shallow cannulating angle improves the probability that a puncturing needle would enter the radial artery at first past cannulation. This would reduce the risk of radial artery spasm as traditionally taught that the first arterial puncture is the best chance of a successful arterial cannulation. The other advantage of a shallow angle of needling is that the opposite arterial wall is further away allowing easier passage of the guidewire whereas a steeper angle is more likely to be associated with difficulty in advancing the wire into the artery, since there is a greater likelihood that the guidewire tip would get caught in the opposite artery wall. Using the above model, the needling tract within the artery is increased by 4.4 times comparing needling angles of 10° with 45°.

1.7.2 Set-Up and Measurements

RayFlow is a 2.5 French (0.84 mm) microcatheter with a balloon-type tapering tip. So long as it is advanced along the pressure wire, it is unlikely to traumatise a coronary artery. A report with a close look at 1,565 coronary arteries of 1,148 patients with 3,398 studies just over 6 years between December 2016 and February 2023, only logged four cases of vascular complications or 0.12% of total studies. These were: 1. Proximal LAD dissection in a prior 60% lesion, 2. Ostial RCA with guide catheter induced dissection, 3. Stent thrombosis in an underexpanded stent that was recently implanted, following proximal placement of the RayFlow, and 4. Coronary artery spasm in a mid-vessel due to pressure wire *advances and withdrawals* as was necessary for the technique to obtain infusate (T_i) and mixed (T_m) temperatures [318, 319].

A separate case study in 2017, owing to an early experience, when the flow rate was accidentally set at 120 mL/min, the safety 600 PSI pump feature did not kick in; resulting in a spontaneous coronary artery dissection (SCAD)-like lesion corresponding to the jet-outlets in mid LAD of a 65-year-old woman, which fortunately settled with conservative management [320]. The pump pressure should be set at no more than 500 PSI (34 bar), which is enough to cover a flow rate of 30 mL/min at 350 PSI. However, this rate has not been used in our practice. If in doubt when 20 mL/min produces no noticeable hyperaemia, a higher rate at 25 mL/min could be used. This may also suggest significant endothelial dysfunction, in which case this can be confirmed with intravenous adenosine infusion at 140 μg/kg/min.

Care should be taken to prime the RayFlow outside the patient by starting infusion (Fig. 1.4), advancing it inside the guide catheter before stopping the priming infusion. Also it is not advisable to deliver any drugs via the RayFlow. First, this can introduce air, and second, there is high resistance in injecting through the RayFlow with uncertain timing of drug delivery. The pump saline volume should be set to its maximal capacity of 150 mL. This will deplete with multiple studies, if set too low such at 20 mL, the infusion stops automatically during the study when this volume is delivered, or if the study overrun, resulting in an incomplete procedure.

The mixed temperature (T_m) and injectate (T_i) both can be obtained with saline infusion over 15 s each and a single study can be completed within 45 s to allow repeat studies. However, the pump may need to be topped up for more runs especially more than one vessels are assessed. The readings are displayed on the Abbott Coroventis CoroFlow™ interface having selected the *absolute flow* option, and inputting the intended saline infusion rate. It is a good practice to do duplicate studies, if the difference in flow rates is within 10% then move on. Otherwise repeat until consistency is obtained. It is highly unusual to do more than three measurements, but following hyperaemia, it will take at least 3 min for baseline flow to re-established. If the next study is done early, at a lower flow rate, a semi-hyperaemic index will be registered. Also, it is expedient to flush the guide catheter regularly to prevent pressure-damping, re-equalising the aortic pressure (Pa) if there is a drift, and zeroing the thermistor in mid vessel 6–8 cm from RayFlow tip.

Start the infusion pump, it usually takes 15–20 s for T_m to stabilise, pull the pressure wire back to the RayFlow tip, with only the radiopaque floppy segment outside the RayFlow. After 10–15 s to obtain a steady T_i, next stop the saline infusion. The temperature rises back to baseline and complete the recording.

There is no need to observe the temperature fluctuations during saline infusions. At the end of each study, the numbers displayed on the screen are usually adequate, but some adjustments in moving the T_m and T_i cursors to a flatter segment may be necessary although the changes are usually minor. The temperature filter averages the signal every 2 s, a longer sampling run does not improve reproducibility [321].

With the above methodology, our departmental pooled Bland-Altman coefficients of variation of 60 repeat measures are: flow, baseline 11.1%, hyperaemic 8.2%, and resistance, baseline 12.0% and hyperaemic 9.3%—hyperaemic indices appear more repeatable by 3% or one third compared to basal indices, 20 mL/min vs 10 mL/min. Interestingly, in vitro repeatability was flow rate dependent; 15 mL/min 10.7%, 25 mL/min 7.9% and 30 mL/min 5.9%, improving with higher flow rates [110]. This is consistent with our data. But these numbers are not far off systolic BP measurement in the office of 8.0–10% to imply inherent haemodynamic variation, rather than technical measurement errors [322, 323]. Which means that the absolute flow rate obtained with continuous thermodilution is the true reflection of beat-to-beat biological variation.

On the other hand, composite indices introduce both intrinsic variations and extrinsic errors in measurements, compounded and amplified, for example CFR and IMR obtained by bolus thermodilution are in the order of 20–30%, and CFR and MRR by continuous thermodilution are 2–3 times more reproducible at 11–13% [95, 96, 120]. As discussed earlier, while large epidemiological studies using less reproducible techniques produce meaningful inferences about a treatment effect, when applied at a personal level; if a threshold is set, they are associated with unacceptable type I or type II errors, i.e. overdiagnosis of a condition a patient does not have or the other way round. Although the former appears to be a more common issue. Gould is unconvinced that CMD as is currently diagnosed or defined is as common as it is reported in the current medical literature based on his PET data he collected over 17 years in Texas (see Chap 8.3.4) [126].

1.7.3 Procedural Anxiety

Mental and physical stresses are physiologically one and the same due to sympathetic activation, but the former has more pronounced afterload increase through unopposed and generalised α_1-receptor activation by catecholamines, without the moderating effect of vasodilatation in the exercising muscles from local β_2-receptor activation [324]. The heart rate and BP go up, increasing oxygen demand especially in those with coronary artery disease. Thus, angina can occur in some patients. And in those with vascular endothelial dysfunction, the haemodynamic response can be exaggerated because of paradoxical vasoconstriction [325], this is noticeable as diffuse reduction in coronary artery calibre, which is responsive to intracoronary nitroglycerine.

The cardiac catheterisation laboratory is inherently unfamiliar and fear-provoking. On the other hand, *how the heart copes under stress is in itself informative.* BP rises by at least 20–30 mmHg and pulse rate to 100 bpm are not uncommon, which then settle over time. But any tugging and pulling sensation felt by the patient could set these off again. Philosophically and perversely, a fully sedated and beta blocked patient would be denied, having this stress response and how the cardiovascular system responses observed objectively, which might be recurring on a daily basis with symptomatic implications.

In a normal heart, these physiological responses do not affect the coronary physiological indices, but a high basal coronary flow would reduce the CFR. Right atrial pacing studies in animals suggest that tachycardia at 100 bpm increases coronary flow by at least 30% [326]. In humans, during papaverine-induced hyperaemic coronary flow, raising BP with phenylephrine did not alter blood flow and by implication, coronary resistance rose in parallel [327]. Taken together, procedural anxiety could increase both basal blood flow and hyperaemic resistance in susceptible patients, these would reduce CFR and raise IMR or hyperaemic resistance, mimicking CMD (Fig. 1.3).

There is an impulse or Rushmer gradient visible with high fidelity pressure sensing, in which the rapid rise of LV pressure during isovolumic contraction briefly overshoots the high arterial inertia and flings open the aortic valve, first noted in 1964 [328]. This peak, or incisura, is ≤ 5 mmHg above aortic pressure, strangely not discussed in any great detail in most medical textbooks. Although now clearly visible in new pressure transducing system in the modern cardiac catheter laboratory, in contrast with Joseph P. Murgo's use of a multisensor catheter to detect simultaneous pressure changes in LV apex and outflow tract, which he started using in February 1972 [329].

Under stress, this impulse gradient can overshoot by 10–15 mmHg, due to increased inotropic cardiac contraction, which can also be induced by β-agonist infusion such as dobutamine, due to high dP/dt or rapid pressure rise against time [329]. Conversely, it can be abolished by phenylephrine infusion that increases systemic vascular resistance (SVR), and in *hypertensives* [330], by increasing arterial inertia the LV has to work against, thus slowing pressure rise. On the other hand, hypertensives with LVH exhibit a mimic from LV mid-cavity obstruction (MCO) [331], and LV outflow tract obstruction (LVOTO) [332], they are physiologically inter-related to intraventricular pressure gradient (IVPG), demonstrable by echocardiography [333].

In older patients with a less compliant LV, LV pressure shows a raised LVEDP > 12 mmHg, induced by mental stress, rising further with hand gripping exercise. The question arises whether the raised LVEDP is a transient phenomenon, although this by itself is a sign of cardiovascular maladaptation suggesting reduced LV diastolic compliance. The threshold leading to clinical diastolic dysfunction and heart failure can be decided by a raised NT-ProBNP ≥ 125 pg/mL [334, 335], and an added outpatient 24-hr ambulatory BP monitoring is helpful to determine whether what was seen in the cardiac catheter laboratory was a stress response or a more sustained reflection of inadequately treated hypertensive heart disease.

To summarise the above pithily and metaphorically:

> *What happens behind a closed door remains hidden. If the door is light, rush out, but if it's weighty, slow down and push harder.*

1.8 Case Examples

1.8.1 Exercise-Induced LBBB

A 58-year-old woman has angina which is clearly reproducible with exertion over the last 6 months. She was previously well and has been on HRT for several years. Her heart was normal on cardiovascular magnetic resonance (CMR) scan and she has non-obstructive coronary arteries on CT coronary angiogram (CTCA). Interestingly, during her exercise treadmill test, as she started stage III of Bruce protocol at 6 min, she was noted to be in LBBB, HR 154 bpm, 163/89 mmHg, and QRS 125 ms; the corresponding figures at rest were HR 80 bpm, 130/70 mmHg and QRS 87 ms. She experienced her usual angina and within 2 min of stopping exercise, she flipped back into narrow complex sinus rhythm, when her HR fell under 100 bpm (Fig. 1.5). During peak exercise, her echocardiogram showed global hypokinesia with an EF of 40%. She has normal C-reactive protein (CRP) level, and she is not overweight with a body mass index (BMI) of 25 (< 30) kg/m^2 and her NT-proBNP is 50 (< 125) pg/mL.

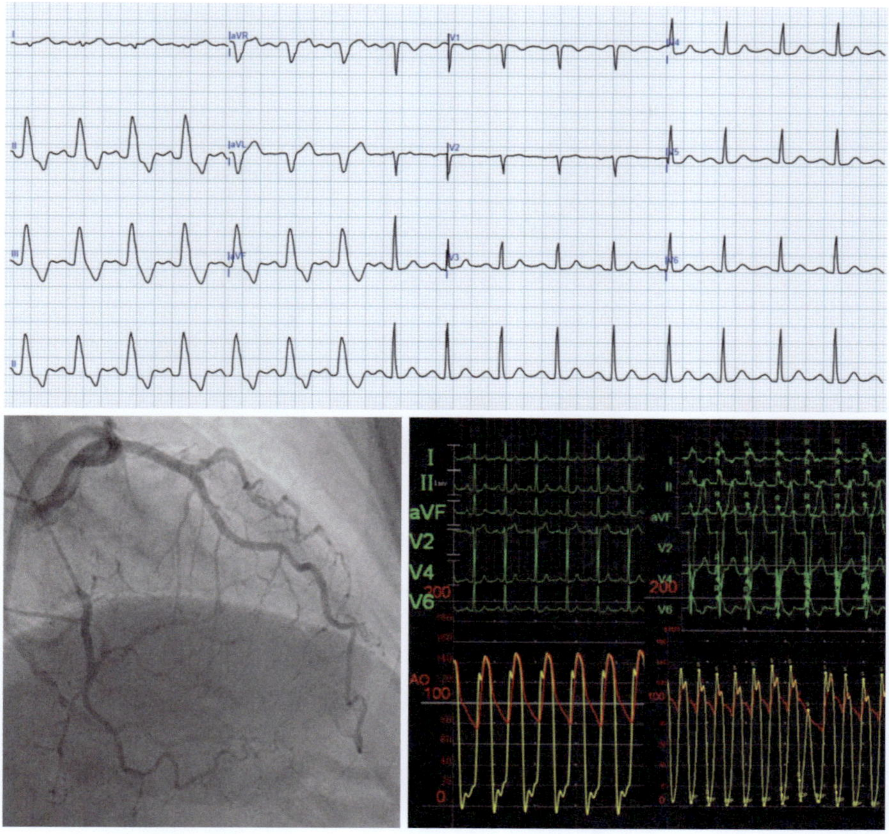

Fig. 1.5 (**Top panel**) ECG during recovery of treadmill test, the exercise-induced LBBB resolved when HR falls under 100 bpm. (**Bottom, left to right panels**) Dual-injection coronary angiogram in right-anterior-oblique (RAO) cranial view that shows unobstructed coronary arteries. ECG, aortic and LV pressure tracings, at rest and during right atrial pacing-induced LBBB. At rest HR 78 bpm and BP 152/80 mmHg, and during LBBB, HR 128 bpm and BP 128/90 mmHg—the rate pressure product (RPP) increases by 30%, a marker of workload and oxygen demand

Procedure Her coronary arteries are disease-free (Fig. 1.5). Nevertheless, her central aortic BP is 140–150 mmHg systolic, with an LVEDP of 15 (< 12) mmHg, which rises to 20 mmHg with handgrip, despite 1.5 mg of midazolam for sedation. With right atrial pacing, she develops angina and LBBB when paced at 128 bpm, her LVEDP falls to under 5 mmHg. There is also a fall in BP, and because of paced HR, the rate pressure product (RPP) increases by 30%; this is a measure of oxygen demand, that should be accompanied with coronary flow increase. However, there is no accompanying rise in coronary flow despite a fall in resistance by 20% (Fig. 1.6). Even when her vasodilatory capacity is normal, and with mildly elevated minimal hyperaemic resistance suggesting that she exhibits impairment of flow augmentation with increased heart rate as is normally expected.

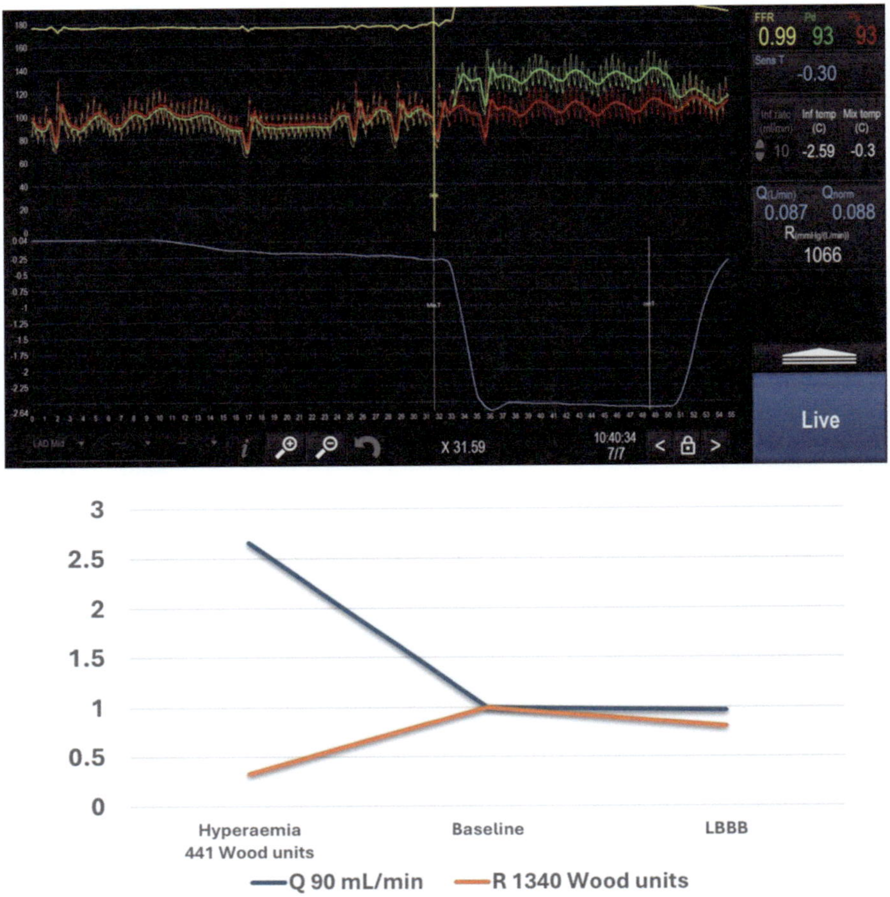

Fig. 1.6 (**Top panel**) Continuous thermodilution estimation of coronary flow, 87 mL/min and resistance 1066 Wood units during right atrial pacing-induced LBBB (**Bottom panel**) Haemodymanic chart of the basal and hyperaemic indices, flow 90, and 239 mL/min, and resistance 1340 and 441 Wood units—thus vasodilatory capacity or CFR is 2.7, and microvascular resistance reserve, MRR 3.0. Similarly, using basal readings as comparators, during LBBB, flow is 0.97 and resistance, 0.80. In other words, flow does not increase despite the increased workload and oxygen demand, and in spite of slight fall of resistancfe by 20%

Interpretation This lady has a normal heart but when her BP rises due to procedural anxiety, her LVEDP also rises > 12 mmHg, but in the absence of a raised NT-ProBNP, implying that the raised LVEDP is not sustained during her daily physical activities. Perhaps this is due to age-related diastolic LV dysfunction. In addition, she has normal coronary microvascular function (CFR 2.7, MRR 3.0 and Rμ 441 (reactive BP) Wood units). Animal and human atrial-pacing studies suggest that tachycardia augments coronary flow by one third from baseline [336]. This is not observed in this woman who has rate-induced LBBB. Thus, LBBB causes supply demand mismatch during exercise, due to her inability to mount an increase in her coronary flow in general, not just focal ischaemia in the dyssynchronous LV septum as is generally believed [337], as a mechanism for her angina. Permanent left bundle branch (LBB): Pacing has emerged as a physiological resynchronisation approach, potentially normalising coronary haemodynamics, and it has been advocated if medical treatment fails [338–340].

1.8.2 Vasoreactive Hypertensive Heart

A 54-year-old man has had angina for 4 years, occurring at night, at rest and on exertion. He is overweight with a BMI of 36 kg/m^2 and has obstructive sleep apnoea (OSA). His use of continuous positive airway pressure (CPAP) to sleep with, has markedly reduced his nighttime angina. He has diabetes, hypertension and hyperlipidaemia, having smoked cigarettes since his teenage years for 25 years, before stopping about 15 years ago. He has chronic obstructive pulmonary disease (COPD) with infective exacerbations requiring ITU treatment on 3 occasions over the last 6 months. His previous diagnostic coronary angiogram undertaken in his local hospital 3 years ago revealed unobstructed coronary arteries. Hence, he has been treated for microvascular angina with bisoprolol, isosorbide mononitrate, ivabradine, nicorandil and ranolazine, as well as ramipril, spironolactone and atorvastatin. Despite the empirical polypharmacy, he has continued to be highly symptomatic. Therefore, the referral for coronary physiology is indicated.

Procedure His coronary arteries are smooth and unobstructed, but with generalised *coronary slow flow phenomenon* (CSFP). It takes about 6 heartbeats for the contrast to reach the LAD apex from the 6 French guide catheter tip.

Next the LV is studied: the LVEDP is raised, at 15 mmHg, both at rest and with handgrip (Fig. 1.7). LV angiogram shows thickened LV with LV mid cavity obstruction (MCO) and there is a pullback gradient of 10–20 mmHg with a central aortic BP of 160/90 mmHg.

With the pressure wire in distal LAD, the Pd/Pa is 0.95 and RFR, 0.94 (> 0.89). Bolus thermodilution is undertaken with escalating doses of IC adenosine (Table 1.1). The CFR is normal but with an elevated IMR; there is an adenosine dose-dependent increase in CFR and reduction in IMR. Next, continuous thermodilution is performed, starting with saline infusion at 20 mL/min to induce hyperaemia. This is repeated 3 times to get 2 close results, and the third study indices are used. With the saline rate reduced to 10 mL/min, for basal figures; this is repeated 4 times to get consistent results: the first two are likely to be from a continuing but dissipating hyperaemic state. Again, the CFR and MRR are normal, but there are consistently raised basal and hyperaemic resistances.

Low doses of acetylcholine (ACh) cause a dose-dependent increase in epicardial vasospasm (Fig. 1.8). With ACh 2 μg, the flow reduces by 27% and resistance increases by 41%, without obstructive coronary artery, Pd/Pa 0.96 which implies resistance to flow at the *microvasculature* as is generally believed, or due to spasm

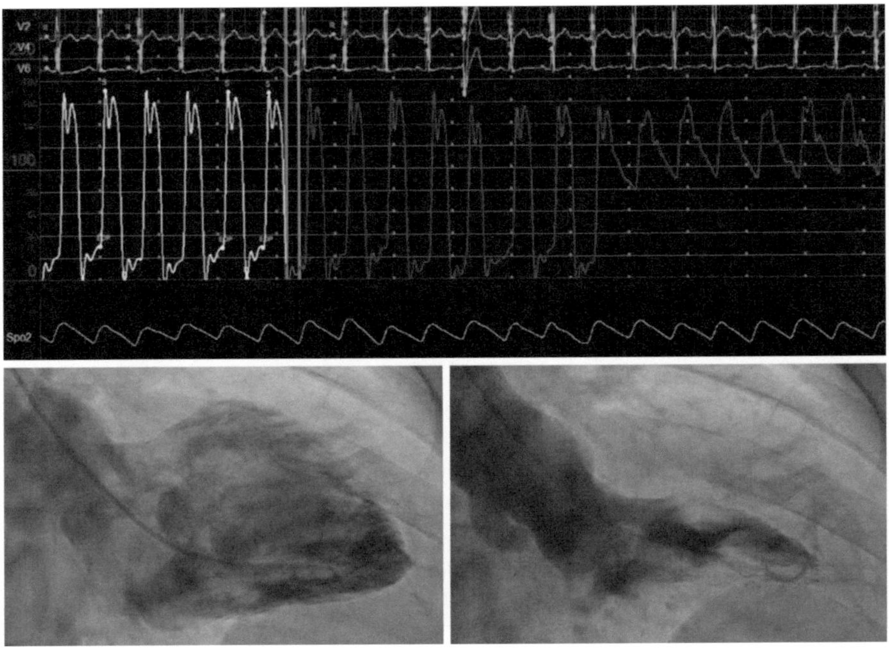

Fig. 1.7 (**Top panel**) LV pressure tracing with pullback of the pigtail catheter from LV apex, along the LV to the aorta. Note the elevated LVEDP, measurable at end-inspiration of 15 mmHg. There is overshoot of pre-aortic valve opening LV incisura reaching 170 mmHg, the systolic LV pressures falls slightly across the LV into the aorta—160 mmHg. (**Bottom, left to right panels**) LV in distaole and systole—impression of LVH and MCO

Table 1.1 Adenosine dose-dependency of hyperaemia and repeated measures

Thermodilution				
Bolus		CFR	IMR	MRR
IC adenosine	200 μg	3.9	38	3.8
	600 μg	4.6	27	5.4
	1000 μg	5.1	22	5.8
Continuous		**3.9**	**27**	**4.0**
		Q, mL/min	**R, Wood units**	
Saline infusion	20 mL/min	216	504	
	Hyperaermic	259	426	
		218	**534**	
	10 mL/min	120	1054	
	Rest	65	1901	
		47	2688	
		56	**2123**	**ΔQ**
IC acetylcholine	2 μg	41	2988	0.73
	20 μg	52	2448	0.93
IC verapamil	1000 μg	110	1007	1.96
IC acetylcholine	20 μg	65	1691	1.16

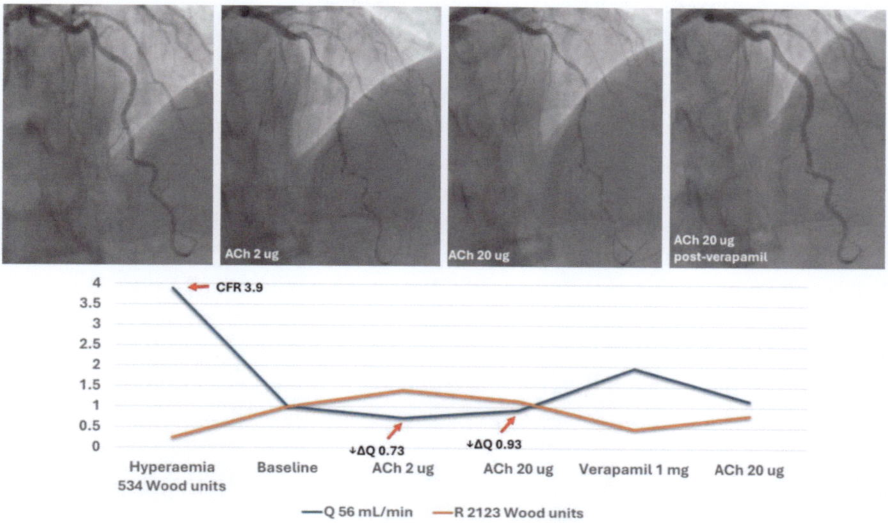

Fig. 1.8 (**Top, left to right panels**) LAD with CSFP that takes 6 heartbeats to reach the apex, low doses of ACh cause epicardial vasospasm, preventable by verapamil pre-treatment. (**Bottom, left to right panels**) Haemodynamic indices at baseline, during hyperaemia and in response to drugs. There is normal vasodilatory capacity, CFR 3.9 and MRR 4.0, but elevated basal and hyperaemic resistance; 2123 and 534 Wood units. ACh 2 μg causes a fall in flow with diffuse epicardial vasospasm. ACh 20 μg provokes more severe epicardial vasospasm without further fall in flow which suggests that the microvascular vasodilatory capacity is intact. Verapamil doubles the flow and prevents epicardial vasospasm with ACh 20 μg rechallenge

of the small vessels which does not need to be occlusive (see case 3). A tenfold dose increase in ACh at 20 μg causes generalised vasospasm especially in distal vessels. But, without a fall in Pd/Pa, 0.95 and without worsening flow suggesting that autoregulatory microvasculature swings into action to maintain flow, overcoming the epicardial vasospasm. Verapamil doubles flow and prevented epicardial vasospasm with ACh 20 μg rechallenge, but flow is still under 1.5, the definition for microvascular endothelial dysfunction.

Interpretation This man does not have obstructive coronary artery disease despite his multiple coronary risk factors. He has uncontrolled hypertension; this is expressed as LVH with MCO, raised LVEDP and coronary resistance—*hypertensive heart disease*. His NT-ProBNP post-procedure is 72 (< 125) ng/L which means his LVEDP does not stay high. In addition, he has increased epicardial and microvascular reactivity indicative of *global endothelial dysfunction* on a background of preserved microvascular vasodilatory capacity. This is another demonstration of CSFP as rheological in nature and not due to CMD. The focus for him is to lose weight, improve his diabetic control and hypertension management.

1.8.3 MINOCA and Epicardial Vasospasm

A 42-year-old Caucasian woman was admitted with a troponin negative chest pain to St George's hospital. She has been diagnosed with vasospastic or Prinzmetal angina on double calcium channel blockers of diltiazem and amlodipine. Despite which she has experienced increasing breakthrough angina after a relatively calm period over the Christmas and new year festive season. Her angina diagnosis was on the basis of her admission to a local hospital 8 months prior. She led a stressful jet-setting and high impact professional life. Following a crescendo of chest pain, she was hospitalised with an anterior myocardial infarction. Her coronary angiogram found a signet ring in the left anterior descending (LAD) artery just before the second diagonal (D2) branch with general reduction in distal vessel calibre (Fig. 1.9).

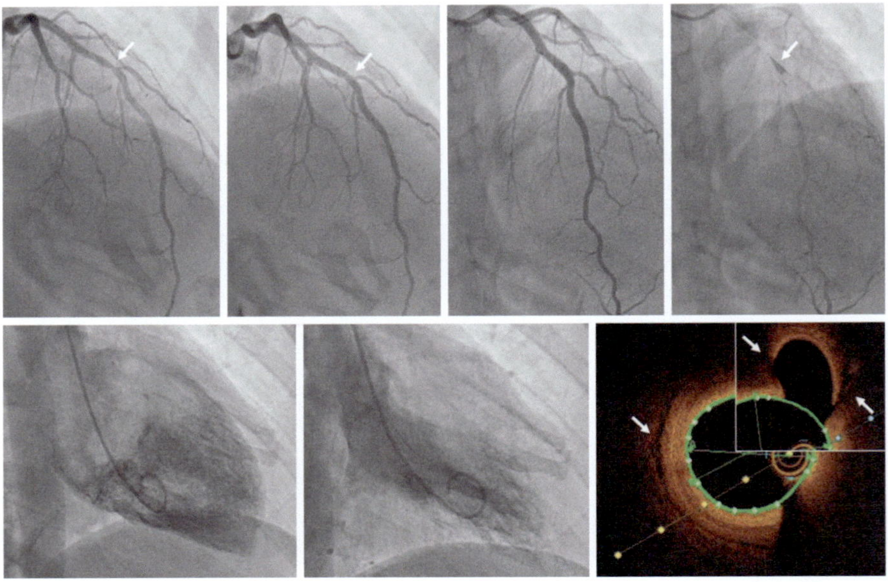

Fig. 1.9 (**Top, left to right panels**) First coronary angiogram shows a discrete ring-like lesion (*arrow*) just before second diagonal (D2) branch in the left anterior descending (LAD) artery, which improves following intracoronary nitroglycerine (*arrow*). On day 2, the repeat coronary angiogram reveals *increased LAD calibe* where the original lesion is, where contrast appears to linger (*arrow*). (**Bottom, left to right panels**) Left vetricular angiogram in diastole and systole, note the mild hypokinesia, but near normal, in the mid to apical anterior wall. The optical coherence tomography (OCT) at just beyond the first septal branch with "subtle" intimomedial circumferential hypodensity which could indicate a split along the tissue plane, and (*inset*) at the origin of the first diagonal branch there are signal dropouts which can be caused by 3 things, (1) Guidewire, but its shadow is accounted for on the opposite vessel wall, (2) Fresh red thrombi which absorb and disperse the OCT signals, none are seen, and finally, (3) True dissection, common at bifurcation junctions where haemodynamic wall stress predominates, especially in the setting of a "non-compliant" artery due to endothelial dysfunction. Howerer, this OCT appearance at side branch origin is usually a normal finding. A pinhole rupture case example is presented in Chap. 5—case 4

Intracoronary nitroglycerine (GTN) vasodilated the lesion as well as the rest of the coronary artery—demonstrating a primary vasospastic event. However, because of continuing symptoms, she was brought back to the cardiac catheter laboratory for intracoronary imaging with optical coherence tomography (OCT) looking for a plaque rupture; if this was present then it could be sealed with a stent. This was not found thus sealing instead the diagnosis of vasospastic angina and myocardial infarction with non-obstructive coronary arteries (MINOCA). Over the next few months, she was titrated up her medication; the dosing of her diltiazem was limited by first degree atrioventricular block with 180 mg mane and 120 mg nocte, amlodipine 5 mg was added in addition to long-acting isosorbide mononitrate 60 mg od and nicorandil 10 mg od. She described her chest pain as a pressure-like sensation, radiating up her left shoulder and down her left arm. GTN's effect was variable. It could take up to 10 min to work. She was premenopausal, has endometriosis on a progesterone-based coil, has asthma on steroids (fluticasone and beclomethasone) inhalers, previous duodenal ulcer maintained on omeprazole 20 mg od and has had complex partial epilepsy since the age of 26; her last seizure was 12 years ago, she continued on levetiracetam 750 mg, and she has been started on atorvastatin 40 mg od for its pleiotropic effect.

While in the coronary care unit, she continued to have chest pain despite intravenous GTN. Her repeated troponins were normal and her electrocardiograms (ECG) static, but with an obvious J-point notch in the inferolateral leads, signifying benign early repolarisation (BER). She had a repeat coronary angiogram with the view to undertake a comprehensive coronary physiology, having been off her vasodilators for 24 hours since admission.

Procedure Her LV function is normal on LV angiogram, with an LVEDP of 5 mmHg, not rising with handgrip, and a central aortic BP of 100/60 mmHg (Fig. 1.10). Her coronary angiogram shows unobstructed coronary arteries with smooth lumen; without obvious plaques, contrast injections down her left coronary artery, however, are associated with peaking of T-wave in the inferior leads and T-wave inversion in the anteroseptal leads, which, in her case are associated with chest pain. Continuous thermodilution is undertaken; the basal and hyperaemic indices are estimated in duplicates: flow 96/90 mL/min and 225/253 mL/min, and resistance 834/883 Wood units and 316/290 Wood units. Using the repeat values, her coronary flow reserve, CFR, is 2.8 and microvascular resistance reserve, MRR, 3.0. Acetylcholine (ACh) is given in escalating doses—2, 20, 100 and 200 μg (Fig. 1.11). There is a *biphasic response to ACh* in flow, with initial flow reduction *presumably* due to transient microvascular spasm followed by moderate epicardial vasospasm, but accompanied by flow > 50% and chest pain. Verapamil abolishes this, and with ACh 200 μg rechallenge, interestingly it blunts the flow observed earlier. Adenosine 1 mg bolus causes similar chest pain. Her contemporaneous thyroid function tests, NT-proBNP, C-reactive protein, follicle stimulating hormone (FSH), luteinising hormone (FSH) and oestradiol [725, (<1461) pmol/l] are all normal.

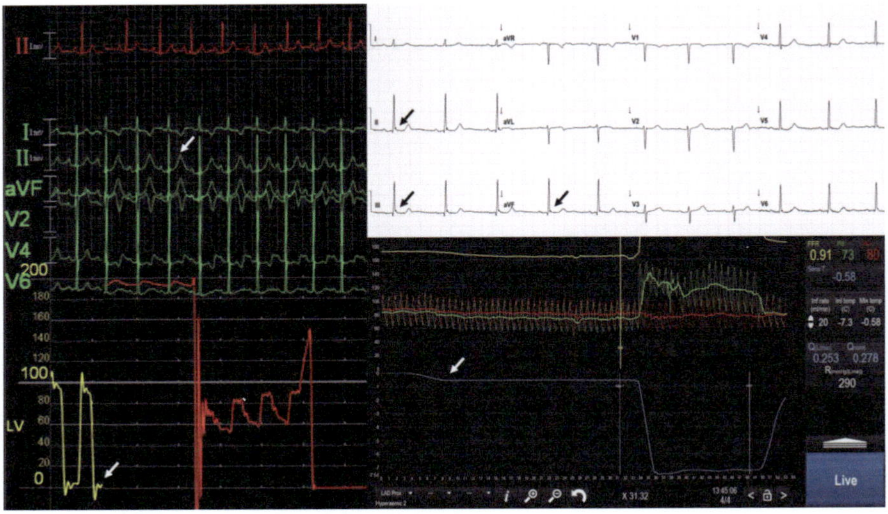

Fig. 1.10 (**Left, top to bottom panels**) Momentary electrocardiographic (ECG) T-wave peaking (*arrow*) and T-wave inversion in inferior and anterior precordial leads respectively, with contrast, saline and adenosine. Left ventricular and aortic pressures are normal (*arrow*). (**Right, top and bottom panels**) The 12-lead ECG shows normal sinus rhytmn with a J-point notch in II, III, aVF and V4-6 (*arrows*). Continuous thermodilution in the left anterior descending (LAD) artery with saline infusion via the RayFlow microcatheter at the rate of 20 mL/min, causing hyperaemia—steady state is achieved within 10 s (*arrow*) demonstrating a normal microvasculture

Her 24-h Holter performed 2 months following hospital discharge picks up no significant cardiac arrhythmias. Her stress perfusion CMR undertaken 1 month off drug treatment reveals a normal heart with no scar, fibrosis or infarct.

Interpretation This woman developed unstable angina culminating with a MINOCA, which on closer inspection was likely due to a limited coronary artery dissection at the LAD/D1 bifurcation, because of a "stiff" artery from endothelial dysfunction, precipitating a transiently occlusive coronary vasospasm, quintessentially a Prinzmetal event, often seen in young men who smoke, as originally described in 1959 [236].

Despite aggressive vasodilators with 2 classes of calcium channel blockers, oral nitrates and nicorandil, she continued to be symptomatic. Her ECG did not show "sharkfin" ST elevation during pain, her LAD has healed and her coronary physiology study demonstrates a relatively high flow and low resistance at baseline, in spite of which she has spare vasodilatory capacity which implies that she has normal coronary microvascular function. ACh induces only "moderate" non-occlusive LAD vasospasm at the highest dose of 200 μg, without flow reduction, but enhanced flow, yet she is symptomatic, and this is reproduced with adenosine, making it possible that she has *non-ischaemic angina from hyperaemia*.

The question is why this young premenopausal woman replete with oestrogen has epicardial endothelial dysfunction, whether this is related to her inhaled

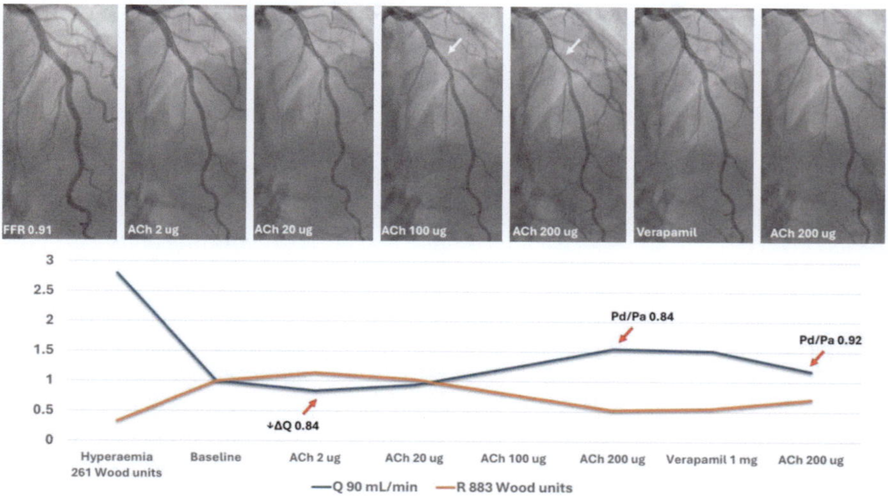

Fig. 1.11 (**Top, left to right panels**) Left anterior descending (LAD) artery, at baseline, it is smooth and widely patent. With acetylcholine (ACh), increasing doses cause a reduction in calibre, and at 200 μg, the segment which was previously dissected becomes moderately vasospastic, more so compared with 100 μg (*arrows*), and this is preventable with verapamil pre-treatment. (**Bottom**) Continuous thermodilution during basal, hyperaemia, ACh and following verapamil. Note that low-dose ACh 2 μg reduces flow and increases resistance with general reduction in epicardial coronary calibre (*arrow*), and the flow rises with higher ACh doses that instead precipitate mid LAD segmental vasospasm, at ACh 200 μg, the flow increases by 55% (> 50%, *arrow*), suggesting intact microvascular endothelial function. There is a moderate fall in distal-to-aortic pressure ratio, Pd/Pa to 0.84, which is reversed by verapamil and with verapamil on board, ACh 200 μg rechallenge does not reduce the LAD calibre further, Pd/Pa stays high at 0.92, **although the flow paradoxically falls** (*arrow*). With ACh 2/20/100/200 μg, the respective Pd/Pa, fractional flow and resistance are—0.94/0.93/0.93/**0.84**; 0.84/0.94/1.24/**1.55**; and 1.14/1.03/0.78/**0.53**

steroids, although this has never been documented in the medical literature, unlike oral steroids, albeit indirectly [341]. There is a biphasic response to ACh—low-dose *microvascular spasm* and high-dose *epicardial vasospasm*. The early fall in flow with ACh 2 μg in the absence of epicardial vasospasm ≥ 90%, in practice, is attributed to microvascular spasm according to guidelines [342]. However, in principle it could be due to a general reduction in distal vessel calibre. As discussed earlier, as per Hagen-Poiseuille's inverse power equation, a small vessel with 2 mm calibre has a resistance of 105 Wood units, when it constricts to 1 mm, the resistance rises to 1778 Wood units, a 17-fold rise in resistance, without the need to vasoconstrict the microvasculature ≤ 500 μm to reduce flow, or recruit proximal and mid epicardial vasospasm (the pressure wire Pd/Pa stays high at 6 cm from RayFlow tip). Conceptually, this appears logical; the early small change in calibre of small vessels from *first contact with ACh* reduces flow, followed by microvascular correction or autoregulation to counteract it, and microvascular endothelial function at a higher ACh dose further increases flow. This is a common pattern, seen in **case 2** earlier and **case 5** later, as a sign of epicardial endothelial dysfunction.

Ishihara et al. [343] in 1997 and Oldenburg et al. [344] in 2000 reported that verapamil 1 mg optimally and safely vasodilated the LAD in humans with little incremental gain at a higher dose of 2 mg, with a 43–46% mean increase in coronary blood flow velocity measured using the Doppler wire, against 131% with papaverine 10 mg, a hyperaemic dose for LAD. Oldenburg et al. [345] a year later further described that verapamil 1 mg injected down the LAD was associated with lactate release in the coronary sinus, which meant shunting to glycolytic anaerobic metabolism or myocardial ischaemia, despite higher blood flow; the higher the flow the greater the lactate release in 52 patients, two-thirds of whom had unobstructed coronary arteries. One proposed mechanism was that pre-arteriolar vasodilatation raised capillary hydrostatic pressure, precipitating interstitial oedema via amplified plasma filtration. This can potentially cause subendocardial ischaemia.

Calcium channel blockers are well known to cause peripheral interstitial oedema. In the rat cremaster muscle (groin muscle around the spermatic cord) microvascular model, diltiazem augmented interstitial filtration through an enhanced postcapillary venular permeability, while for verapamil, it was through elevated capillary hydrostatic pressure [346]. Verapamil, by blocking L-type Ca^{2+}-channels, transiently decreased regional contractility, induced dyskinesia, and produced non-ischaemic ST elevation in open-chest canine hearts, which lasted under 5 min [347]. In contrast, because acetylcholine-evoked endothelial NO release does not principally depend on L-type Ca^{2+} channels, verapamil does not materially inhibit ACh-mediated NO-dependent vasodilation [348, 349]. Nevertheless, high-dose verapamil modestly attenuates ACh-induced, endothelium-derived hyperpolarising factor (EDHF) which at most translates into 10–20% flow reduction [350]. The endothelial cells at the myo-endothelial junction (endothelial cellular projection to muscle cell across the internal elastic lamina) are replete with Ca^{2+}-activated K^+ channels, which are triggered by an ACh-M_3-receptor/IP_3-mediated Ca^{2+} surge from the endoplasmic reticulum (intracellular Ca^{2+} release) and via *endothelial L-type Ca^{2+} channels* (influx of extracellular Ca^{2+}). The resulting K^+ efflux hyperpolarises the endothelial cell, and that voltage spreads through myo-endothelial gap junctions to the smooth muscle, causing vasodilation [351]. Verapamil blocks endothelial L-type Ca^{2+} channels, reducing endothelial Ca^{2+} entry and thus attenuates this EDHF-mediated response. In other words, verapamil contributes to "endothelial dysfunction", but this is usually masked by its dominant relaxation of vascular smooth muscle cells. In CMD, this effect may become important [352], and theoretically, nicorandil can overcome it by donating NO and directly opening K^+ channels [353].

Thus, the large reduction in flow with ACh in this case, before and after verapamil is likely to be a non-pharmacological interaction, neither through the negative inotropic effect of verapamil raising LVEDP as this is a short-lived event. Making altered microvascular transcapillary homeostasis in the presence of endothelial dysfunction an attractive hypothesis. This will be discussed later.

The above studies suggest that verapamil 1 mg is able to recruit about a third of the vasodilatory range. In this case, the phenomenon of verapamil's negating of microvascular endothelial function, i.e. it prevents ACh-induced epicardial vasospasm, yet it abolishes ACh-provoked flow increase at the microvascular level, is intriguing—from the same baseline; therefore, this is the *opposite of masking,* where the "vascular smooth muscle cells" are dilated by verapamil, thus they could not be further dilated by ACh—in which case the flow should not fall precipitously with ACh rechallenge. The recommendation that vasodilators are withheld before spasm testing with ACh is to uncover inherent or underlying vasoreactivity which is otherwise blunted by treatment. Although this is a reasonable theoretical consideration based on observational studies, but without cross-over experimental underpinning [354], especially since vasoreactivity could change over time with reproducibility as low as 29% in some repeat-testing series, even among patients who remained untreated between tests [355]. Moreover, giving upfront intraarterial verapamil as a radial artery antispasmodic agent does not interfere with ACh spasm testing in the coronary artery [305].

The **Verapamil-attenuated ACh response** has previously been noted [356], but it is not inevitable [357], neither does it reduce hyperaemic flow (see case 4). It is a complex sequence of events which does not have a name, perhaps aptly be called, the "**Oldenburg Paradox**", since the paradoxical coronary ischaemia with verapamil was first described by Olaf Oldenburg and his colleagues in 2001 [345]. Just to recap, in this case:

1. Hyperaemia	→	Q ↑181%	R ↓71%
2. ACh 200 μg	→	Q ↑55%	R ↓47%
3. Verapamil 1 mg	→	Q ↑52%	R ↓44%
4. ACh 200 μg rechallenge	→	Q ↑18% (Δ ↓37% before Verapamil)	R ↓29%

This effect might explain calcium channel blockers' lack of efficacy in CMD [234, 358]. In this lady, since ACh does not provoke clinical epicardial vasospasm, and the flow response to verapamil is blunted (52%, < 100%), she has a trial off all her cardiac medication and was reviewed 4 months later in the outpatient clinic; this has not led to an increase in her symptomatology.

1.8.4 Non-ischaemic Hyperaemic Angina

A 53-year-year old South Asian women has typical angina, starting mostly at rest over the last 7 months—left sided, with radiation up her neck and down her left arm, which could last for over 30 minutes, with variable response to sublingual nitroglycerine spray. And she has been seen in the emergency department repeatedly with troponin negative chest pain. Her ECG showed non-specific inferolateral ST sagging. She took multivitamins, including vitamin D and is treated for hypercholesterolaemia. She has no diabetes or hypertension, has never smoked, and is premenopausal with a normal weight, BMI 24 kg/m^2. One year before her chest pain began, she started having postprandial crampy upper abdominal pain, severe enough to double up and roll on the floor. Extensive upper gastrointestinal investigations failed to find a cause, and antispasmodics did not seem to help. Instead, she was treated with an

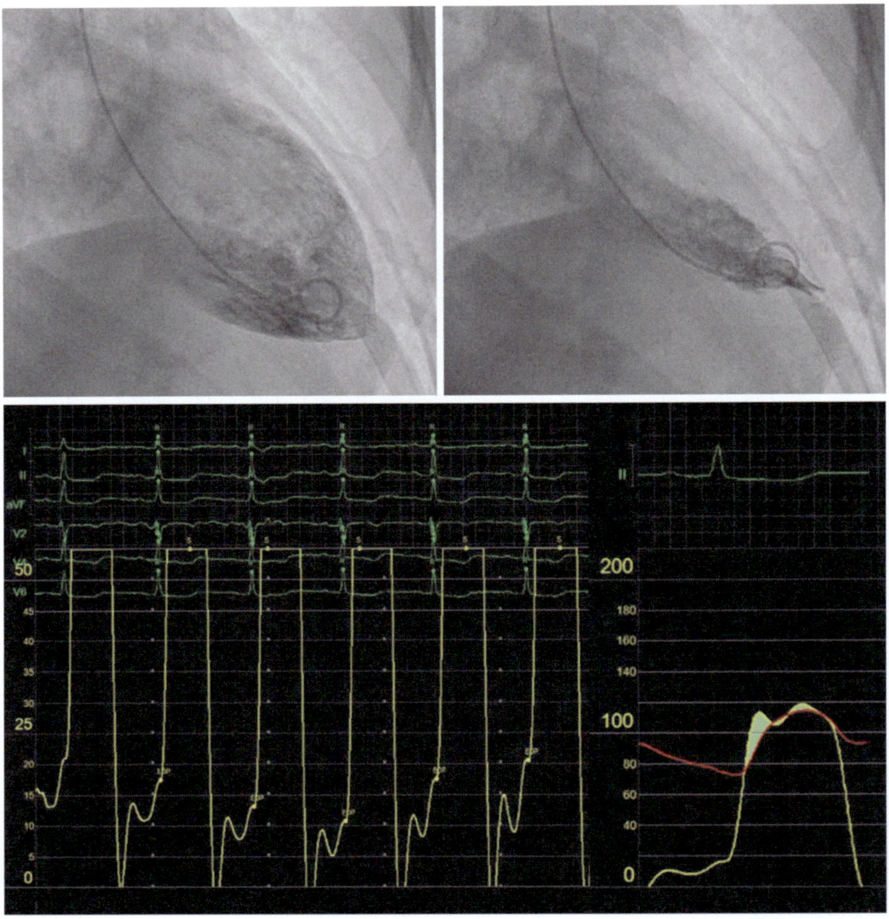

Fig. 1.12 (**Top, left to right panels**) Left vetricular angiogram in diastole and systole, note the systolic apical diverticulum—can be a sign of pressure overload. (**Bottom, left to right panels**) Left ventricular end-diastolic pressure (LVEDP) rising to as high as 20 mmHg, and matched peak systolic blood pressure (BP) in the left ventricle and aorta, implying no intraventricular obstruction or aortic stenosis, and BP being normal—no increased systemic arterial afterload

opioid, tramadol 50 mg twice a day. In one of her hospitalisations, she had an echocardiogram that showed a normal heart. Her adenosine stress perfusion CMR undertaken 6 months ago was also normal. She has undilated LA, no LVH and EF 70%, ESVI 19 (14–33) mL/m^2, SVI 44 (37–62) mL/m^2 and VAC 0.42 (0.6–1.0).

Procedure Her LV is studied first: she has normal contractility, LVEDP 12–15 mmHg and it rises to over 15 mmHg with handgrip with a central aortic BP of 110/60 mmHg (Fig. 1.12), without a significant pressure gradient across the aortic valve. The coronary arteries are smooth and unobstructed. Interestingly, contrast injections are

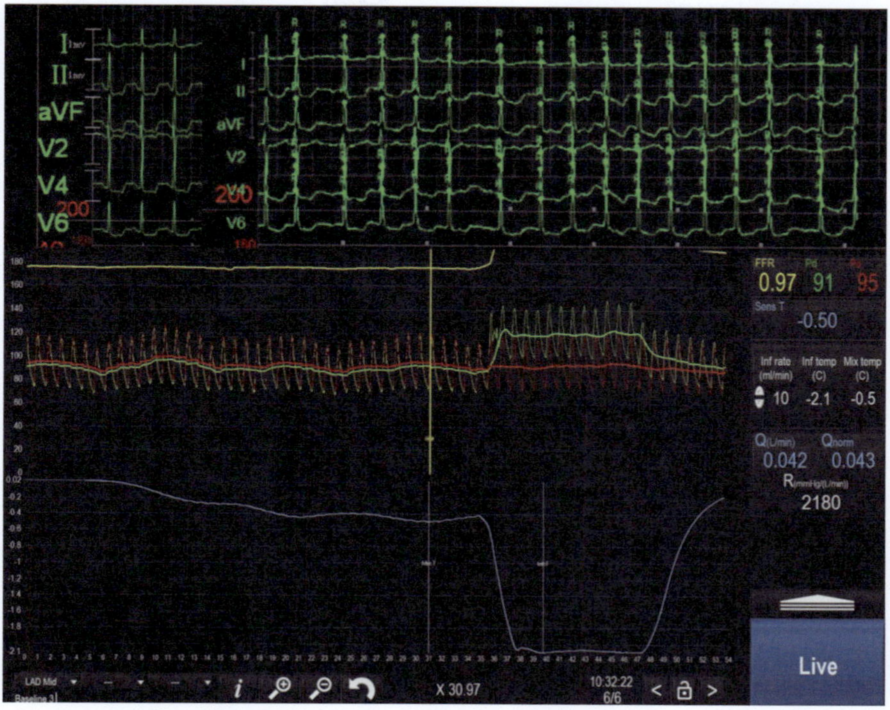

Fig. 1.13 (**Top, left to right panels**) Electrocardiographic ST depression with chest pain with contrast injectrion, and atrial fibrillation with high-dose acetylcholine that does not cause bradycardia and dropped beats. (**Bottom**) Basal flow repeated 3 times with saline infusion at the rate of 10 mL/min for consistency, the flow is low and resistance is high at rest

associated with chest pain and increased ST depression (Fig. 1.13). Continuous thermodilution is undertaken to the LAD. The basal indices are repeated 3 times for consistency; flow 49, 40 and **42** mL/min, resistance 1880, 2324 and **2180** Wood units: hyperaemic indices; flow 164 and **167** mL/min, and resistance 486 and **464** Wood units. The last respective estimates are used to derive CFR, which is 4.0 and MRR 4.7. Escalating doses of ACh are given—2, 20, 100 and 200 μg; these increase flow > 50%. The last doses are associated with typical chest pain and ECG ST depression; with the last dose, a transient run of atrial fibrillation (AF) occurs. Verapamil 1 mg doubles the flow, without sequelae, but when rechallenged with ACh 200 μg, chest pain and ECG ST depression are reproduced, again, with a short run of AF. While she is in AF, IC adenosine 1 mg is given which produces similar level hyperaemic flow as is induced with 20 mL/min saline infusion. Despite quadrupling the flow, the symptom and sign continue (Fig. 1.14).

Interpretation This woman has clear-cut and classical angina, albeit not effort-related, with a lingering duration. *Since she develops chest pain and ECG ST depression with ACh, without epicardial vasospasm, that is a definite proof that she*

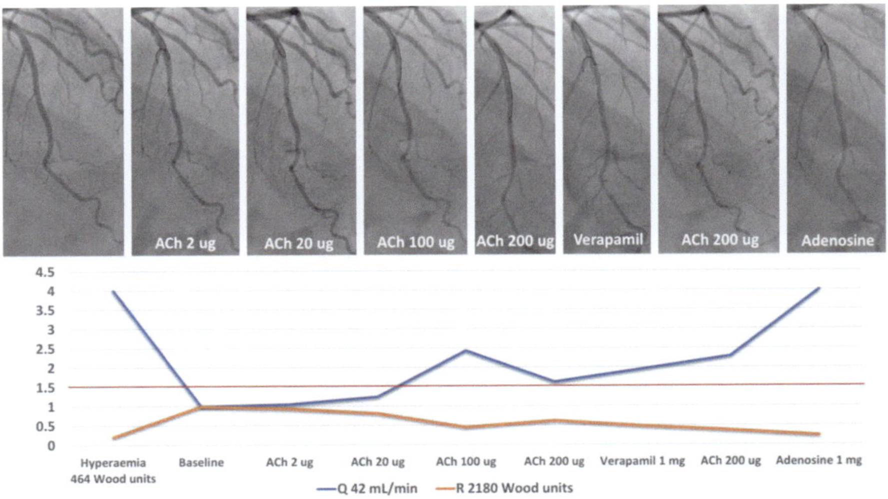

Fig. 1.14 (**Top, left to right panels**) Left anterior descending (LAD) artery, flow is brisk and maintained without significant change in epicardial calibre in response to increasing doses of acetylcholine and other drugs given intracoronarily. (**Bottom**) Haemodymanic plot of changes in flow and resistance as multiples of the basal values. There is low flow and high resistance in the resting state, but with normal vasodilatgory capacity and above 50% rise in flow with acetylcholine suggesting intact microvascular endothelial function

has microvascular spasm, despite not having slow coronary flow phenomenon (CSFP). But thinking it through, a more complicated picture emerges. She has a structurally and functionally normal heart on both echocardiogram and CMR. However, she has a supranormal EF with low VAC—to generate her cardiac output, she depletes her end-systolic LV reserve. Is there a restriction in her filling her LV? During her procedure, she has raised LVEDP without systolic or diastolic LV dysfunction, without LV intracavity gradient or systemic hypertension, and she has raised coronary resistance—more at rest (low flow state) than during hyperaemia.

On the other hand, her coronary vasodilatory capacity is preserved, together with epicardial and microvascular endothelial function. Cardiac "constraint" could be due to (1) extra pericardial compression, (2) pericardial constriction, and (3) intra pericardial restraint. In her case, contrast, ACh and adenosine all caused chest pain and ST depression—these agents cause vasodilatation.

One oft-quoted mechanism for microvascular angina, why functional ischaemia such as that with dobutamine stress echocardiogram is not usually elicited is that the ischaemia is patchy, due to flow diversion, or steal away from the ischaemic areas. Although the ST depression is usually *impressive and global*, more indicative of a large myocardium in peril, than islets of cardiac tissue devoid of blood supply. In addition, coronary sinus lactate extraction is commonly normal. Finally, in this case, pre-treatment with verapamil did not modify the effects of ACh suggesting that this "microvascular spasm" is not functional, yet not structural—seemingly paradoxical. Perhaps there could be an analogy with migraine—the headache is due

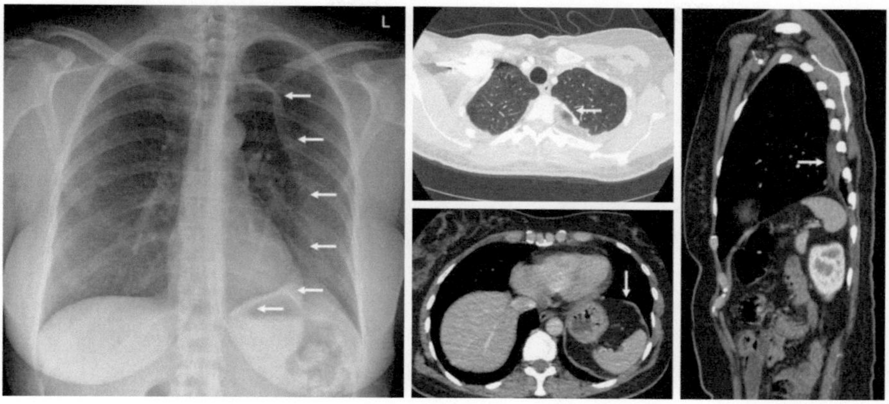

Fig. 1.15 (**Left panel**) Chest X-Ray with a left-sided mid thoracic linear opacity. (**Middle and left panels, clockwise**) Close to spine there, is a bifid intrathoracic rib which continues as a fibrous band that is tethered to the dome of an eventrated left hemidiaphragm (stomach and spleen visible) which pushes the heart forward; the mass effect is at 5 o'oclock behind the heart (*arrows*)

to vasodilation of brain blood vessels within a confined space, bounded by the skull. Can hyperaemic angina where there is cardiac constraint be a "migraine of the heart" (see Chap. 8.3.4 for more indepth discussion)?

In summary, this woman has a constrained heart with a triad of low flow, high LVEDP and raised coronary resistance; hyperaemia appears to cause "non-ischaemic" angina with ST depression. She has left hemidiaphragmatic eventration (Fig. 1.15). *Her CT thorax reveals a left-sided intrathoracic rib coursing down close to the spine with fibrous extension tethered into the dome of the eventrated left hemidiaphragm.*

Diaphragms are underappreciated in cardiology. There are cases whereby diaphragmatic herniation of abdominal organs into the thorax causes mass effect by compressing the cardiac chambers, resulting in a low cardiac output state precipitating syncope [359–361]. Under normal circumstances, the diaphragms increase venous return and preload and reduce afterload by generating negative intrathoracic pressure (−3 mmHg), transmitting this into the pericardium, lowering pericardial constraint, and redistributing splanchnic blood volume centrally [362]. In other words, a "chest compression-esque" feature during cardiopulmonary resuscitation.

It has been demonstrated that cardiac output is increased when the left diaphragm is paced during cardiac surgery [363], and a pilot study in synchronised bilateral diaphragmatic pacing translates into clinical benefits in heart failure in the short term [364]. It is therefore logical to surmise that this woman with a non-functioning eventrated left hemidiaphragm could explain her coronary physiology through a mass effect as extracardiac constraint and, equally, a possible cause for her unexplained postprandial abdominal pain.

Breathing has profound effects on the cardiovascular system; the heart rate and blood pressure vary throughout the respiratory cycle, which could be exaggerated with either Valsalva maneuver, or its reverse, the Mueller manoeuvrer. It is tempting to speculate that slow deep diaphragmatic breathing followed by pursed-lips expiration, as practiced widely in cardiac rehabilitation reduce coronary resistance and promote coronary flow, at least there is a theoretical basis for this.

Breathing exercises could reduce coronary resistance and increase preload, thus enhancing coronary flow and cardiac output by generating diaphragmatic negative intrathoracic pressure that is transmitted to the pericardium, reducing constraint and afterload in extracardiac vessels—the so-called respiratory pump during chest compression, a BP of 60 mmHg can be generated [365]. Indeed, there are small studies suggesting that breathing exercises reduce angina and increase exercise capacity [366].

1.8.5 PCOS, Hypertension and Myocardial Bridging

A 44-year-old Caucasian woman has had chest pain dating back to 16 years but was experiencing more symptoms, culminating with her presenting to the emergency department twice over the last 6 months. Interesting, she was noted to have inverted P in limb leads I and II during these admissions. She was on diltiazem 240/120 mg daytime and nighttime dosing, ramipril 10 mg od and ivabradine 5 mg bd, as well as atorvastatin 20 mg for hyperlipidaemia. She was diagnosed with hypertension at the age of 13, but without an obvious secondary cause identified in the specialist hypertension clinic. With the above regimen, her home and clinic BP appeared elevated, last self-measured at 150/98 mmHg. She was told that she has polycystic ovaries but does not require any specific management. She is overweight with a BMI of 37 kg/m^2 and her periods have been irregular and heavy. She has fibroadenoma but not endometriosis. Her recent hormonal profile suggests that she is premenopausal; oestradiol is 410 (< 1461) pmol/L, FSH is < 25 IU/L, and her prolactin has been noted to be as high as 698 (102–496) mIU/L, but not consistently so; a repeated blood sampling gives a lower value at 388.

Her chest pain is classically angina in its description but not exertional; it has woken her up from sleep at two o'clock in the early hours of the morning. Otherwise, the onset is unpredictable, usually at rest but more noticeable when her heart rate is above 100 bpm. She is getting the pain three times a week. Her CTCA, undertaken when she was 35, found a short segment of myocardial bridging in the mid LAD beyond the diagonal branch. A contemporaneous echocardiogram then revealed a normal heart. The following year her CMR found a structurally and functionally normal heart, EF 68%, without LA dilatation or LVH, and VAC 0.48 (0.6–1.0). At 39 she had an exercise stress echocardiogram where she exercised for 8 min 30 s on Bruce protocol treadmill, HR 87 to 170 bpm (94% predicted and 10 Mets) and BP 138/75 to 160/85 mmHg—at rest and at peak exercise respectively. She stopped the treadmill test because of fatigue; there were no ischaemic ECG changes nor inducible cardiac ischaemia on echocardiogram on a background of a normal heart. Prior to her coronary physiology study, although her office BP was high, she had a 24-hr

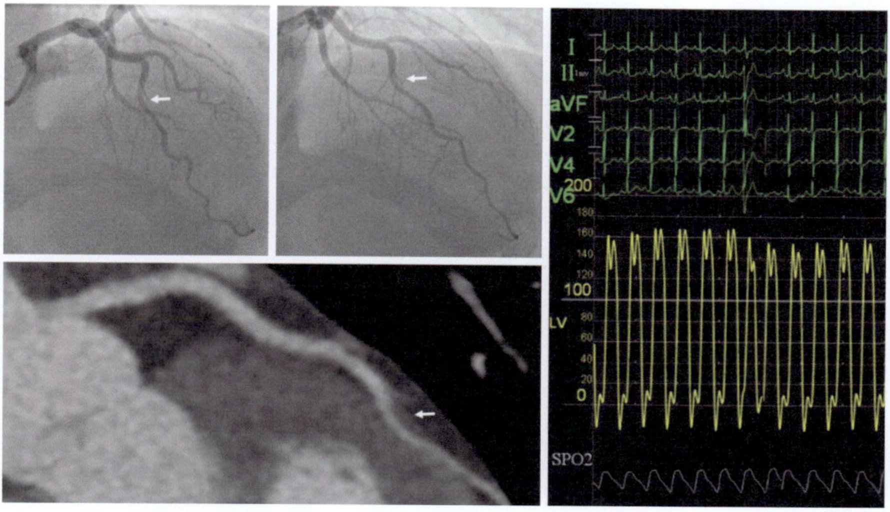

Fig. 1.16 (**Top, left to right panels**) The LAD in systole and distole, the *arrows* point to the myocardial bridging segment, which corresponds to the CTCA (**Bottom, left panel**). (**Right panel**) LV pressure and reactive hypertension, the LVEDP < 12 mmHg despite BP > 160 mmHg

ambulatory BP monitor (ABPM) which returned a daytime mean of 123/78 mmHg and a normal nighttime dip by 26%, mean 91/56 mmHg—which means she is prone to a white coat effect or reactive BP rise in response to stress. Her 5-day ECG Holter revealed 21 atrial ectopics and four episodes of drop beats with Wenckebach at night in the setting of mean daytime HR of 68 bpm.

Procedure Her coronary arteries are unobstructed; the LAD in the mid vessel after the diagonal branch has a "kinked and tethered" appearance and mid to distal tortuosity (Fig. 1.16). This corresponds to her CTCA finding of a short tunnelled LAD 9 years prior. The LV function is normal, LVEDP 5 mmHg despite a reactively high BP of up to 170 mmHg systolic—note the prominent LV pressure incisura before the aortic valve opens. This means procedural anxiety is causing increased peripheral vascular resistance at a HR of about 100 bpm.

With the pressure wire down the LAD, the Pd/Pa is 0.91. The hyperaemic indices are obtained four times to obtain consistency (Table 1.2). Together with the basal indices that are repeated twice, the CFR is 3.1 and MRR 3.8, the basal and hyperaemic resistance are 413 and 1553 Wood units respectively. She is given IV dobutamine, sequentially increased to 20 μg/kg/min, her coronary flow is estimated when her heart rates are 120 and 149 bpm, there is no reduction in flow, but a doubling at peak dose, and the Pd/Pa does not fall under 0.80 (Fig. 1.17, Table 1.2). Her coronary flow is also measured during escalating doses of ACh and verapamil. The flow falls with ACh 2 μg but picks up with higher ACh doses. She does not develop chest pain, ECG changes or significant angiographic epicardial vasoconstriction and Pd/Pa is consistently non-ischaemic but does fall with ACh.

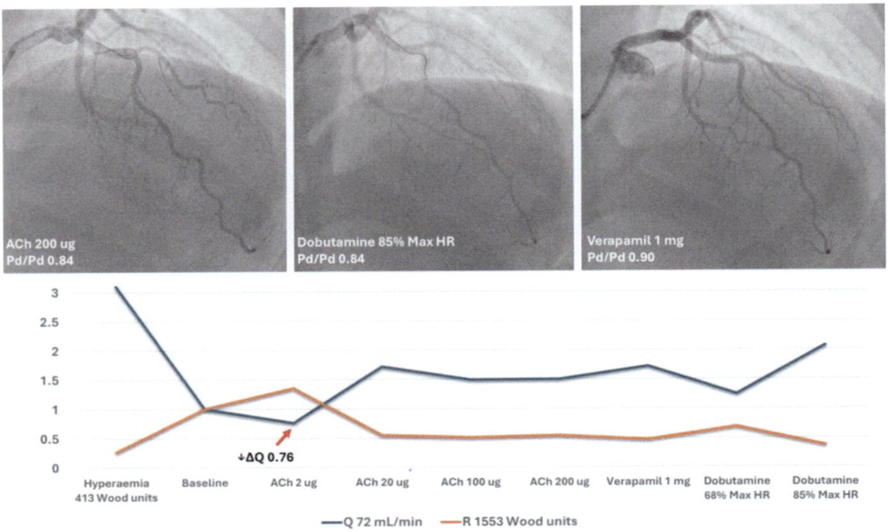

Fig. 1.17 (**Top, left to right panels**) The LAD in response to acetylcholine (ACh) 200 μg, during dobutamine stress with maximal heart response at 85% predicted and following verapamil 1 mg—none are associated with angiographic epicardial vasospasm or significnat flow limitation on Pd/Pa. (**Bottom**) Haemodynamic response to saline hyperaemia, ACh, verapamil and dobutamine. There is an initial subtle epicardial vasospasm and a fall in flow with low-dose ACh 2 μg, with normal flow responses at higher ACh (20, 100 and 200 μg) doses despite reduction in LAD calibre (Pd/Pa 0.96, 0.93, 0.81 and 0.84), and doubling of flow with dobutamine suggesting that the myocardial bridge is not contributory to her symptomn

Table 1.2 Myocardial bridge, dobutamine, and coronary flow

Continuous thermodilution				
		Q, mL/min	R, Wood units	
Saline infusion	20 mL/min	162	552	
		188	489	
		241	379	
		223	**413**	
	10 mL/min	69	1573	
	CFR 3.1	**72**	**1553**	MRR 3.8
				ΔQ
IC acetylcholine	2 μg	55	2096	**0.76**
	20 μg	124	852	1.72
	100 μg	107	799	1.49
	200 μg	108	844	1.50
IC verapamil	1000 μg	124	738	1.72
IV Dobutamine	HR 68%	89	1075	1.24
20 μg/kg/min	HR 85%	149	580	2.07

Interpretation This premenopausal woman has non-obstructive coronary arteries with non-flow limiting muscle bridging, a heart that has both normal systolic and diastolic function. She has preserved coronary vasodilatory capacity and intact microvascular endothelial function, but *epicardial endothelial dysfunction*, as evidenced by reduced Pd/Pa with ACh but not with verapamil implying a level of vasoconstriction in response to ACh. She has *hypertension*, procedural anxiety increased her BP and this translated into raised coronary resistance. The *epicardial vasospasm* with low-dose ACh appears to be a common feature in PCOS. In this case ACh-induced a *biphasic response*, flow falls at low dose and rises at higher doses. Although she does not have a formal diagnosis of PCOS, she has been told she has polycystic ovaries, she is overweight, has hypertension, hyperlipidaemia and mild hyperprolactinaemia, albeit not sustained and an LH/FSH ratio > 2 (2.7, repeated 2.9) potentially implying increased GnRH pulsatility [367].

These are features within the PCOS spectrum. The diltiazem she took was likely to be the cause of her observed low atrium ectopy with inverted P in her limb leads [368]. Her drug treatment was rationalised, switching her from diltiazem to nebivolol which would reduce her HR and BP, sympathetic overactivity and address her epicardial endothelial dysfunction. Her ivabradine was discontinued. Weight lost would be essential to address the cardiometabolic sequelae [369]. Finally and in general, with better understanding and recognition of PCOS which is a complex multi-disciplinary metabolic endocrine condition affecting women of reproductive age, more targeted management could be implemented at an early stage [370].

1.8.6 LBBB and Exercise Intolerance

A 74-year-old Caucasian woman has limiting exercise tolerance with unobstructed coronary arteries and without overt LV systolic dysfunction. She has hypertension, hyperlipidaemia, LBBB with trifascicular block and a QRS of 153 ms, and she has had multiple coronary procedures. In a formal treadmill exercise undertaken 4 months ago, she had to stop after 1 min because of breathlessness and angina. However, she was able to mount a heart rate response from 86 to 117 bpm suggesting that she did not have chronotropic incompetence. Her CMR done a month earlier, was artefactual with degraded pictures because of difficulty with breath-holding. Nevertheless, broadly her LV appeared preserved with an EF of 59% and a normal volume-derived ventriculo-arterial coupling (VAC) of 0.69 (0.6–1.0, ESVI 25 mL/m^2 / SVI 36 mL/m^2, BMI 29 kg/m^2). But her NT-ProBNP was elevated at 238 (< 125) pmol/mL one month ago.

She had attended the emergency department repeatedly for her symptoms. This was despite her empirical treatment with a polypharmacy of amlodipine 5 mg od, Bisoprolol 7.5 mg od, Irbesartan 150 mg od, Nicorandil 10 mg od and Ranolazine 375 mg bd.

She underwent six coronary procedures over the years: a stent to her proximal left anterior descending (LAD) artery across the diagonal branch when she was 55, and another stent to her mid right coronary artery (RCA) at 61; followed by a coronary angiogram when she was 63, when she was admitted with a troponin negative chest pain. The LAD and RCA stents were patent; there appeared to be ostial stenosis in the large anomalous circumflex (Cx) artery which came off the proximal RCA. She had right radial artery spasm during the procedure coupled with subclavian grip which made catheter manipulation challenging. On a separate sitting during the same admission, she was restudied via the right femoral artery. With selective cannulation of the anomalous Cx, the ostium was found to be widely open, and a pressure wire study to the stent-trapped diagonal branch gave an FFR of 0.88 (> 0.80). She had a further coronary angiogram the following year which again found non-obstructive coronary arteries. Her LBBB preceded all the procedures.

She had stress echocardiograms with variable results over the years. At 63 with dobutamine (93% maximal HR) it found moderate Cx territory ischaemia, at 66 she managed 3 min on the treadmill (81% maximal HR), her echocardiogram found an EF of 40–45%, improving to 50% with mild LAD territory ischaemia, and at 71 with dobutamine (95% maximal HR), EF 45–50%, this revealed no inducible ischaemia, and VAC 1.2 (0.6–1.0) which would suggest LV systolic dysfunction, and average E/e' 15 (< 8), implying diastolic dysfunction. But without LA dilatation or LVH. In view of her recurrent symptoms she was admitted for a coronary physiology study.

Procedure Because of prior difficulty with the radial access, the procedure is undertaken with the right femoral approach. The femoral artery is cannulated using ultrasound guidance with a 4 French sheath and then a sheathless off-the-shelf 5 French XB3.5 guide catheter is inserted with a 4 French MPA2 diagnostic catheter as an introducer to intubate the left coronary artery. This keeps the femoral puncture a 4 French-sized access to allow easy post-procedural haemostasis (Fig. 1.18).

The LV is studied, the LVEDP is 12–13 mmHg, not rising with handgrip, the central aortic BP is 163/67 mmHg. The coronary arteries, including the RCA arising Cx, as well as the stents are unobstructed (Fig. 1.19). With the pressure wire down the distal LAD, the Pd/Pa is 0.95. Continuous thermodilution is performed, with the following hyperaemic (repeated ×2) and basal (repeated ×3) indices; flow 169 and **160** mL/min and 81, 54 and **54** mL, and resistance 556 and **554** Wood units, and 1271, 1905 and **1937** Wood units—CFR 3.0 and MRR 3.5.

Dobutamine infusion is given at 5 μg/kg/min, and the infusion rate is doubled every 3 minutes, up to 20 μg/kg/min, followed by a bolus dose of atropine 300 μg (Fig. 1.19). There is a rise in flow with the first dose of 5 μg/kg/min, 1.8-fold, with a dose-dependent fall with higher doses, 1.72, 1.61 and 1.26 compared to baseline, with rising coronary resistance, the heart rate rises only following atropine with a fall in BP. This is associated with her typical chest tightness.

Interpretation This woman has had two decades of symptomatology and multiple coronary procedures culminating with the diagnosis of ANOCA. She has unobstructed coronary arteries, albeit with an anomalous Cx that arises from the RCA and not the aorta; therefore, intramural compression is not an issue for her. This usually is the mechanism for flow restriction in the anomalous coronary artery as demonstrated by Paolo Angelini [371]. She has mild LV systolic and diastolic

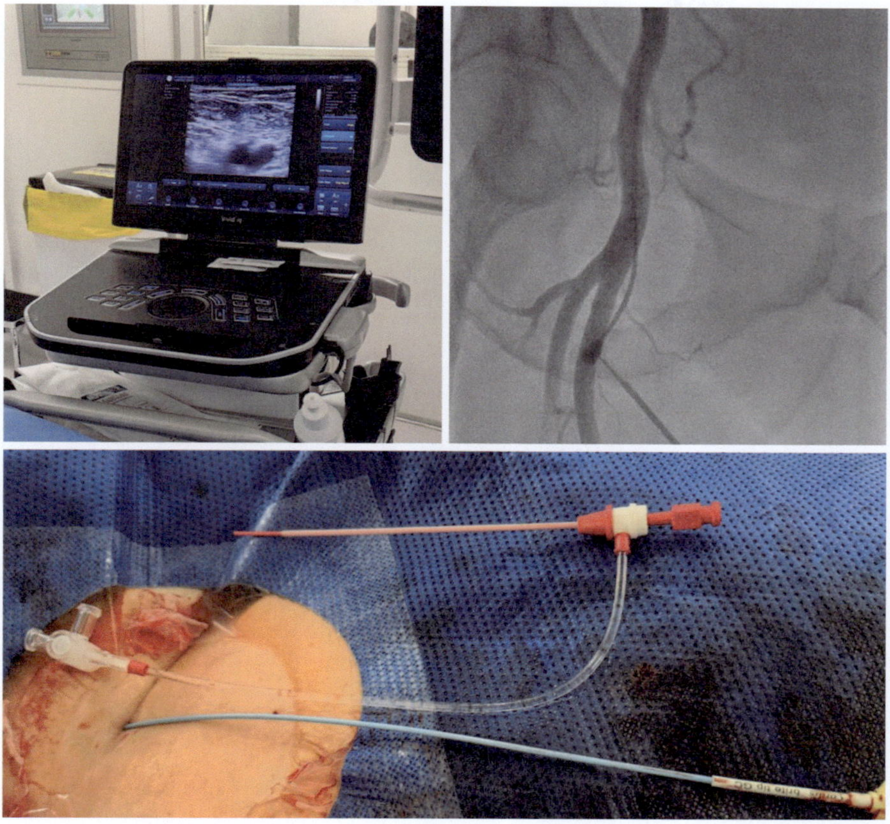

Fig. 1.18 (**Top, left to right panels**) Ultrasound-guided cannulation of the right femoral artery with a 4 French sheath, the femoral angiogram shows an acceptable entry site. (**Bottom panel**) Sheathlessly introduced 5 French guide catheter in situ. After the procedure, the 4 French femorral sheath on top is swapped in to await an activated clotting time (ACT) of under 150 s before the sheath is puilled. Generally a 10 min manual grroin compression is necessary to achieve haemostasis

dysfunction associated with a raised NT-ProBNP which indicates that she has elevated LVEDP on a daily basis. Her vasodilatory capacity is preserved, and she has elevated coronary resistance which would be in line with her hypertension. The fact that dobutamine stress in her case is associated with falling absolute flow would suggest that her LV becomes dysfunctional due to LBBB-related dyssynchrony raising both her LVEDP and resistances. This contrasts with non-invasive studies which report a normal or reduced LV septal flow but hyperperfusion of the LV lateral wall during exercise, creating a somewhat counterintuitive functional flow reduction in the dyssynchronous septum due to LBBB [372, 373].

She has “true” LBBB as evidenced by *notching* in the R in I and aVL, an indicator that she could benefit from pacing [374]. There are emerging data to suggest that left bundle branch pacing (LBBP) in the setting of mild LV dysfunction would be

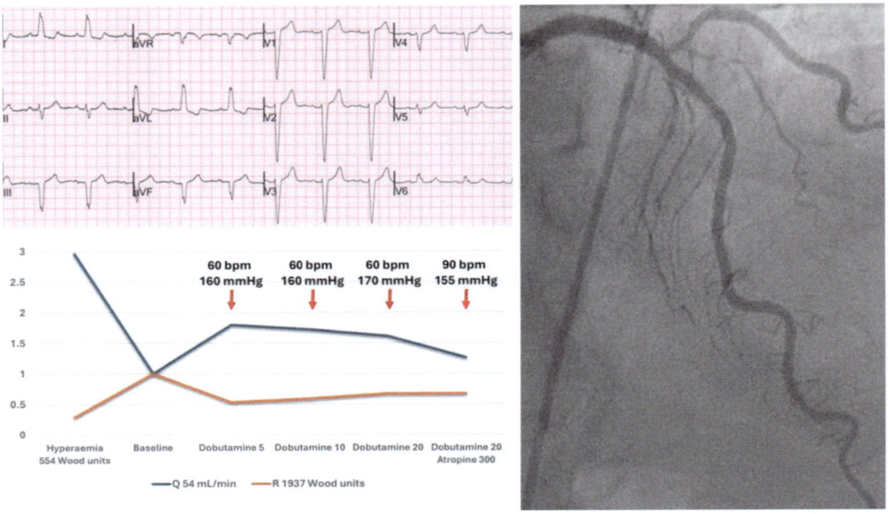

Fig. 1.19 (**Top, left to right panels**) The ECG shows LBBB with a QRS of 153 ms with left anterior hemniblock (left axis deviation) and borderline first degree heart block. Left main coronary artery leading to the LAD with stent across the diagonal banch with mild-to-moderate diffuse instent restenosis and an absent Cx. (**Left bottom**) Haemodynamic indices in response to saline hyperaemia and to escalating doses of dobutamine followed by atropine. Note the falling flow with higher doses of dobutamine causing a demand-supply mismatch

beneficial [339, 375], and even with preserved LV, so-called painful LBBB with intractable angina could respond to pacing too [338, 376].

On the other hand, permanent right ventricular pacing-induced LBBB can give rise to angina (Chap. 2) [377, 378] and LV dysfunction in 25% of patients followed up over 2–5 years [379, 380]. This case highlights the discordance of a normal vasodilatory capacity not translated into increasing flow with stress; this may be a common phenomenon in the presence of exercise-induced LV dysfunction in LBBB. Also, use of bolus thermodilution in LBBB has led to misdiagnosis for coronary microvascular dysfunction (CMD) [119]. LBBP was first described in 2017 by Weijian Huang from Wenzhou, Zhejiang, China, as a single case report in the *Canadian Journal of Cardiology* [381]. Eight years on, this publication has already been cited 827 times. LBBP is transforming pacing practice with randomised control trials emerging and is breaking the usual twenty-year rule for a new idea to achieve widespread adoption. It is a pacing technique that is physiological with two leads; it normalises conduction and is much cheaper than the traditional cardiac resynchronisation therapy (CRT) of biventricular pacing. With rapidly accumulating evidence for LBBP, it is not hard to predict that it will become standard of care for symptomatic LBBB when drug treatment fails.

References

1. O'Malley CD. Andreas Vesalius of Brussels, 1514–1564. Berkeley and Los Angeles: University of California Press; 1964.
2. Fernel J. De naturali parte medicinae. Paris: Simon de Colines; 1542.
3. Compier AH. Rhazes in the renaissance of Andreas Vesalius. Med Hist. 2012;56(1):3–25. https://doi.org/10.1017/s0025727300000259.
4. Vesalius A. Paraphrasis in nonum librum Rhazae medici Arabis clarissimi ad regem Almansorem, de singularum corporis partium affectuum curatione. Louvain: Rutger Rescius; 1537.
5. Cunningham A. The anatomical renaissance: the resurrection of the anatomical projects of the ancients. Cambridge: Cambridge University Press; 1997.
6. Rhazes ABMiZ. Continens Rasis (Liber Continens). Latin edition ed. Venice: Ottaviano Scoto.
7. Vesalius A. De Humani Corporis Fabrica. Basel: Johannes Oporinus; 1543.
8. Tsien T-H. Paper and printing. In: Needham J, editor. Science and civilisation in China. Cambridge: Cambridge University Press; 1985. p. 38–49.
9. Eisenstein EL. The printing revolution in early modern Europe. 2nd ed. Cambridge: Cambridge University Press; 2012.
10. Gottlieb LS. Andreas Vesalius 1514-1564: Quadricentenary of the death of the founder of modern anatomy. Arch Intern Med. 1964;114(2):294–5. https://doi.org/10.1001/archinte.1964.03860080144015.
11. Disraeli B. Speech on the reform bill. Edinburgh Address; 2023.
12. González Grueso FD. El Mío Cid y Aragorn. Biblioteca Virtual Miguel de Cervantes; 2004.
13. Vesalius A. Anatomicarum Gabrielis Fallopii Observationum Examen. Venice: Vincentius Luchinus; 1564.
14. Harvey W, Leake CD. Exercitatio anatomica de motu cordis et sanguinis in animalibus. Springfield: Thomas; 1928.
15. Karamanou M, Stefanadis C, Tsoucalas G, Laios K, Androutsos G. Galen's (130-201 AD) conceptions of the heart. Hell J Cardiol. 2015;56(3):197–200.
16. Pearce JMS. Malpighi and the discovery of capillaries. Eur Neurol. 2007;58(4):253–5. https://doi.org/10.1159/000107974.
17. Hales S. Statical essays: volume I. Vegetable Staticks: or, an account of some statical experiments on the sap in vegetables. 1st ed. London: W. Innys and R. Manby; 1727.
18. Hales S. Statical essays: volume II. Haemastaticks: or, an account of some Hydraulick and hydrostatical experiments on the blood and blood-vessels of animals. 1st ed. London: W. Innys and R. Manby; 1733.
19. Branthwaite MA, Bradley RD. Measurement of cardiac output by thermal dilution in man. J Appl Physiol. 1968;24(3):434–8. https://doi.org/10.1152/jappl.1968.24.3.434.
20. Forrester JS, Ganz W, Diamond G, McHugh T, Chonette DW, Swan HJC. Thermodilution cardiac output determination with a single flow-directed catheter. Am Heart J. 1972;83(3):306–11. https://doi.org/10.1016/0002-8703(72)90429-2.
21. Ganz W, Donoso R, Marcus HS, Forrester JS, Swan HJC. A new technique for measurement of cardiac output by thermodilution in man. Am J Cardiol. 1971;27(4):392–6. https://doi.org/10.1016/0002-9149(71)90436-X.
22. Argueta EE, Paniagua D. Thermodilution cardiac output: a concept over 250 years in the making. Cardiol Rev. 2019;27(3):138–44. https://doi.org/10.1097/crd.0000000000000223.
23. Hamilton WF, Moore JW, Kinsman JM, Spurling RG. Studies on the circulation. Am J Physiol Legacy Content. 1932;99(3):534–51. https://doi.org/10.1152/ajplegacy.1932.99.3.534.
24. Stewart GN. Researches on the circulation time and on the influences which affect it. J Physiol. 1897;22(3):159–83. https://doi.org/10.1113/jphysiol.1897.sp000684.
25. Lim PO. Angina with coronary microvascular dysfunction and its physiological assessment: a review with cases. Br J Cardiol. 2022;29(2):13. https://doi.org/10.5837/bjc.2022.013.

26. United States Holocaust Memorial M: Deportation of Hungarian Jews. https://encyclopedia.ushmm.org/content/en/timeline-event/holocaust/1942-1945/deportation-of-hungarian-jews (2025)
27. Froně A, Ganz V. Measurement of flow in single blood vessels including cardiac output by local Thermodilution. Circ Res. 1960;8(1):175–82. https://doi.org/10.1161/01.RES.8.1.175.
28. Ganz V, Fronek A. The action of nitroglycerin on coronary and systemic haemodynamics and on the oxygen metabolism of the myocardium. Cor Vasa. 1961;3:107–19.
29. Lategola M, Rahn H. A self-guiding catheter for cardiac and pulmonary arterial catheterization and occlusion. Proc Soc Exp Biol Med. 1953;84(3):667–8. https://doi.org/10.3181/00379727-84-20745.
30. University of California San Diego. Department of S. In Memoriam: Dr. Arnost Fronek, MD, PhD; 2025.
31. Forrester JS. A tale of serendipity, ingenuity, and chance: 50th anniversary of creation of the Swan-Ganz catheter. J Am Coll Cardiol. 2019;74(1):100–3. https://doi.org/10.1016/j.jacc.2019.04.050.
32. Berry D. William (Vilem) Ganz, 1919-2009, cardiologist and co-inventor of the Swan-Ganz catheter which revolutionized cardiovascular investigations. Eur Heart J. 2011;32(6):660–1.
33. Stern S. William Ganz: from refugee to world fame. Cardiol J. 2010;17(6):650–1.
34. Ganz W, Tamura K, Marcus HS, Donoso R, Yoshida S, Swan HJC. Measurement of coronary sinus blood flow by continuous Thermodilution in man. Circulation. 1971;44(2):181–95. https://doi.org/10.1161/01.CIR.44.2.181.
35. Bagger JP. Coronary sinus blood flow determination by the thermodilution technique: influence of catheter position and respiration. Cardiovasc Res. 1985;19(1):27–31. https://doi.org/10.1093/cvr/19.1.27.
36. Langenberg CJM, Pietersen HG, Geskes G, Wagenmakers AJM, Soeters PB, Durieux M. Coronary sinus catheter placement: assessment of placement criteria and cardiac complications. Chest. 2003;124(4):1259–65. https://doi.org/10.1378/chest.124.4.1259.
37. Emanuelsson H, Dohnal M, Lamm C, Tenerz L. Initial experiences with a miniaturized pressure transducer during coronary angioplasty. Catheter Cardiovasc Diagn. 1991;24(2):137–43. https://doi.org/10.1002/ccd.1810240213.
38. Meier P, Zierler KL. On the theory of the indicator-dilution method for measurement of blood flow and volume. J Appl Physiol. 1954;6(12):731–44. https://doi.org/10.1152/jappl.1954.6.12.731.
39. Zierler KL. Theoretical basis of indicator-dilution methods for measuring flow and volume. Circ Res. 1962;10(3):393–407. https://doi.org/10.1161/01.RES.10.3.393.
40. Gould KL, Lipscomb K, Hamilton GW. Physiologic basis for assessing critical coronary stenosis: instantaneous flow response and regional distribution during coronary hyperemia as measures of coronary flow reserve. Am J Cardiol. 1974;33(1):87–94. https://doi.org/10.1016/0002-9149(74)90743-7.
41. Vogel R, LeFree M, Bates E, O'Neill W, Foster R, Kirlin P, et al. Application of digital techniques to selective coronary arteriography: use of myocardial contrast appearance time to measure coronary flow reserve. Am Heart J. 1984;107(1):153–64. https://doi.org/10.1016/0002-8703(84)90150-9.
42. Pijls NH, Aengevaeren WR, Uijen GJ, Hoevelaken A, Pijnenburg T, van Leeuwen K, et al. Concept of maximal flow ratio for immediate evaluation of percutaneous transluminal coronary angioplasty result by videodensitometry. Circulation. 1991;83(3):854–65. https://doi.org/10.1161/01.cir.83.3.854.
43. Pijls NH, Uijen GJ, Hoevelaken A, Arts T, Aengevaeren WR, Bos HS, et al. Mean transit time for the assessment of myocardial perfusion by videodensitometry. Circulation. 1990;81(4):1331–40. https://doi.org/10.1161/01.cir.81.4.1331.
44. Pijls NH, Uijen GJ, Hoevelaken A, Pijnenburg T, van Leeuwen KL, Fast JH, et al. Mean transit time for videodensitometric assessment of myocardial perfusion and the concept of maximal flow ratio: a validation study in the intact dog and a pilot study in man. Int J Card Imaging. 1990;5(2–3):191–202. https://doi.org/10.1007/BF01833988.

45. Pijls NH, Uijen GJ, Pijnenburg T, van Leeuwen K, Aengevaeren WR, Barth JD, et al. Reproducibility of mean transit time for maximal myocardial flow assessment by videodensitometry. Int J Card Imaging. 1990;6(2):101–8. https://doi.org/10.1007/BF02398893.
46. Pijls NHJ. Journey into the Discovery of Coronary Physiology: 20 Years of FFR. Imaging & Physiology Summit. Seoul, Korea: Imaging & Physiology Summit; 2015.
47. Pijls NH, van Son JA, Kirkeeide RL, De Bruyne B, Gould KL. Experimental basis of determining maximum coronary, myocardial, and collateral blood flow by pressure measurements for assessing functional stenosis severity before and after percutaneous transluminal coronary angioplasty. Circulation. 1993;87(4):1354–67. https://doi.org/10.1161/01.CIR.87.4.1354.
48. Pijls NHJ, de Bruyne B. Coronary pressure. Dordrecht: Springer Science+Business Media; 2000.
49. Gould KL, Kirkeeide RL, Buchi M. Coronary flow reserve as a physiologic measure of stenosis severity. J Am Coll Cardiol. 1990;15(2):459–74. https://doi.org/10.1016/s0735-1097(10)80078-6.
50. Gould KL, Kitkungvan D, Johnson NP, Nguyen T, Kirkeeide R, Bui L, et al. Mortality prediction by quantitative PET perfusion expressed as coronary flow capacity with and without revascularization. JACC Cardiovasc Imaging. 2021;14(5):1020–34. https://doi.org/10.1016/j.jcmg.2020.08.040.
51. Knuuti J, Saraste A. Quantitative PET perfusion imaging: how to interpret the results? JACC Cardiovasc Imaging. 2021;14(5):1035–7. https://doi.org/10.1016/j.jcmg.2020.10.020.
52. Young DF, Tsai FY. Flow characteristics in models of arterial stenoses – I. Steady flow. J Biomech. 1973;6(4):395–410. https://doi.org/10.1016/0021-9290(73)90099-7.
53. Young DF, Tsai FY. Flow characteristics in models of arterial stenoses. II. Unsteady flow. J Biomech. 1973;6(5):547–59. https://doi.org/10.1016/0021-9290(73)90012-2.
54. De Bruyne B, Pijls NH, Paulus WJ, Vantrimpont PJ, Sys SU, Heyndrickx GR. Transstenotic coronary pressure gradient measurement in humans: in vitro and in vivo evaluation of a new pressure monitoring angioplasty guide wire. J Am Coll Cardiol. 1993;22(1):119–26. https://doi.org/10.1016/0735-1097(93)90825-l.
55. Kirkeeide RL, Gould KL, Parsel L. Assessment of coronary stenoses by myocardial perfusion imaging during pharmacologic coronary vasodilation. VII. Validation of coronary flow reserve as a single integrated functional measure of stenosis severity reflecting all its geometric dimensions. J Am Coll Cardiol. 1986;7(1):103–13. https://doi.org/10.1016/s0735-1097(86)80266-2.
56. Frank O. Die Grundform des arteriellen Pulses. Erste Abhandlung: Mathematische Analyse. Z Biol. 1899;37:483–526.
57. Guyton AC. Textbook of medical physiology. Philadelphia: W. B. Saunders; 1956.
58. Sutera SP, Skalak R. The history of Poiseuille's law. Annu Rev Fluid Mech. 1993;25:1–20. https://doi.org/10.1146/annurev.fl.25.010193.000245.
59. Knowlton FP, Starling EH. The influence of variations in temperature and blood-pressure on the performance of the isolated mammalian heart. J Physiol. 1912;44(3):206–19. https://doi.org/10.1113/jphysiol.1912.sp001511.
60. Badeer HS, Hicks JW. Hemodynamics of vascular 'waterfall': is the analogy justified? Respir Physiol. 1992;87(2):205–17. https://doi.org/10.1016/0034-5687(92)90060-A.
61. Holt JP. The collapse factor in the measurement of venous pressure. Am J Physiol Legacy Content. 1941;134(2):292–9. https://doi.org/10.1152/ajplegacy.1941.134.2.292.
62. Permutt S, Bromberger-Barnea B, Bane HN. Alveolar pressure, pulmonary venous pressure, and the vascular waterfall. Med Thorac. 1962;19:239–60. https://doi.org/10.1159/000192224.
63. Foley MJ, Rajkumar CA, Ahmed-Jushuf F, Simader FA, Chotai S, Pathimagaraj RH, et al. Coronary sinus reducer for the treatment of refractory angina (ORBITA-COSMIC): a randomised, placebo-controlled trial. Lancet. 2024;403(10436):1543–53. https://doi.org/10.1016/S0140-6736(24)00256-3.
64. Dole WP, Alexander GM, Campbell AB, Hixson EL, Bishop VS. Interpretation and physiological significance of diastolic coronary artery pressure-flow relationships in the canine coronary bed. Circ Res. 1984;55(2):215–26. https://doi.org/10.1161/01.res.55.2.215.

65. Pantely GA, Ladley HD, Bristow JD. Low zero-flow pressure and minimal capacitance effect on diastolic coronary arterial pressure-flow relationships during maximum vasodilation in swine. Circulation. 1984;70(3):485–94. https://doi.org/10.1161/01.cir.70.3.485.
66. Seiler C. Assessment and impact of the human coronary collateral circulation on myocardial ischemia and outcome. Circ Cardiovasc Interv. 2013;6(6):719–28. https://doi.org/10.1161/CIRCINTERVENTIONS.113.000555.
67. Yamamoto K, Ito H, Iwakura K, Shintani Y, Masuyama T, Hori M, et al. Pressure-derived collateral flow index as a parameter of microvascular dysfunction in acute myocardial infarction. J Am Coll Cardiol. 2001;38(5):1383–9. https://doi.org/10.1016/s0735-1097(01)01585-6.
68. Meier P, Schirmer SH, Lansky AJ, Timmis A, Pitt B, Seiler C. The collateral circulation of the heart. BMC Med. 2013;11(1):143. https://doi.org/10.1186/1741-7015-11-143.
69. Pijls NH, De Bruyne B, Peels K, Van Der Voort PH, Bonnier HJ, Bartunek JKJJ, et al. Measurement of fractional flow reserve to assess the functional severity of coronary-artery stenoses. N Engl J Med. 1996;334(26):1703–8. https://doi.org/10.1056/NEJM199606273342604.
70. Hu X, Zhang J, Yang S, Jiang J, Peng X, Lu D, et al. Angiography-derived fractional flow reserve versus intravascular ultrasound to guide percutaneous coronary intervention in patients with coronary artery disease (FLAVOUR II): a multicentre, randomised, non-inferiority trial. Lancet. 2025;405(10488):1491–504. https://doi.org/10.1016/S0140-6736(25)00504-5.
71. Flanagan L. My journey with ischemia and nonobstructed coronary arteries. Circ Cardiovasc Qual Outcomes. 2022;15(7):e008745. https://doi.org/10.1161/circoutcomes.121.008745.
72. Phillips B, Hansen C, Stevens M. The fallibility of the female heart: a patient's perspective. JACC: Case Rep. 2025;30(4):102965. https://doi.org/10.1016/j.jaccas.2024.102965.
73. Tavella R, Beltrame JF. Shortcomings in managing patients with ischemia with nonobstructed coronary arteries. Circ Cardiovasc Qual Outcomes. 2022;15(7):e008746. https://doi.org/10.1161/circoutcomes.122.008746.
74. Schreuder JJ, Castiglioni A, Donelli A, Maisano F, Jansen JR, Hanania R, et al. Automatic intraaortic balloon pump timing using an intrabeat dicrotic notch prediction algorithm. Ann Thorac Surg. 2005;79(3):1017–22. https://doi.org/10.1016/j.athoracsur.2004.07.074.
75. Chen CH, Fetics B, Nevo E, Rochitte CE, Chiou KR, Ding PA, et al. Noninvasive single-beat determination of left ventricular end-systolic elastance in humans. J Am Coll Cardiol. 2001;38(7):2028–34. https://doi.org/10.1016/s0735-1097(01)01651-5.
76. Hébert JL, Lecarpentier Y, Zamani K, Coirault C, Daccache G, Chemla D. Relation between aortic dicrotic notch pressure and mean aortic pressure in adults. Am J Cardiol. 1995;76(4):301–6. https://doi.org/10.1016/s0002-9149(99)80086-1.
77. White KC, Quick L, Durkin Z, McCullough J, Laupland KB, Blank S, et al. Mean arterial pressure in critically ill adults receiving vasopressors: a multicentre, observational study. Crit Care Resusc. 2025;27(1):100103. https://doi.org/10.1016/j.ccrj.2025.100103.
78. Berne RM. Regulation of coronary blood flow. Physiol Rev. 1964;44(1):1–29. https://doi.org/10.1152/physrev.1964.44.1.1.
79. Mahendiran T, Collet C, Bruyne BD. Coronary-artery autoregulation with increasing stenosis. N Engl J Med. 2024;390(21):2030–2. https://doi.org/10.1056/NEJMc2402216.
80. Bruyne BD, Fearon WF, Pijls NHJ, Barbato E, Tonino P, Piroth Z, et al. Fractional flow reserve–guided PCI for stable coronary artery disease. N Engl J Med. 2014;371(13):1208–17. https://doi.org/10.1056/NEJMoa1408758.
81. Al-Lamee R, Thompson D, Dehbi HM, Sen S, Tang K, Davies J, et al. Percutaneous coronary intervention in stable angina (ORBITA): a double-blind, randomised controlled trial. Lancet. 2018;391(10115):31–40. https://doi.org/10.1016/s0140-6736(17)32714-9.
82. Johnson NP, Kirkeeide RL, Gould KL. History and development of coronary flow reserve and fractional flow reserve for clinical applications. Interven Cardiol Clin. 2015;4(4):397–410. https://doi.org/10.1016/j.iccl.2015.06.001.
83. Seto AH, Kern MJ. Should CFR be routinely measured in the Cath lab? J Am Coll Cardiol Intv. 2022;15(10):1057–9. https://doi.org/10.1016/j.jcin.2022.03.028.

84. van de Hoef TP, Lee JM, Boerhout CKM, de Waard GA, Jung J-H, Lee SH, et al. Combined assessment of FFR and CFR for decision making in coronary revascularization: from the multicenter international ILIAS registry. J Am Coll Cardiol Intv. 2022;15(10):1047–56. https://doi.org/10.1016/j.jcin.2022.03.016.
85. van de Hoef TP, van Lavieren MA, Damman P, Delewi R, Piek MA, Chamuleau SA, et al. Physiological basis and long-term clinical outcome of discordance between fractional flow reserve and coronary flow velocity reserve in coronary stenoses of intermediate severity. Circ Cardiovasc Interv. 2014;7(3):301–11. https://doi.org/10.1161/circinterventions.113.001049.
86. Cook CM, Jeremias A, Petraco R, Sen S, Nijjer S, Shun-Shin MJ, et al. Fractional flow reserve/instantaneous wave-free ratio discordance in Angiographically intermediate coronary Stenoses: an analysis using Doppler-derived coronary flow measurements. J Am Coll Cardiol Intv. 2017;10(24):2514–24. https://doi.org/10.1016/j.jcin.2017.09.021.
87. Murai T, Stegehuis VE, van de Hoef TP, Wijntjens GWM, Hoshino M, Kanaji Y, et al. Coronary flow capacity to identify stenosis associated with coronary flow improvement after revascularization: a combined analysis from DEFINE FLOW and IDEAL. J Am Heart Assoc. 2020;9(14):e016130. https://doi.org/10.1161/jaha.120.016130.
88. Garcia D, Harbaoui B, van de Hoef TP, Meuwissen M, Nijjer SS, Echavarria-Pinto M, et al. Relationship between FFR, CFR and coronary microvascular resistance – practical implications for FFR-guided percutaneous coronary intervention. PLoS One. 2019;14(1):e0208612. https://doi.org/10.1371/journal.pone.0208612.
89. Tas A, Alan Y, Kara Tas I, Umman S, Parker KH, van de Hoef T, et al. The impact of high microvascular resistance on coronary wave energetics depends on coronary microvascular functionality. Eur Heart J Open. 2025:oeaf050. https://doi.org/10.1093/ehjopen/oeaf050.
90. Tas A, Alan Y, Ozcan A, Parker KH, van de Hoef T, Sezer M, et al. Ventricular-coronary interaction delay is associated with discordance between fractional flow reserve and coronary flow Reserve in Intermediate Coronary Stenoses. Am J Cardiol. 2025;248:80–8. https://doi.org/10.1016/j.amjcard.2025.04.003.
91. Hoffman JI, Buckberg GD. The myocardial oxygen supply:demand index revisited. J Am Heart Assoc. 2014;3(1):e000285. https://doi.org/10.1161/jaha.113.000285.
92. Xie H, Gao L, Fan F, Gong Y, Zhang Y. Research Progress and clinical value of subendocardial viability ratio. J Am Heart Assoc. 2024;13(6):e032614. https://doi.org/10.1161/jaha.123.032614.
93. De Bruyne B, Pijls NH, Smith L, Wievegg M, Heyndrickx GR. Coronary thermodilution to assess flow reserve: experimental validation. Circulation. 2001;104(17):2003–6. https://doi.org/10.1161/hc4201.099223.
94. Bruyne BD, Pijls NHJ, Gallinoro E, Candreva A, Fournier S, Keulards DCJ, et al. Microvascular resistance Reserve for Assessment of coronary microvascular function. J Am Coll Cardiol. 2021;78(15):1541–9. https://doi.org/10.1016/j.jacc.2021.08.017.
95. Gallinoro E, Bertolone Dario T, Mizukami T, Paolisso P, Bermpeis K, Munhoz D, et al. Continuous vs bolus Thermodilution to assess microvascular resistance reserve. J Am Coll Cardiol Intv. 2023;16(22):2767–77. https://doi.org/10.1016/j.jcin.2023.09.027.
96. Jansen TPJ, de Vos A, Paradies V, Dimitriu-Leen A, Crooijmans C, Elias-Smale S, et al. Continuous versus bolus Thermodilution-derived coronary flow reserve and microvascular resistance reserve and their association with angina and quality of life in patients with angina and nonobstructive coronaries: a head-to-head comparison. J Am Heart Assoc. 2023;12(16):e030480. https://doi.org/10.1161/jaha.123.030480.
97. Aarnoudse W, van den Berg P, van de Vosse F, Geven M, Rutten M, Van Turnhout M, et al. Myocardial resistance assessed by guidewire-based pressure-temperature measurement: in vitro validation. Catheter Cardiovasc Interv. 2004;62(1):56–63. https://doi.org/10.1002/ccd.10793.
98. Fearon WF, Aarnoudse W, Pijls NH, De Bruyne B, Balsam LB, Cooke DT, et al. Microvascular resistance is not influenced by epicardial coronary artery stenosis severity:

experimental validation. Circulation. 2004;109(19):2269–72. https://doi.org/10.1161/01.Cir.0000128669.99355.Cb.
99. Fearon WF, Balsam LB, Farouque HMO, Robbins RC, Fitzgerald PJ, Yock PG, et al. Novel index for invasively assessing the coronary microcirculation. Circulation. 2003;107(25):3129–32. https://doi.org/10.1161/01.CIR.0000080700.98607.D1.
100. Ng MK, Yeung AC, Fearon WF. Invasive assessment of the coronary microcirculation: superior reproducibility and less hemodynamic dependence of index of microcirculatory resistance compared with coronary flow reserve. Circulation. 2006;113(17):2054–61. https://doi.org/10.1161/circulationaha.105.603522.
101. Yong AS, Layland J, Fearon WF, Ho M, Shah MG, Daniels D, et al. Calculation of the index of microcirculatory resistance without coronary wedge pressure measurement in the presence of Epicardial stenosis. J Am Coll Cardiol Intv. 2013;6(1):53–8. https://doi.org/10.1016/j.jcin.2012.08.019.
102. Ford TJ, Stanley B, Good R, Rocchiccioli P, McEntegart M, Watkins S, et al. Stratified medical therapy using invasive coronary function testing in angina. J Am Coll Cardiol. 2018;72(23_Part_A):2841–55. https://doi.org/10.1016/j.jacc.2018.09.006.
103. Ford TJ, Stanley B, Sidik N, Good R, Rocchiccioli P, McEntegart M, et al. 1-year outcomes of angina management guided by invasive coronary function testing (CorMicA). J Am Coll Cardiol Intv. 2020;13(1):33–45. https://doi.org/10.1016/j.jcin.2019.11.001.
104. Taqueti VR. Treating coronary microvascular dysfunction as the "culprit" lesion in patients with refractory angina: lessons from CorMicA at 1 year. J Am Coll Cardiol Intv. 2020;13(1):46–8. https://doi.org/10.1016/j.jcin.2019.12.001.
105. Sidik NP, Stanley B, Sykes R, Morrow AJ, Bradley CP, McDermott M, et al. Invasive endotyping in patients with angina and no obstructive coronary artery disease: a randomized controlled trial. Circulation. 2024;149(1):7–23. https://doi.org/10.1161/CIRCULATIONAHA.123.064751.
106. Taqueti VR. Prevalence of abnormal coronary function in patients with angina and no obstructive coronary artery disease on coronary computed tomography angiography: insights from the CorCTA trial. Circulation. 2024;149(1):24–7. https://doi.org/10.1161/circulationaha.123.066571.
107. Lim PO. Is bolus-Thermodilution reliable in defining coronary microvascular dysfunction? JACC Cardiovasc Imaging. 2023;16(7):993. https://doi.org/10.1016/j.jcmg.2023.03.025.
108. Lim PO. Is index of microvascular resistance of Sisyphean utility in Takotsubo syndrome? ESC Heart Fail. 2024;11(6):4438–40. https://doi.org/10.1002/ehf2.14943.
109. Kodeboina M, Nagumo S, Munhoz D, Sonck J, Mileva N, Gallinoro E, et al. Simplified assessment of the index of microvascular resistance. J Interv Cardiol. 2021;2021:9971874. https://doi.org/10.1155/2021/9971874.
110. van't Veer M, Adjedj J, Wijnbergen IF, Toth GG, Rutten MCM, Barbato E, et al. Novel monorail infusion catheter for volumetric coronary blood flow measurement in humans: in vitro validation. EuroIntervention. 2016;12(6):701–7. https://doi.org/10.4244/eijv12i6a114.
111. Adjedj J, Picard F, Collet C, Bruneval P, Fournier S, Bize A, et al. Intracoronary saline-induced hyperemia during coronary Thermodilution measurements of absolute coronary blood flow: an animal mechanistic study. J Am Heart Assoc. 2020;9(15):e015793. https://doi.org/10.1161/JAHA.120.015793.
112. De Bruyne B, Adjedj J, Xaplanteris P, Ferrara A, Mo Y, Penicka M, et al. Saline-Induced Coronary Hyperemia. Circulation: Cardiovascular Interventions. 2017;10(4):e004719. https://doi.org/10.1161/CIRCINTERVENTIONS.116.004719.
113. Minten L, et al. Optimization of absolute coronary blood flow measurements to assess microvascular function: in vivo validation of hyperemia and higher infusion speeds. Circ Cardiovasc Interv. 2024;17(7):e013860. https://doi.org/10.1161/CIRCINTERVENTIONS.123.013860.
114. Grancini L, Diana D, Centola A, Monizzi G, Mastrangelo A, Olivares P, et al. The SALINE technique for the treatment of the no-reflow phenomenon during percutaneous coronary intervention in STEMI. J Clin Med. 2023;12(6) https://doi.org/10.3390/jcm12062405.

115. Gallinoro E, Candreva A, Fernandez-Peregrina E, Bailleul E, Meeus P, Sonck J, et al. Saline-induced coronary hyperemia with continuous intracoronary thermodilution is mediated by intravascular hemolysis. Atherosclerosis. 2022;352:46–52. https://doi.org/10.1016/j.atherosclerosis.2022.05.011.
116. Paolisso P, Gallinoro E, Candreva A, Bermpeis K, Fabbricatore D, Esposito G, et al. 389 microvascular dysfunction in patients with type II diabetes mellitus: invasive assessment of absolute coronary blood flow and microvascular resistance reserve. Eur Heart J Suppl. 2021;23(Supplement_G) https://doi.org/10.1093/eurheartj/suab136.005.
117. Blaustein MP, Lederer WJ. Sodium/calcium exchange: its physiological implications. Physiol Rev. 1999;79(3):763–854. https://doi.org/10.1152/physrev.1999.79.3.763.
118. Gallinoro E , Candreva A, Colaiori I, Kodeboina M, Fournier S, Nelis O, Di Gioia G, Sonck J, van 't Veer M, Pijls N H J, Collet C, De Bruyne B. Thermodilution-derived volumetric resting coronary blood flow measurement in humans. EuroIntervention. 2021;17(8):e672–e679. https://doi.org/10.4244/EIJ-D-20-01092.
119. Inoue N, Joko Y, Morikawa S. Possible involvement of coronary microvascular dysfunction in painful left bundle branch block. JACC: Case Rep. 2023;23:102008. https://doi.org/10.1016/j.jaccas.2023.102008.
120. Gallinoro E, Bertolone DT, Fernandez-Peregrina E, Paolisso P, Bermpeis K, Esposito G, et al. Reproducibility of bolus versus continuous thermodilution for assessment of coronary microvascular function in patients with ANOCA. EuroIntervention. 2023;19(2):e155–e66. https://doi.org/10.4244/eij-d-22-00772.
121. Belmonte M, Gallinoro E, Pijls NHJ, Bertolone DT, Keulards DCJ, Viscusi MM, et al. Measuring absolute coronary flow and microvascular resistance by Thermodilution: JACC review topic of the week. J Am Coll Cardiol. 2024;83(6):699–709. https://doi.org/10.1016/j.jacc.2023.12.014.
122. de Vos A, Jansen TPJ, et al. Microvascular resistance reserve to assess microvascular dysfunction in ANOCA patients. JACC Cardiovasc Interv. 2023;16(4):470–81. https://doi.org/10.1016/j.jcin.2022.12.012.
123. Jansen TPJ, Crooijmans C, Pijls N, Paradies V, de Vos A, Dimitriu-Leen AC, et al. Effects of age on microvascular function in patients with normal coronary arteries. EuroIntervention. 2024;20(11):e690–e8. https://doi.org/10.4244/eij-d-23-00778.
124. Pijls NHJ, De Bruyne B. The coronary circulation. Coronary pressure. Dordrecht: Springer Netherlands; 2000. p. 5–24.
125. Pijls NH, van Son JA, Kirkeeide RL, De Bruyne B, Gould KL. Experimental basis of determining maximum coronary, myocardial, and collateral blood flow by pressure measurements for assessing functional stenosis severity before and after percutaneous transluminal coronary angioplasty. Circulation. 1993;87(4):1354–67. https://doi.org/10.1161/01.cir.87.4.1354.
126. Johnson NP, Gould KL. Subendocardial ischemia: does CMD really exist? Cardiovasc Revasc Med. 2025;71:31–7. https://doi.org/10.1016/j.carrev.2025.01.008.
127. Dalal F, Escobedo Y, Exaire JE, Mixon TA, Al-Azizi K, Kumar D, et al. Evaluation of mid vs distal left anterior descending artery measures in coronary physiology assessment. Cardiovasc Revasc Med. 2024; https://doi.org/10.1016/j.carrev.2024.12.018.
128. Konst RE, Elias-Smale SE, Pellegrini D, Hartzema-Meijer M, van Uden BJC, Jansen TPJ, et al. Absolute coronary blood flow measured by continuous Thermodilution in patients with ischemia and nonobstructive disease. JACC. 2021;77(6):728–41. https://doi.org/10.1016/j.jacc.2020.12.019.
129. Rivero F, Gutiérrez-Barrios A, Gomez-Lara J, Fuentes-Ferrer M, Cuesta J, Keulards DCJ, et al. Coronary microvascular dysfunction assessed by continuous intracoronary thermodilution: a comparative study with index of microvascular resistance. Int J Cardiol. 2021;333:1–7. https://doi.org/10.1016/j.ijcard.2021.03.005.
130. Sipkema P, Takkenberg JJ, Zeeuwe PE, Westerhof N. Left coronary pressure-flow relations of the beating and arrested rabbit heart at different ventricular volumes. Cardiovasc Res. 1998;40(1):88–95. https://doi.org/10.1016/s0008-6363(98)00119-9
131. Bellamy RF. Diastolic coronary artery pressure-flow relations in the dog. Circ Res. 1978;43(1):92–101. https://doi.org/10.1161/01.res.43.1.92.

132. Klocke FJ, Mates RE, Canty JM, Ellis AK. Coronary pressure-flow relationships. Controversial issues and probable implications. Circ Res. 1985;56(3):310–23. https://doi.org/10.1161/01.RES.56.3.310.
133. Spaan JA. Response to the article by Klocke et al. on "coronary pressure-flow relationships: controversial issues and probable implications". Circ Res. 1985;56(6):789–92. https://doi.org/10.1161/01.res.56.6.789.
134. Wackers FJT, Strauss HW, Udelson J, Wackers FJT, Carrio I. The history C. K. Lance Gould, MD (born October 28, 1938). J Nucl Cardiol. 2019;26(6):1841–3. https://doi.org/10.1007/s12350-019-01822-9.
135. Senguttuvan NB, Kovvuri HLR, et al. Inefficient maximal hyperemic response following intravenous adenosine in polycythemia: a first-in-the-world report. J Am Coll Cardiol Intv. 2025; https://doi.org/10.1016/j.jcin.2025.03.021.
136. Skalidis I, Garot P, Antiochos P. Adaptive high microvascular resistance: a diagnostic dilemma in coronary physiology. European Heart Journal Open. 2025; https://doi.org/10.1093/ehjopen/oeaf073.
137. Gould KL, Johnson NP, Roby AE, Bui L, Kitkungvan D, Patel MB, et al. Coronary flow capacity and survival prediction after revascularization: physiological basis and clinical implications. Eur Heart J. 2023;45(3):181–94. https://doi.org/10.1093/eurheartj/ehad579.
138. Gould KL, Johnson NP, Roby AE, Kirkeeide R, Haynie M, Nguyen T, et al. Optimal medical care and coronary flow capacity-guided myocardial revascularization vs usual care for chronic coronary artery disease: the CENTURY trial. Eur Heart J. 2025; https://doi.org/10.1093/eurheartj/ehaf356.
139. Lim PO, MacDonald TM. Step test in hypertension. QJM. 2000;93(11):703–5. https://doi.org/10.1093/qjmed/93.11.703.
140. Newton I. A new and most accurate theory of the moon's motion; whereby all her irregularities may be solved. London: David Gregory; 1702.
141. Mayer T. Lunar tables and correspondence with the board of longitude. Cambridge: Cambridge University Library; 1966.
142. Shindell M. Lunar: a history of the moon in myths, maps + matter. London: Thames & Hudson; 2024.
143. Gillispie CC. Pierre-Simon Laplace, 1749–1827: a life in exact science. Princeton: Princeton University Press; 2018.
144. Watson JD. The double helix. In: Penguin readers, level 6. Harlow: Pearson Education Limited; 2008.
145. Gann A, Witkowski J. The lost correspondence of Francis Crick. Nature. 2010;467(7315):519–24. https://doi.org/10.1038/467519a.
146. Ridley M. Francis Crick: discoverer of the genetic code. Atlas Books; 2006.
147. Pauling L, Corey RB, Branson HR. The structure of proteins: two hydrogen-bonded helical configurations of the polypeptide chain. Proc Natl Acad Sci. 1951;37(4):205–11. https://doi.org/10.1073/pnas.37.4.205.
148. Watson JD, Crick FHC. Letter from James D. Watson and Francis H. C. Crick to Linus Pauling. In: Pauling L, editor.. Cambridge: Oregon State University Libraries, Special Collections & Archives Research Center; 1953.
149. Cochran W, Crick FH, Vand V. The structure of synthetic polypeptides. I. The transform of atoms on a helix. Acta Crystallogr. 1952;5(5):581–6. https://doi.org/10.1107/S0365110X52001635.
150. Crick FHC. Is alpha-keratin a coiled coil? Nature. 1952;170(4334):882–3. https://doi.org/10.1038/170882b0.
151. Crick FHC. The Fourier transform of a coiled-coil. Acta Crystallogr. 1953;6(8–9):685–9. https://doi.org/10.1107/S0365110X53001952.
152. Franklin RE, Gosling RG. Molecular configuration in sodium Thymonucleate. Nature. 1953;171(4356):740–1. https://doi.org/10.1038/171740a0.
153. Dna, Social R. Potted Account of Research on DNA at King's College; 2010.
154. Olby R. The path to the double helix: the discovery of DNA. London: Macmillan Press; 1974.

155. Wilkins MHF, Gosling RG, Seeds WE. Physical studies of nucleic acid. Nucleic acid: an extensible molecule. Nature. 1951;167:759–62.
156. Hamilton LD. DNA: models and reality. Nature. 1968;218:633–7. https://doi.org/10.1038/218633a0.
157. Raju TNK. The Nobel chronicles. Lancet. 1999;354(9173):171. https://doi.org/10.1016/S0140-6736(05)75311-3.
158. Wilkins MHF. I. Ultraviolet dichroism and molecular structure in living cells. II. Electron Microscopy of Nuclear Membranes. Naples: Pubblicazioni della Stazione Zoologica di Napoli, Vol. XXIII, Suppl.; 1951. p. 104–14.
159. Manchester KL. Historical opinion: Erwin Chargaff and his 'rules' for the base composition of DNA: why did he fail to see the possibility of complementarity? Trends Biochem Sci. 2008;33(2):65–70. https://doi.org/10.1016/j.tibs.2007.10.009.
160. Garman EF. Rosalind Franklin 1920–1958. Acta Crystallogr Sect D Struct Biol. 2020;76(7):698–701. https://doi.org/10.1107/S2059798320008827.
161. Centre CA. The Papers of Rosalind Franklin (Reference: FRKN), Churchill Archives Centre Catalogue; 2025.
162. Watson JD, Crick FHC. Molecular structure of nucleic acids: a structure for deoxyribose nucleic acid. Nature. 1953;171(4356):737–8. https://doi.org/10.1038/171737a0.
163. Maddox B. The double helix and the 'wronged heroine'. Nature. 2003;421(6921):407–8. https://doi.org/10.1038/nature01399.
164. Struewing JP, Hartge P, Wacholder S, Baker SM, Berlin M, McAdams M, et al. The risk of cancer associated with specific mutations of BRCA1 and BRCA2 among Ashkenazi Jews. N Engl J Med. 1997;336(20):1401–8. https://doi.org/10.1056/nejm199705153362001.
165. Sutton B. The story behind Photograph 51; 2023.
166. Malone J. X-rays for medical imaging: radiation protection, governance and ethics over 125 years. Phys Med. 2020;79:47–64. https://doi.org/10.1016/j.ejmp.2020.09.012.
167. Jayatilake R. Rosalind Franklin: Neliti Face of Science 007. https://breakthrough.neliti.com/rosalind-franklin/ (2023)
168. Franklin RE. Influence of the bonding electrons on the scattering of X-rays by carbon. Nature. 1950;165(4185):71. https://doi.org/10.1038/165071a0.
169. Cobb M, Comfort N. What Rosalind Franklin truly contributed to the discovery of DNA's structure. Nature. 2023;616(7958):657–60. https://doi.org/10.1038/d41586-023-01313-5.
170. O'Connor E, McGowan J, McCarthy CGP, Amini A, Grogan H, Fitzpatrick DA. Whole genome sequence of the commercially relevant mushroom strain Agaricus bisporus var. bisporus ARP23. G3 Genes|Genomes|Genetics. 2019;9(10):3057–66. https://doi.org/10.1534/g3.119.400563.
171. Ball P. Lab's labour's lost. Nature. 2015;525(7570):454–5.
172. Nature E. Rosalind Franklin: celebrating an inspirational legacy. Nature. 2020;583:492.
173. Klug A. The discovery of the DNA double helix. J Mol Biol. 2004;335(1):3–26. https://doi.org/10.1016/j.jmb.2003.11.015.
174. Franklin RE, Gosling RG. The structure of sodium thymonucleate fibres. I. The influence of water content. Acta Crystallogr. 1953;6(8–9):673–7. https://doi.org/10.1107/S0365110X53001939.
175. Franklin RE, Gosling RG. The structure of sodium thymonucleate fibres. II. The cylindrically symmetrical Patterson function. Acta Crystallogr. 1953;6(8–9):678–85. https://doi.org/10.1107/S0365110X53001940.
176. Franklin RE, Gosling RG. The structure of sodium thymonucleate fibres. III. The three-dimensional Patterson function. Acta Crystallogr. 1955;8(3):151–6. https://doi.org/10.1107/S0365110X55000595.
177. Moran L. Watson & Crick Nature Paper (1953). Sandwalk Blog; 2007.
178. Watson JD, Crick FHC. The complementary structure of deoxyribonucleic acid. Proc R Soc Lond A Math Phys Eng Sci. 1953;223:79–96.
179. Perutz MF, Wilkins MHF, Watson JD. DNA Helix. Science. 1969;164(3887):1537–9. https://doi.org/10.1126/science.164.3887.1537.

180. Chargaff E. A quick climb up Mount Olympus: the double helix. A personal account of the discovery of the structure of DNA. Science. 1968;159(3822):1448.
181. Perutz MF. I wish I'd made you angry earlier: essays on science, scientists, and humanity. Plainview: Cold Spring Harbor Laboratory Press; 1998.
182. Wilkins M. The third man of the double helix: the autobiography of Maurice Wilkins. Oxford: Oxford University Press; 2003.
183. Glynn J. Remembering my sister Rosalind Franklin. Lancet. 2012;379(9821):1094–5. https://doi.org/10.1016/S0140-6736(12)60452-8.
184. Crick FHC. What mad pursuit? A personal view of scientific discovery. New York: Basic Books; 1988.
185. Wilkins MH, Stokes AR, Wilson HR. Molecular structure of deoxypentose nucleic acids. Nature. 1953;171(4356):738–40. https://doi.org/10.1038/171738a0.
186. Moreland D, Jones P. Emil Fischer's sample collection. Bull Hist Chem. 2016;41:12–8. https://doi.org/10.70359/bhc2016v041p012.
187. Secrist JA. Nucleoside and nucleotide nomenclature. Curr Protoc Nucleic Acid Chem. 2000:A.1D–A.D.3.
188. Frixione E, Ruiz-Zamarripa L. The "scientific catastrophe" in nucleic acids research that boosted molecular biology. J Biol Chem. 2019;294(7):2249–55. https://doi.org/10.1074/jbc.CL119.007397.
189. De Marco C, Charron T, Rousseau G. Adenosine in acute myocardial infarction-associated reperfusion injury: does it still have a role? Front Pharmacol. 2022;13 https://doi.org/10.3389/fphar.2022.856747.
190. Wilson RF, Wyche K, Christensen BV, Zimmer S, Laxson DD. Effects of adenosine on human coronary arterial circulation. Circulation. 1990;82(5):1595–606. https://doi.org/10.1161/01.CIR.82.5.1595.
191. Achenbach S, Rudolph T, Rieber J, Eggebrecht H, Richardt G, Schmitz T, et al. Performing and interpreting fractional flow reserve measurements in clinical practice: an expert consensus document. Interv Cardiol. 2017;12(2):97–109. https://doi.org/10.15420/icr.2017:13:2.
192. Schlundt C, Bietau C, Klinghammer L, Wiedemann R, Rittger H, Ludwig J, et al. Comparison of intracoronary versus intravenous administration of adenosine for measurement of coronary fractional flow reserve. Circ Cardiovasc Interv. 2015;8(5) https://doi.org/10.1161/circinterventions.114.001781.
193. Dalal F, Escobedo Y, Exaire JE, Mixon TA, Al-Azizi K, Kumar YD, et al. Evaluation of intravenous versus intracoronary adenosine in coronary reactivity testing. Am J Cardiol. 2025;234:9–13. https://doi.org/10.1016/j.amjcard.2024.10.011.
194. Jong CB, Lu TS, Yan-Tyng Liu P, Hsieh MY, Meng SW, Huang CC, et al. High dose escalation of intracoronary adenosine in the assessment of fractional flow reserve: a retrospective cohort study. PLoS One. 2020;15(10):e0240699. https://doi.org/10.1371/journal.pone.0240699.
195. Verdoia M, Erbetta R, Sagazio E, Barbieri L, Negro F, Suryapranata H, et al. Impact of increasing dose of intracoronary adenosine on peak hyperemia duration during fractional flow reserve assessment. Int J Cardiol. 2019;284:16–21. https://doi.org/10.1016/j.ijcard.2018.09.088.
196. Pietzsch J. Speed read: deciphering life's enigma code. NobelPrizeorg; 2022.
197. Bernal JD. Dr Rosalind E. Franklin. Nature. 1958;182(4629):154. https://doi.org/10.1038/182154a0.
198. Klug A. Rosalind Franklin and the discovery of the structure of DNA. Nature. 1968;219(5156):808–10. https://doi.org/10.1038/219808a0.
199. Klug A. Rosalind Franklin and the double helix. Nature. 1974;248(5451):787–8. https://doi.org/10.1038/248787a0.
200. Ehrenberg W, Spear WE. X-ray micro-radiography of biological specimens. Nature. 1951;168(4273):513–4. https://doi.org/10.1038/168513b0.
201. Chivers T. Everything is predictable: how Bayes' remarkable theorem explains the world. London: Weidenfeld & Nicolson; 2023.

202. Orlin B. Change is the only constant: the wisdom of calculus in a madcap world. New York: Scribner; 2018.
203. Weiss JL, Frederiksen JW, Weisfeldt ML. Hemodynamic determinants of the time-course of fall in canine left ventricular pressure. J Clin Invest. 1976;58(3):751–60. https://doi.org/10.1172/JCI108522.
204. Herberg U, Linden K, Dewald O, Gatzweiler E, Seehase M, Duerr GD, et al. 3D real-time echocardiography combined with mini pressure wire generate reliable pressure-volume loops in small hearts. PLoS One. 2016;11(10):e0165397. https://doi.org/10.1371/journal.pone.0165397.
205. Yoshizane T, Kawamura I, Kawasaki M, Tanaka R, Minatoguchi S, Nagaya M, et al. Validation by cardiac catheterization of noninvasive estimation of time constant of left ventricular pressure decline as an index of relaxation by speckle tracking echocardiography. Am J Cardiol. 2018;121(12):1645–51. https://doi.org/10.1016/j.amjcard.2018.02.061.
206. Nagueh SF, Smiseth OA, Appleton CP, Byrd BF, et al. Recommendations for the evaluation of left ventricular diastolic function by echocardiography: an update from the American Society of Echocardiography and the European Association of Cardiovascular Imaging. J Am Soc Echocardiogr. 2016;29(4):277–314. https://doi.org/10.1016/j.echo.2016.01.011.
207. Hald A. The method of averages by Tobias Mayer, 1750. In: A history of mathematical statistics from 1750 to 1930. New York: Wiley; 1998.
208. Bayes T. An essay towards solving a problem in the doctrine of chances. Philos Trans R Soc Lond. 1763;53:370–418.
209. Laplace P-S. A philosophical essay on probabilities. New York: Cosimo Classics; 2007.
210. Berkowitz AR, Cook DJ. Leibniz–Bouvet Correspondence; 2018.
211. Lim PO. Acute myocardial infarction with non-obstructive coronary artery disease due to plaque erosion treated with balloon-occluded thrombolysis. Eur Heart J Case Rep. 2024;8(9):ytae461. https://doi.org/10.1093/ehjcr/ytae461.
212. Lim PO. Gruntzig's coronary angioplasty, revisited, modified and improved. Acta Cardiol. 2024;79(7):852–3. https://doi.org/10.1080/00015385.2024.2391140.
213. Lim PO. Grüntzig's technique, relearnt. Br J Cardiol. 2024;31:123–5. https://doi.org/10.5837/bjc.2024.042.
214. Lim PO. Stent, balloon and hybrid in de novo PCI: could the whole be greater than the sum of its parts? Br J Cardiol. 2023;30(4):37. https://doi.org/10.5837/bjc.2023.037.
215. Cole GD, Nowbar AN, Mielewczik M, Shun-Shin MJ, Francis DP. Frequency of discrepancies in retracted clinical trial reports versus unretracted reports: blinded case-control study. BMJ. 2015;351:h4708. https://doi.org/10.1136/bmj.h4708.
216. Doshi P. Ticagrelor doubts: inaccuracies uncovered in key studies for AstraZeneca's billion dollar drug. BMJ. 2025;389:r1201. https://doi.org/10.1136/bmj.r1201.
217. Henderson RA, Pocock SJ, Clayton TC, Knight R, Fox KA, Julian DG, et al. Seven-year outcome in the RITA-2 trial: coronary angioplasty versus medical therapy. J Am Coll Cardiol. 2003;42(7):1161–70. https://doi.org/10.1016/s0735-1097(03)00951-3.
218. Hartley A, Shah M, Nowbar AN, Rajkumar C, Howard JP, Francis DP. Key opinion leaders' guide to spinning a disappointing clinical trial result. BMJ. 2018;363:k5207. https://doi.org/10.1136/bmj.k5207.
219. Jureidini J, McHenry LB. The illusion of evidence based medicine. BMJ. 2022;376:o702. https://doi.org/10.1136/bmj.o702.
220. Lammers D, Richman J, Holcomb JB, Jansen JO. Use of Bayesian statistics to reanalyze data from the pragmatic randomized optimal platelet and plasma ratios trial. JAMA Netw Open. 2023;6(2):e230421. https://doi.org/10.1001/jamanetworkopen.2023.0421.
221. Gunn-Sandell LB, Bedrick EJ, Hutchins JL, Berg AA, Kaizer AM, Carlson NE. A practical guide to adopting Bayesian analyses in clinical research. J Clin Transl Sci. 2024;8(1):e3. https://doi.org/10.1017/cts.2023.689.
222. Armero C, Rodríguez A, Hernández J. A brief look into Bayesian statistics in cardiology data analysis. REC Interv Cardiol (English Edition). 2022;4 https://doi.org/10.24875/RECICE.M22000288.

223. Iglesias JF, Muller O, Heg D, Roffi M, Kurz DJ, Moarof I, et al. Biodegradable polymer sirolimus-eluting stents versus durable polymer everolimus-eluting stents in patients with ST-segment elevation myocardial infarction (BIOSTEMI): a single-blind, prospective, randomised superiority trial. Lancet. 2019;394(10205):1243–53. https://doi.org/10.1016/S0140-6736(19)31877-X.
224. Pilgrim T, Heg D, Roffi M, Tüller D, Muller O, Vuilliomenet A, et al. Ultrathin strut biodegradable polymer sirolimus-eluting stent versus durable polymer everolimus-eluting stent for percutaneous coronary revascularisation (BIOSCIENCE): a randomised, single-blind, non-inferiority trial. Lancet. 2014;384(9960):2111–22. https://doi.org/10.1016/S0140-6736(14)61038-2.
225. Madhavan MV, Howard JP, Naqvi A, Ben-Yehuda O, Redfors B, Prasad M, et al. Long-term follow-up after ultrathin vs. conventional 2nd-generation drug-eluting stents: a systematic review and meta-analysis of randomized controlled trials. Eur Heart J. 2021;42(27):2643–54. https://doi.org/10.1093/eurheartj/ehab280.
226. Heberden W. Some account of a disorder of the breast. Med Trans R Coll Physicians Lond. 1772;2:59–67.
227. Sinha A, Dutta U, Demir OM, De Silva K, Ellis H, Belford S, et al. Rethinking false positive exercise electrocardiographic stress tests by assessing coronary microvascular function. J Am Coll Cardiol. 2024;83(2):291–9. https://doi.org/10.1016/j.jacc.2023.10.034.
228. Beltrame JF, La S, Marathe J. Clinical utility of the humble exercise ECG stress test. JACC. 2024;83(2):300–2. https://doi.org/10.1016/j.jacc.2023.10.036.
229. Dimitriadis K, Pyrpyris N, Tsioufis K. Exercise electrocardiographic stress test for diagnosing coronary microvascular dysfunction. J Am Coll Cardiol. 2024;83(20):e189–e. https://doi.org/10.1016/j.jacc.2024.02.048.
230. Escárcega RO, Singh K, Chazal RA, Wood MJ. Exercise stress testing specificity in patients with ANOCA. JACC. 2024;83(20):e187–e8. https://doi.org/10.1016/j.jacc.2024.02.049.
231. Miner SES, Blair JA, McCarthy MC, Nield LE. The complex and incomplete relationship between exercise stress testing and coronary microvascular dysfunction. J Am Coll Cardiol. 2024;83(20):e193–e4. https://doi.org/10.1016/j.jacc.2024.02.047.
232. Waksman O, Chitturi KR, Case BC, Hashim HD, Waksman R. False reassurance. J Am Coll Cardiol. 2024;83(20):e191–e. https://doi.org/10.1016/j.jacc.2024.02.046.
233. Seitz A, Morár N, Pirozzolo G, Athanasiadis A, Bekeredjian R, Sechtem U, et al. Prognostic implications of coronary artery stenosis and coronary spasm in patients with stable angina: 5-year follow-up of the abnormal COronary VAsomotion in patients with stable angina and unobstructed coronary arteries (ACOVA) study. Coron Artery Dis. 2020;31(6):530–7. https://doi.org/10.1097/mca.0000000000000876.
234. Jansen TPJ, Konst RE, de Vos A, Paradies V, Teerenstra S, van den Oord SCH, et al. Efficacy of diltiazem to improve coronary vasomotor dysfunction in ANOCA: the EDIT-CMD randomized clinical trial. JACC Cardiovasc Imaging. 2022;15(8):1473–84. https://doi.org/10.1016/j.jcmg.2022.03.012.
235. Rinaldi R, Russo M, Occhipinti G, Laudani C, Torre I, Colucci M, et al. Sex-related differences in the prognostic role of acetylcholine provocation testing. J Am Heart Assoc. 2025;14(5):e037942. https://doi.org/10.1161/JAHA.124.037942.
236. Prinzmetal M, Ekmekci A, Toyoshima H, Kwoczynski JK. Angina pectoris: III. Demonstration of a chemical origin of ST deviation in classic angina pectoris, its variant form, early myocardial infarction, and some noncardiac conditions preliminary report. Am J Cardiol. 1959;3(3):276–93. https://doi.org/10.1016/0002-9149(59)90212-7.
237. Montone RA, Niccoli G, Fracassi F, Russo M, Gurgoglione F, Cammà G, et al. Patients with acute myocardial infarction and non-obstructive coronary arteries: safety and prognostic relevance of invasive coronary provocative tests. Eur Heart J. 2018;39(2):91–8. https://doi.org/10.1093/eurheartj/ehx667.
238. Lim PO. Angina: the ischemic triad. Am J Cardiol. 2024;223:118–9. https://doi.org/10.1016/j.amjcard.2024.05.023.

239. Buzzi A. Claude Bernard on cardiac catheterization. Am J Cardiol. 1959;4(3):405–9. https://doi.org/10.1016/0002-9149(59)90057-8.
240. Chauveau J-B-A, Marey É-J. Détermination graphique des rapports du choc du cœur avec les mouvements des oreillettes et des ventricules: expérience faite à l'aide d'un appareil enregistreur (sphygmographe). CR Hebd Seances Acad Sci. 1861;53:622–5.
241. Fye WB. Jean-Baptiste Auguste Chauveau. Clin Cardiol. 2003;26(7):351–3. https://doi.org/10.1002/clc.4950260712.
242. Frank O. On the dynamics of cardiac muscle. Am Heart J. 1959;58(2):282–317. https://doi.org/10.1016/0002-8703(59)90345-X.
243. Lewis T. The mechanism and graphic registration of the heart beat, vol. xx. New York: P. B. Hoeber; 1921. p. 452.
244. Bers DM, Borlaug BA. Mechanisms of cardiac contraction and relaxation. In: Libby P, Bonow RO, Mann DL, Tomaselli GF, Bhatt DL, Solomon SD, editors. Braunwald's heart disease: a textbook of cardiovascular medicine. 12th ed. Philadelphia: Elsevier; 2021. p. 889–912.
245. Wiggers CJ. Studies on the consecutive phases of the cardiac cycle. Am J Physiol Legacy Content. 1921;56(3):415–38. https://doi.org/10.1152/ajplegacy.1921.56.3.415.
246. Katz AM. Ernest Henry Starling, his predecessors, and the "law of the heart". Circulation. 2002;106(23):2986–92. https://doi.org/10.1161/01.CIR.0000040594.96123.55.
247. Starling EH. The Linacre lecture on the law of the heart. Longmans, Green, & Company; 1918.
248. Elzinga G. "Starling's law of the heart" a historical misinterpretation. Basic Res Cardiol. 1989;84(1):1–4. https://doi.org/10.1007/BF01906997.
249. Fenn WO. A quantitative comparison between the energy liberated and the work performed by the isolated sartorius muscle of the frog. J Physiol. 1923;58(2–3):175–203. https://doi.org/10.1113/jphysiol.1923.sp002115.
250. Tagami T, Kuwamoto K, Watanabe A, Unemoto K, Yokobori S, Matsumoto G, et al. Optimal range of global end-diastolic volume for fluid management after aneurysmal subarachnoid hemorrhage: a multicenter prospective cohort study. Crit Care Med. 2014;42(6):1348–56. https://doi.org/10.1097/CCM.0000000000000163.
251. Walley KR. Left ventricular function: time-varying elastance and left ventricular aortic coupling. Crit Care. 2016;20:270. https://doi.org/10.1186/s13054-016-1439-6.
252. Fukuda N, Terui T, Ohtsuki I, et al. Titin and troponin: central players in the frank-starling mechanism of the heart. Curr Cardiol Rev. 2009;5(2):119–24. https://doi.org/10.2174/157340309788166714.
253. Lim HS. Law of the heart. In: Hemodynamic physiology in advanced heart failure and cardiogenic shock. Cham: Springer Nature Switzerland; 2024. p. 3–23.
254. Monroe RG, Gamble WJ, CG LF, Kumar AE, Stark J, Sanders GL, et al. The Anrep effect reconsidered. J Clin Invest. 1972;51(10):2573–83. https://doi.org/10.1172/jci107074.
255. Azzalini L, Seth M, Sukul D, Arora DS, Chattahi J, Osman A, et al. Impact of left ventricular end-diastolic pressure on the outcomes of patients undergoing percutaneous coronary intervention. Am J Cardiol. 2022;185:107–14. https://doi.org/10.1016/j.amjcard.2022.09.007.
256. Planer D, Mehran R, Witzenbichler B, Guagliumi G, Peruga JZ, Brodie BR, et al. Prognostic utility of left ventricular end-diastolic pressure in patients with ST-segment elevation myocardial infarction undergoing primary percutaneous coronary intervention. Am J Cardiol. 2011;108(8):1068–74. https://doi.org/10.1016/j.amjcard.2011.06.007.
257. Suga H, Sagawa K. Instantaneous pressure-volume relationships and their ratio in the excised, supported canine left ventricle. Circ Res. 1974;35(1):117–26.
258. Feng L, Lin Z, Ji Y, Lim PO. Post-infarct lateral extension-Brody effect or stent thrombosis? J Electrocardiol. 2025;91:154014. https://doi.org/10.1016/j.jelectrocard.2025.154014.
259. Kass DA, Chen CH, Curry C, Talbot M, Berger R, Fetics B, et al. Improved left ventricular mechanics from acute VDD pacing in patients with dilated cardiomyopathy and ventricular conduction delay. Circulation. 1999;99(12):1567–73. https://doi.org/10.1161/01.cir.99.12.1567.

260. Sunagawa K, Maughan WL, Burkhoff D, Sagawa K. Left ventricular interaction with arterial load studied in isolated canine ventricle. Am J Phys. 1983;245(5 Pt 1):H773–80. https://doi.org/10.1152/ajpheart.1983.245.5.H773.
261. Fraser AG. Ventricular–arterial coupling – clinical tools and diagnostic indications. ESC/EAE Echocardiographic Imaging Course. Bucharest, Romania: European Society of Cardiology; 2020.
262. Redfield MM, Jacobsen SJ, Borlaug BA, Rodeheffer RJ, Kass DA. Age- and gender-related ventricular-vascular stiffening: a community-based study. Circulation. 2005;112(15):2254–62. https://doi.org/10.1161/circulationaha.105.541078.
263. Segev A, Ishay RT-B, Metra M, Maor E, Freimark D, Younis A, et al. Heart failure with supranormal ejection fraction: clinical characteristics and outcomes compared to mildly reduced and preserved ejection fraction. Clin Res Cardiol. 2025;114(5):665–75. https://doi.org/10.1007/s00392-025-02620-9.
264. Nguyen M, Berhoud V, Bartamian L, Martin A, Ellouze O, Bouhemad B, et al. Agreement between different non-invasive methods of ventricular elastance assessment for the monitoring of ventricular–arterial coupling in intensive care. J Clin Monit Comput. 2020;34(5):893–901. https://doi.org/10.1007/s10877-019-00397-7.
265. Lower R. Tractatus de Corde: item de Motu & Colore Sanguinis, et Chyli in eum transitu. Rotterdam: Arnold Leers; 1669.
266. Torrent-Guasp F. El Ciclo Cardiaco: Consideraciones críticas sobre la interpretación clásica y nuevas ideas sobre el mismo. Madrid: Editorial Diana; 1954.
267. Torrent-Guasp F, Kocica MJ, Corno A, Komeda M, Cox J, Flotats A, et al. Systolic ventricular filling. Eur J Cardiothorac Surg. 2004;25(3):376–86. https://doi.org/10.1016/j.ejcts.2003.12.020.
268. The Man Who Unfolded a Thousand Hearts. El hombre que desplegó mil corazones. Spain: Media 3.14, Desmesura Films; 2008.
269. Ballester M, Ferreira A, Carreras F. The myocardial band. Heart Fail Clin. 2008;4(3):261–72. https://doi.org/10.1016/j.hfc.2008.02.011.
270. Cosín Aguilar J. Francisco Torrent-Guasp 1931-2005. Revista Española de Cardiología (English Edition). 2005;58(6):611–764. https://doi.org/10.1016/S1885-5857(06)60260-0.
271. Kocica MJ, Corno AF, Carreras-Costa F, Ballester-Rodes M, Moghbel MC, Cueva CN, et al. The helical ventricular myocardial band: global, three-dimensional, functional architecture of the ventricular myocardium. Eur J Cardiothorac Surg. 2006;29(Suppl 1):S21–40. https://doi.org/10.1016/j.ejcts.2006.03.011.
272. Torrent-Guasp F. La estructuración macroscópica del miocardio ventricular. Rev Esp Cardiol. 1980;33(3):265–87.
273. Trainini JC, Herreros J. El explorador del corazón: biografía de Francisco Torrent-Guasp. 1st ed. Ciudad Autónoma de Buenos Aires: Biblos; 2019.
274. Buckberg GD, Clemente C, Cox JL, Coghlan HC, Castella M, Torrent-Guasp F, et al. The structure and function of the helical heart and its buttress wrapping. IV. Concepts of dynamic function from the Normal macroscopic helical structure. Semin Thorac Cardiovasc Surg. 2001;13(4):342–57. https://doi.org/10.1053/stcs.2001.29956.
275. Trainini J, Beraudo M, Alejandro T, Mario W, Jesús V, Jorge L, et al. Why is the heart helical. J Anat. 2025;10:1–17. https://doi.org/10.52338/tjoa.2025.4670.
276. Torrent-Guasp F. Estructura y funcion del corazon. Rev Esp Cardiol. 1998;51(2):91–102. https://doi.org/10.1016/s0300-8932(98)74718-9.
277. Baroni M, Pedrotti P, Nava S, Giannattasio C, Roghi A. Cardiac magnetic resonance imaging of left ventricular apical hypoplasia in two complex congenital clinical syndromes. Circ J. 2014;78(6):1507–9. https://doi.org/10.1253/circj.cj-13-1555.
278. Fernandez-Valls M, Srichai MB, Stillman AE, White RD. Isolated left ventricular apical hypoplasia: a new congenital anomaly described with cardiac tomography. Heart. 2004;90(5):552–5. https://doi.org/10.1136/hrt.2003.010637.

279. Hu SY, Meng C, Ku LZ, Yan H, Lu YF, Wang L, et al. Isolated left ventricular apical hypoplasia: a case report. JRSM Cardiovasc Dis. 2025;14:20480040251325379. https://doi.org/10.1177/20480040251325379.
280. Román R, Anchante H, Menacho K, Medina F. Isolated left ventricular apical hypoplasia: case report. Eur Heart J Case Rep. 2023;7(2):ytad046. https://doi.org/10.1093/ehjcr/ytad046.
281. Brusamolino M, Oliveró R, González V, Rodriguez-Palomares JF, Pontone G. Multimodal imaging evaluation and follow-up of a congenital left ventricular aneurysm. CJC Open. 2025; https://doi.org/10.1016/j.cjco.2025.06.002.
282. Ohlow MA. Congenital left ventricular aneurysms and diverticula: an entity in search of an identity. J Geriatr Cardiol. 2017;14(12):750–62. https://doi.org/10.11909/j.issn.1671-5411.2017.12.005.
283. Ohlow MA, von Korn H, Lauer B. Characteristics and outcome of congenital left ventricular aneurysm and diverticulum: analysis of 809 cases published since 1816. Int J Cardiol. 2015;185:34–45. https://doi.org/10.1016/j.ijcard.2015.03.050.
284. Torrent-Guasp F, Buckberg GD, Clemente C, Cox JL, Coghlan HC, Gharib M. The structure and function of the helical heart and its buttress wrapping. I. The normal macroscopic structure of the heart. Semin Thorac Cardiovasc Surg. 2001;13(4):301–19. https://doi.org/10.1053/stcs.2001.29953.
285. Buckberg GD, Hoffman JIE, Coghlan HC, Nanda NC. Ventricular structure–function relations in health and disease: part I. The normal heart. Eur J Cardiothorac Surg. 2014;47(4):587–601. https://doi.org/10.1093/ejcts/ezu278.
286. Smith HJ, Kent KM, Epstein SE. Relationship between regional contractile function and S-T segment elevation after experimental coronary artery occlusion in the dog. Cardiovasc Res. 1978;12(7):444–8. https://doi.org/10.1093/cvr/12.7.444.
287. Spotnitz HM. Macro design, structure, and mechanics of the left ventricle. J Thorac Cardiovasc Surg. 2000;119(5):1053–77. https://doi.org/10.1016/S0022-5223(00)70106-1.
288. Gould KL, Johnson NP, Narula J. Reply: is bolus-Thermodilution reliable in defining coronary microvascular dysfunction? JACC Cardiovasc Imaging. 2023;16(7):994–5. https://doi.org/10.1016/j.jcmg.2023.04.010.
289. Gould KL, Johnson NP, Narula J. Microvascular dysfunction or diffuse Epicardial CAD with Normal stress vasodilation. JACC Cardiovasc Imaging. 2023;16(4):549–52. https://doi.org/10.1016/j.jcmg.2022.10.029.
290. Schindler TH, Fearon WF, Pelletier-Galarneau M, Ambrosio G, Sechtem U, Ruddy TD, et al. Myocardial perfusion PET for the detection and reporting of coronary microvascular dysfunction: a JACC: cardiovascular imaging expert panel statement. JACC Cardiovasc Imaging. 2023;16(4):536–48. https://doi.org/10.1016/j.jcmg.2022.12.015.
291. Panting JR, Gatehouse PD, Yang GZ, Grothues F, Firmin DN, Collins P, et al. Abnormal subendocardial perfusion in cardiac syndrome X detected by cardiovascular magnetic resonance imaging. N Engl J Med. 2002;346(25):1948–53. https://doi.org/10.1056/NEJMoa012369.
292. Camaioni C, Knott KD, Augusto JB, Seraphim A, Rosmini S, Ricci F, et al. Inline perfusion mapping provides insights into the disease mechanism in hypertrophic cardiomyopathy. Heart. 2020;106(11):824–9. https://doi.org/10.1136/heartjnl-2019-315848.
293. Yamada A, Ishida M, Kitagawa K, Sakuma H. Assessment of myocardial ischemia using stress perfusion cardiovascular magnetic resonance. Cardiovasc Imaging Asia. 2018;2(2):65–75.
294. Mehta PK, Goykhman P, Thomson LE, Shufelt C, Wei J, Yang Y, et al. Ranolazine improves angina in women with evidence of myocardial ischemia but no obstructive coronary artery disease. JACC Cardiovasc Imaging. 2011;4(5):514–22. https://doi.org/10.1016/j.jcmg.2011.03.007.
295. Joung S, Wei J, Nelson MD, Aldiwani H, Shufelt C, Tamarappoo B, et al. Progression of coronary microvascular dysfunction to heart failure with preserved ejection fraction: a case report. J Med Case Rep. 2019;13(1):134. https://doi.org/10.1186/s13256-019-2074-z.
296. Morrow A, Young R, Abraham GR, Hoole S, Greenwood JP, Arnold JR, et al. Zibotentan in microvascular angina: a randomized, placebo-controlled, crossover trial. Circulation. 2024;150(21):1671–83. https://doi.org/10.1161/CIRCULATIONAHA.124.069901.

297. Rahman H, Scannell CM, Demir OM, Ryan M, McConkey H, Ellis H, et al. High-resolution cardiac magnetic resonance imaging techniques for the identification of coronary microvascular dysfunction. JACC Cardiovasc Imaging. 2021;14(5):978–86. https://doi.org/10.1016/j.jcmg.2020.10.015.
298. Thomson LE, Wei J, Agarwal M, Haft-Baradaran A, Shufelt C, Mehta PK, et al. Cardiac magnetic resonance myocardial perfusion reserve index is reduced in women with coronary microvascular dysfunction. A National Heart, Lung, and Blood Institute-sponsored study from the women's ischemia syndrome evaluation. Circ Cardiovasc Imaging. 2015;8(4) https://doi.org/10.1161/circimaging.114.002481.
299. Vink CEM, Borodzicz-Jazdzyk S, de Jong EAM, Woudstra J, van de Hoef TP, Chamuleau SAJ, et al. Quantitative perfusion by cardiac magnetic resonance imaging reveals compromised myocardial perfusion in patients with angina with non-obstructive coronary artery disease. Clin Res Cardiol. 2025; https://doi.org/10.1007/s00392-025-02606-7.
300. Karamitsos TD. RETRACTED: mapping the future of myocardial ischemia testing with cardiac magnetic resonance∗. JACC. 2018;71(9):980–2. https://doi.org/10.1016/j.jacc.2017.12.047.
301. Liu A, Wijesurendra RS, Liu JM, Forfar JC, Channon KM, Jerosch-Herold M, et al. Diagnosis of microvascular angina using cardiac magnetic resonance. J Am Coll Cardiol. 2018;71(9):969–79. https://doi.org/10.1016/j.jacc.2017.12.046.
302. Bradley CP, Orchard V, McKinley G, Heggie R, Wu O, Good R, et al. The coronary microvascular angina cardiovascular magnetic resonance imaging trial: rationale and design. Am Heart J. 2023;265:213–24. https://doi.org/10.1016/j.ahj.2023.08.067.
303. Kunadian V, Chieffo A, Camici PG, Berry C, Escaned J, Maas AHEM, et al. An EAPCI expert consensus document on Ischaemia with non-obstructive coronary arteries in collaboration with European Society of Cardiology Working Group on coronary pathophysiology microcirculation endorsed by coronary vasomotor disorders international study group. Eur Heart J. 2020;41(37):3504–20. https://doi.org/10.1093/eurheartj/ehaa503.
304. Ajmal M, Widmer RJ, Corban MT. Evaluation of coronary microvascular and endothelial function in the cardiac catheterization laboratory. Curr Treat Options Cardiovasc Med. 2023;25(7):219–32. https://doi.org/10.1007/s11936-023-00989-2.
305. Schäufele T, Nobre Menezes M, Schulte Steinberg B, Hubert A, Martínez Pereyra V, Arndt H, et al. Effects of radial artery spasm prophylaxis on intracoronary vasomotor responses during acetylcholine spasm provocation testing. Int J Cardiol. 2025;419 https://doi.org/10.1016/j.ijcard.2024.132703.
306. Olaru M-M, Lim PO. Sheath tip radial artery disruption as a mechanism for forearm hematoma: insights from the distal radial artery approach. Roman J Cardiol. 2024;34(1):50–5. https://doi.org/10.2478/rjc-2024-0006.
307. Korngold EC, Westerdahl DE, Ullery BW. Left distal radial artery access-site Pseudoaneurysm treated with open surgical repair. J Soc Cardiovasc Angiogr Interv. 2023;2(5) https://doi.org/10.1016/j.jscai.2023.101047.
308. Yamazaki D, Makabe S, Yuzurihara M. Rare complication of distal radial artery puncture: arteriovenous fistula formation following percutaneous coronary intervention. Cureus. 2025;17(2):e79541. https://doi.org/10.7759/cureus.79541.
309. Wolowczyk L, Williams AJ, Donovan KL, Gibbons CP. The snuffbox arteriovenous fistula for vascular access. Eur J Vasc Endovasc Surg. 2000;19(1):70–6. https://doi.org/10.1053/ejvs.1999.0969.
310. Babunashvili A, Dundua D. Recanalization and reuse of early occluded radial artery within 6 days after previous transradial diagnostic procedure. Catheter Cardiovasc Interv. 2011;77(4):530–6. https://doi.org/10.1002/ccd.22846.
311. Kiemeneij F, Burzotta F, Fajadet J. Thirty years of transradial coronary interventions. EuroIntervention. 2022;18(1):19–21. https://doi.org/10.4244/eij-e-22-00009.
312. Kiemeneij F. Left distal transradial access in the anatomical snuffbox for coronary angiography (ldTRA) and interventions (ldTRI). EuroIntervention. 2017;13(7):851–7. https://doi.org/10.4244/eij-d-17-00079.

313. Roh JW, Kim Y, Lee OH, Im E, Cho DK, Choi D, et al. The learning curve of the distal radial access for coronary intervention. Sci Rep. 2021;11(1):13217. https://doi.org/10.1038/s41598-021-92742-7.
314. Ferreira-Martins J, Lim PO. Two-step distal radial artery cannulation for challenging radial anatomies. Cardiology. 2021;146(2):144–50. https://doi.org/10.1159/000510293.
315. Lim PO. Transradial Catheter Kink – take a grip. Catheter Cardiovasc Interv. 2025; https://doi.org/10.1002/ccd.31582.
316. Lim PO, Elghamry Z. Heparin-free distal radial artery approach to cardiac catheterisation and the small radial recurrent artery. Br J Cardiol. 2021;28(3):39. https://doi.org/10.5837/bjc.2021.039.
317. Will M, Weiss TW, Weber M, Kwok CS, Borovac JA, Lamm G, et al. Left vs. right radial approach for coronary catheterization: relation to age and severe aortic stenosis. Front Cardiovasc Med. 2022;9 https://doi.org/10.3389/fcvm.2022.1022415.
318. Keulards DCJ, et al. Safety of absolute coronary flow and microvascular resistance measurements by thermodilution. EuroIntervention. 2021;17(3):229–32. https://doi.org/10.4244/EIJ-D-20-00074.
319. Seki R, Keulards DCJ, Gutierrez-Barrios A, Fawaz S, Mahendiran T, Bertolone DT, et al. Safety of continuous coronary Thermodilution measurements. JACC Cardiovasc Interv. 2023;16(22):2794–6. https://doi.org/10.1016/j.jcin.2023.09.030.
320. García-Guimaraes M, Rivero F, Cuesta J, Alfonso F. Iatrogenic coronary artery dissection induced during invasive absolute coronary blood flow measurement: optical coherence tomography findings. EuroIntervention. 2017;13(3):364–5. https://doi.org/10.4244/eij-d-17-00048.
321. Fawaz S, Munhoz D, Mahendiran T, Gallinoro E, Mizukami T, Khan SA, et al. Assessing the impact of prolonged averaging of coronary continuous Thermodilution traces. Diagnostics. 2024;14(3):285.
322. Marshall TP. Blood pressure variability: the challenge of variation. Am J Hypertens. 2008;21(1):3–4. https://doi.org/10.1038/ajh.2007.20.
323. Warren RE, Marshall T, Padfield PL, Chrubasik S. Variability of office, 24-hour ambulatory, and self-monitored blood pressure measurements. Br J Gen Pract. 2010;60(578):675–80. https://doi.org/10.3399/bjgp10X515403.
324. Sara JDS, Toya T, Ahmad A, Clark MM, Gilliam WP, Lerman LO, et al. Mental stress and its effects on vascular health. Mayo Clin Proc. 2022;97(5):951–90. https://doi.org/10.1016/j.mayocp.2022.02.004.
325. Kop WJ, Krantz DS, Howell RH, Ferguson MA, Papademetriou V, Lu D, et al. Effects of mental stress on coronary epicardial vasomotion and flow velocity in coronary artery disease: relationship with hemodynamic stress responses1. J Am Coll Cardiol. 2001;37(5):1359–66. https://doi.org/10.1016/S0735-1097(01)01136-6.
326. Vatner SF, Higgins CB, Franklin D, Braunwald E. Role of tachycardia in mediating the coronary hemodynamic response to severe exercise. J Appl Physiol. 1972;32(3):380–5. https://doi.org/10.1152/jappl.1972.32.3.380.
327. Rossen JD, Winniford MD. Effect of increases in heart rate and arterial pressure on coronary flow reserve in humans. J Am Coll Cardiol. 1993;21(2):343–8. https://doi.org/10.1016/0735-1097(93)90673-O.
328. Rushmer RF. Initial ventricular impulse. A potential key to cardiac evaluation. Circulation. 1964;29:268–83. https://doi.org/10.1161/01.cir.29.2.268.
329. Pasipoularides A, Murgo JP, Miller JW, Craig WE. Nonobstructive left ventricular ejection pressure gradients in man. Circ Res. 1987;61(2):220–7. https://doi.org/10.1161/01.res.61.2.220.
330. Ohba I, Otsuji Y, Shiki K, Hamasaki S, Minagoe S, Tei C. Different effects of propranolol, phenylephrine, and saline volume loading on catecholamine-induced left ventricular outflow tract obstruction in acute coronary syndrome. Int Heart J. 2006;47(2):287–95. https://doi.org/10.1536/ihj.47.287.
331. Harrison MR, Grigsby CG, Souther SK, Smith MD, DeMaria AN. Midventricular obstruction associated with chronic systemic hypertension and severe left ventricular hypertrophy. Am J Cardiol. 1991;68(8):761–5. https://doi.org/10.1016/0002-9149(91)90650-A.

332. Pasipoularides A. Clinical assesment of ventricular ejection dynamics with and without outflow obstruction. J Am Coll Cardiol. 1990;15(4):859–82. https://doi.org/10.1016/0735-1097(90)90287-Y.
333. Yotti R. What is the relevance of an intraventricular ejection pressure gradient induced by exercise. Revista Española de Cardiología (English Edition). 2004;57(12):1133–256. https://doi.org/10.1016/S1885-5857(06)60205-3.
334. Birrell H, Isles C, Fersia O, Anwar M, Mondoa C, McFadyen A. Assessment of the diagnostic value of NT-proBNP in heart failure with preserved ejection fraction. Br J Cardiol. 2024;31(1):002. https://doi.org/10.5837/bjc.2024.002.
335. Tcheugui JB, Zhang S, McEvoy JW, Ndumele CE, Hoogeveen RC, Coresh J, et al. Elevated NT-ProBNP as a cardiovascular disease risk equivalent: evidence from the atherosclerosis risk in communities (ARIC) study. Am J Med. 2022;135(12):1461–7. https://doi.org/10.1016/j.amjmed.2022.07.012.
336. Kyriakides ZS, Kolettis TM, Kremastinos D. Cardiac pacing and coronary hemodynamics. Prog Cardiovasc Dis. 1999;41(6):471–80. https://doi.org/10.1016/s0033-0620(99)70023-x.
337. Degtiarova G, Claus P, Duchenne J, Schramm G, Nuyts J, Verberne HJ, et al. Impact of left bundle branch block on myocardial perfusion and metabolism: a positron emission tomography study. J Nucl Cardiol. 2021;28(4):1730–9. https://doi.org/10.1007/s12350-019-01900-y.
338. Czuriga D, Lim PO. Cardiac resynchronization therapy relieves intractable angina due to exercise-induced left bundle branch block without left ventricular systolic dysfunction: a detailed Case study. J Cardiovasc Electrophysiol. 2016;27(5):609–12. https://doi.org/10.1111/jce.12911.
339. Huang W, Su L, Wu S, Xu L, Xiao F, Zhou X, et al. A novel pacing strategy with low and stable output: pacing the left bundle branch immediately beyond the conduction block. Can J Cardiol. 2017;33(12):1736. https://doi.org/10.1016/j.cjca.2017.09.013.
340. Tandon K, Lakey J, Shvilkin A. A case of self-diagnosed painful left bundle branch block. HeartRhythm Case Rep. 2021;7(12):812–5. https://doi.org/10.1016/j.hrcr.2021.09.005.
341. Pujades-Rodriguez M, Morgan AW, Cubbon RM, Wu J. Dose-dependent oral glucocorticoid cardiovascular risks in people with immune-mediated inflammatory diseases: a population-based cohort study. PLoS Med. 2020;17(12):e1003432. https://doi.org/10.1371/journal.pmed.1003432.
342. Ong P, Camici PG, Beltrame JF, Crea F, Shimokawa H, Sechtem U, et al. International standardization of diagnostic criteria for microvascular angina. Int J Cardiol. 2018;250:16–20. https://doi.org/10.1016/j.ijcard.2017.08.068.
343. Ishihara M, Sato H, Tateishi H, Kawagoe T, Shimatani Y, Kurisu S, et al. Effects of various doses of intracoronary verapamil on coronary resistance vessels in humans. Jpn Circ J. 1997;61(9):755–61. https://doi.org/10.1253/jcj.61.755.
344. Oldenburg O, Eggebrecht H, Herrmann J, Naber CK, Haude M, Erbel R, et al. Dose-dependent effects of intracoronary verapamil on systemic and coronary hemodynamics. Cardiovasc Drugs Ther. 2000;14(6):651–5. https://doi.org/10.1023/a:1007823116491.
345. Oldenburg O, Eggebrecht H, Gutersohn A, Schaar J, Brauck K, Haude M, et al. Myocardial lactate release after intracoronary verapamil application in humans: acute effects of intracoronary verapamil on systemic and coronary hemodynamics, myocardial metabolism, and norepinephrine levels. Cardiovasc Drugs Ther. 2001;15(1):55–61. https://doi.org/10.1023/a:1011162818809.
346. Gustafsson D. Microvascular mechanisms involved in calcium antagonist edema formation. J Cardiovasc Pharmacol. 1987;10:S121–S31.
347. Shimada M, Nakamura Y, Iwanaga S, Asakura K, Hori S, Hattori S, et al. Nonischemic ST-segment elevation induced by negative inotropic agents. Jpn Circ J. 1999;63(8):610–6. https://doi.org/10.1253/jcj.63.610.
348. Tran Q-K, Ohashi K, Watanabe H. Calcium signalling in endothelial cells. Cardiovasc Res. 2000;48(1):13–22. https://doi.org/10.1016/s0008-6363(00)00172-3.

349. Versari D, Virdis A, Ghiadoni L, Daghini E, Duranti E, Masi S, et al. Effect of verapamil, trandolapril and their combination on vascular function and structure in essential hypertensive patients. Atherosclerosis. 2009;205(1):214–20. https://doi.org/10.1016/j.atherosclerosis.2008.11.023.
350. Jiang Z-G, Shi X-R, Guan B-C, Zhao H, Yang Y-Q. Dihydropyridines inhibit acetylcholine-induced hyperpolarization in Cochlear artery via blockade of intermediate-conductance calcium-activated potassium channels. J Pharmacol Exp Ther. 2007;320(2):544–51. https://doi.org/10.1124/jpet.106.115212.
351. Garland CJ, Dora KA. Hyperpolarization and the endothelium. Curr Opin Physio. 2023;34:100674. https://doi.org/10.1016/j.cophys.2023.100674.
352. Zhang Z, Li X, He J, Wang S, Wang J, Liu J, et al. Molecular mechanisms of endothelial dysfunction in coronary microcirculation dysfunction. J Thromb Thrombolysis. 2023;56(3):388–97. https://doi.org/10.1007/s11239-023-02862-2.
353. Sheng JZ, Ella S, Davis MJ, Hill MA, Braun AP. Openers of SKCa and IKCa channels enhance agonist-evoked endothelial nitric oxide synthesis and arteriolar vasodilation. FASEB J. 2009;23(4):1138–45. https://doi.org/10.1096/fj.08-120451.
354. Kurabayashi M, Asano M, Shimura T, Suzuki H, Aoyagi H, Yamauchi Y, et al. Ultra-long acting calcium channel blockers may decrease accuracy of the acetylcholine provocation test. Int J Cardiol. 2017;236:71–5. https://doi.org/10.1016/j.ijcard.2017.02.123.
355. Sueda S, Kurokawa K, Sakaue T, Ikeda S. What is the meaning of provoked spasm phenotypes by vasoreactivity testing? J Cardiol. 2024;83(1):1–7. https://doi.org/10.1016/j.jjcc.2023.06.013.
356. Lim PO. Takayasu arteritis and stent always end in tears. Eur Heart J Case Rep. 2023;7(9):ytad421. https://doi.org/10.1093/ehjcr/ytad421.
357. Lim PO. What causes cocaine-related coronary slow flow phenomenon? IHJ Cardiovasc Rep. 2024;8(1):36–9. https://doi.org/10.1016/j.ihjcvr.2024.04.003.
358. Sütsch G, Oechslin E, Mayer I, Hess OM. Effect of diltiazem on coronary flow reserve in patients with microvascular angina. Int J Cardiol. 1995;52(2):135–43. https://doi.org/10.1016/0167-5273(95)02458-9.
359. AlHazmi H, Bahadur AY, AlAhmadi K, Bahadur OY. Syncope: atypical presentation of diaphragmatic hernia. Cureus. 2024;16(1):e51715. https://doi.org/10.7759/cureus.51715.
360. Deveer M, Beydilli H, Cullu N, Sivrioglu AK. Diaphragmatic eventration presenting with sudden dyspnoea. BMJ Case Rep. 2013; https://doi.org/10.1136/bcr-2013-008613.
361. Yildiz A, Tuncez A, Demirkan B, Guray Y. An unusual cause of syncope: diaphragmatic hernia. Echocardiography. 2013;30(5):E136–7. https://doi.org/10.1111/echo.12150.
362. Salah HM, Goldberg LR, Molinger J, Felker GM, Applefeld W, Rassaf T, et al. Diaphragmatic function in cardiovascular disease: JACC review topic of the week. J Am Coll Cardiol. 2022;80(17):1647–59. https://doi.org/10.1016/j.jacc.2022.08.760.
363. Roos M, Kobza R, Jamshidi P, Bauer P, Resink T, Schlaepfer R, et al. Improved cardiac performance through pacing-induced diaphragmatic stimulation: a novel electrophysiological approach in heart failure management? Europace. 2009;11(2):191–9. https://doi.org/10.1093/europace/eun377.
364. Zuber M, Young R, Shaburishvili T, Rudenko K, Demyanchuk V, Jorbenadze A, et al. First in human VisONE heart failure study: asymptomatic diaphragmatic stimulation for chronic heart failure: one month results. J Card Fail. 2019;25(8, Supplement):S183. https://doi.org/10.1016/j.cardfail.2019.07.517.
365. Convertino VA. Mechanisms of inspiration that modulate cardiovascular control: the other side of breathing. J Appl Physiol. 2019;127(5):1187–96. https://doi.org/10.1152/japplphysiol.00050.2019.
366. Akkus O, Huzmeli I, Seker T, Bekler O, Sen F, Kaypakli O, et al. Effectiveness of device-guided breathing in chronic coronary syndrome: a randomized controlled study. Acta Cardiol Sin. 2023;39(5):720–32. https://doi.org/10.6515/acs.202309_39(5).20230306e.

367. Merza WM, Yaseen AK, Mahmood MA. FSH, LH, lipid and adipokines in polycystic ovary syndrome: clinical biochemistry insights for diagnosis and management. J Steroid Biochem Mol Biol. 2025;251:106773. https://doi.org/10.1016/j.jsbmb.2025.106773.
368. Faber B. Serial electrocardiograms show acute onset of inverted P waves in a 62-year-old-male with chest pain: a Case report. Int J Paramed. 2024:133–40. https://doi.org/10.56068/ZMXE2675.
369. Romeo S, Vidal-Puig A, Husain M, Ahima R, Arca M, Bhatt DL, et al. Clinical staging to guide management of metabolic disorders and their sequelae: a European atherosclerosis society consensus statement. Eur Heart J. 2025:ehaf314. https://doi.org/10.1093/eurheartj/ehaf314.
370. Zhou K, Lou C, Chang P-H, Jiang J, Zhao Y, Chang H-M, et al. Promising drugs for PCOS: targeting metabolic and endocrine dysfunctions. Nat Rev Endocrinol. 2025; https://doi.org/10.1038/s41574-025-01121-z.
371. Lim PO. Paolo Angelini's legacy in the study of and treatment for anomalous coronary arteries. Tex Heart Inst J. 2023;50(6) https://doi.org/10.14503/THIJ-23-8351.
372. Koepfli P, Wyss CA, Gaemperli O, Siegrist PT, Klainguti M, Schepis T, et al. Left bundle branch block causes relative but not absolute septal underperfusion during exercise. Eur Heart J. 2009;30(24):2993–9. https://doi.org/10.1093/eurheartj/ehp372.
373. Skalidis EI, Kochiadakis GE, Koukouraki SI, Parthenakis FI, Karkavitsas NS, Vardas PE. Phasic coronary flow pattern and flow reserve in patients with left bundle branch block and normal coronary arteries. J Am Coll Cardiol. 1999;33(5):1338–46. https://doi.org/10.1016/S0735-1097(98)00698-6.
374. Tan NY, Witt CM, Oh JK, Cha Y-M. Left Bundle Branch Block. Circ Arrhythm Electrophysiol. 2020;13(4):e008239. https://doi.org/10.1161/CIRCEP.119.008239.
375. Ye Y, Chen X, He L, Wu S, Su L, He J, et al. Left bundle branch pacing for heart failure and left bundle branch block patients with mildly reduced and preserved left ventricular ejection fraction. Can J Cardiol. 2023;39(11):1598–607. https://doi.org/10.1016/j.cjca.2023.08.034.
376. Garg A, Master V, Ellenbogen KA, Padala SK. Painful left bundle branch block syndrome successfully treated with left bundle branch area pacing. JACC Case Rep. 2020;2(4):568–71. https://doi.org/10.1016/j.jaccas.2019.11.081.
377. Mishina T, Inoue N, Morikawa S. Evaluation of right ventricular pacing-induced coronary microvascular dysfunction using guide wire-based sensor technology: a case report. Eur Heart J Case Rep. 2025;9(2) https://doi.org/10.1093/ehjcr/ytaf022.
378. Parollo M, Zucchelli G, Santoro MG, Barletta V, Paperini L, Bongiorni MG. His-bundle pacing to treat an unusual case of chest pain after pacemaker implant. J Cardiol Cases. 2022;25(5):272–4. https://doi.org/10.1016/j.jccase.2021.11.002.
379. Abdin A, Yalin K, Napp A, Gramlich M, Marx N, Schuett K. Incidence and predictors of pacemaker induced cardiomyopathy: a single-center experience. J Electrocardiol. 2019;57 https://doi.org/10.1016/j.jelectrocard.2019.08.016.
380. Chopra M, Hsieh J-C, Mueller W, Braunstein E, Beldner S, Mitra R, et al. Incidence of pacing-induced cardiomyopathy: left bundle branch area pacing versus leadless pacing. J Interv Card Electrophysiol. 2025:1–8. https://doi.org/10.1007/s10840-025-02048-1.
381. Huang W, Su L , Wu S , Xu L, Xiao F , Zhou X , Ellenbogen KA. A novel pacing strategy with low and stable output: pacing the left bundle branch immediately beyond the conduction block. Can J Cardiol. 2017;33(12):1736.e1–1736.e3. https://doi.org/10.1016/j.cjca.2017.09.013

Part II

Chapter 2
Paced Heart

Abstract Permanent right ventricular pacing with left bundle branch block (LBBB) morphology is associated with pacing-induced cardiomyopathy, and it is reversible with pacing upgrade, with the left ventricle (LV) resynchronised. It can also cause angina in the absence of epicardial coronary artery disease (ANOCA) and LV systolic dysfunction (LVSD). A 55-year-old woman with ANOCA, obesity and a right ventricle apical pacemaker with 100% pacing rate in LBBB shows how LV dyssynchrony affects coronary flow. During atrial-synchronised RV pacing, raising the heart rate from 120 to 150 bpm drives her left anterior descending (LAD) artery flow ratios down from 1.58 to 1.13, while microvascular resistance rises proportionally from 0.38 to 0.84, compared with baseline coronary haemodynamics, using continuous thermodilution. When the LV is paced directly from the septum via the LAD pressure wire as a pacing lead with an external pulse generator at 120 bpm, the LAD flow climbs 15% over that of RV pacing at the same heart rate despite a lower blood pressure and expends less vasodilatory reserve. In simple terms, RV pacing is 25% less energy efficient in generating an equivalent level coronary flow in the LAD, and LBBB causes ischaemia due to failure of coronary flow to augment to meet demand, constrained by rising resistance. It is a global phenomenon than a localised ischaemia in the LV septum—the distinction between an inefficient heart generating less coronary flow generally versus a circumscribed dyssynchronous septal compression. The former is a more compelling mechanism for LBBB-induced LVSD, especially that painful LBBB is relatively rare.

2.1 Introduction

The first chapter describes two LBBB cases, one was fixed (Chap. 1—1.8.6) and another was exercise-induced (Chap. 1—1.8.1). In both cases, although vasodilatory capacity is demonstrably intact, coronary flow fails to increase with heart rate, raising the prospect that angina in LBBB is due to supply demand mismatch even in the absence of coronary artery disease. This throws into question the oft-quoted

P. O. Lim, *Coronary Thermodilution*,
https://doi.org/10.1007/978-3-032-10734-3_2

localised ischaemia in the septum due to LV dyssynchrony. Instead, an alternative proposal involves a more generalised electromechanical inefficiency in generating coronary sufficiency. This chapter completes the triptych of LBBB, when a patient received a permanent pacemaker with the ventricular lead in RV apex, resulting in an LBBB morphology as is expected.

RV-paced LBBB is a mimic, not a true LBBB from intrinsic conduction defect; the prominent “M” in I, aVL and V1 is not seen; instead it is a single spike [1]. In addition to a superior axis with negative R-wave from inferior leads of II, III and aVF, and not the left axis deviation as usually observed. The pacing impulse starts in the RV apex, sweeping to the LV bases, which interestingly abolishes LV mid cavity or outflow tract obstruction. However, it gives rise to a small instantaneous LV to aortic gradient due to a delay in LV pressure to peak [2].

2.2 Case

A 55-year-old woman of South Asian descent was admitted with chest pain 5 years ago in the setting of 2:1 atrioventricular (AV) block (Fig. 2.1). Her coronary angiogram, echocardiogram and cardiovascular magnetic resonance (CMR) scan all showed a normal heart with unobstructed coronary arteries. Her CMR revealed an ejection fraction (EF) of 68% with an end-systolic volume index (ESVI) of 21 (14–33) mL/m^2 and stroke volume index (SVI) of 45 (37–62) mL/m^2, giving her a ventriculo-arterial coupling (VAC) of 0.47 (0.6–1.0). It also showed no left atrial (LA) dilatation, left ventricular hypertrophy (LVH), infarction, scar or fibrosis. At the time her body mass index (BMI) was 32.4 kg/m^2. Other than asthma on salbutamol and montelukast inhalers she has no other comorbidities. Lyme disease was excluded by serology.

A dual-chamber permanent pacemaker (PPM) was implanted; it was a challenging procedure with difficulty in crossing the tricuspid valve and poor sensing in the LV septum. Hence the RV apex was paced with active V lead fixation, with a 5 mV sensing, and the right atrial appendage was actively fixed with the A lead.

She described her angina as a central chest heaviness with radiation down her left arm, reproducibly precipitated by physical exercise and mental stress. Her Bruce protocol exercise stress echocardiogram 1 year post-PPM (4 years ago) when she was admitted with a troponin negative chest pain; she had to stop after 3 min and 36 s due to fatigue; HR 85 to 153 bpm (at 91% predicted maximal HR) and BP 152/88 to 164/86 mmHg. There was no evidence of inducible cardiac ischaemia on echocardiogram. Her BMI had increased to 36.4 kg/m^2. She was for the first time noted to be fully V-paced with an LBBB morphology. Four months prior, when she was reviewed in the outpatient clinic she had her own sinus rhythm with a narrow complex QRS duration of 81 ms. She was treated with ivabradine 5 mg bd and ranolazine 500 mg bd.

Her angina persisted and she was admitted again to the hospital 10 months prior to her coronary physiology study below. Her ECG showed RV pacing with LBBB

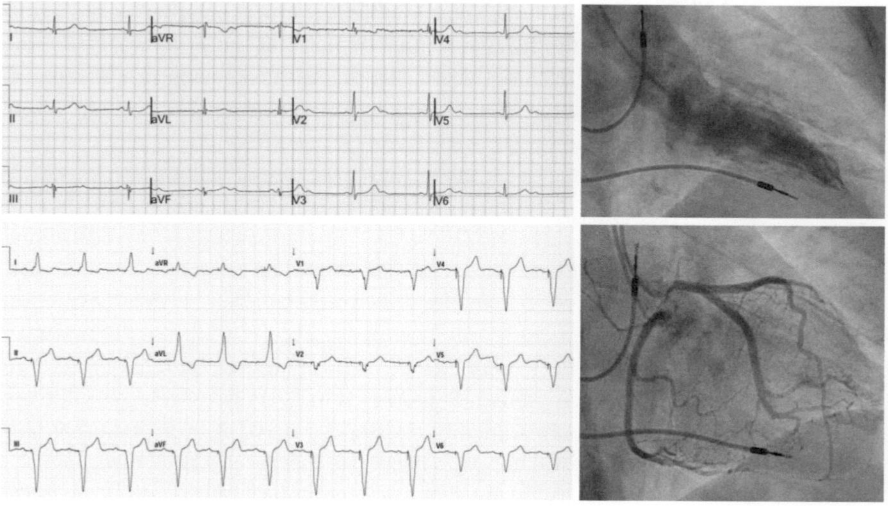

Fig. 2.1 (**Left, top and bottom panels**) ECG 5 years ago that shows 2:1 Mobitz type II atrioventricular block at 45 bpm, and intraventricular conduction defect (IVCD) due to His-Purkinje disease, with a QRS of 97 ms, early R/S transition (R > S already in V2) giving an anterior, leftward and horizontal heart, plus low-voltage complexes (especially in limb leads) to suggest obesity and abdominal adiposity; at the time her BMI was 32.4 kg/m^2. ECG at presentation to the emergency department 10 months before her coronary physiology study, A-sense and RV-paced LBBB morphology with distinct QS or rS in V1 with broad monophasic R in I and aVL with a slurred upstroke, and note that the lateral precordial V4-V6 are *predominantly negative* rather than showing the expected tall R. This, together with a superior frontal axis, indicates a pacing site low in the RV apex, directing the major depolarisation vector upward and posteriorly. There is global ST discordance (upright T where QRS negative and vice versa), the QRS duration is 171 ms. (**Right, top and bottom panels**) LV angiogram with normal LV systolic function, with the A and V leads in situ. Corresponding coronary angiogram via dual injections of right and left coronary arteries which are unobstructed

morphology, with a QRS interval of 171 ms. An updated echocardiogram revealed LV apical dyssynchrony with an appearance of hypokinesia, EF 59%, and aortic valve sclerosis with a peak gradient of 8.4 mmHg—which has developed over the years.

Procedure A bi-distal radial approach is used with 5 French sheaths. Her left ventricle (LV) is studied first. The left ventricular end-diastolic pressure (LVEDP) is elevated 15–25 mmHg with an HR of 100 bpm despite midazolam 1 mg IV. LV angiogram shows no wall motion abnormalities, EF 60% (Fig. 2.1). With the pressure wire in the LV to interrogate the LV pressure-time derivatives: maximum +dP/dt (index of contractility) is 1850 (>1200) mmHg/s, minimum –dP/dt (index of relaxation), –1932 (–1100) mmHg/s, and Weiss' Tau, τ (time constant of relaxation) 0.03 s (0.05) (Fig. 2.2). These suggest normal systolic contractility and **active** diastolic relaxation but elevated LVEDP, likely from reduced **passive** compliance. There is a 13 mmHg aortic valvular gradient which is in accord with her echocardiographic assessment.

The coronary arteries are unobstructed (Fig. 2.1). With the pressure wire in distal LAD, the distal-to-aortic pressure ratio (Pd/Pa) is 0.92–0.94. Continuous thermodilution is undertaken in the LAD. Hyperaemic flow is obtained with 20 mL/min saline infusion through the RayFlow microcatheter in the proximal LAD, the flow, Q is 204, repeated **205** mL/min, and when the saline infusion rate is reduced to 10 mL/min for basal flow, it is 115, and repeated **113** mL/min. The corresponding hyperaemic and basal resistance are 406, **413**, 795 and **739** Wood units. Hence, using the consistent duplicates as baseline and hyperaemic values, the coronary flow reserve (CFR) is 1.8 (< 2.0), microvascular resistance reserve (MRR) is 1.79 (≤ 2.1) and calculated IMR is 21 (413/20, < 25). She appears to be vasodilated at baseline, high flow and low resistance at rest. This could be related to her tachycardia of 100 bpm, at a heart rate of 70 bpm; her flow would be 30% less or 205/79 = 2.6, CFR *corrected* for tachycardia.

She is next paced via her PPM with atrial synchrony at a heart rate of 120, 140 and 150 bpm. The respective incremental increases in LAD flow from baseline are 1.58, 1.48 and 1.13, and the corresponding resistances are 0.38, 0.60 and 0.84; falling coronary flow with rising resistance as heart rate increases with RV pacing.

Finally, direct LV pacing is instituted with a unipolar configuration, negative (black, cathodal) clip at the LAD *pressure wire*, while the positive (red, anodal) clip is connected to an indifferent subcutaneous electrode (green needle inserted at the left wrist under local anaesthesia) [3, 4]. The pacing rate is at 120 bpm with 10 Volts with an external generator (Fig. 2.2)—this simulates septal pacing with ECG

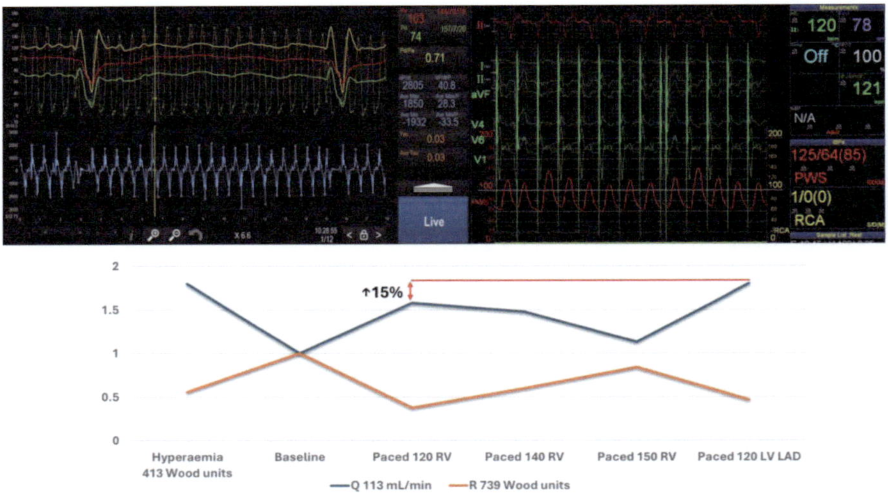

Fig. 2.2 -time (**Top, left panel**) Aorto-LV pressure and dP/dt. There is a 13 mmHg gradient due to aortic sclerosis, and the LV pressure-time derivatives, ±dP/dt suggest normal systolic and intrinsic diastolic function, but elevated LVEDP due to passive LV non-compliance, which might be related to obesity. (**Bottom**) Coronary haemodynamics in response to saline hypereamia and pacing, the low CFR or reduced vasodilatory capacity is likely caused by baseline tachycardia, but also there could be an element of obesity-related pericardial constraint, the hyperaemic resistance is mildly elevated. AV synchronised pacing is associated with rate-related decreasing flow and rising resistance (280, 443 and 619 Wood units at 120/140/150 bpm respectively). Isolated pacing of the LV at a corresponding 120 bpm is associated with 15% increase in coronary flow at the same heart rate during RV pacing. (**Top, right panel**) Pacing the LV via the LAD pressure wire, the ECG morphology changes, with tall and broad positive QRS in V6 and negative QRS in V1

reversal of morphology; QRS is upright in V6 and downward in V1. Despite loss of atrial synchrony, LAD flow increases 1.8-fold and resistance falls by 53% from baseline, whereas compared with AV synchronised RV pacing with LBBB morphology, there is an incremental increase in 15% flow, beyond the > 10% theoretical measurement error to suggest that this is a real electrophysiological finding.

Interpretation This woman with high BMI within the obesity range has unobstructed coronary arteries, normal systolic and inherent diastolic LV function, but raised LVEDP and borderline increased coronary resistance (≥ 400 Wood units) from reduced LV diastolic compliance which is likely to be obesity-related extracardiac constraint. Her high EF with low VAC would support this. Three key findings from her coronary physiology study are evident:

1. A tachycardia-induced baseline high flow and low resistance state, giving her a *functionally restricted vasodilatory capacity.*
2. While in A-sense and RV pacing with LBBB morphology, her coronary flow failed to augment with rising resistance, which means *LV dyssynchrony increases microvascular resistance.*
3. When the LV is paced directly, at an equivalent rate of 120 bpm, there is a 15% gain in coronary flow, with fractional resistance from baseline of 0.47 vs 0.38; BP 125/64 vs 140/60 mmHg. In other words, a synchronised LV is associated with increased coronary flow not through falling resistance, in contrary to a dyssynchronous LV that works harder and uses up more of its vasodilatory reserve to augment coronary flow, i.e. at HR 120 bpm; RV pace Q 179 mL/min, R 280 Wood units and SBP 140 mmHg vs LV pace Q 206 mL/min, R 346 Wood units and SBP 120 mmHg.

Using the rate-pressure product (RPP = HR·SBP) as surrogate for oxygen demand, metabolic-cost efficiency, E = Q/RPP, or flow delivered per unit RPP:

$$E_{RV} = 179/(120 \times 140) = 0.01065$$
$$E_{LV} = 206/(120 \times 120) = 0.01431$$

$$\frac{E_{LV}}{E_{RV}} = \frac{0.01431}{0.01065} \approx 1.34$$

Therefore, direct LV pacing, even without atrial synchrony, delivers 34% more coronary flow for each unit of rate-pressure product than RV pacing. The inverse is that, with RV pace, the heart needs 25% more RPP or oxygen to generate an equivalent flow. Another way to look at this is flow per unit resistance, to command the same LAD flow rate; LV pace dilates the microvasculature 7% less, leaving for a higher untapped vasodilatory reserve.

This woman's contemporaneous NT-ProBNP is 281 (< 125) pg/mL consistent with her raised LVEDP; oestradiol < 55 pmol/L, FSH 38 (> 25) IU/L and LH 33 (> 15) IU/L—in line with a postmenopausal state; and HbA1c 38 (20–41) mmol/mol, which meant that she is not diabetic despite a BMI of 35.6 kg/m^2 at the time of her procedure.

2.3 Discussion

The case illustrates a postmenopausal woman with **obesity** and likely pericardial constraint (see next chapter), with initial supranormal EF using up the end-systolic LV reserve, hence low VAC accounting for the raised LVEDP and mildly increased coronary resistance, and **RV pace with LBBB morphology** which renders the heart inefficient in augmenting coronary flow with rising metabolic demand. Her angina may have a dual mechanism working synergistically in tandem. A canine experimental model suggests that LBBB on its own does not raise LVEDP, but disproportionately elevates early diastolic pressure with high pacing rates of 120-180 bpm [5]. Conceivably, this pressure is transmitted to the lungs causing breathlessness and increases coronary resistance impeding flow. However, the raised LVEDP at rest in this report would point to a separate pathology—obesity.

Obesity is associated with AV block and conduction abnormalities; it nearly doubles the risk, but to some extent this is mediated through coronary artery disease and hypertension in the UK population [6]. This is confirmed in other populations too [7]. There are multiple reasons why this happens. Chief amongst which is direct fat infiltration of the AV node, His bundle and proximal bundle branches, and fat between the myocytes, stretches the tissue and causes pressure-induced atrophy and adverse remodelling [8]. Cells within the epicardial and perinodal adipose tissue secrete a whole host of mediators called adipokines (leptin, adiponectin, resistin/visfatin, TNF-α, IL-6, etc.) which in excess lead to inflammation, fibrosis, as well as being arrhythmogenic and interfering with normal electrical conduction. Also, obstructive sleep apnoea (OSA) is highly prevalent in obesity. Apnoeic episodes provoke surges in vagal tone and intermittent hypoxaemia; bradyarrhythmias and second-degree AV block are potentially treatable with continuous positive airway pressure (CPAP) [9].

Patients with isolated LBBB with a normal heart or mild LVSD, in a third of cases, develop heart failure within 5 years [10, 11]. Cardiac resynchronisation therapy (CRT) was initially worked out on the basis of improved cardiac work using the LV pressure-volume (PV) loop testing different pacing sites, pacing the coronary sinus; impulse activation from the lateral wall appeared to be beneficial in shifting the PV loop to the left and down and unfolding the shoulder in the systolic isovolumic contraction upstroke, thus boosting stroke work [12]. Underpinned by haemodynamic physiology, CRT in LBBB has been trialled and received ESC Class I/IIa indication for QRS $\geq$ 150/130 ms and EF $\leq$ 35%; about 10% improved their EF > 50% with CRT [13, 14]. Normalising the conduction physiology with direct pacing of the left bundle, with LBBP, can narrow QRS by 30 ms, and in some series, normalised cardiac function in half of the cohorts [15, 16]. Early indication of head-to-head HeartSync-LBBP RCT suggests that two-lead LBBP outperforms three-lead CRT [17], and other trials are in the pipeline [18].

LV dyssynchrony with LBBB morphology as a result of RV pace shares the same adverse physiology as native LBBB, with 10–20% of patients developing LVSD between 3 and 5 years [19, 20]. In a follow-up series of 55 patients with AF and pacing who underwent AV nodal ablation, therefore converted to 100% RV pace, half of the patients over 5 years developed LVSD. *This is the most direct evidence that sustained LV dyssynchrony is harmful to the heart* [21]. There is a general acceptance for this, and gradual shift away from RV pace, if practicable. In the woman described here, an attempt was made to pace the LV septum 5 years ago, but the orientation of her heart made it difficult. This might be related to her obesity, making her septum more horizontal in a rotated heart. In the setting of pacing-induced LVSD, the simplest solution, in the absence of venous occlusion, is to add a coronary sinus lead to upgrade the system to a CRT [22].

With the advent of LBBP, despite it having been described only in 2017 [23]; being a physiological pacing approach, increasingly it is permissively adopted for all-comers regardless of LV function [24–26]. Also, this drive for a high septal lead placement needed for LBBP has improved the technical skillset, making obesity no longer a barrier for procedural success [27]. As for the case described in this report, ESC guidelines recommend pacemaker upgrade if the RV pace is ≥ 20%, but the LVSD has to be at least moderate, which excludes her because she has a normal EF with 100% RV pace. She was symptomatic with angina, breathlessness and exercise intolerance. Given the high incidence of ensuing LVSD, waiting for this to happen before offering her a system upgrade appears perverse.

Angina due to RV pace is surprisingly underreported in the medical literature in contrast to deterioration in LV systolic function [28, 29]. There are three obvious reasons: 1. Most patients have low rates of pacing, 2. Many patients have concomitant coronary artery disease and 3. Lack of novelty value for publication. Parollo et al. [30] in 2022 reported a 63-year-old man who had a previous CABG, whose angina was triggered during his 10% of RV pacing periods, subsequently confirmed with a formal lab-based multisite pacing to elicit his angina. When his pacemaker was upgraded to a CRT, with the LV lead inserted into the His bundle, his angina resolved with pacing shifting from RV to LV.

It is unclear, despite the high rates of LVSD with RV pace, why pacing-induced cardiomyopathy is not more universal, even with 100% RV pace. The mechanism for LBBB-related LVSD is not yet completely clarified. But it is tempting to speculate that it could be ischaemic in nature, akin to tachycardia-induced cardiomyopathy [31]. In echocardiographic Doppler LAD studies, when the RV apex was paced, there was a reduction in flow velocities in dogs and humans [32, 33].

Mishina et al. [29] in 2025 hypothesised that angina due to RV pace might partly be related to CMD as they defined with bolus thermodilution (CFR < 2.0 and/or IMR ≥ 25). They reported a 53-year-woman with an RV pace of 15% and a QRS duration of 146 ms when paced. The coronary haemodynamics at rest in native rhythm and with unipolar RV pace at 110 bpm were LAD, CFR **2.4** vs 1.5 and IMR **19** vs 27 and RCA, CFR **3.8** vs 2.2 and IMR **30** vs 32. Thus, when she was not pacing with her own native narrow QRS of 54 ms, there was *discordance* of CFR/IMR between LAD and RCA (CMD in RCA with high CFR), and during RV pace, the IMR rose in LAD (became CMD) but not RCA (already CMD). As highlighted in the previous chapter, the up to 30% coefficient of variation with bolus thermodilution renders this technique uninterpretable, when repeated in the same artery and between artery comparisons. But the broad conclusion in Mishina et al.'s case could be that RV pace *expends the coronary vasodilatory reserve, but this does not equate CMD, instead it is normal physiology*. In contrast, with the current report, RV pace increases LAD flow at rest in the setting of baseline tachycardia, but it fails to augment it with increasing heart rate due to rising resistance, and coupled with high LVEDP related to obesity, and it causes angina despite absence of CMD. Thus, LBBB creates a vicious circle, and it reduces stress coronary flow which then depresses cardiac function, leading to LVSD which impairs coronary flow compounded by LBBB. Put simply, obesity unmasks the deleterious effect of RV-paced LBBB in this woman. Finally, the fact that LBBP normalises the LV would suggest that LVSD in LBBB is partly a global ischaemic process.

References

1. Tan NY, Witt CM, Oh JK, Cha Y-M. Left Bundle Branch Block. Circ Arrhythm Electrophysiol. 2020;13(4):e008239. https://doi.org/10.1161/CIRCEP.119.008239.
2. Bank AJ, Gage RM, Burns KV. Right ventricular pacing, mechanical dyssynchrony, and heart failure. J Cardiovasc Transl Res. 2012;5(2):219–31. https://doi.org/10.1007/s12265-011-9341-8.
3. Javid R, Wassef N, Wheatcroft SB, Tayebjee MH. Coronary guidewires in temporary cardiac pacing and assessment of myocardial viability: current perspectives and future directions. J Clin Med. 2023;12(22):6976.
4. Heinroth KM, Stabenow I, Moldenhauer I, et al. Temporary transcoronary pacing by coated guidewires. Clin Res Cardiol. 2006;95(4):206–11. https://doi.org/10.1007/s00392-006-0361-3.
5. Andersen ØS, Krogh MR, Boe E, Storsten P, Aalen JM, Larsen CK, Skulstad H, Odland HH, Smiseth OA, Remme EW. Left bundle branch block increases left ventricular diastolic pressure during tachycardia due to incomplete relaxation. J Appl Physiol. 2020;128(4):729–38. https://doi.org/10.1152/japplphysiol.01002.2018
6. Chi X, Zhang N, Zhang L, et al. Effects of body mass index and blood pressure on atrioventricular block: two-sample mendelian randomization. Heart Rhythm. 2024;21(2):174–83. https://doi.org/10.1016/j.hrthm.2023.10.024.
7. Liu H, Li X, Liu P, et al. Obesity and physical inactivity are associated with increased risks of cardiac conduction disease: a report from the Kailuan cohort study. NPJ Cardiov Health. 2024;1(1):9. https://doi.org/10.1038/s44325-024-00008-8.
8. Ernault AC, Meijborg VMF, Coronel R. Modulation of cardiac Arrhythmogenesis by Epicardial adipose tissue: JACC state-of-the-art review. J Am Coll Cardiol. 2021;78(17):1730–45. https://doi.org/10.1016/j.jacc.2021.08.037.
9. Maeno K-i, Kasai A, Setsuda M, et al. Advanced atrioventricular block induced by obstructive sleep apnea before oxygen desaturation. Heart Vessel. 2009;24(3):236–40. https://doi.org/10.1007/s00380-008-1113-2.
10. Sze E, Dunning A, Loring Z, et al. Comparison of incidence of left ventricular systolic dysfunction among patients with left bundle branch block versus those with normal QRS duration. Am J Cardiol. 2017;120(11):1990–7. https://doi.org/10.1016/j.amjcard.2017.08.003.
11. Witt CM, Wu G, Yang D, et al. Outcomes with left bundle branch block and mildly to moderately reduced left ventricular function. JACC Heart Failure. 2016;4(11):897–903. https://doi.org/10.1016/j.jchf.2016.07.002.
12. Delnoy PPHM, Ottervanger JP, Oude Luttikhuis H, et al. Pressure–volume loop analysis during implantation of biventricular pacemaker/cardiac resynchronization therapy device to

optimize right and left ventricular pacing sites. Eur Heart J. 2009;30(7):797–804. https://doi.org/10.1093/eurheartj/ehp011.
13. de Vere F, Wijesuriya N, Howell S, et al. Optimizing outcomes from cardiac resynchronization therapy: what do recent data and insights say? Expert Rev Cardiovasc Ther. 2024;22(12):663–80. https://doi.org/10.1080/14779072.2024.2445246.
14. Schiavone M, Arosio R, Valenza S, et al. Cardiac resynchronization therapy: present and future. Eur Heart J Suppl. 2023;25(Supplement_C):C227–C33. https://doi.org/10.1093/eurheartjsupp/suad046.
15. Vijayaraman P, Sharma PS, Cano Ó, et al. Comparison of left bundle branch area pacing and biventricular pacing in candidates for resynchronization therapy. JACC. 2023;82(3):228–41. https://doi.org/10.1016/j.jacc.2023.05.006.
16. Li X, Qiu C, Xie R, et al. Left bundle branch area pacing delivery of cardiac resynchronization therapy and comparison with biventricular pacing. ESC Heart Failure. 2020;7(4):1711–22. https://doi.org/10.1002/ehf2.12731.
17. Chen X, Zhang L, Xu W, Huang J, Dong M, editors. HeartSync-LBBP trial interim results: left bundle branch pacing versus biventricular pacing in chronic systolic heart failure with left bundle branch block. European Heart Rhythm Association Congress (EHRA) 2025, Late-Breaking Science Session. Vienna, Austria; 2025
18. Wang Y, Zhu H, Hou X, et al. Randomized trial of left bundle branch vs biventricular pacing for cardiac resynchronization therapy. JACC. 2022;80(13):1205–16. https://doi.org/10.1016/j.jacc.2022.07.019.
19. Kiehl EL, Makki T, Kumar R, et al. Incidence and predictors of right ventricular pacing-induced cardiomyopathy in patients with complete atrioventricular block and preserved left ventricular systolic function. Heart Rhythm. 2016;13(12):2272–8. https://doi.org/10.1016/j.hrthm.2016.09.027.
20. Somma V, Ha FJ, Palmer S, Mohamed U, Agarwal S. Pacing-induced cardiomyopathy: a systematic review and meta-analysis of definition, prevalence, risk factors, and management. Heart Rhythm. 2023;20(2):282–90. https://doi.org/10.1016/j.hrthm.2022.09.019.
21. Tops LF, Schalij MJ, Holman ER, et al. Right ventricular pacing can induce ventricular Dyssynchrony in patients with atrial fibrillation after atrioventricular node ablation. J Am Coll Cardiol. 2006;48(8):1642–8. https://doi.org/10.1016/j.jacc.2006.05.072.
22. Kaza N, Htun V, Miyazawa A, et al. Upgrading right ventricular pacemakers to biventricular pacing or conduction system pacing: a systematic review and meta-analysis. EP Europace. 2022;25(3):1077–86. https://doi.org/10.1093/europace/euac188.
23. Huang W, Su L, Wu S, et al. A novel pacing strategy with low and stable output: pacing the left bundle branch immediately beyond the conduction block. Can J Cardiol. 2017;33(12):1736. https://doi.org/10.1016/j.cjca.2017.09.013.
24. Ye Y, Chen X, He L, et al. Left bundle branch pacing for heart failure and left bundle branch block patients with mildly reduced and preserved left ventricular ejection fraction. Can J Cardiol. 2023;39(11):1598–607. https://doi.org/10.1016/j.cjca.2023.08.034.
25. Yu GI, Kim TH, Cho YH, et al. Left bundle branch area pacing in mildly reduced heart failure: a systematic literature review and meta-analysis. Clin Cardiol. 2023;46(7):713–20. https://doi.org/10.1002/clc.24028.
26. Zeng J, He C, Zou F, et al. Early left bundle branch pacing in heart failure with mildly reduced ejection fraction and left bundle branch block. Heart Rhythm. 2023;20(10):1436–44. https://doi.org/10.1016/j.hrthm.2023.07.063.
27. Jastrzębski M, Kiełbasa G, Cano O, et al. Left bundle branch area pacing outcomes: the multicentre European MELOS study. Eur Heart J. 2022;43(40):4161–73. https://doi.org/10.1093/eurheartj/ehac445.
28. Patel AK, Yap VU, Thomsen JH. Adverse effects of right ventricular pacing in a patient with aortic stenosis, hemodynamic documentation and management. Chest. 1977;72(1):103–5. https://doi.org/10.1378/chest.72.1.103.

29. Mishina T, Inoue N, Morikawa S. Evaluation of right ventricular pacing-induced coronary microvascular dysfunction using guide wire-based sensor technology: a case report. Eur Heart J Case Rep. 2025;9(2). https://doi.org/10.1093/ehjcr/ytaf022.
30. Parollo M, Zucchelli G, Santoro MG, et al. His-bundle pacing to treat an unusual case of chest pain after pacemaker implant. J Cardiol Cases. 2022;25(5):272–4. https://doi.org/10.1016/j.jccase.2021.11.002.
31. Kim DY, Kim SH, Ryu K-H. Tachycardia induced cardiomyopathy. Korean Circ J. 2019;49(9):808–17. https://doi.org/10.4070/kcj.2019.0199.
32. Fang F, Jin Z-N, Li H-Y, et al. Left anterior descending coronary artery flow impaired by right ventricular apical pacing: the role of systolic dyssynchrony. Int J Cardiol. 2014;176(1):80–5. https://doi.org/10.1016/j.ijcard.2014.06.037.
33. Lu J, Li W, Fu Y, et al. Hemodynamic changes in left anterior descending coronary artery and anterior interventricular vein during right ventricular apical pacing: a Doppler ultrasound study in open chest beagles. PLoS One. 2013;8(6):e67196. https://doi.org/10.1371/journal.pone.0067196.

Chapter 3
Constraint Heart

Abstract Angina with non-obstructive coronary arteries (ANOCA) predominates in women, believed to be due to (1) vasoreactivity, especially that of the microvasculature and (2) flow autoregulatory failure from restricted or expended microvascular vasodilatory reserve. As yet these classifications have not yielded a homogeneous grouping with predictable outcome to drug therapy. Most of these women have a structurally and functionally normal heart on imaging studies, which begs the question—could their angina be due to extracardiac factors? This chapter describes six women with tentative polycystic ovary syndrome (PCOS) background and angina. They appeared to share either in part or in total, features of left ventricular and coronary haemodynamics, which are potentially generalisable; a triad of (1) raised left ventricular end-diastolic pressure (LVEDP) and coronary resistance, (2) reduced or expended vasodilatory reserve, and (3) microvascular reactivity, which are consistent with the diagnosis of coronary microvascular dysfunction (CMD). However, what is usually regarded as isolated microvascular spasm to acetylcholine-provocation does not automatically translate to responsiveness to calcium channel blockers and nitrates. Thus, raising the prospect that the dramatic findings in the cardiac catheter laboratory, characterised by slowing of coronary flow, chest pain and ECG changes; though clearly pathological, counterintuitively may in fact not vasospastic in nature, but to a greater extent due to subendocardial extravascular compression of the microvasculature, which could be the hitherto underrecognised, but postulated underlying mechanism of ANOCA.

3.1 Introduction

Angina is due to a mismatch of fuel supply to and energy demand from the heart. Adenosine, a metabolic by-product, activating the A_1 receptor triggers the mental perception of angina, travelling up sympathetic afferents via the spinal cord and separately along the vagus nerve, but it has a short half-life of about 10 s [1]. Therefore, it does not linger as a metabolite. In contrast, in women with a structurally normal heart and unobstructed coronary arteries, the angina has a lingering quality, which often lasts

P. O. Lim, *Coronary Thermodilution*,
https://doi.org/10.1007/978-3-032-10734-3_3

over 30 min, long after any trigger has passed, first described nearly 60 years ago [2, 3]. And they generally do not immediately, partially or not at all, responsive to nitrates (GTN) [4–6], neither to L-type calcium channel blockers [7–10], nor to selective endothelin-1 inhibitors [11, 12], or exhibit a consistent response to fasudil, an inhibitor of cytosolic Rho kinase (ROCK) that prevents phosphorylation and calcium-sensitisation of the myosin light chain in vascular smooth muscle cells (VSMCs) [13]. Since all these known vasospastic and mechanistic pathways are exhaustively tested, there must be a persistent ischaemic process that is slow to resolve. This must be mechanical in nature; could it be the myocardial interstitial milieu, once disrupted, that takes time to re-equilibrate? Has it something to do with vascular endothelial dysfunction cascade that leads to increased capillary permeability between endothelial cell junctions?

In practice, there are three modes by which angina can occur; epicardial coronary artery disease, epicardial and/or microvascular spasm, and vasodilatory restriction [14]. In premenopausal women, in the absence of coronary risk factors, such as smoking, diabetes, hypercholesterolaemia and hypertension; oestrogen maintains a healthy vascular endothelium, preventing coronary atherosclerosis and epicardial vasospasm [15]. Coronary microvascular spasm that is provoked by acetylcholine in the cardiac catheter laboratory, first reported by Mohri et al. in 1998 [9, 16–19], can still occur, but this is should episodic, a more predictable effort-related angina implies impairment of coronary autoregulation—could this be due extracardiac compression [20, 21]?

3.2 Cases

3.2.1 Cardiac Standstill

A 32-year-old Caucasian woman with three hospitalisations for troponin negative chest pain over a two-year period was admitted for a one-stop coronary angiogram and physiology study. Her chest pain was mostly postprandial in the evening, sharp and dull, lasting for hours. For this reason she had a gastroscopy that found a hiatus hernia with antral gastritis, but omeprazole, a proton pump inhibitor, had not helped. She has polycystic ovary syndrome (PCOS), on metformin 500 mg once a day, and hypothyroidism on thyroxine 50 μg once a day, with a body mass index (BMI) of 38 (≥ 30) kg/m^2.

Her exercise stress echocardiogram (ESE) with contrast that was performed 6 months earlier showed a structurally and functionally normal heart with an ejection fraction (EF) of 65%. She was able to exercise for *10 min* on the Bruce protocol treadmill test with normal haemodynamics, rest and peak heart rate (HR) and blood pressure (BP); 90 to 180 bpm (95% predicted, 220-age), and 116/67 to 180/90 mmHg. She stopped exercising because of fatigue and exhibited no electrocardiographic, neither echocardiographic evidence of cardiac ischaemia. On apical 4 chamber view of her left ventricle, her body-surface-indexed end-systolic volume (ESVI) was 15 mL/m^2 and stroke volume index (SVI) was 39 mL/m^2; thus ventriculo-arterial coupling (VAC) was low at 0.38 (0.6–1.0).

Procedure This is undertaken via the right distal radial artery with a 4 Fr system, upsizing to a 5Fr EBU3.5 guide inserted sheathlessly, using a 4 Fr MPA2 catheter as a railroad-introducer, following midazolam 0.5 mg for sedation. As expected, her coronary arteries are disease-free, and her left ventricular angiogram shows no wall motion abnormalities. Bolus thermodilution is carried out in the left anterior descending (LAD) artery. With the pressure wire in distal LAD, the distal-to-aortic pressure ratio (Pd/Pa) is 0.95, and rest full-cycle ratio (RFR) is 0.93 (> 0.89), suggesting no flow limitation.

With intravenous adenosine given at 140 μg/kg/min over 1 min (HR 110 to 120 bpm), the fractional flow reserve (FFR) is 0.92 (> 0.80), coronary flow reserve (CFR) 1.6, index of microvascular resistance (IMR) 11, and microvascular resistance reserve (MRR) 1.6. Acetylcholine (ACh) 2 μg is associated with slowing of flow (Fig. 3.1). Bolus thermodilution is repeated after ACh 20 μg, flow (CFR) fractionally falls to 0.7 or 30% reduction, and IMR rose to 37, with further slowing of flow. With ACh 100 μg, her flow ceases and she goes into ventricular standstill. Fortunately, intracoronary nitroglycerine (GTN) 200 μg reverses the no reflow within 20 seconds. Repeat coronary angiogram shows no left main coronary dissection.

Her cardiovascular magnetic resonance (CMR) scan one month later showed no structural or functional abnormalities, EF 61%, other than a low SVI 39 (43–67) mL/m^2, VAC 0.64 (0.6–1.0); repeated 9 months later with adenosine stress perfusion given at 140 μg/kg/min for 3 min (HR 85 to 117 bpm without a change in BP 125/87 mmHg)—EF 59% with low SVI 35 (43–67) mL/m^2, VAC 0.69 (0.6–1.0); first-pass stress perfusion imaging revealed *mild circumferential subendocardial delay in contrast washout in all left ventricular levels*, consistent with coronary microvascular dysfunction (CMD). Her ESE was repeated 28 months from her coronary physiology, and she lost 7 kg in weight, bringing her BMI down to 35 kg/m^2. She was able to complete *12 min* of Bruce protocol treadmill exercise and had stopped because of fatigue, again with normal haemodynamics; rest HR and peak BP; 90 to 176 bpm (95% predicted), and 129/85 to 174/96 mmHg—without demonstrable

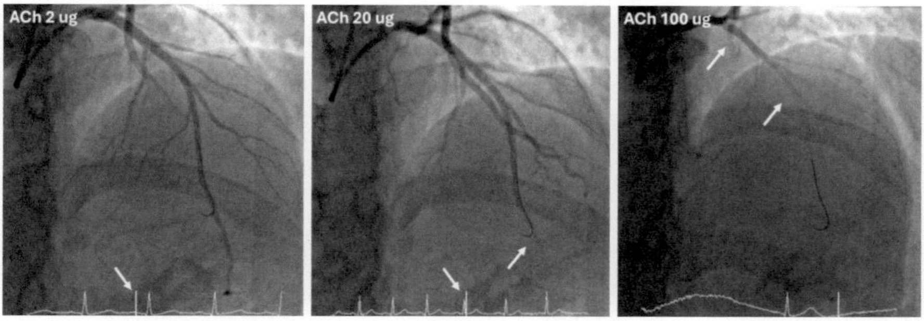

Fig. 3.1 **(Left to right panels)** Unobstructed coronary arteries, acetylcholine (ACh) 2 μg slows flow down the left anterior descending (LAD) artery, reaching the left ventricular apex at about two heart beats (*arrow*), with ACh 20 μg; the LAD flow does not reach the apex after 3 heart beats (*arrows*), and ACh 100 μg causes "no reflow" from intense microvascular spasm (*arrows*) and ventricular standstill, rapidly reversible with intracoronary nitroglycerine

electrocardiographic, nor echocardiographic cardiac ischaemia; EF 62%, VAC 0.62 (0.6–1.0). Her angina has reduced in frequency on low-dose diltiazem 90 mg once a day.

Interpretation This young woman with PCOS, who is overweight, has no diabetes, but she has ACh-induced microvascular vasospasm, without reduction in her functional capacity, although losing weight appears to increase her exercise tolerance by 2 min on treadmill. The only consistent but subtle echocardiogram and CMR feature is the low VAC; whether there is an element of pericardial constraint, she increases her stroke volume through depleting her left ventricular end-systolic volumetric reserve.

Her low CFR suggests expended vasodilatory capacity, in the context of low IMR, i.e. functional coronary microvascular dysfunction (CMD). In other words, she is vasodilated at baseline and has high basal flow. Working backward and converting IMR of 11 x 20 to 220 Wood units of hyperaemic minimal resistance using Ohm's equation, hyperaemic flow = Pd/Resistance—(76/220)X1000 = 345 ml/min; divided it by a CFR of 1.6 gives a resting flow of 230 ml/min which is 2–3 times the expected normal basal flow rate. Since bolus thermodilution is known to overestimate flow, this conceivably could be taken as that she is in a high flow and low resistance state at baseline. This would be categorised as *functional CMD* (CFR 1.6 and IMR 11; also see case 2 in Chap. 9) and ACh in her case at low dose of 20 µg causes significant coronary flow slowing and reduction of 30% (CFR 0.7 and IMR 37) from baseline due to *isolated microvascular spasm*. It is important to note that losing 8% of her body weight over three years boosted her exercise tolerance.

3.2.2 *Stiff Heart*

A 44-year-old South Asian nulliparous woman complained of exertional angina and breathlessness, associated with a cough. She has a strong family history of premature coronary artery disease—her two brothers and both parents had coronary artery disease before 50. Her untreated cholesterol was only mildly elevated, not quite at a familial hypercholestrolaemic level; LDL cholesterol 2.78 (< 3.0) mmol/L and total cholesterol 5.3 (< 5.0) mmol/L. The rest of her biochemistry and hormonal profile were normal, including blood counts, electrolytes and thyroid function; oestradiol at 404 (> 92) pmol/L, N-terminal pro-B-type natriuretic peptide, NT-ProBNP < 50 (< 125) pg/mL, and C-reactive protein, CRP 16 (< 3) mg/L. She is a non-smoker, has no hypertension, nor diabetes. Nevertheless, she has a whole host of health challenges; polycystic ovary syndrome (PCOS), uterine fibroids, endometriosis, adenomyosis, vitamin D deficiency, osteopenia, erosive gastritis, recurrent helicobacter pylori infection, hiatus hernia, fibromyalgia and chronic fatigue syndrome.

She repeatedly presented to the emergency department with troponin-negative chest pain over the years; last time was 14 months ago, and she was referred to the cardiology clinic for assessment. She was previously extensively investigated, and her CT coronary angiogram 7 years prior was normal, which was organised by the rapid access chest pain clinic. Her dobutamine stress echocardiogram the following year when she was 37, with an adequate heart rate response of 85% age-predicted (76 to 156 bpm), she was symptom-free during the test, there were no electrocardiographic changes of note, and no demonstrable echocardiographic ischaemia; her EF rose from 60 to 80% at peak heart rate. Her heart was structurally normal.

Eight months ago, she had a repeat stress echocardiogram, this time with a treadmill test. She was able to exercise for *9 min* on the Bruce protocol. Her HR response was 67 to 160 bpm, thus achieving 90% predicted maximum HR for her age, and her BP at rest was 128/81 mmHg, rising to 150/81 mmHg at peak exercise. She stopped exercising because of fatigue and there was no electrocardiographic nor echocardiographic evidence of inducible cardiac ischaemia. Her baseline EF was 66.7%. She has no LVH, LV mass index (LVMI) 62 (44–88) g/m^2, apical 4-chamber left atrial volume index (LAVI) 25.8 (16–34) ml/m^2, average E/e' 7.28 (< 8), and ventriculo-arterial coupling (VAC = end systolic volume index, ESVI/SVI, stroke volume index) was 0.51 (0.6–1.0). She has gained 8 kg in weight between the two stress echocardiograms to 74 kg giving her a body mass index (BM) of 32 (≥ 30) kg/m^2; this was also reflected in her electrocardiograms over the period (Fig. 3.2).

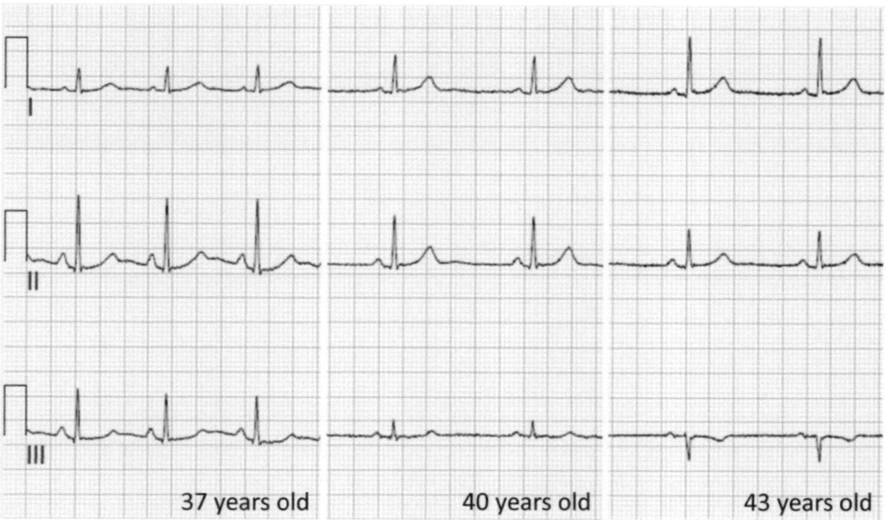

Fig. 3.2 -wave (**Left to right panels**) Note the increase in R in lead I, whereas it becomes S with T-wave inversion in lead III over time, suggesting that weight gain through abdominal visceral adiposity and diaphragmatic elevation has lifted the base of the heart, rotating it counterclockwise along the QRS axis from 71° to 47° and then to 11° to become more horizontal. As the P-wave axis has 70°, 58° and 51°, the size of atrial P in lead III diminishes with the ST concavity of atrial repolarisation

Procedure Her coronary arteries are unobstructed (Fig. 3.3) and LV angiogram reveals no wall motion abnormalities. The left ventricular end-diastolic pressure (LVEDP) is over 15 mmHg without central aortic hypertension, at 130/70 mmHg. Continuous thermodilution is undertaken in the LAD. The respective basal and hyperaemic indices are flow 75, 164 ml/L, and resistance 1356, 546 Wood units. Therefore, the coronary flow reserve, CFR, is 2.1, and microvascular resistance reserve, MRR, is 2.5. Escalating doses of ACh (2, 20, 100 μg) are given with reduction in flow, fractionally from baseline—0.64, 0.69 and 0.72, associated with dropped heart beats and transient peaking of T, as well as ST depression in anteroseptal leads associated with angina.

Importantly, no epicardial vasospasm is seen suggesting isolated ACh-provoked microvascular spasm. Verapamil 1 mg is given; this returns flow to baseline, and a second dose is given, increasing flow by 15% from baseline. ACh 100 μg is given as a rechallenge and the flow falls by 10% from baseline with symptoms. Finally, nitroglycerine (GTN) 200 μg is given without improvement in flow that is reduced by ACh. This is repeated and flow rises by 20% above baseline.

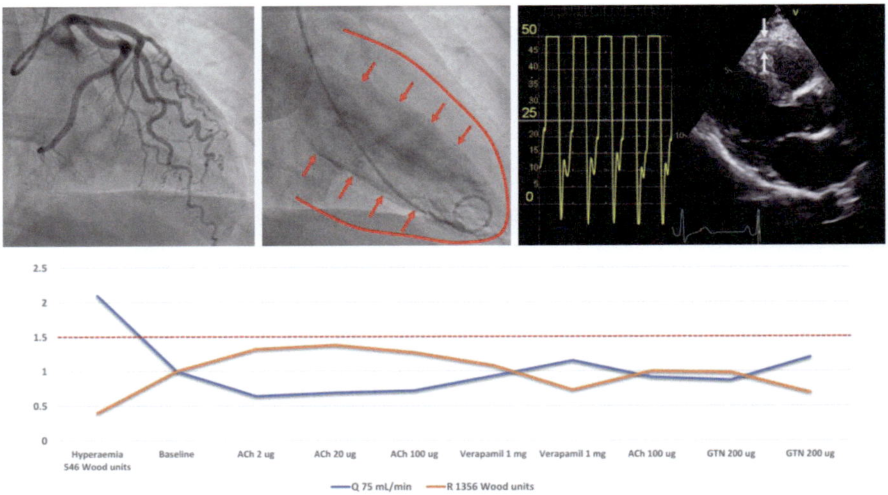

Fig. 3.3 (**Top, left to right panels**) Unobstructed coronary arteries, with the pressure wire in distal left anterior descending (LAD) artery; the distal-to-aortic pressure ratio, Pd/Pa, is 0.95 and rest full-cycle ratio, RFR, is 0.93 (> 0.89). The left ventricular angiogram reveals normal contractility, but the left ventricular end-diastolic pressure, LVEDP, is consistently over 15 mmHg, averaging at about 20 mmHg. Echocardiographic measurement of epicardial adipose tissue (EAT), which is 10 (> 7) mm. (**Bottom panel**) The vasodilatory range is restricted at hyperaemia with a coronary flow reserve, CFR, of 2.1. Acetylcholine at increasing doses is associated with flow reduction and rising resistance, in the absence of epicardial vasospasm, suggesting microvascular spasm, especially that peaking of anteroseptal T occurs with angina. Interestingly her response to verapamil and GTN is limited

Interpretation This premenopausal woman has angina and breathlessness despite a structurally normal heart on echocardiogram, without objective ischaemia demonstrable both by dobutamine 7 years ago and by exercise more recently. There are however 3 interesting subtle echocardiographic features, 1. EF > 65%, 2. VAC < 0.5, and epicardial adipose tissue (EAT) thickness > 7 mm. However, her NT-ProBNP is not elevated. Otherwise, she would fulfil the diagnosis of heart failure with supranormal ejection fraction, HFsnEF. It may be that she is at an early spectrum of the disease process, without sustained LVEDP elevation, or her obesity masks the NT-ProBNP rise via increased clearance by adipose tissue, reduced production through altered myocardial stress response, or dissipated in an expanded blood volume.

She has *restricted coronary vasodilatory range* (CFR 2.1), *raised hyperaemic resistance* (546 Wood units) and ACh-provoked isolated *microvascular spasm* without attendant epicardial vasospasm; **verapamil and GTN responses are blunted**. ACh rechallenge after verapamil does not stop her angina. All in all, from the coronary physiology point of view, she has a structurally stiff heart, akin to *pericardial constraint*—high LVEDP and low VAC—her stroke volume is maintained by depleting the contractile reserve with lower "residual" left ventricular end systolic volume.

3.2.3 Vaping

A 24-year-old Caucasian woman complained of exertional chest pain, located centrally with radiation down her left breast, occasionally occurring at rest, and sometimes with an emotional trigger. She has had multiple hospitalisations with her chest pain, which were all troponin negative. Her dobutamine stress echocardiogram and CT coronary angiogram were normal. She is a non-smoker, but she vapes, and has had a deep vein thrombosis followed by pulmonary embolism after a knee surgery 7 years previously, treated with subcutaneous heparin. She was diagnosed with PCOS in her teenage years, and this was revisited a couple of a years ago, and confirmed with an abdominal ultrasound as part of an investigation for irregular periods. For her PCOS, she takes metformin 500 mg once a day and has antidepressant-induced hyperprolactinaemia. She has a BMI of 37 ($\geq$ 30) kg/m^2.

Procedure She has unobstructed coronary arteries, and continuous thermodilution is undertaken to her LAD. With the pressure wire in distal LAD, the Pd/Pa is 0.96. The following basal and hyperaemic indices are obtained; flow 80 and 240 mL/min, and resistance 1090 and 322 Wood units—CFR 3.0 and MRR 3.4. ACh 2 μg induces mild epicardial vasospasm without significant change in flow from baseline, fractionally at 1.04 (Fig. 3.4). With ACh 20 μg, she develops significant and diffuse mid to distal LAD vasospasm associated with chest pain, but flow actually increases by 60%. *Verapamil 1 mg reverses the LAD vasospasm* with similar level of increase in flow, as with ACh 20 μg. When rechallenged with ACh 20 μg, the previously noted epicardial vasospasm is attenuated, and flow doubles.

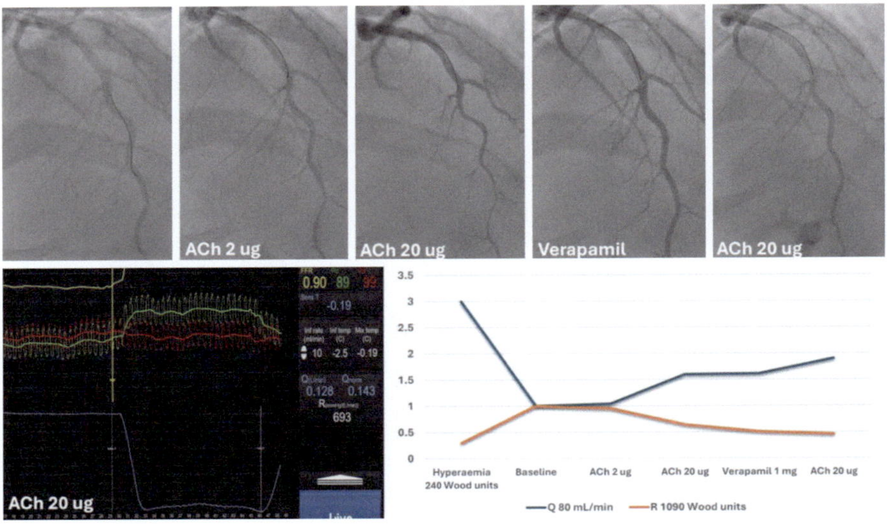

Fig. 3.4 (Top, left to right panels) Unobstructed left anterior descending (LAD) artery with dose-dependent acetylcholine (ACh) induced mid to distal vasospasm that is ameliorated by verapamil pre-treatment. **(Bottom, left to right panels)** Continuous thermodilution following ACh 20 μg, even though there is significant LAD vasospasm, the competent microvasculature with intact endothelial function raises flow in response to ACh, showing a discordant response to ACh, and the chart plots her haemodynamic indices in response to hyperaemia and drugs

Interpretation This young woman has preserved vasodilatory capacity with normal microvascular resistance and endothelial function, but she has *ACh-induced LAD vasospasm*, which is dose dependent, and it is amelioratable by verapamil pre-treatment, which facilitates flow increase with ACh. Put in another way, ACh-provoked diffuse epicardial vasospasm blunts ACh-induced microvascular vasodilation, i.e. differential ACh effect between epicardial coronary artery and the microvasculature. This woman therefore has quintessential epicardial endothelial dysfunction which is an unusual finding in a young premenopausal woman, but it is likely related to nicotine exposure from vaping and her PCOS.

3.2.4 Pericardial Effusion

A 62-year-old South Asian woman with exertional angina and breathlessness has a structurally and functionally normal heart on dobutamine stress echocardiogram, as well as on perfusion CMR. She however has a small rim of chronic and persistent circumferential pericardial effusion measuring 0.5 cm, without overt features of constriction, but averaged E/e’ of 8.24 (< 8), suggesting LV diastolic dysfunction. She is a non-smoker, has no hypertension, nor diabetes, but is treated for hyperlipidaemia, and has had PCOS plus endometriosis in her 20s—currently on oestrogen replacement therapy and is not overweight, with a BMI of 22 kg/m². In addition, she has 3 cm hiatus hernia proven on gastroscopy, and this is treated with a proton pump inhibitor; she has mild kidney dysfunction with an eGFR of 41 (> 60) mL/min/1.73 m² and Raynaud's disease with long-standing hypochromic and microcytic anaemia, managed with iron infusions. Her NT-ProBNP was elevated at 230 (< 125) pg/mL as was her CRP over the last 2 years, 51–311 (< 10) mg/L.

Procedure In view of her Raynaud's disease, the coronary physiology is undertaken via the right femoral approach with a 4 French sheath, upsizing sheathlessly to a 5 French EBU3.5 for left coronary artery cannulation. Her central aortic BP is 100/70 mmHg and LVEDP 10 mmHg, not rising with handgrip. She has unobstructed coronary arteries, and continuous thermodilution is performed on the LAD (Fig. 3.5). With the pressure wire in the distal LAD, the Pd/Pa is 0.95 and RFR is 0.92 (> 0.89), confirming no epicardial flow limitation.

The respective basal and hyperaemic indices are flow 50 and 90 mL/min, and 1689 and 837 Wood units—CFR 1.8 and MRR 2.0. Escalating ACh (2, 20 and 100 μg) doses are associated with initial flow reduction, but the flow increases as coronary slow flow phenomenon (CSFP) becomes more obvious, culminating with chest pain, ST elevation and hypotension half-way through the ACh 200 μg

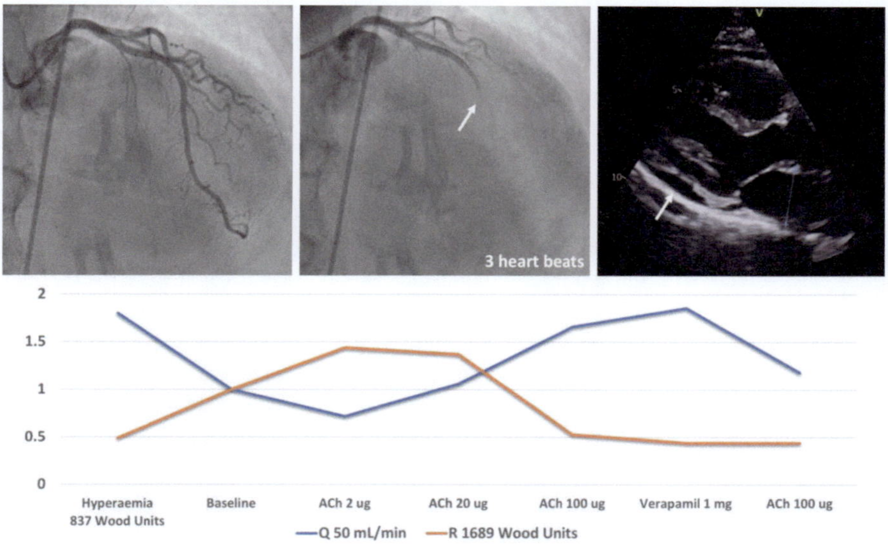

Fig. 3.5 **(Top, left to right panels)** Unobstructed left anterior descending (LAD) artery and symptomatic coronary slow flow phenomenon (CSFP) with acetylcholine (ACh) 100 μg rechallenge, even after verapamil 1 mg pre-treatment—the *arrow* shows flow in mid LAD after 3 heart beats. The echocardiogram shows the rim of pericardial effusion (*arrow*). **(Bottom panel)** Continuous thermodilution chart plots the haemodynamic indices in response to hyperaemia and drugs. Note the reduced vasodilatory range and high coronary resistance both at rest and during hyperaemia, with a biphasic flow response to increasing doses of ACh. Interestingly, verapamil pre-treatment does not overcome the ACh-provoked microvascular spasm

slow IC bolus. She is given nitroglycerine 200 μg, followed by pre-treatment with verapamil 1 mg, which did not alter the deleterious ACh 100 μg rechallenge.

Interpretation This postmenopausal woman on oestrogen replacement therapy, with remote PCOS history, who is lean, has unobstructed coronary arteries and a normal heart but exhibits restricted vasodilatory capacity, raised coronary resistance, and discordantly, preserved epicardial and biphasic microvascular endothelial function. She has clear-cut *ACh-provoked microvascular spasm* **resistant to verapamil pre-treatment** and *CMD* (CFR 1.8, hyperaemic resistance 837 Wood units). This may be due in part to pericardial effusion (raised NT-ProBNP but low BP and LVEDP during the procedure) and a yet undefined systemic inflammatory condition (persistently raised CRP).

3.2.5 Bariatric Surgery

A 64-year-old woman of South Asian origin has chest pain after eating. She has had PCOS since she was 15; her obesity is complicated by diabetes with neuropathy and nephropathy, managed with gastric bypass and insulin. She unfortunately develops dumping syndrome, requiring frequent small meals. Her BMI is now 30 (< 30) kg/m^2. She has no hypertension, nor hyperlipidaemia, but suffers from fibromyalgia treated with buprenorphine patch. Her dobutamine stress echocardiogram performed 6 months previously showed a structurally and functionally normal heart with an EF of 60%, rising to 80% at peak stress, HR at 87% (75 to 136 bpm) predicted, with controlled BP (137/90 to 140/76 mmHg), and a VAC of 0.61 (0.6–1.0).

Procedure As expected, she has unobstructed coronary arteries (Fig. 3.6) and her LV has normal contractility without wall motion abnormalities, LVEDP 10 mmHg, not rising with handgrip and central aortic BP 120/80 mmHg. Bolus thermodilution is initially undertaken, with intracoronary adenosine 200 μg; the FFR is 0.92, CFR 4.7 and IMR 9. For confirmation of these normal values, continuous thermodilution is next carried out, and the basal and hyperaemic indices are as follows: flow 82 and 202 ml/min, and resistance 1109 and 382 Wood units—CFR 2.5 and MRR 2.9. These are normal values. Increasing doses of ACh are given. For the 3 doses of 2, 20 and 100 μg, these are associated with flow hovering at or under the basal level, but with 200 μg, she develops CSFP and pain despite increase in flow by 57%. Pre-treatment with verapamil 1 mg does not prevent the CSFP with ACh rechallenge, instead paradoxically abolishes the earlier ACh-related flow augmentation.

Interpretation Interestingly, this lady with PCOS associated with multiple comorbidities has a normal heart, bar-isolated *microvascular spasm* with high-dose ACh; whether this is the cause of her postprandial chest pain is unclear. Importantly, verapamil does appear to be effective under the circumstance.

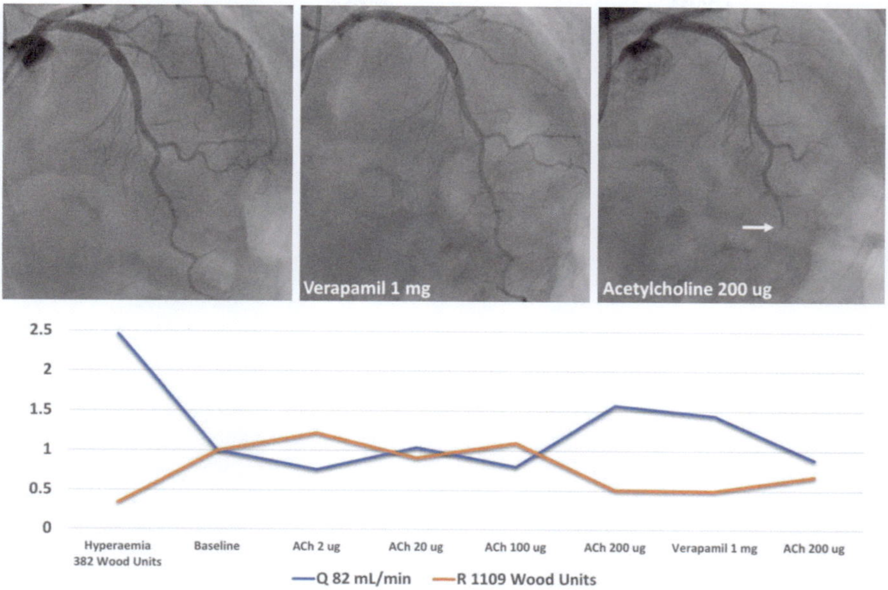

Fig. 3.6 **(Top, left to right panels**) Unobstructed left anterior descending (LAD) artery, and symptomatic coronary slow flow phenomenon (CSFP) with acetylcholine (ACh) 200 μg rechallenge, even after verapamil 1 mg pre-treatment—the *arrow* shows flow in mid LAD after 3 heart beats. **(Bottom panel**) Continuous thermodilution chart plots the haemodynamic indices in response to hyperaemia and drugs. Note the preserved vasodilatory range and normal coronary resistance both at rest and during hyperaemia, with a blunted or reduced flow response to increasing doses of ACh, culminating with chest pain and CSFP with ACh 200 μg. Interestingly, verapamil pre-treatment does not overcome the ACh-provoked microvascular spasm

3.2.6 Constraint Heart

A 64-year old Caucasian woman complained of an exertional angina which she had for four months and was typical in description—which did not occur at rest or at night; at the time she was assessed in the rapid access chest pain clinic seven months previously. She is overweight, with a BMI of 32 (≥ 30) kg/m^2, has hypothyroidism, gastro-oesophageal reflux disease and hyperlipidaemia. When she was 35, she attempted IVF for pregnancy and had two ovarian cysts removed, followed by abdominal endometrial ablation for endometriosis. Because of menopausal symptoms, she was started on Evorel Conti 50 (Oestradiol hemihydrate 50 μg and Norethisterone acetate 170 μg) patches x2/week from the age of 57.

She had a diagnostic coronary angiogram three weeks later that showed unobstructed coronary arteries with a degree of CSFP noted. She was prescribed nebivolol 2.5 mg, which has improved her angina. Both her echocardiogram and treadmill exercise were performed the following two months. The former showed a normal heart, EF 69%, and

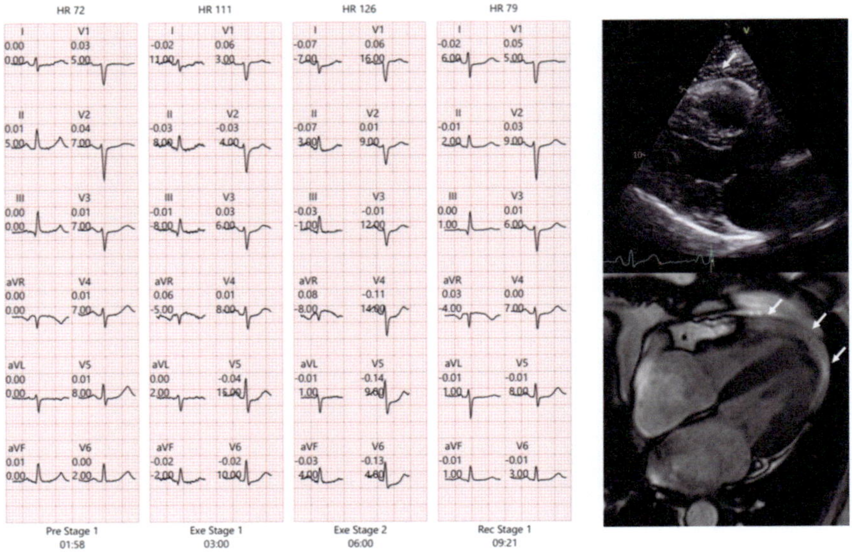

Fig. 3.7 (**Left panel**) Bruce protocol treadmill test that shows exercise-induced lateral V4–6 ST depression. (**Right, upper and lower panels**) Parasternal long-axis view of echocardiogram, at end-systole, epicardial adipose tissue (EAT) as highlighted by the *arrow*. CMR in four-chamber view showing that the LV apex is capped with epicardial adipose tissue (EAT), pointed by the *arrows*

the latter; she stopped the Bruce protocol treadmill exercise after *8 min* and 16 s at 104% maximal predicted HR, because of chest pain and light-headedness; HR 78 to 164 bpm and BP 124/68 to 154/58 mmHg; there was lateral ST depression from Stage II (Fig. 3.7).

A week later she had her perfusion CMR which also found a normal heart with a supranormal EF of 67% (> 65%), without LA dilatation, LVH, fibrosis, infarction or inducible ischaemia detected; ESVI 21 (13–31) mL/m^2, SVI 43 (36–60) mL/m^2 and VAC 0.49 (0.6–1.0).

Procedure Her distal left radial artery with a 5 French system is used to access her LV (Fig. 3.8). Resting central aortic systolic BP is 140 mmHg, LVEDP 22 mmHg; with handgrip the BP rises to 160 mmHg with a small corresponding elevation in LVEDP 25 mmHg; max +dP/dt (index of contractility)1448 (> 1200 [22]) mmHg/s, min -dP/dt (index of relaxation) -1419 (< −1100 [23]) mmHg/s and Weiss' Tau, τ (time constant of relaxation) 0.04 (< 0.05) s. [24, 25]). LV angiogram reveals no wall motion abnormalities.

Her coronary arteries are unobstructed. With the pressure wire down the distal LAD, the Pd/Pa is 0.96 and RFR 0.94 (> 0.89). Continuous thermodilution is undertaken, initially with hyperaemic saline infusion through the RayFlow microcatheter at the rate of 20 mL/min; this is associated with bradycardia and hypotension. Nevertheless, the study is completed within 1 min; flow, Q 83 mL/min and minimal resistance, R 635 Wood units. The saline rate is reduced to 15 mL/min and duplicate

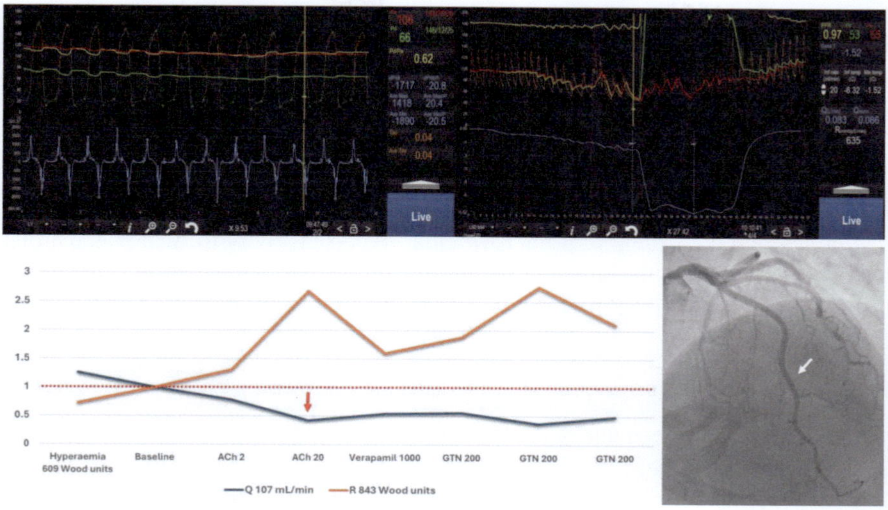

Fig. 3.8 (**Top, left to right panels**) Simultaneous aortic and LV pressures, handgrip raises the systolic BP from 140 to 160 mmHg, the max and min ±dP/dt, and Weiss' Tau, τ are all within normal limits. Saline hyperaemia at 20 mL/min is not tolerated well with bradycardia and hypotension; 140 to 80 mmHg systolic, despite which, the coronary resistance is elevated > 500 Wood units. (**Bottom, left to right panels**) Haemodynamic indices at hyperaemia, rest and in response to ACh, verapamil and GTN. The low CFR is due to baseline vasodilation, if the flow is 60, instead of 107 mL/min, against a hyperaemic flow of 135 mL/min, then the CFR will be 2.25, it becomes normal but still, the range is restricted. ACh at low doses cause reduction in flow > 50% (*arrow*) which appears not to be responsive to either verapamil or GTN. The *arrow* points to the LAD segment after three heart beats of coronary slow flow phenomenon (CSFP) with ACh

measurements are undertaken; Q 114 and **135** mL/min, and R 771 and **609** Wood units. Baseline indices are also obtained in duplicates; Q 101 and **107** mL/min, and R 856 and **843** Wood units—using the repeat indices, CFR 1.26, MRR 1.38 and IMR 30 (609/20).

ACh 2 and 20 μg cause increasing CSFP associated with chest pain, in addition to drop heart beats; flow falls ↓22% and ↓58%, respectively, with rising resistance, without evident epicardial vasospasm. Verapamil 1 mg causes transient Wenckebach phenomenon with lengthening PR and non-conducted P every three beats; neither verapamil alone (↓54% of resting flow) nor GTN 200 μg given in triplicate (↓56, ↓37 and ↓49% of baseline flow) is associated with an increase in flow.

Interpretation This woman has unobstructed coronary arteries with a structurally normal heart. In addition, her systolic and diastolic LV function are both preserved, but with significantly raised LVEDP and hyperaemic coronary resistance, and resting high flow with low resistance giving a low CFR and MRR. This may be contributed partly by her nebivolol which was not interrupted prior to the study. Further, she exhibits ACh hypersensitivity by developing isolated *microvascular spasm* which appears to be resistant to both verapamil and GTN.

Her contemporaneous NT-ProBNP is 168 (< 125) pg/mL, oestradiol 73 (HRT 100–250) pmol/L, sex hormone binding globulin, SHBG 30 (27.1–128) nmol/L, free oestradiol Index 73/30 = 2.4 (1–3), and testosterone < 1.39 (0.7–2.09) nmol/L. *The low CFR/MRR and high coronary resistance would place her firmly in the CMD category.* And in the context of high EF and low VAC, she fulfils the diagnosis of HFsnEF. But this is a mimic; in this case, it is due to an extracardiac constraint, likely to be by the pericardium. The unifying diagnosis which explains both the pericardial constraint with microvascular hypersensitivity to ACh is epicardial adipose tissue (EAT). Its bulk contributes to a pressure effect within the pericardial space [26–33], and EAT paracrine-related inflammation causes endothelial dysfunction [34–36].

The lack of immediate reversal of '*microvascular spasm*' with either verapamil or GTN suggests a non-arteriolar or VSMC spasm phenomenon; high LVEDP causes a pre-existing subendocardial compression, and ACh, through its coupling with capillary endothelial M_3 muscarinic receptor, promotes endothelial leakage or capillary permeability of plasma ultrafiltrates (water, electrolytes and small proteins); increasing myocardial interstitial pressure, causing postcapillary venular compression, raising microvascular resistance, thus impeding flow are observed as CSFP. The vasodilators could in fact exacerbate the interstitial homeostatic pressure because with them the flow deteriorates, until the status quo recurs with gradual resorption or re-equilibration of the excess fluid in the interstitial space by intraluminal oncotic pressure and lymphatic clearance. This *hypothetical chain of events* potentially explains the hallmark of ANOCA with its lingering angina beyond 30 mins long after a trigger has long dissipated—a primary interstitial-pressure-driven mechanism [37]. For verapamil, through its selective arteriolar over venular dilatation increases capillary filtration pressure, hence permeability, and GTN, by reducing venular pressure makes worse the "waterfall" effect in keeping postcapillary venules collapsed during diastole, as per Starling resistor's model [38]. This also explains why GTN's effect in ANOCA is highly variable.

3.3 Discussion

The 6 cases of putative PCOS discussed in this chapter represent a roughly 10% procedural caseload over 12 months, suggesting that it is relatively common among women with ANOCA. The general estimate of PCOS is in the order 10–15% prevalence in women of reproductive age [39]. They are further summarised (Table 3.1). There are three pertinent observations. **First**, coronary vasoreactivity occurs across the PCOS spectrum; premenopausal, and menopause with, or without oestrogen replacement therapy. Implying that despite oestrogen being a powerful endothelium-dependent vasodilator, it could be overcome by other factors, increasing their overall vasoreactive tendency. **Second**, they all have a structurally normal heart, without demonstrable cardiac ischaemia or chest pain on non-invasive tests, apart from Case 6, and without objective exercise intolerance; all those who were tested achieved their

Table 3.1 Coronary physiology in polycystic ovary syndrome

Case	Age	BMI	Comorbidities	[c]Epicardial Adipose Tissue	Vasodilatory Capacity (CFR)	Coronary Resistance (Wood units)	Vasoreactivity (ACh)	Verapamil
1[a]	32	38	Hiatus hernia, gastritis and *hypothyroidism*	++	Reduced 1.6 (baseline high flow, low resistance)	Normal 11 (IMR)	Microvascular spasm	+++ with GTN in restoring flow
2	44	32	Hiatus hernia, gastritis, fibromyalgia, chronic fatigue syndrome, helicobacter pylori infections and endometriosis	+++ (CMR +++)	Restricted 2.1 (baseline normal flow, high resistance)	Raised[b] 546 Raised LVEDP	Microvascular spasm	+ Blunted response, with GTN too
3	24	37	Vaping	No local data	Normal 3.0	Normal 240	Epicardial vasospasm	+++ restored vessel calibre
4	62	22	Hiatus hernia, Raynaud's disease, anaemia and pericardial effusion. On oestrogen replacement therapy	+/++ 1 cm and pericardial effusion	Reduced 1.8 (baseline low flow, high resistance)	Raised[b] 837	Microvascular spasm	+++ Increased flow but did not prevent slow flow with ACh rechallenge
5	64	30	Diabetes on insulin, fibromyalgia and gastric bypass with dumping syndrome	+++	Normal 2.5	Normal 382	Microvascular spasm	++ Increased flow but did not prevent slow flow with ACh rechallenge
6	64	32	Hiatus hernia, gastritis, *hypothyroidism* and endometriosis	+++ (CMR +++)	Reduced 1.3 (baseline high flow, low resistance)	Raised[b] 609 Raised LVEDP	Microvascular spasm	No response, same with GTN

[a]Standard bolus thermodilution with intravenous adenosine given at 140 μg/kg/min for a minute. Not confirmed with repeated measures, nor continuous thermodilution. See text for further discussions. Ventricular standstill with ACh, responsive to GTN

[b]Increased coronary resistance without systemic hypertension

[c]Post hoc subjective quantification on echocardiogram

target heart rates with formal exercise testing (Cases 1, 2 and 6). **Third**, calcium channel blockers, in these cases, specifically IC verapamil, appear not to be effective in preventing ACh-induced microvascular spasm. The exception is the young woman who vapes; her diffuse epicardial vasospasm is likely due to endothelial dysfunction from exposure to nicotine and PCOS, abrogating the vascular protection of her endogenous oestrogen [40].

3.3.1 Microvascular Spasm

There are four interconnected mechanisms for unopposed vasoconstrictive predisposition in PCOS. In brief, PCOS is associated with centrally driven ovarian and adrenal overproduction of androgens, such as testosterone. These are pro-inflammatory hormones essential for overcoming tissue injury and infection—through multiple pathways, *suppressing endothelial nitric oxide synthase (eNOS)* in the vascular endothelium, reducing nitric oxide (NO) bioavailability, thus tilting in favour of vasoconstriction. As well as *sympathetic nervous activation*, and through *androgen receptor activation in vascular smooth muscle cells (VSMC)*, promoting calcium influx and contraction, and lastly, *insulin resistance that encourages endothelin-1 (ET-1) production* in vascular endothelium, through insulin receptor triggering from increased circulating insulin.

Interestingly, therapeutically targeting insulin resistance can overcome most of the PCOS features, suggesting that it is the major root cause for the development of PCOS, in those with genetic predisposition and become overweight, giving rise to excess circulating non-esterified fatty acid (NEFA) or free fatty acid (FFA), which is partly responsible for the *cardiometabolic syndrome* in the first place, including insulin resistance [41]. This purports to be the origin of at least three-quarter cases of PCOS, the rest, so-called non-obese PCOS phenotype can occur through other means, such as hypothalamic-pituitary-ovarian (HPO) axis dysfunction, or adrenal hyperandrogenism.

As yet there is no direct evidence that cardiac catheter laboratory-based demonstration of coronary vasoreactivity correlates with daily symptoms. Due to the invasive nature of administering IC ACh in a large population of healthy controls, to derive normal ranges, whether this can be an incidental finding for a given subject, when it occurs this cannot be discounted. Further, from hypertension research, the only people whose BP do not rise with age are those who live in rural mountainous areas on a subsistence diet, which made the newer hypertension guidelines to lower the treatment target for systolic BP to < 130 mmHg [42, 43]. In other words, it is likely that "subclinical" vasoreactivity is highly prevalent in the general population. However, the assumed connection between lab-based demonstration of vasoreactivity with ACh and daily symptomatic burden is intuitive and *per se notum*. This can be quite dramatic with contrast-induced "no reflow" (Fig. 3.9), which has previously been reported [44]. This phenomenon is usually disregarded as air embolism [45].

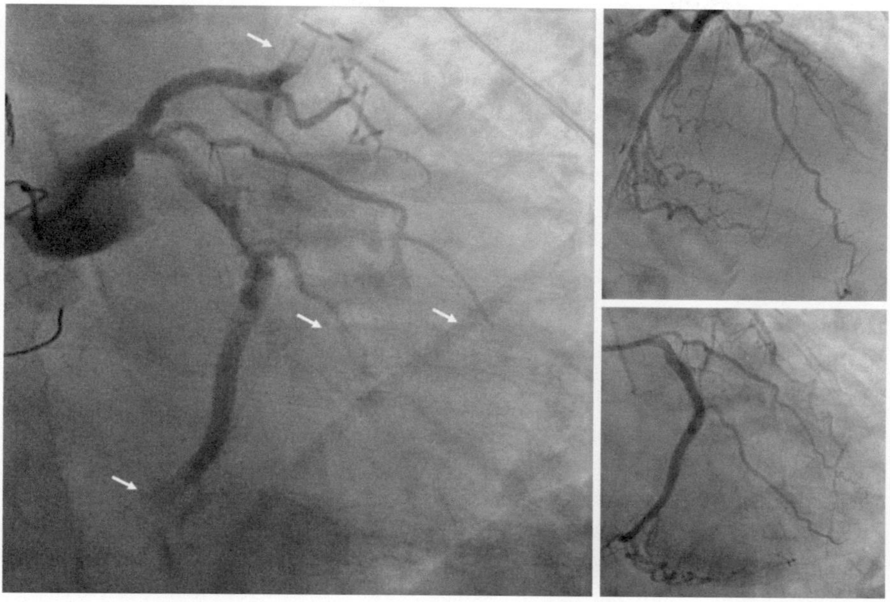

Fig. 3.9 Cardiac arrest with coronary angiogram. A 77-year-old Caucasian woman who had graft failures 12 years after her cardiac surgery at 48, treated with stentings to her mid-left anterior descending (LAD) and circumflex (Cx) arteries 18 years and 9 years, respectively. Her stents remained non-restenotic with three follow-up coronary angiograms in the intervening years for anginal exacerbations. Prior to her current procedure she has had 7 procedures, but on this occasion, the first contrast injection down her left coronary artery was associated with generalised no reflow (**Left panel**)—top *arrow* points to the Boston Taxus 2.5x24 mm stent silhouette and Medtronic Resolute Integrity 3.0x26 mm in Cx, and she drifted into pulseless electrical activity (PEA) requiring chest compressions. Intracoronary 1 mg adrenaline was given with restoration of coronary flow that shows widely patent and unobstructed coronary arteries without significant instent restenoses in both stents (**right, top and bottom panels**). She was also given intravenous 200 mg of hydrocortisone in case this was contrast allergy. There was no evidence of intraluminal filling defects to suggest clots embolization, and air bubbles are usually visible angiographically with rapid clearance and transient electrocardiographic changes—sustained haemodynamic compromise is unusual. This woman made an uneventful recovery. She continued to be highly symptomatic with a reduction of her EF (55 to 45%) over 2 years with LBBB and a QRS of 160 mm; she was referred for conduction system pacing (Chap. 1, 1.8.1 and 1.8.6; and Chap. 2 for LBBB coronary physiology)

On a historical note, the first inadvertent selective coronary angiogram was undertaken by Mason F. Sones (1918–1985) in 1958, in Cleveland Clinic, Ohio. It was a contrast injection into the right coronary artery (RCA) of a 26-year-old man with rheumatic heart disease undergoing work-up for valvular cardiac surgery. Sones used a National Institute of Health (NIH) multiple purpose catheter with side holes, with a lower dye load and a reduced pressure setting on the contrast injector. As he withdrew the catheter from left ventricle into aorta to gauge the degree of aortic regurgitation, the catheter whiplashed into the RCA ostium and opacified the vessel [46]. The patient rapidly went in ventricular standstill—he did his famous shout, "Cough, cough, cough…". It was fortunately quirky that this patient had *contrast-induced coronary microvascular spasm* which is usually short-lasting and self-terminating. Had he gone into ventricular fibrillation (VF) instead, as it was widely believed to be the case at the time, that selective coronary angiogram should never be attempted, and the defibrillator was not yet invented; this patient dying of VF meant that selective coronary angiography would indeed be banned with this as a cautionary tale. Percutaneous coronary intervention (PCI) as we are familiar with today could not be done. And the later development of CT coronary angiogram (CTCA) would be awaited, but unquestionably it will dominate future cardiology practice, since this modality now combines structure, function and physiology and is advancing rapidly to the high level of resolution, capable of assessing pericoronary adipose tissue (PCAT) [47] and myocardial stress perfusion [48].

Masahiro Mohri in 1998 first put together a case series of 29 patients with ACh-induced microvascular spasm, with a mean age 63 years (range 54–68) and 20/29 (69%) were women, with fairly conventional frequency of coronary risk factors—17% had LVH [18]. All, but one woman, were postmenopausal, and none were on oestrogen replacement therapy. Escalating ACh 10 μg, 30 μg and 100 μg were given over 30 seconds down the LAD, producing either chest pain or ischaemic ECG in 2, 5 and 19 subjects in a dose-dependent manner with the respective doses, and a single RCA case; it was positive at ACh 5 μg. These changes rapidly resolved with 1 mg of IC isosorbide dinitrate. Of the 11 patients who had coronary sinus lactate sampling, about 50% had lactate spillover, or a reduced lactate extraction ratio (LER) of < 10%, implying switching to anaerobic glycolysis, and 82% (9/11) developed ischaemic ECG changes. *Two patients had chest pain and ECG changes during cardiac catheterisation, before ACh challenge.* In practice, this is common with contrast injected down the coronary arteries but could be an underrecognized marker for microvascular dysfunction that requires further exploration (Fig. 3.9).

Juan Carlos Kaski's accompanying editorial questions the usefulness of coronary sinus lactate sampling [16]. Harvey G. Kemp Jr., who originally coined the term, "syndrome X" in his assessment of an earlier atrial-pacing study in 10 patients with ANOCA, noted that 50% of subjects also had an LER of < 10%, while their cardiac output increased with falling LVEDP, as expected in normal subjects [49, 50]. Interestingly, a similar pacing study in 16 young men aged 18–27 also found that 50% had an LER of < 10% during the procedure, done 2 decades before [51]. *This means that reduced lactate extraction in coronary sinus has limited clinical utility, if the confirmatory result is only a flip of the coin.* Nevertheless, cardiac ischaemia can truly occur in the absence of significant epicardial coronary artery disease, although luminal atherosclerotic burden of < 50% by definition, thus small vessel disease corresponding to a single coronary artery territory is hard to exclude, but in most, cardiac function is curiously not affected [52, 53]. As non-invasive cardiac imaging techniques continue to improve, these will allow better patient characterisation and selection, to reduce subject heterogeneity for future research [54–57].

In response to the Mohri's report, Kausar and Adams astutely surmised that *cardiac syndrome X* and *metabolic syndrome X* are one and the same, or are "common sobriquet", [17]. PCOS, in its fully fledged form, embodies all the features of *cardiometabolic syndrome*; insulin resistance, abdominal obesity, dyslipidaemia, hypertension, and hyperglycaemia. However, microvascular spasm's clinico-aetiological correlation is less well defined. Although it is thought to be responsible for takotsubo syndrome (TTS), or stress cardiomyopathy, secondary to a transient surge of catecholamines, in response to emotional, or physical stress. But TTS occurs mostly in lean postmenopausal women, and not obese women with PCOS where microvascular spasm is demonstrably more prevalent, as is seen in this case series.

There appears to be a clear distinction from epicardial vasospasm, where calcium channel blockade is highly effective; it is not so with microvascular spasm—***verapamil pre-treatment paradoxically potentiates ACh-induced flow reduction*** [58]. This phenomenon has also been noted with nitroglycerine pre-treatment [59]. This observation underpins the findings of EDIT-CMD study, where 6 weeks' diltiazem treatment was inefficacious in patients with ANOCA due to a combination of CMD and vasoreactivity. In fact, it unmasked microvascular spasm, and unexpectedly reduceed coronary flow, more so in patients with structural CMD, i.e. those with low CFR and high IMR [7, 9]. Nevertheless, questioning calcium channel blockade's cornerstone role in the management of ANOCA is controversial [7, 10, 60, 61]. However, another small-sized pilot study found no improvement in the quality of life with diltiazem after 3 months' treatment, despite its efficacy in reducing epicardial vasospasm [62]. In kidney and skin, L-type calcium channel blockers (e.g. diltiazem and amlodipine), by lowering arteriolar tone produce glomerular hypertension [63, 64] and ankle oedema [65] respectively, which is akin to *opening up the floodgates to the capillary beds*; these are worse if the systemic BP is not controlled. In the heart, this may, coupled with endothelial dysfunction, which makes the capillaries leaky via glycocalyx degradation [66], raising the capillary hydrostatic pressure can drive fluid into the myocardial interstitium, increasing the tissue pressure, and compounded by high LVEDP, can collapse the microvasculature (in particular the postcapillary venules) leading to the above observation. This has been observed in hypertrophic cardiomyopathy [67], which is demonstrable on stress perfusion CMR as a ring-shaped subendocardial perfusion defect in 90% of cases [68]. The same was first reported in CMD (cardiac syndrome X) over twenty years ago, which has reappeared as a non-invasive marker for CMD (**Case 1**) [11, 69–71].

On the other hand, nebivolol appears to be favourable, which has been shown to dilate the microvasculature through β_3-adrenoreceptor activation of endothelial nitric oxide pathway *in vitro* [72]. Another potential microvascular therapeutic target, endothelin-A receptor blockade, with the highly selective zibotentan in the Prize study, failed to reduce angina nor improve exercise tolerance, despite increased LV subendocardial perfusion on CMR at rest, but not at hyperaemia [11]. There is a great deal of subject heterogeneity between studies, or unlike epicardial stenosis, microvascular dysfunction requires further fine-tuning in its aetiopathological definition. Furthermore, obesity is rarely factored in, in studies involving coronary vasoreactivity, but it is thought to be an independent predictive factor, albeit a favourable one, according to a Korea Registry where it was defined as a BMI of ≥ 23 kg/m^2 in an east Asian population [73, 74]. Unfortunately, these studies were mostly with patients with high atherosclerotic burden and concomitant multiple coronary risk factors, with superadded vasoreactivity, therefore not strictly extrapolatable to PCOS patients [52].

3.3.2 Coronary Microvascular Dysfunction

The left ventricular EF is a unitless ratio, a blunt, incomplete and inclusive measure with poor correlation with actual cardiac function, be it systolic or diastolic, as defined by the pressure-volume loop—that is why there is a plethora of patient classifications with heart failure of varying EF percentiles [75]. For example, a super fit athlete with eccentric LV remodelling can have a low EF [76]. When end-systolic volume (ESV) is factored in, EF loses its independent prognostic value [77–80]. Nevertheless, EF does carry a U-shaped long-term outcome. In those with a supra-normal (sn) EF of >65%, there is nearly doubling of mortality over 20 years [81, 82]. This group coupled with symptoms of heart failure (HFsnEF), together with those with preserved (p) EF > 50% (HFpEF); there is a phenotypic cardiometabolic continuum, with a subgroup having excessive epicardial adipose tissue (EAT) [33, 83–85]. This is defined by a thickness of 5–9 mm, measurable using echocardiographic parasternal long-axis view, aligning with the aortic annulus, during systole. In general, 75% of EAT overlies the right ventricle (RV), potentially causing ventriculo-arterial decoupling, i.e. restricting RV diastolic filling, therefore not matching pulmonary afterload. Thus, EAT is an emerging therapeutic target; it is also a marker of systemic inflammation, an independent outcome measure, and can externally restraint the left heart via ventricular interdependence, leading to left ventricular diastolic dysfunction and reduction in exercise capacity [30–33, 36, 86, 87]. The fact that pericardiectomy improves cardiac haemodynamics in this group proves that EAT does cause pericardial constraint that is reversible [26]. This is relevant to case 2, as a novel cause of functional CMD, which has been christened as obese phenotype of HFpEF [31, 84, 86].

The four cases with CMD (Cases 1, 2, 4 and 6) have a structurally normal heart on CMR. Importantly, without LVH and left atrial dilation, which means a functional, rather than a structural vasodilatory restriction. Microvascular spasm is a functional cause of CMD. Albeit transient, it requires energy and cannot be sustained. *It should not be associated with increased LVEDP nor high coronary resistance.* Unless these patients have increased afterload, such as systemic hypertension, aortic stenosis, or left ventricular mid cavity or outflow obstruction. Other rare causes of ANOCA are the exercise-induced left bundle branch block (LBBB, Chap. 1) and left atrial hypertension (EILAH), but while the former responses to cardiac resynchronisation therapy via pacing [88–91], the latter does not benefit from iatrogenic left to right atrial shunting with interatrial shunt device (IASD) [92, 93].

The least expected cause of CMD is extracardiac constraint, which would explain the resting elevation in LVEDP and increased coronary resistance in these cases. Consistent with this hypothesis, stroke volume in these patients were low, generated not by left ventricular dilatation, but by depleting LV end-systolic volume reserve—they potentially have a low EVSI/SVI; this ratio incidentally corresponds to ventriculo-arterial coupling (VAC). And they undercouple between LV and afterload, when under stress, explaining the perceived exercise intolerance. The Mayo Clinic group has elegantly demonstrated that *surgical pericardiectomy* in patients with comparable characteristics as those described here lowers pulmonary capillary wedge pressure (PCWP, analogous to LVEDP) with volume loading and symptomatic improvement at 6 months [28, 29].

3.3.3 Women's Cardiovascular Health

Medicine had been the province and remit of men across the ages. However, there is increasing representation of women in cardiology; 16% of consultants are female; they make up over 60% of medical students, and about a third of heart specialist trainees in the UK in 2021 [94]. With greater representation as doctors comes more general and holistic focus on women's unmet medical needs. There are recent calls to action after surveying the gaps in gender-specific knowledge and a push to implement more streamlined and equitable healthcare access to all women [95, 96]. Considering a pioneering female doctor was the Bristol-born Elizabeth Blackwell (1821–1910), who was 11 when her family immigrated to New York, and she qualified from Geneva Medical College in 1849, which is now State University of New York (SUNY) Upstate Medical University [97]. She was inspired by a young close family friend dying following a protracted gynaecological illness, who confided in her that she wished she had been cared for by a lady doctor. The ban for women entering medicine at the time was partly due to puritanical concern of exposing the delicate gender to human anatomy, especially that of reproductive organs, leading to moral collapse. In the event, she gave up teaching as was a common profession for women then and applied to be admitted into the medical school at 26. The Dean of faculty, Charles A. Lee, asked 129 male students to vote on her entry, which they thought was a joke, and unanimously balloted in her favour, only to be taken aback when she actually turned up for class as the 130th student, and graduated a couple of years later.

Blackwell was a clinical observer at today's Queen Elizabeth Hospital in Birmingham and St Thomas' Hospital in London and visited the Hunterian museum, chaperoned by a family friend, Charles Plevins. Before spending 4 months at La Maternité in Paris learning midwifery and obstetrics. She unfortunately contracted gonorrhoea from a newborn which blinded her left eye, thus ending her surgical aspiration. Next, she spent 18 months at St. Bartholomew's Hospital in London where among her clinical activities she was tutored by James Paget (1814–1899) in pathological anatomy. She went on to promote medical education and healthcare for women, and published her book, *Pioneer Work in Opening the Medical Profession to Women: Autobiographical Sketches* in 1895 [98].

In contrast, Harriot K. Hunt's (1805–1875) admission to Harvard Medical School in Boston in 1847 and 1850 was blackballed by the male students there. She, at 28, instead pursued homeopathic medicine and plant-based natural remedies under the tutelage of an English couple, Richard D. Mott and his wife, Elizabeth. Mott had earlier treated her younger sister by 3 years, who presumably had tuberculosis with wholesome diet, rest and exercise, a more holistic approach—with better outcome than could be achieved by conventional doctors. So to speak, the standard treatment for tuberculosis at the time was strict diet, bloodletting and cold therapy, as was the case of poet John Keats (1795–1821), who incidentally was a trained physician. His early demise at 25 was likely to have been contributed by his intensive medical therapy [99]. With benefits of hindsight, weakening the host is not the best way to deal with any bacterial infection. The Female Medical College of Pennsylvania, founded in 1850, presently Drexel University College of Medicine, awarded Hunt an honorary doctorate in medicine in 1853. Like Blackwell, she provided a more compassionate care for women and advocated for women's rights.

An even earlier and well-documented female doctor was the Prussian Dorothea C. Erxleben (1715–1762), who was home taught by her father. To make ends meet to support her large family, she practiced medicine without a licence by taking over her father's practice when he died in 1747, and she was 32. She was sued for malpractice following the death of a patient by 3 local doctors in 1753, and King Frederick the Great adjudicated the case. In fact, in 1740, he exempted her brother who was a medical student from conscription, as she petitioned, and granted her wish to study medicine at 26, but further stipulated that she must be accompanied by her brother when attending classes. Unfortunately, he dropped out from his medical studies, and she married her cousin's widower with 5 kids, adding 4 more of her own. Thus, she did not attend the University of Halle as she had intended, but continued with self-study. This time round, the King decreed in 1754 that she needed to pass her medical examination and submit a dissertation. She did both and was granted her medical degree the same year, aged 38, but died 8 years later of breast cancer in her hometown, Quedlinburg, a UNESCO World Heritage Site in today's Germany [100].

William Heberden the Elder (1710–1801) gave a presentation describing *angina pectoris* in 1768 at the Royal College of Physicians; this was based on his experience of over 20 years' practice at St George's Hospital, sited at Hyde Park Corner, at the time in London. The population in the city then was under 200,000. He saw one such patient per year. These, he observed, were fat middle-aged men with short necks, mostly from upper strata of society. Mainly clerics and doctors, and their lifespan, were limited to no more than 10 years from symptomatic onset. As exemplified by Heberden's surgical colleague at St George's Hospital, John Hunter (1728–1793), who suffered from angina and collapsed during a heated boardroom dispute [101]. Incidentally, Blackwell visited Hunter's Museum in May 1849 [98]. In other words, coronary artery disease in "men" is a relatively modern disease. In comparison, "angina", likely in women, was described in the "Yellow Court Scripture of Eleven Organs" printed in 848 AD by Hù Yin, a Taoist female doctor who lived during the reign of Táng dynasty (618–907 AD) Emperor Lǐ Chén (b.

810, r. 846–859 AD)—this *strong pain around the chest, radiating to the shoulder, the upper abdomen, the back and the arms*, the tongue which is linked to the heart loses it taste and shrinks. Breathing exercises were prescribed, as well as avoiding spicy foods [102]. These recommendations are not without physiological basis: modern cardiac rehabilitation supports the use of breathing techniques to reduce heart rate and enhance coronary perfusion via parasympathetic activation [103], Hyperventilation-Breath Hold (HVBH—30–35 breaths in one minute followed by end-expiratory breath-hold) produces profound hypercapnic hyperaemia within 20–30 s comparable to that of adenosine [104], and capsaicin has been shown to paradoxically provoke coronary artery spasm when there is systemic inflammation, which may be obesity-related [105].

There were female doctors throughout China's history, caring for women in royal households; some became entangled in palace intrigues and even more working as uncredited partner doctors to their husbands [102]. Of note, in Míng dynasty China (1368–1644), there was Tán Yúnxiàn (1461–1554) who probably was the first well-documented female doctor in her own right, in recorded history. That being said, there existed a medical school in Salerno, in medieval Italy around 900 AD, which admitted women, but no reliable biographical history is extant [106]. Tán was born in Wúxī, which is next to Sūzhōu, close to Shànghǎi, by the Yangtze river delta in Jiāngsū province, south of Běijīng by 581 miles. In Tán's era, medicine was learnt by rote, reading the classics, and by apprenticeship, the skills passed down within the family. For example, Tán's great grandfather married into the Huáng family that had been doctors for generations in Nánjīng. His son, Tán's grandfather, Tán Fù became both a scholar and a renowned physician and had written an immortal' nourishing formulary [107]. Tán lost her mother young, while her father was a busy civil servant in charge of Láizhōu, a county city in Shāndōng province, having passed the imperial exam obtaining the top rank Jīnshì degree; she was essentially raised, nurtured and tutored by her paternal grandparents. They came to live in as extended family later in their lives and gifted her their precious medical tools and manuals. She was grief-stricken for 7 months when her grandmother died and found it hard to get off the bed, until one day in a dream her grandmother appeared and instructed her to the relevant medical text, where she found her cure. This damascene conversion gave her the courage and confidence to practice medicine outside her own immediate household, independently [108].

Female patients were seen with them behind curtain and only their arms stretched out through the veil were available for examination, where their pulses were palpated by male physicians. Unsurprisingly, Tán specialised in women's health. She took detailed personal history and astutely guessed that stresses from family circumstances and husband-wife dynamics were often the *causa mali* of these women's ailments [102]. This "psychosocial adversity" has now been recognised as a major amplifier of cardiovascular risk factors in women [109]. Women who did not want to be seen by male doctors came streaming by in large numbers to consult her. She practiced herbal medicine and moxibustion, in the guise of Hunt, only about 400 years earlier. Her book, entitled, *Miscellaneous Records of a Female Doctor*, written in 1510 with an autobiographical preface, novelly described in detail, 31 women she saw, with successful outcomes, while referencing tried and tested treatment strategies and herbal remedies from others before her—recognisably a "modern-style" medical case reporting [107]. She lived contemporaneously with Leonardo da Vinci (1452–1519), Michelangelo Buonarroti (1475–1564) and Andreas Vesalius (1514–1564) during the European renaissance—where they were sketching accurate human anatomy through dissections. And Hippocrates' (460–370 BC) four humours' theory of blood, phlegm, yellow and black biles was being practised, with dominant bloodletting and purging. In contrast, the Chinese worked on and continue to work on the conceptual circulation of blood within the body and "qi" energy on the body surface; when their flow is obstructed is when sickness arises. For example, instead of bloodletting, they drained "dampness" via kidney diuresis and sweating, such as with herbal sauna, which to some extent these practices accord with modern science [110, 111].

While a modern-equivalent diagnosis cannot be precisely attributed to any single case described by Tán, some she followed up for 11 years, there is an overarching theme of overeating, obesity, menstrual irregularities, infertility, anxiety, grief, palpitations, chest tightness and breathlessness. In that era, a rotund and rounded figure for a woman was considered fortunate and also a sign prosperity. Thus, it was almost a certainty that she would have dealt with ANOCA, Takostubo syndrome (TTS) or stress cardiomyopathy and PCOS. The fact that Tán lived to 93 (or 96, added 3 extra years as per Chinese convention), more than double the average lifespan for a women of her time, was a testament to the effectiveness of her natural remedies. We are just beginning to explore foods as nutraceuticals and their effects on the microbiome; these might be keys to healthier and longer life [112]. Indeed, the World Health Organization (WHO) regards certain aspects of traditional practices as complementary to modern healthcare.

With advanced biochemical techniques and pharmaceutical analyses, there is a convergence of traditional and modern medicine. Many powerful drugs clinically used are derived from animal, plant, bacteria and fungus, such as *heparin* as an anticoagulant from pig's guts used during invasive coronary procedures; *aspirin* was originally purified from willow tree bark used as an antiplatelet to allow coronary stent implantation; *sirolimus* (rapamycin) in drug-eluting stent (DES) used to prevent instent restenosis (ISR) was initially isolated from Easter island (Rapa Nui) soil sample containing streptococcus hygroscopicus; and *simvastatin* used to lower cholesterol was derived from the fungus aspergillus terreus. One herbal remedy Tán used a lot of in her text was fu ling, or poria cocos, literally in Latin for porous coconut, both in shape and size, or wolfiporia extensa. It is a sclerotium, which is a compact mass of hardened fungal mycelium, and in this case it grows underground by the roots of pine trees. Similar to the truffle, only that truffle is the fruiting body with spores as opposed to a tuberous sclerotium which in effect is a dormant fungus, to survive harsh environmental conditions, and to sprout when the weather improves—it is saprophytic or recycles rotting dead wood. The sclerotium is taken as part of a concoction or added to foods; it purportedly has multitude of actions; prebiotic, diuretic, anxiolytic, antidiabetic, anti-ischaemic, antioxidant and anti-inflammatory properties—Pachymic acid's triterpenoid extract is undergoing preclinical studies for its antitumour properties [113]. Another herb, the sweet mugwort, or artemisia annua, used by Tán for moxibustion, from which the compound artemisinin was isolated by Tú Yòuyou (b. 1930), won her the Nobel prize for Medicine or Physiology is 2015; it is used to treat multi-drug resistant malaria [114]. Her breakthrough came after reading Gē Hóng's (284–364 AD) *Handbook of Prescriptions for Emergencies* from the Eastern Jìn Dynasty (317–420 AD) that he used *cold extraction* of crushed leaves with water to treat fever—Tú used ether, as artemisinin is heat sensitive and would be destroyed by boiling. When added to porridge, it was used by Sòng dynasty's (960–1279) celebrated poet, Sū Dōngpō's (1037–1101) wife, Wáng Rùnzhī (1048–1093) to treat a sick ox with septic furuncles, which was reportedly untreatable by a veterinarian in February 1082 [115]. Modern-day analyses suggest that derivatives of artemisinin are effective against a broad spectrum of pathogens, including methicillin-resistant staphylococcus aureus (MRSA) [116].

Fudan University's team in Shànghǎi in 2016 reported a novel approach to reduce obesity—by browning of white fat and dissipating it via thermogenesis, or heat production [117]. They screened 3000 compounds and a semisynthetic derivative artemisinin, artemether (ATM), differentiated preadipose cells from multiple body sites into brown adipose tissue (BAT). These cells have small fat droplets with high density of mitochondria involved in utilising these as local fuel, turning them into burnt energy. In contrast, white adipose tissue (WAT), which essentially a reservoir for triglyceride as a single large fatty droplet within each adipocyte, is found under subcutaneous tissue; it viscerally pads organs and spills over to cause non-alcoholic fatty liver disease (NAFLD) and pancreatic steatosis. The chain of events through subsequent excessive release of free fatty acid (FFA) is thought to be one mechanism by which PCOS is triggered. They further confirmed similar efficacy with other artemisinin derivatives, including dihydroartemisinin (DHA), the active metabolite of artemisinin *in vivo*. Injecting ATM subcutaneously into the groin fat pads and peritoneum of fat fed and obese mice produced the desired effects as postulated. In addition, appetite suppression via the brain stem satiety centre in the mode of tumour-induced "cachexia" was elucidated by others using the FDA-approved artemisinin-derivative, artesunate, which is clinically used to treat malaria, in mice as well as in monkeys [118].

The Shànghǎi group followed up their use of artemisinin in PCOS [119, 120]. This is through its enhanced degradation of cytochrome P450 family 11 subfamily A member 1 (CYP11A1), a key enzyme involved in androgenesis in ovaries and adrenals. When ATM was co-administered with dehydroepiandrosterone (DHEA) to mice, the rise in testosterone was abated and PCOS-like features in the ovary did not developed. Further, ATM was used in rats given insulin and human chorionic gonadotropin (hCG) injections which normally induce PCOS; this was avoided and they retained their fertility. In view of these positive findings, a pilot clinical study was conducted in 19 women with PCOS and mean age of 28 and BMI of 23 (> 23, definition of Asian obesity). These patients had menstrual irregularities, with ultrasound evidence of ovarian cysts, each with ≥ 12, and diameter < 10 mm, and elevated testosterone > 1.67 nmol/L—Rotterdam PCOS diagnostic criteria. Each was treated with DHA 40 mg three times a day over a 12-week period. Testosterone was significantly reduced as was anti-Müllerian hormone (AMH), which correlated with follicular growth; thus there was a corresponding reduction in ovarian cysts on ultrasound, as well as normalisation of their menstrual cycle. Nevertheless, DHA has a very short half-life, requiring daily multiple dosings. Therefore, more works are needed, to find a longer-acting preparation—the authors suggested a skin patch, and a definitive clinical trial. All these perhaps will take at least another 15 years, to prove that this treatment option is viable.

3.3.4 Polycystic Ovary Syndrome

Irving F. Stein (1887–1976) and Michael L. Leventhal (1901–1971) in Chicago used pneumoroentgenography followed by laparotomy in 1929 in young women with infertility and oligomenorrhoea to examine their ovaries and found them to be bulky and polycystic [121]. Carbon dioxide, 1 litre, insufflated at 80 mmHg through uterus into patent fallopian tubes and then peritoneum in cases 4 to 6 of their report, followed by 2 mL lipoidol contrast to assess the reproductive tract under fluoroscopy. They presented 7 cases; only one was thin with acne, the rest were overweight and hirsute, and one had a goitre. Surgical debulking of ovaries appeared to restore menstrual regularity in all, and *case 1* had a couple of babies, which meant that the ovarian cysts drove the Stein-Leventhal syndrome, while recognising that it was likely to be centrally or pituitarily related. Although the first description of polycystic ovaries was 40 years before and ovarian wedge resection undertaken 30 years earlier, Stein and Leventhal's paper in 1935 put together an eponymous syndrome, linking polycystic ovaries with clinical features, investigations, surgical treatment, and outcome up to 4 years. They completed follow-up of 69 patients over 27 years, with restoration of fertility in 87% [122]. However, the surgical option has been superseded by modern drug therapy. Nevertheless, they were pioneers of the trans-uterine peritoneal pneumographic technique from 10 years earlier to their paper in 1935, which allowed for safe radiographic visualisation of the ovaries in obese women, where direct blind abdominal puncture could be risky [123], before the advent of ultrasound in 1981 [124].

PCOS is variously defined over the years [125], but conservatively it affects more than 1 in 10 women with high prevalence within the family [126]. A clustering among parents and siblings makes it a heritable condition although as yet, no single gene defect has been found, like the Plakophilin-2 (PKP2) gene in arrhythmogenic right ventricular cardiomyopathy (ARVC) (Chap. 9—case 3). A women with PCOS has a 1-in-5 likelihood of having another first degree women relative with the condition. The hallmark of "mainstream" PCOS is insulin resistance [127]—inducing this with high fat feeding produces PCOS-like features in animals used as a model for research. Conversely, drugs which target this directly or indirectly are effective therapies such as metformin, pioglitazone and, more recently, sodium-glucose cotransporter type 2 inhibitors (SGLT2i) [128]. Fascinatingly, men in family with a woman with PCOS appear to share many of the phenotypic features of

PCOS—insulin resistance, obesity, hyperlipidaemia and raised anti-Müllerian hormone (AMH), plus premature "androgenic" frontal balding. There appears a Baker's hypothesis scenario occurring, in that, a woman born of mother with PCOS and gestational diabetes has double the risk of developing PCOS, i.e. nearly 1 in 2, suggesting *in utero* programming from hyperinsulinemia [129], which appears to be ameliorated with use of metformin during pregnancy, at least for childhood obesity [130]. On the other hand, there may be an equally significant role of suboptimal high caloric dietary habits within the family. Therefore, whether PCOS occurs in a woman is multifaceted, with interaction of "nature-and-nurture" factors, once initiated, becomes self-perpetuating.

PCOS is identified as a major health issue for premenopausal women, even as they transition into menopause. Although it is not obviously associated with mortality excess, it imparts significant morbidity burden with more cardiovascular risk factors and reduced quality of life [131–133]. For example, compared with about a 6% rate of diabetes in the general population, their prevalence of diabetes is 6–7 times higher as they age [134]. From the cases described here, they have increased coronary microvascular vasoreactivity. Interestingly, intracoronary verapamil appears to facilitate, instead of negating it—as described earlier. In other words, verapamil pretreatment reduces coronary flow increase with ACh. If this is generalisable, it could explain the negative trials of calcium channel blockers in CMD [9, 62]. PCOS with its insulin resistance, hyperandrogenism, obesity and systemic inflammation is associated with endothelin-1 (ET-1) upregulation. However, there are dual ET-1 receptors—**ET-A** in the vascular smooth muscles and **ET-B** in the endothelium. The former causes vasoconstriction and the latter causes vasodilatation via the NO pathway—the net balance of ET-1 effect on vascular tone is therefore hard to predict. And a recent RCT with ET-A receptor blockade in CMD showed lack of efficacy [11]. Nevertheless, it appears that in PCOS, androgens inhibit the vasodilatory response of ET-B receptor, which is potentiated by oestrogen, as demonstrated in the dermal microvasculature [135, 136]. And forearm blood flow response to ACh is blunted, suggesting systemic peripheral vascular endothelial dysfunction [137].

3.3.5 Epicardial Adipose Tissue

Ontologically, epicardial adipose tissue (EAT) is a subset of brown fat descended from splanchnopleuric mesoderm in common with visceral abdominal fat. It has thermogenic potential, keeping the embryonic heart warm by releasing heat. In contrast to other adipose tissues, which are separated from the organs by fascial planes, and have their own feeding vessels, *EAT adheres directly to the coronary arteries and is integrated within the myocardial microvasculature*, which means that there is a bidirectional crosstalk and near-site paracrine secretion from the EAT into the coronary microvasculature [138].

Postnatally, EAT shifts from a purely thermogenic role to three main tasks: energy regulation, mechanical support, and myocardial remodelling. Since the heart's primary fuel is free fatty acid (FFA), it provides ready access to a source of energy supply in particular during exercise and ischaemia, and it secretes adipokines (e.g. adiponectin, omentin and leptin), adrenomedullin and cytokines that regulate cardiac metabolism, inflammation and vascular tone, inhibiting myocardial fibrosis and support tissue repair, respectively. EAT cushions coronary arteries from torsion during cardiac contraction and its viscoelastic properties absorb hemodynamic stress, reducing vascular shear forces. EAT disappears with systolic heart failure.

However, when there is **excess** EAT, *it switches to an inflammatory mode* by upregulating TGF-β which increases pericardial fibrosis and stiffness, *LV diastolic dysfunction*, arrhythmogenic remodeling of atria precipitating AF and secretes high levels of inflammatory cytokines, such as IL-6, TNF-α, ten to fifty times that of other adipose tissue, weight for weight, and increased adipokines inhibit eNOS, causing *endothelial dysfunction.*

EAT also has high density of type 1 and 2 β-adrenergic receptors; hence it is sensitive to sympathetic stimulation, and catecholamines couple with β_1-adrenergic receptor by releasing FFAs and glycerol, and β_2-adrenergic receptor which mediates inflammation.

In the context of PCOS, apart from the above, as EAT expresses androgen and mineralocorticoid receptors, it hypertrophies under PCOS-driven hyperandrogenism [139], and hyperaldosteronism is prevalent in hypertension [140, 141]. The bulk of EAT with a stiffened pericardium causes pericardial constraint [86, 142], while the EAT-related mediators, such as IL-6 and TNF-α, and superoxide radicals inhibit eNOS and scavenge NO [143]. Under such a vasoreactive milieu, where there is no NO "brake", ACh instead binds directly to type 3 Muscarinic receptors of the VSMC causing epicardial or microvascular spasm.

In letrozole-induced mouse model of PCOS, by inhibiting ovarian aromatase (CYP19A1) in granulosa cells, therefore shunting oestrogen production to hyperandrogenism, which in turn drives fat deposition and its inflammation, which then releases excess adipokines, TNF-α in particular amplifies the PCOS features in a vicious cycle [144]. This self-reinforcing forward pathway can be interrupted by inhibiting TNF-α with etanercept, an immunoglobulin-based decoy receptor that mops up the excess TNF-α, a drug that is used to treat inflammatory joint and skin diseases such as psoriasis and ankylosing spondylitis. There is a limited human trial in facilitating IVF in 100 women aged 20–40 with PCOS, resulting 48% vs 38% successful pregnancies, thus achieving parity with general IVF outcome [145]. PCOS contributes to a third of women, and if anovulatory, three quarters of those attending infertility clinics [39]. However, etanercept's immunological modulation and potentially serious infection and neurological side effects make it an unlikely candidate for further human studies in PCOS.

The obvious question is what can be done about EAT; the clear answer is weight management, but most of these patients are mildly or moderately obese ($BMI \leq 35\ kg/m^2$) where surgery is not indicated. Diet and exercise though effective in shedding up to 10% of body weight within the first six months, after two years over 50% relapsed [146]. On the other hand, Glucagon-like peptide-1 receptor agonists (GLP-1 RA) are now available (such as semaglutide and tirzepatide) which enable weight loss of 10–20% reduction in body weight under trial conditions and is ideally suited for obese patients with diabetes [147, 148]. However, their effectiveness depends on continuing use, as discontinuation typically leads to partial or complete weight regain. This is still an evolving situation.

One unintended treatment that also reduces EAT within 3–6 months is low-dose thyroxine, at 25–50 μg. Subclinical hypothyroidism is associated with increased EAT [149–152]. Thyroid function test is part of routine care, and if the thyroid stimulating hormone (TSH) is elevated, thyroxine should be considered and titrated based on TSH response. Low-dose thyroxine increases the metabolic activity of EAT (potentially similar to "browning") and increases heart rate by 5–10 bpm [153, 154]. EAT is analogous to a lithium battery pack for the smartphone, as the charge depletes with use, so is the EAT reduced with increased heart rate. Short-term, low-dose thyroxine is generally not associated with AF or bone loss, especially when carefully monitored. Somewhat counterintuitively, beta blockers as a group is first-line treatment for angina, and it causes weight gain [155, 156], and by implication EAT deposition, which may be detrimental to obese patients with EAT-related pericardial constraint. Although third-generation vasodilating beta blockers such as nebivolol [157] or carvedilol have better metabolic profile, and the former at least in vitro, through β_3-receptor adrenergic agonism browns fats and causes lipolysis [158, 159]. Nevertheless, short-duration low-dose thyroxine could be studied as a potential treatment for obese patients with EAT-related pericardial constraint, which may open up a new therapeutic avenue.

3.3.6 Starling's Hypothesis

Ernest H. Starling (1866–1927)'s *Law of the Heart* is well known to cardiologists and intensivists, but nearly twenty years before, in 1896, he published his seminal work on capillary forces at Guy's Hospital Medical School where he undertook his undergraduate studies and obtained his MD in 1890 [160]. He demonstrated that isotonic fluids are absorbed directly by blood vessels throughout the body, driven not by lymphatic uptake or backward filtration, but by the oncotic (colloid osmotic) pressure of plasma proteins. Quantifying serum proteins' osmotic pressure at approximately 25 mm Hg, he showed how the precise balance between capillary *hydrostatic pressure* and plasma *oncotic pressure* governs fluid exchange and maintains the volume of circulating blood.

The classic pressure sequence—arterioles (30 mmHg) → capillaries → venules (15 mmHg) illustrates this balance: in the **proximal** capillary segment, filtration pressure exceeds oncotic pressure, driving fluid into the interstitium, whereas in the **distal** segment, declining hydrostatic pressure allows oncotic pressure to dominate, drawing fluid back into the capillary lumen before it reaches the venules. Transcapillary pressure difference:

$$\Delta P = Pc - Pi - \sigma(\pi c - \pi i)$$

P_c = capillary (hydrostatic) pressure (30 mmHg); P_i = interstitial hydrostatic pressure (14.9 ± 3.1 mmHg) end-diastole [161]; π_c = capillary oncotic (colloid) pressure (26–28 mmHg) [162]; π_i = interstitial oncotic pressure (14 mmHg) [163]; σ = the reflection coefficient quantifies how "leaky" the capillary wall is to plasma proteins; 0 to 1; σ = 1 means the barrier is perfect: no proteins cross, σ = 0 means totally leaky: proteins equilibrate freely, so there's no oncotic pull, causing tissue oedema and rising interstitial pressure. In the heart with continuous and non-fenestrated capillaries, σ = 0.9–1.0, where σ (π_c − π_i) pulls the fluid back into the capillaries [164].

$$\Delta P = 30 - 14.9 - 0.9 \times (26 - 14) = 4.3\text{mmHg}$$

$$Jv = Kf \cdot \Delta P(\text{mL}/\text{min})$$

J_v—Net fluid movement and K_f—filtration coefficient (surface area x hydraulic conductivity, L_p) = 0.35 mL/min/mmHg/100 g (heart microvascular filtration coefficient) [163].

$$Jv = 0.35 \times 4.3 = 1.5\text{mL}/\text{min}/100\text{g}$$

This interstitial fluid is absorbed into the lymphatic system, and the heart is highly resistant to tissue oedema under normal circumstances, the lymphatic flow, $Q_l \propto P_i$; it can take in x5–10 resting flow (0.1–0.5 mL/min/100 g, but when $J_v > Q_{l(max)}$, transudate occurs causing tissue oedema.

Glycocalyx was first described by John. H. Luft in 1966, when he visualised a "sugar husk" lining on capillary endothelium via electron microscope the endothelial glycocalyx that forms a carbohydrate-rich, negatively charged mesh that governs fluid exchange across capillaries in rat intestinal mucosa [165]. In the revised Starling model, the oncotic pressure difference across this glycocalyx layer opposes, but never reverses filtration at the distal capillaries juxtaposing the venules, so that fluid filtered out at the arteriolar end is not reabsorbed at the postcapillary venular end but instead returns to the circulation via lymphatics (the "no absorption" rule) [166]. When the glycocalyx is damaged, by inflammatory mediators, ischaemia–reperfusion, hyperglycaemia, or sepsis, it undergoes shedding of proteoglycans and glycosaminoglycans, disrupting its barrier function, markedly increasing capillary permeability to protein and water, and driving interstitial oedema [167]. With *glycocalyx degradation* secondary to endothelial dysfunction in mind, consider these:

1. Verapamil, by dilating arterioles, raises capillary hydrostatic pressure, P_c and thus increases ΔP proportionally → higher J_v. High-dose GTN ≥ 100 μg dilating both arterioles and venules potentially has the same effect.
2. Acetylcholine acting on a dysfunctional endothelium increases hydraulic conductivity (L_p or K_f), and capillaries become leakier to both fluid and protein → interstitial oncotic pressure (π_i) climbs → further increases ΔP.

3. Pericardial constraint, fixed-volume sac → any fluid accumulation instantly elevates P_i and compresses lymphatics and its collecting vessels → reduces Q_l, even as J_v is rising.
4. Postcapillary venules collapse more readily than capillaries because their wall-thickness-to-radius ratio (w/r) is low, giving them a low "critical closing pressure" ($P_{cc} < 5$ mmHg, $P_i > P_c$ mirroring LVEDP) [168]. According to Laplace's Law, $P_{cc} \propto w / r$, so a thinner-walled vessel with a larger lumen will collapse at a lower intraluminal pressure when extrinsic forces rise [168]. Capillaries, by contrast, have a relatively thick basal lamina, pericyte support, and a smaller radius, so their w/r is higher, and they resist collapse under the same external pressure. *Postcapillary venular collapse* is a matter of course during the cardiac cycle, but when it occurs during diastole as the coronary fills is when microvascular resistance rises disproportionately. An analogy is right atrial and ventricle collapse in cardiac tamponade in diastole [169].

Over minutes to hours, the "oedematous" microvasculature finds a new steady state: elevated P_i and π_i reduce ΔP back towards zero, so J_v falls until it again equals the (now reduced) Q_l, and net filtration resumes at a new, higher pressure equilibrium. This "perfect storm" can explain the exercise and emotional trigger of angina and the slow resolution of angina long after the anginal trigger has passed and the lack of efficacy of vasodilators in addressing a *mechanical problem*, giving a rational reason why beta blockers could work.

References

1. Lagerqvist B, Sylvén C, Beermann B, Helmius G, Waldenström A. Intracoronary adenosine causes angina pectoris like pain—an inquiry into the nature of visceral pain. Cardiovasc Res. 1990;24(8):609–13. https://doi.org/10.1093/cvr/24.8.609.
2. Kemp HG Jr, Vokonas PS, Cohn PF, Gorlin R. The anginal syndrome associated with normal coronary arteriograms. Report of a six year experience. Am J Med. 1973;54(6):735–42. https://doi.org/10.1016/0002-9343(73)90060-0.
3. Likoff W, Segal BL, Kasparian H. Paradox of Normal selective coronary arteriograms in patients considered to have unmistakable coronary heart disease. N Engl J Med. 1967;276(19):1063–6. https://doi.org/10.1056/NEJM196705112761904.
4. Beltrame JF, Horowitz JD. Why do nitrates have limited efficacy in coronary microvessels? Cardiovasc Drugs Ther. 2013;27(3):187–8. https://doi.org/10.1007/s10557-013-6454-0.
5. Bugiardini R, Borghi A, Pozzati A, et al. The paradox of nitrates in patients with angina pectoris and angiographically normal coronary arteries. Am J Cardiol. 1993;72(3):343–7. https://doi.org/10.1016/0002-9149(93)90683-4.
6. Russo G, Di Franco A, Lamendola P, et al. Lack of effect of nitrates on exercise stress test results in patients with microvascular angina. Cardiovasc Drugs Ther. 2013;27(3):229–34. https://doi.org/10.1007/s10557-013-6439-z.
7. Beneduce A, Leone AM, Berry C, Chieffo A. Coronary vasomotor disorders: one size does not fit all. JACC Cardiovasc Imaging. 2022;15(9):1677–8. https://doi.org/10.1016/j.jcmg.2022.06.019.
8. Jansen TPJ, Damman P, Royen N, Elias-Smale SE. Reply. JACC Cardiovasc Imaging. 2022;15(9):1678–9. https://doi.org/10.1016/j.jcmg.2022.07.005.

9. Jansen TPJ, Konst RE, de Vos A, et al. Efficacy of diltiazem to improve coronary vasomotor dysfunction in ANOCA: the EDIT-CMD randomized clinical trial. JACC Cardiovasc Imaging. 2022;15(8):1473–84. https://doi.org/10.1016/j.jcmg.2022.03.012.
10. Stone PH. Progressive understanding of coronary microvascular disease and vasomotor dysfunction: some answers, more questions∗. JACC Cardiovasc Imaging. 2022;15(8):1485–7. https://doi.org/10.1016/j.jcmg.2022.04.020.
11. Morrow A, Young R, Abraham GR, et al. Zibotentan in microvascular angina: a randomized, placebo-controlled, Crossover Trial. Circulation. 2024;150(21):1671–83. https://doi.org/10.1161/CIRCULATIONAHA.124.069901.
12. Feenstra RGT, Jansen TPJ, Boekholdt MS, et al. Efficacy and safety of the endothelin-1 receptor antagonist macitentan in epicardial and microvascular vasospasm; a proof-of-concept study. IJC Heart Vasc. 2023;47:101238. https://doi.org/10.1016/j.ijcha.2023.101238.
13. Mohri M, Shimokawa H, Hirakawa Y, Masumoto A, Takeshita A. Rho-kinase inhibition with intracoronary fasudil prevents myocardial ischemia in patients with coronary microvascular spasm. JACC. 2003;41(1):15–9. https://doi.org/10.1016/S0735-1097(02)02632-3.
14. Lim PO. Angina: the ischemic triad. Am J Cardiol. 2024;223:118–9. https://doi.org/10.1016/j.amjcard.2024.05.023.
15. SenthilKumar G, Katunaric B, Bordas-Murphy H, Sarvaideo J, Freed JK. Estrogen and the vascular endothelium: the unanswered questions. Endocrinology. 2023;164(6). https://doi.org/10.1210/endocr/bqad079.
16. Kaski JC. Chest pain and normal coronary arteriograms: role of "microvascular spasm". Lancet. 1998;351(9110):1144–5. https://doi.org/10.1016/s0140-6736(98)22016-2.
17. Kausar SA, Adams S. Coronary microvascular spasm and angina pectoris. Lancet 1998;351(9118):1817. https://doi.org/10.1016/S0140-6736(05)78786-9.
18. Mohri M, Koyanagi M, Egashira K, et al. Angina pectoris caused by coronary microvascular spasm. Lancet. 1998;351(9110):1165–9. https://doi.org/10.1016/S0140-6736(97)07329-7.
19. Mohri M, Takeshita A. Coronary microvascular disease in humans. Jpn Heart J. 1999;40(2):97–108. https://doi.org/10.1536/jhj.40.97.
20. Iacobellis G, Bianco AC. Epicardial adipose tissue: emerging physiological, pathophysiological and clinical features. Trends Endocrinol Metab. 2011;22(11):450–7. https://doi.org/10.1016/j.tem.2011.07.003.
21. Ito T, Niwa A, Yokoi M, et al. Relationship between Epicardial fat volume and coronary microvascular dysfunction. Circ Rep. 2025:advpub. https://doi.org/10.1253/circrep.CR-25-0073.
22. Camm AJ, Lüscher TF, Serruys PW. The ESC textbook of cardiovascular medicine. Oxford: Blackwell Publishing; 2006.
23. How to diagnose diastolic heart failure. European study group on diastolic heart failure. Eur Heart J. 1998;19(7):990–1003. https://doi.org/10.1053/euhj.1998.1057.
24. Weiss JL, Frederiksen JW, Weisfeldt ML. Hemodynamic determinants of the time-course of fall in canine left ventricular pressure. J Clin Invest. 1976;58(3):751–60. https://doi.org/10.1172/jci108522.
25. Zile MR, Baicu CF, Gaasch WH. Diastolic heart failure–abnormalities in active relaxation and passive stiffness of the left ventricle. N Engl J Med. 2004;350(19):1953–9. https://doi.org/10.1056/NEJMoa032566.
26. Borlaug BA, Carter RE, Melenovsky V, et al. Percutaneous pericardial resection. Circ Heart Fail. 2017;10(4):e003612. https://doi.org/10.1161/CIRCHEARTFAILURE.116.003612.
27. Borlaug BA, Reddy YNV. The role of the pericardium in heart failure: implications for pathophysiology and treatment. JACC: Heart Failure. 2019;7(7):574–85. https://doi.org/10.1016/j.jchf.2019.03.021.
28. Borlaug BA, Schaff HV, Asirvatham SJ, et al. Surgical pericardiotomy to treat heart failure with preserved ejection fraction: a first clinical study. Eur Heart J. 2023;44(44):4719–21. https://doi.org/10.1093/eurheartj/ehad620.
29. Borlaug BA, Strong M. Heart failure solutions. JACC: Basic Transl Sci. 2024;9(4):448–50. https://doi.org/10.1016/j.jacbts.2024.02.010.

30. Koepp KE, Obokata M, YNV R, Olson TP, Borlaug BA. Hemodynamic and functional impact of Epicardial adipose tissue in heart failure with preserved ejection fraction. JACC Heart Fail. 2020;8(8):657–66. https://doi.org/10.1016/j.jchf.2020.04.016.
31. Obokata M, Reddy YNV, Pislaru SV, Melenovsky V, Borlaug BA. Evidence supporting the existence of a distinct obese phenotype of heart failure with preserved ejection fraction. Circulation. 2017;136(1):6–19. https://doi.org/10.1161/circulationaha.116.026807.
32. Packer M, Zile MR, Kramer CM, et al. Tirzepatide for Heart Failure with Preserved Ejection Fraction and Obesity. N Engl J Med. 0(0). https://doi.org/10.1056/NEJMoa2410027.
33. Pugliese NR, Paneni F, Mazzola M, et al. Impact of epicardial adipose tissue on cardiovascular haemodynamics, metabolic profile, and prognosis in heart failure. Eur J Heart Fail. 2021;23(11):1858–71. https://doi.org/10.1002/ejhf.2337.
34. Elsanhoury A, Nelki V, Kelle S, Van Linthout S, Tschöpe C. Epicardial fat expansion in diabetic and obese patients with heart failure and preserved ejection fraction—a specific HFpEF phenotype. Front Cardiovasc Med. 2021;8:720690. https://doi.org/10.3389/fcvm.2021.720690.
35. Mazurek T, Zhang L, Zalewski A, et al. Human Epicardial adipose tissue is a source of inflammatory mediators. Circulation. 2003;108(20):2460–6. https://doi.org/10.1161/01.CIR.0000099542.57313.C5.
36. Packer M. Epicardial adipose tissue may mediate deleterious effects of obesity and inflammation on the myocardium. J Am Coll Cardiol. 2018;71(20):2360–72. https://doi.org/10.1016/j.jacc.2018.03.509.
37. Kaski JC, Crea F, Gersh BJ, Camici PG. Reappraisal of ischemic heart disease. Circulation. 2018;138(14):1463–80. https://doi.org/10.1161/circulationaha.118.031373.
38. Holt JP. THE collapse factor in the measurement of venous pressure. Amer J Physiol Legacy Cont. 1941;134(2):292–9. https://doi.org/10.1152/ajplegacy.1941.134.2.292.
39. Balen A. Overview and definitions of polycystic ovary syndrome and the polycystic ovary. In: Balen A, Franks S, Homburg R, Kehoe S, editors. Current management of polycystic ovary syndrome. London: RCOG Press; 2010. p. 2–12.
40. Cheraghi M, Amiri M, Omidi F, et al. Acute cardiovascular effects of electronic cigarettes: a systematic review and meta-analysis. European Heart J Open. 2024; https://doi.org/10.1093/ehjopen/oeae098.
41. Carreau A-M, Battista M-C, Baillargeon J-P. Insulin resistance and lipotoxicity in PCOS: causes and consequences. In: Pal L, Seifer DB, editors. Polycystic ovary syndrome: current and emerging concepts. Cham: Springer International Publishing; 2022. p. 133–54.
42. He J, Tell GS, Tang YC, Mo PS, He GQ. Effect of migration on blood pressure: the Yi people study. Epidemiology. 1991;2(2):88–97. https://doi.org/10.1097/00001648-199103000-00002.
43. McEvoy JW, McCarthy CP, Bruno RM, et al. ESC guidelines for the management of elevated blood pressure and hypertension. Eur Heart J. 2024;45(38):3912–4018. https://doi.org/10.1093/eurheartj/ehae178.
44. Bolad IA, Khan B, Ghumman W. Contrast-induced coronary no-flow phenomenon: during diagnostic coronary angiography. Tex Heart Inst J. 2011;38(5):600–1. https://www.ncbi.nlm.nih.gov/pubmed/22163148.
45. Heupler FA. Contrast-induced coronary no-flow phenomenon. Tex Heart Inst J. 2012;39(1):162. Author reply. https://www.ncbi.nlm.nih.gov/pubmed/22412261.
46. Cheng TO. First selective coronary arteriogram. Circulation. 2003;107(5):E42–2; author reply E–2. https://doi.org/10.1161/01.cir.0000053958.38681.81.
47. Kahmann J, Nörenberg D, Papavassiliu T, et al. Interrelation of pericoronary adipose tissue texture and coronary artery disease of the left coronary artery in cardiac photon-counting computed tomography. Front Cardiovasc Med. 2024;11. https://doi.org/10.3389/fcvm.2024.1499219.
48. Takafuji M, Kitagawa K, Ishida M, et al. Dynamic CT-perfusion parameters as indicators of microcirculation: investigation in patients without obstructive coronary artery disease. Clin Radiol. 2024; https://doi.org/10.1016/j.crad.2024.106766.

49. Arbogast R, Bourassa MG. Myocardial function during atrial pacing in patients with angina pectoris and normal coronary arteriograms: comparison with patients having significant coronary artery disease. Am J Cardiol. 1973;32(3):257–63. https://doi.org/10.1016/S0002-9149(73)80130-4.
50. Kemp HG Jr. Left ventricular function in patients with the anginal syndrome and normal coronary arteriograms. Am J Cardiol. 1973;32(3):375–6. https://doi.org/10.1016/S0002-9149(73)80150-X.
51. Gertz EW, Wisneski JA, Neese R, et al. Myocardial lactate extraction: multi-determined metabolic function. Circulation. 1980;61(2):256–61. https://doi.org/10.1161/01.cir.61.2.256.
52. Ang DT, Carberry J, Ford TJ, et al. Coronary microvascular function and atherosclerotic plaque burden in ischaemia and no obstructive coronary arteries: a secondary analysis of the CorMicA trial. Heart. 2024:heartjnl–2024–324677. https://doi.org/10.1136/heartjnl-2024-324677.
53. Magarian GJ, Palac R, Reinhart S. Syndrome of diminished vasodilator reserve of the coronary microcirculation (microvascular angina or syndrome X): diagnosis by combined atrial pacing and thallium 201 imaging–a case report. Angiology. 1990;41(8):667–72. https://doi.org/10.1177/000331979004100813.
54. Schindler TH, Fearon WF, Pelletier-Galarneau M, et al. Myocardial perfusion PET for the detection and reporting of coronary microvascular dysfunction: a JACC: cardiovascular imaging expert panel statement. JACC Cardiovasc Imaging. 2023;16(4):536–48. https://doi.org/10.1016/j.jcmg.2022.12.015.
55. Lim PO. Is bolus-Thermodilution reliable in defining coronary microvascular dysfunction? JACC Cardiovasc Imaging. 2023;16(7):993. https://doi.org/10.1016/j.jcmg.2023.03.025.
56. Gould KL, Johnson NP, Narula J. Reply: Is Bolus-Thermodilution Reliable in Defining Coronary Microvascular Dysfunction? JACC Cardiovasc Imaging. 2023;16(7):994–5. https://doi.org/10.1016/j.jcmg.2023.04.010.
57. Gould KL, Johnson NP, Narula J. Microvascular dysfunction or diffuse Epicardial CAD with Normal stress vasodilation. JACC Cardiovasc Imaging. 2023;16(4):549–52. https://doi.org/10.1016/j.jcmg.2022.10.029.
58. Lim PO. Takayasu arteritis and stent always end in tears. European Heart J Case Rep. 2023;7(9). https://doi.org/10.1093/ehjcr/ytad421.
59. Seitz A, Feenstra RGT, Konst RE, et al. Acetylcholine rechallenge. J Am Coll Cardiol Intv. 2022;15(1):65–75. https://doi.org/10.1016/j.jcin.2021.10.003.
60. Kim HL, Jo SH. Current evidence on long-term prognostic factors in vasospastic angina. J Clin Med. 2021;10(18) https://doi.org/10.3390/jcm10184270.
61. Rahman H, Sinha A, Demir OM, Perera D. EDIT-CMD: are we comparing apples with oranges? JACC Cardiovasc Imaging. 2022;15(9):1674–6. https://doi.org/10.1016/j.jcmg.2022.04.027.
62. Kook H, Hong SJ, Yang K-S, et al. Comparison of nebivolol versus diltiazem in improving coronary artery spasm and quality of life in patients with hypertension and vasospastic angina: a prospective, randomized, double-blind pilot study. PLoS One. 2020;15(9):e0239039. https://doi.org/10.1371/journal.pone.0239039.
63. Carmines PK, Navar LG. Disparate effects of ca channel blockade on afferent and efferent arteriolar responses to ANG II. American Journal of Physiology-Renal Physiology. 1989;256(6):F1015–F20. https://doi.org/10.1152/ajprenal.1989.256.6.F1015.
64. Hayashi K, Homma K, Wakino S, et al. T-type ca channel blockade as a determinant of kidney protection. Keio J Med. 2010;59(3):84–95. https://doi.org/10.2302/kjm.59.84.
65. de la Sierra A. Mitigation of calcium channel blocker-related oedema in hypertension by antagonists of the renin-angiotensin system. J Hum Hypertens. 2009;23(8):503–11. https://doi.org/10.1038/jhh.2008.157.
66. Reitsma S, Slaaf DW, Vink H, van Zandvoort MAMJ, oude Egbrink MGA. The endothelial glycocalyx: composition, functions, and visualization. Pflugers Arch - European J Physiol. 2007;454(3):345–59. https://doi.org/10.1007/s00424-007-0212-8.

67. Takemura G, Takatsu Y, Fujiwara H. Luminal narrowing of coronary capillaries in human hypertrophic hearts: an ultrastructural morphometrical study using endomyocardial biopsy specimens. Heart. 1998;79(1):78–85. https://doi.org/10.1136/hrt.79.1.78.
68. Kim EK, Lee S-C, Chang S-A, et al. Prevalence and clinical significance of cardiovascular magnetic resonance adenosine stress-induced myocardial perfusion defect in hypertrophic cardiomyopathy. J Cardiovasc Magn Reson. 2020;22(1):30. https://doi.org/10.1186/s12968-020-00623-1.
69. Foley MJ, Rajkumar CA, Ahmed-Jushuf F, et al. Coronary sinus reducer for the treatment of refractory angina (ORBITA-COSMIC): a randomised, placebo-controlled trial. Lancet. 2024;403(10436):1543–53. https://doi.org/10.1016/S0140-6736(24)00256-3.
70. Im DJ, Hong SJ, Park E-A, et al. Guidelines for cardiovascular magnetic resonance imaging from the Korean Society of Cardiovascular Imaging (KOSCI) - part 3: perfusion, delayed enhancement, and T1- and T2 mapping. Investig Magn Reson Imaging. 2020;24(1):1–20. https://doi.org/10.13104/imri.2020.24.1.1.
71. Panting JR, Gatehouse PD, Yang GZ, et al. Abnormal subendocardial perfusion in cardiac syndrome X detected by cardiovascular magnetic resonance imaging. N Engl J Med. 2002;346(25):1948–53. https://doi.org/10.1056/NEJMoa012369.
72. Dessy C, Saliez J, Ghisdal P, et al. Endothelial β3-Adrenoreceptors Mediate Nitric Oxide–Dependent Vasorelaxation of Coronary Microvessels in Response to the Third-Generation β-Blocker Nebivolol. Circulation. 2005;112(8):1198–205. https://doi.org/10.1161/CIRCULATIONAHA.104.532960.
73. Fabrizio R, Behzad B, Mirnabi P, et al. Familial risk of vasospastic angina: a nationwide family study in Sweden. Open Heart. 2023;10(2):e002504. https://doi.org/10.1136/openhrt-2023-002504.
74. Lee MH, Jo SH, Kwon S, et al. Impact of overweight/obesity on clinical outcomes of patient with vasospastic angina: from the vasospastic angina in Korea registry. Sci Rep. 2020;10(1):4954. https://doi.org/10.1038/s41598-020-61947-7.
75. Kerkhof PLM, Peace RA, Handly N. Ratiology and a complementary class of metrics for cardiovascular investigations. Physiology. 2019;34(4):250–63. https://doi.org/10.1152/physiol.00056.2018.
76. Claessen G, De Bosscher R, Janssens K, et al. Reduced ejection fraction in elite endurance athletes: clinical and genetic overlap with dilated cardiomyopathy. Circulation. 2024;149(18):1405–15. https://doi.org/10.1161/CIRCULATIONAHA.122.063777.
77. Kato M, Kitada S, Kawada Y, et al. Left ventricular end-systolic volume is a reliable predictor of new-onset heart failure with preserved left ventricular ejection fraction. Cardiol Res Pract. 2020;2020:3106012. https://doi.org/10.1155/2020/3106012.
78. Kerkhof PLM, Heyndrickx GR. Case report on the importance of longitudinal analysis of left ventricular end-systolic volume, rather than ejection fraction, in a heart transplant patient. Eur Heart J Case Rep. 2021;5(6):ytab146. https://doi.org/10.1093/ehjcr/ytab146.
79. Turakhia MP, McManus DD, Whooley MA, Schiller NB. Increase in end-systolic volume after exercise independently predicts mortality in patients with coronary heart disease: data from the heart and soul study. Eur Heart J. 2009;30(20):2478–84. https://doi.org/10.1093/eurheartj/ehp270.
80. White HD, Norris RM, Brown MA, et al. Left ventricular end-systolic volume as the major determinant of survival after recovery from myocardial infarction. Circulation. 1987;76(1):44–51. https://doi.org/10.1161/01.CIR.76.1.44.
81. Chang H-C, Tseng C-H, Huang W-M, et al. Supranormal left ventricular ejection fraction, concentric remodeling, and long-term survival. JACC: Asia. 2024; https://doi.org/10.1016/j.jacasi.2024.08.020.
82. Wehner GJ, Jing L, Haggerty CM, et al. Routinely reported ejection fraction and mortality in clinical practice: where does the nadir of risk lie? Eur Heart J. 2020;41(12):1249–57. https://doi.org/10.1093/eurheartj/ehz550.

83. Jin X, Hung C-L, Tay WT, et al. Epicardial adipose tissue related to left atrial and ventricular function in heart failure with preserved versus reduced and mildly reduced ejection fraction. Eur J Heart Fail. 2022;24(8):1346–56. https://doi.org/10.1002/ejhf.2513.
84. Kitzman DW, Lam CSP. Obese heart failure with preserved ejection fraction phenotype. Circulation. 2017;136(1):20–3. https://doi.org/10.1161/CIRCULATIONAHA.117.028365.
85. Venkateshvaran A, Faxen UL, Hage C, et al. Association of epicardial adipose tissue with proteomics, coronary flow reserve, cardiac structure and function, and quality of life in heart failure with preserved ejection fraction: insights from the PROMIS-HFpEF study. Eur J Heart Fail. 2022;24(12):2251–60. https://doi.org/10.1002/ejhf.2709.
86. Crum Y, Hoendermis ES, van Veldhuisen DJ, et al. Epicardial adipose tissue and pericardial constraint in heart failure with preserved ejection fraction. ESC Heart Failure. 2024;11(3):1698–706. https://doi.org/10.1002/ehf2.14739.
87. Gorter TM, van Woerden G, Rienstra M, et al. Epicardial adipose tissue and invasive hemodynamics in heart failure with preserved ejection fraction. JACC Heart Fail. 2020;8(8):667–76. https://doi.org/10.1016/j.jchf.2020.06.003.
88. Cerantola M, Frankel DS, Callans DJ, Santangeli P, Schaller RD. Left bundle branch area pacing for the treatment of painful left bundle branch block syndrome. HeartRhythm Case Rep. 2023;9(2):121–5. https://doi.org/10.1016/j.hrcr.2022.12.003.
89. Czuriga D, Lim PO. Cardiac resynchronization therapy relieves intractable angina due to exercise-induced left bundle branch block without left ventricular systolic dysfunction: a detailed case study. J Cardiovasc Electrophysiol. 2016;27(5):609–12. https://doi.org/10.1111/jce.12911.
90. Hofer D, Anwer S, Tanner FC, et al. Improved symptoms, exercise capacity, and homogeneity of cardiac deformation through conduction system pacing in a patient with symptomatic left bundle branch block. HeartRhythm Case Rep. 2023;9(1):43–7. https://doi.org/10.1016/j.hrcr.2022.10.013.
91. Oladunjoye OO, Oladunjoye AO, Oladiran O, et al. Persistent exertional chest pain in a Marathon runner: exercise-induced, painful, left bundle branch block syndrome treated with his-bundle pacing. Mayo Clin Proceed Innov Quality Outcomes. 2019;3(2):226–30. https://doi.org/10.1016/j.mayocpiqo.2019.03.008.
92. Litwin SE, Komtebedde J, Hu M, et al. Exercise-induced left atrial hypertension in heart failure with preserved ejection fraction. JACC: Heart Failure. 2023;11(8, Part 2):1103–17. https://doi.org/10.1016/j.jchf.2023.01.030.
93. Maurer MS, Rosenblum HR. Difficult diagnoses are often undertreated: the case of HFpEF with exercise-induced left atrial hypertension∗. JACC Heart Fail. 2023;11(8, Part 2):1118–20. https://doi.org/10.1016/j.jchf.2023.02.010.
94. Portwood C. Reasons and resolutions for gender inequality among cardiologists and cardiology trainees. Br J Cardiol. 2023;30(2):13. https://doi.org/10.5837/bjc.2023.013.
95. Tayal U, Pompei G, Wilkinson I, et al. Advancing the access to cardiovascular diagnosis and treatment among women with cardiovascular disease: a joint British cardiovascular societies' consensus document. Heart. 2024;110(22):e4–e. https://doi.org/10.1136/heartjnl-2024-324625.
96. Vogel B, Acevedo M, Appelman Y, et al. The lancet women and cardiovascular disease commission: reducing the global burden by 2030. Lancet. 2021;397(10292):2385–438. https://doi.org/10.1016/S0140-6736(21)00684-X.
97. Porter D. Three 19th-century women doctors: Elizabeth Blackwell, Mary Walker, and Sarah Loguen Fraser. JAMA. 2008;300(18):2182–3. https://doi.org/10.1001/jama.2008.590.
98. Blackwell E. Pioneer work in opening the medical profession to women: autobiographical sketches. London/New York: Longmans, Green, and Co; 1895. p. 276.
99. Smith H. John Keats: poet, patient, physician. Rev Infect Dis. 1984;6(3):390–404. https://doi.org/10.1093/clinids/6.3.390.

100. Steger F. Importance of learning from the model: Dorothea Erxleben (1715–1762), the first graduated female doctor in Germany. Droit, Santé et Société. 2018;N° 3–4(3):71–75. https://doi.org/10.3917/dsso.053.0071.
101. O'Brien JC. My surgical heroes. Proc (Bayl Univ Med Cent). 2013;26(1):67–75. https://doi.org/10.1080/08998280.2013.11928924.
102. Santilli E. Female Doctors in Ancient China: Comparative Studies Through Literature and Science. In: Healthcare Policies and Systems in Europe and China. p. 285–301.
103. Sugimoto T, Sugiyama K, Matsumura K, et al. Effects of consciously controlled slow breathing on cardiac parasympathetic nervous activity postexercise in young healthy males. Clin Physiol Funct Imaging. 2025;45(2):e70007. https://doi.org/10.1111/cpf.70007.
104. Shergill S, Hillier E, Velvet A, Budgeon CA, Moafi A, Elshibly M, England R, Parke KS, Wormleighton JV, Adlam D, Hothi SS, Ladwiniec A, Friedrich MG, McCann GP, Arnold JR. Vasoactive breathing manoeuvres as an effective coronary vasodilator in patients with suspected coronary artery disease: a prospective comparative oxygenation-sensitive CMR study. Eur Heart J Imaging Methods Pract. 2025. https://doi.org/10.1093/ehjimp/qyaf141
105. Munjuluri S, Wilkerson DA, Sooch G, et al. Capsaicin and TRPV1 channels in the cardiovascular system: the role of inflammation. Cells. 2021;11(1). https://doi.org/10.3390/cells11010018.
106. Ferraris ZABA FVAMD. The women of Salerno: contribution to the origins of surgery from medieval Italy. Ann Thorac Surg. 1997;64(6):1855–7. https://doi.org/10.1016/S0003-4975(97)01079-5.
107. Tan Y, Wilcox L, Lu Y. Miscellaneous Records of Female Doctor. Portland, Oregon: The Chinese Medical Database; 2015. p. 175.
108. A female doctor's life and work: Preface and postfaces to a book by Tan Yunxian 談允賢 (1461–1556). In: Ebrey PB, Zhang CE, Yao P, editors. Chinese autobiographical writing. An anthology of personal accounts: University of Washington Press; 2023. p. 135–140.
109. Ebong IA, Quesada O, Fonkoue IT, et al. The role of psychosocial stress on cardiovascular disease in women: JACC state-of-the-art review. J Am Coll Cardiol. 2024;84(3):298–314. https://doi.org/10.1016/j.jacc.2024.05.016.
110. Akinniyi G, Lee J, Kim H, Lee JG, Yang I. A medicinal halophyte Ipomoea pes-caprae (Linn.) R. Br.: a review of its botany, traditional uses, Phytochemistry, and bioactivity. Mar Drugs. 2022;20(5). https://doi.org/10.3390/md20050329.
111. Källström M, Soveri I, Oldgren J, et al. Effects of sauna bath on heart failure: a systematic review and meta-analysis. Clin Cardiol. 2018;41(11):1491–501. https://doi.org/10.1002/clc.23077.
112. Meegaswatte H, Speer K, McKune AJ, Naumovski N. Functional foods and nutraceuticals for the Management of Cardiovascular Disease Risk in postmenopausal women. RCM. 2024;25(12). https://doi.org/10.31083/j.rcm2512460.
113. Wei C, Wang H, Sun X, et al. Pharmacological profiles and therapeutic applications of pachymic acid (review). Exp Ther Med. 2022;24(3):547. https://doi.org/10.3892/etm.2022.11484.
114. Zheng WR, Li EC, Peng S, Wang XS. Tu Youyou winning the Nobel prize: ethical research on the value and safety of traditional Chinese medicine. Bioethics. 2020;34(2):166–71. https://doi.org/10.1111/bioe.12456.
115. Su S. Letter to Zhang Dun (章惇) [与章子厚书]. Collected Works of Su Shi (《苏东坡集》 or 《东坡全集》)1082.
116. Wang P, Zeng Y, Liu J, et al. Antimicrobial and anti-biofilm effects of dihydroartemisinin-loaded chitosan nanoparticles against methicillin-resistant Staphylococcus aureus. Microb Pathog. 2025;199:107208. https://doi.org/10.1016/j.micpath.2024.107208.
117. Lu P, Zhang F-c, Qian S-w, et al. Artemisinin derivatives prevent obesity by inducing browning of WAT and enhancing BAT function. Cell Res. 2016;26(10):1169–72. https://doi.org/10.1038/cr.2016.108.

118. Guo X, Asthana P, Zhai L, et al. Artesunate treats obesity in male mice and non-human primates through GDF15/GFRAL signalling axis. Nat Commun. 2024;15(1):1034. https://doi.org/10.1038/s41467-024-45452-3.
119. Liu Y, Jiang JJ, Du SY, et al. Artemisinins ameliorate polycystic ovarian syndrome by mediating LONP1-CYP11A1 interaction. Science. 2024;384(6701):eadk5382. https://doi.org/10.1126/science.adk5382.
120. Stener-Victorin E. Remedy hope for polycystic ovary syndrome. Science. 2024;384(6701):1174–5. https://doi.org/10.1126/science.adq0328.
121. Stein IF, Leventhal ML. Amenorrhea associated with bilateral polycystic ovaries. Am J Obstet Gynecol. 1935;29(2):181–91. https://doi.org/10.1016/S0002-9378(15)30642-6.
122. Adashi EY, Cibula D, Peterson M, Azziz R. The polycystic ovary syndrome: the first 150 years of study. F&S Reports. 2023;4(1):2–18. https://doi.org/10.1016/j.xfre.2022.12.002.
123. Stein IF, Arens RA. IODIZED oil and pneumoperitoneum combined in gynecologic diagnosis: preliminary report. JAMA J Am Med Assoc. 1926;87(16):1299. https://doi.org/10.1001/jama.1926.92680160002013b.
124. Swanson M, Sauerbrei EE, Cooperberg PL. Medical implications of ultrasonically detected polycystic ovaries. J Clin Ultrasound. 1981;9(5):219–22. https://doi.org/10.1002/jcu.1870090504.
125. Azziz R. How polycystic ovary syndrome came into its own. F&S Science. 2021;2(1):2–10. https://doi.org/10.1016/j.xfss.2020.12.007.
126. Lafci NG, Yilmaz B, Yildiz BO. PCOS – the many faces of a disorder in women and men. J Endocrinol Investig 2024. https://doi.org/10.1007/s40618-024-02512-1, J Endocrinol Invest.
127. Burghen GA, Givens JR, Kitabchi AE. Correlation of Hyperandrogenism with Hyperinsulinism in polycystic ovarian disease*. J Clin Endocrinol Metab. 1980;50(1):113–6. https://doi.org/10.1210/jcem-50-1-113.
128. Mrabet HE, Ben Salem H, Ach T, Ben Abdelkarim A, Alaya W. Effects of SGLT-2 inhibitors on clinical and biological hyperandrogenism and menstruation irregularities in patients with polycystic ovary syndrome: a systematic review of randomized trials. SAGE Open Med. 2024;12:20503121241308997. https://doi.org/10.1177/20503121241308997.
129. Chen X, Koivuaho E, Piltonen TT, Gissler M, Lavebratt C. Association of maternal polycystic ovary syndrome or anovulatory infertility with obesity and diabetes in offspring: a population-based cohort study. Hum Reprod. 2021;36(8):2345–57. https://doi.org/10.1093/humrep/deab112.
130. Fornes R, Simin J, Nguyen MH, et al. Pregnancy, perinatal and childhood outcomes in women with and without polycystic ovary syndrome and metformin during pregnancy: a nationwide population-based study. Reprod Biol Endocrinol. 2022;20(1):30. https://doi.org/10.1186/s12958-022-00905-6.
131. Glintborg D, Rubin KH, Nybo M, Abrahamsen B, Andersen M. Cardiovascular disease in a nationwide population of Danish women with polycystic ovary syndrome. Cardiovasc Diabetol. 2018;17(1):37. https://doi.org/10.1186/s12933-018-0680-5.
132. Zhao L, Zhu Z, Lou H, et al. Polycystic ovary syndrome (PCOS) and the risk of coronary heart disease (CHD): a meta-analysis. Oncotarget. 2016;7(23):33715–21. https://doi.org/10.18632/oncotarget.9553.
133. de Groot PC, Dekkers OM, Romijn JA, Dieben SW, Helmerhorst FM. PCOS, coronary heart disease, stroke and the influence of obesity: a systematic review and meta-analysis. Hum Reprod Update. 2011;17(4):495–500. https://doi.org/10.1093/humupd/dmr001.
134. Sharma S, Mahajan N. Polycystic ovarian syndrome and menopause in forty plus women. J Midlife Health. 2021;12(1):3–7. https://doi.org/10.4103/jmh.jmh_8_21.
135. Moreau KL, LE DB. The role of androgens in microvascular endothelial dysfunction in polycystic ovary syndrome: does size matter? J Physiol. 2019;597(11):2829–30. https://doi.org/10.1113/jp277961.

136. Usselman CW, Yarovinsky TO, Steele FE, et al. Androgens drive microvascular endothelial dysfunction in women with polycystic ovary syndrome: role of the endothelin B receptor. J Physiol. 2019;597(11):2853–65. https://doi.org/10.1113/jp277756.
137. Lakhani K, Leonard A, Seifalian AM, Hardiman P. Microvascular dysfunction in women with polycystic ovary syndrome. Hum Reprod. 2005;20(11):3219–24. https://doi.org/10.1093/humrep/dei199.
138. Iacobellis G. Physiology and Cardioprotection of the Epicardial adipose tissue. In: Iacobellis G, editor. Epicardial Adipose Tissue: From Cell to Clinic. Cham: Springer; 2020. p. 9–17.
139. Aydogdu A, Uckaya G, Tasci I, et al. The relationship of epicardial adipose tissue thickness to clinical and biochemical features in women with polycystic ovary syndrome. Endocr J. 2012;59(6):509–16. https://doi.org/10.1507/endocrj.EJ11-0328.
140. Lim PO, Rodgers P, Cardale K, Watson AD, MacDonald TM. Potentially high prevalence of primary aldosteronism in a primary-care population. Lancet 1999;353(9146):40. https://doi.org/10.1016/S0140-6736(05)74868-6.
141. Petramala L, Concistrè A, Iannucci G, Letizia C. Adrenal Secretome and Epicardial Adipose Tissue. In: Iacobellis G, editor. Epicardial Adipose Tissue: From Cell to Clinic. Cham: Springer International Publishing; 2020. p. 167–72.
142. Timóteo AT, Barbas Albuquerque F, Lacerda Teixeira B. Pericardium, epicardial adipose tissue, and heart failure with preserved ejection fraction: pathophysiology, quantification and treatment target11All authors take responsibility for all aspects of the reliability and freedom from bias of the data presented and their discussed interpretation. Int J Cardiol. 2024;412:132303. https://doi.org/10.1016/j.ijcard.2024.132303.
143. Rabkin SW. Epicardial adipose tissue and reactive oxygen species. In: Laher I, editor. Systems biology of free radicals and antioxidants. Berlin/Heidelberg: Springer; 2014. p. 1021–30.
144. Stener-Victorin E, Padmanabhan V, Walters KA, et al. Animal models to understand the etiology and pathophysiology of polycystic ovary syndrome. Endocr Rev. 2020;41(4). https://doi.org/10.1210/endrev/bnaa010.
145. Liang J-x, Zhang Y, Xiao C-h, et al. Application value of tumor necrosis factor inhibitors in in vitro fertilization-embryo transfer in infertile women with polycystic ovary syndrome. BMC Pregnancy Childbirth. 2023;23(1):247. https://doi.org/10.1186/s12884-023-05546-0.
146. Wadden TA, Webb VL, Moran CH, Bailer BA. Lifestyle modification for obesity. Circulation. 2012;125(9):1157–70. https://doi.org/10.1161/CIRCULATIONAHA.111.039453.
147. Westermeier F, Fisman EZ. Glucagon-like peptide-1 receptor agonists (GLP-1RAs) and cardiometabolic protection: historical development and future challenges. Cardiovasc Diabetol. 2025;24(1):44. https://doi.org/10.1186/s12933-025-02608-9.
148. Yao H, Zhang A, Li D, et al. Comparative effectiveness of GLP-1 receptor agonists on glycaemic control, body weight, and lipid profile for type 2 diabetes: systematic review and network meta-analysis. BMJ. 2024;384:e076410. https://doi.org/10.1136/bmj-2023-076410.
149. Belen E, Değirmencioğlu A, Zencirci E, et al. The association between subclinical hypothyroidism and Epicardial adipose tissue thickness. Korean Circ J. 2015;45(3):210–5. https://doi.org/10.4070/kcj.2015.45.3.210.
150. Closs C, Vargas-Uricoechea H, Schwarzstein D, et al. Relationship of subclinical hypothyroidism on Epicardial adipose tissue: a systematic review and meta-analysis. Curr Probl Cardiol. 2023;48(7):101674. https://doi.org/10.1016/j.cpcardiol.2023.101674.
151. Sayin I, Erkan AF, Ekici B, et al. Thickening of the epicardial adipose tissue can be alleviated by thyroid hormone replacement therapy in patients with subclinical hypothyroidism. Kardiol Pol. 2016;74(12):1492–8. https://doi.org/10.5603/KP.a2016.0053.
152. Yazıcı D, Özben B, Toprak A, et al. Effects of restoration of the euthyroid state on epicardial adipose tissue and carotid intima media thickness in subclinical hypothyroid patients. Endocrine. 2015;48(3):909–15. https://doi.org/10.1007/s12020-014-0372-1.
153. Biondi B, Palmieri EA, Klain M, et al. Subclinical hyperthyroidism: clinical features and treatment options. Eur J Endocrinol. 2005;152(1):1–9. https://doi.org/10.1530/eje.1.01809.

154. Razvi S, Ingoe L, Keeka G, et al. The beneficial effect of L-thyroxine on cardiovascular risk factors, endothelial function, and quality of life in subclinical hypothyroidism: randomized, crossover trial. J Clin Endocrinol Metab. 2007;92(5):1715–23. https://doi.org/10.1210/jc.2006-1869.
155. Messerli FH, Bell DS, Fonseca V, et al. Body weight changes with beta-blocker use: results from GEMINI. Am J Med. 2007;120(7):610–5. https://doi.org/10.1016/j.amjmed.2006.10.017.
156. Sharma AM, Pischon T, Hardt S, Kunz I, Luft FC. Hypothesis: Beta-adrenergic receptor blockers and weight gain: a systematic analysis. Hypertension 2001;37(2):250–254. https://doi.org/10.1161/01.hyp.37.2.250.
157. Tzemos N, Lim PO, MacDonald TM. Nebivolol reverses endothelial dysfunction in essential hypertension: a randomized, double-blind, crossover study. Circulation. 2001;104(5):511–4. https://doi.org/10.1161/hc3001.094207.
158. Bordicchia M, Pocognoli A, D'Anzeo M, et al. Nebivolol induces, via β3 adrenergic receptor, lipolysis, uncoupling protein 1, and reduction of lipid droplet size in human adipocytes. J Hypertens. 2014;32(2):389–96. https://doi.org/10.1097/hjh.0000000000000024.
159. Ozyıldız AG, Eroglu S, Bal U, et al. Effects of carvedilol compared to Nebivolol on insulin resistance and lipid profile in patients with essential hypertension. J Cardiovasc Pharmacol Ther. 2017;22(1):65–70. https://doi.org/10.1177/1074248416644987.
160. Starling EH. On the absorption of fluids from the connective tissue spaces. J Physiol. 1896;19(4):311–26.
161. Laine GA, Allen SJ. Left ventricular myocardial edema. Lymph flow, interstitial fibrosis, and cardiac function. Circ Res. 1991;68(6):1713–21. https://doi.org/10.1161/01.RES.68.6.1713.
162. Olson KR. CIRCULATION | circulatory system design: roles and principles. In: Farrell AP, editor. Encyclopedia of fish physiology. San Diego: Academic; 2011. p. 977–83.
163. Mehlhorn U, Geissler HJ, Laine GA, Allen SJ. Myocardial fluid balance. Eur J Cardiothorac Surg. 2001;20(6):1220–30. https://doi.org/10.1016/s1010-7940(01)01031-4.
164. Kedem O, Katchalsky A. Thermodynamic analysis of the permeability of biological membranes to non-electrolytes. Biochim Biophys Acta. 1958;27:229–46. https://doi.org/10.1016/0006-3002(58)90330-5.
165. Luft JH. Fine structures of capillary and endocapillary layer as revealed by ruthenium red. Fed Proc. 1966;25(6):1773–83. https://pubmed.ncbi.nlm.nih.gov/5927412/.
166. Woodcock TE, Woodcock TM. Revised Starling equation and the glycocalyx model of transvascular fluid exchange: an improved paradigm for prescribing intravenous fluid therapy. BJA: Br J Anaesth. 2012;108(3):384–94. https://doi.org/10.1093/bja/aer515.
167. VanTeeffelen JW, Brands J, Stroes ES, Vink H. Endothelial Glycocalyx: sweet shield of blood vessels. Trends Cardiovasc Med. 2007;17(3):101–5. https://doi.org/10.1016/j.tcm.2007.02.002.
168. Pinsky MR, García MIM, Dubin A. Significance of critical closing pressures (starling resistors) in arterial circulation. Crit Care. 2024;28(1):127. https://doi.org/10.1186/s13054-024-04912-4.
169. Shabetai R. Cardiac Tamponade. In: The pericardium. New York: Springer Science+Business Media; 2013. p. 121–66.

Chapter 4
Euphoric Heart

Abstract Coronary slow flow phenomenon (CSFP) is present if it takes more than three heart beats for contrast media, when injected down a coronary artery, to pass from catheter tip to distal vessel. This is under non-emergent conditions in the cardiac catheter laboratory, and it is visually dramatic in an otherwise asymptomatic patient under study. It makes intuitive sense to attribute this to a restriction of blood flow into the myocardial microvasculature, therefore delaying dye transit, because of coronary microvascular dysfunction (CMD). However, there is a clear distinction between contrast and blood clearance; while the former is delayed, the latter may not be. Using continuous thermodilution in a series of patients with angina and non-obstructive coronary arteries (ANOCA), including two habitual recreational drug users (cocaine and cannabis), CSFP is consistently associated with a vasoreactive epicardial coronary artery, i.e. endothelial dysfunction, but it bears neither noticeable relationship with epicardial artery calibre nor microvascular function. Hence, it is possible to conclude by process of elimination that unprovoked CSFP is purely a rheological manifestation, due to an interaction between the contrast media and a dysfunctional epicardial artery that has a "sticky" vessel wall, likely with glycocalyx degradation which is a hallmark feature of endothelial dysfunction. Hypothetically, when present, CSFP can be altered by changing contrast viscosities via dilutions.

4.1 Introduction

How fast the resulting contrast flow down a disobliterated coronary artery following systemic thrombolysis carries prognostic information; this is classified according to Thrombolysis in Myocardial Infarction (TIMI) score of 0, I, II and III based on angiographic assessment [1]. Zero means no flow, I—contrast does not flow distally beyond the occlusion, II—slow but does traverse the whole length of artery, and III—normal flow. TIMI III flow is associated with the smallest infarct size on cardiac imaging studies, and this obviously relates to microvascular obstruction due to clots and myocardial interstitial oedema [2, 3]. This is also observed during coronary angioplasty, when the angiographic contrast flow slows following balloon

P. O. Lim, *Coronary Thermodilution*,
https://doi.org/10.1007/978-3-032-10734-3_4

dilatation or stent placement, termed, “no reflow”, ≤ TIMI II, due to distal embolisation of clots or atherosclerotic debris causing microvascular spasm or plugging of the microvasculature [4, 5].

On the other hand, in stable patients undergoing a diagnostic coronary angiogram, in general about 1% and up to 5–7% in those with unobstructed coronary arteries where coronary slow flow phenomenon is seen, first described in 1972 by Tambe et al. [6–9]. There is speculation that this is due to increased resistance to flow, due to coronary microvascular dysfunction (CMD), and has been described as a syndrome [10], making it a *distinct diagnostic entity* for angina with non-obstructive coronary arteries (ANOCA) [11]. In this chapter, patients who had CSFP underwent detailed coronary physiology study to assess whether it is associated with quantitative microvascular function by measuring coronary flow using continuous thermodilution.

4.2 Cases

4.2.1 Exploding Head

A 52-year-old Caucasian woman was referred to the coronary physiology clinic for assessment. She has had chest pain for many years, but this has become worse during Covid-19 lockdown in 2020. Her chest pain was exertional, as well as occurring at rest. She described the pain as starting in the chest and then rapidly radiated up to her head, giving her an explosive headache. Her neurologist gave her the diagnosis of *exploding head syndrome*, or *cardiac cephalgia*. Her daycase *diagnostic coronary angiogram* 5 months prior found smooth and unobstructed arteries, but with CSFP. Two weeks following her procedure she had an outpatient echocardiogram that found a normal heart with an ejection fraction (EF) of 60–65%, without noticeable wall motion abnormalities, left atrial dilatation, left ventricular hypertrophy (LVH) or diastolic dysfunction (E/e’ 7.7, < 8). Her treadmill exercise stress echocardiogram performed in the following three weeks, in which she did 7 min, stopping because of fatigue rather than chest pain—her pulse and BP at rest were 73 bpm and 123/83 mmHg, and at peak effort, 125 bpm and 135/80 mmHg, corresponding to 74%, under the 85% of predicted maximal heart rate, thus submaximal. There were no significant ECG changes of note, but at baseline she had reduced EF to 50–55%, new hypokinesia in apical anterior wall, that deteriorated to involve 4/17 mid apical anteroseptum and anterolateral segments—unexpected findings. Again, she did not have left atrial dilatation or LVH, end-systolic volume index, ESVI 36 (10–38) mL/m^2, stroke volume index, SVI 31 (30–59) mL/m^2, ventriculo-arterial coupling, VAC 1.2 (0.5–1.0) and E/E’ 14.9 (< 8). Her body mass index (BMI) was 35 kg/m^2. On the other hand, her cardiovascular magnetic resonance (CMR) scan 3 months later revealed a normal heart, both structurally and functionally, without scar, fibrosis or infarct, EF 62%, ESVI 30 (14–33) mL/m^2, SVI 49 (37–62) mL/m^2, VAC 0.6 (0.5–1.0)—a mysteriously normalised heart. Both her parents died of cardiac causes before their sixties. She is a chronic smoker, albeit 4 cigarettes a day despite her asthma, she has irritable bowel syndrome, congenital absence of right kidney, and has become menopausal 18 months earlier.

Procedure In view of her persistent symptoms, she is admitted for cardiac catheterisation. Her left ventricle is initially studied, and the left ventricular end-diastolic pressures (LVEDP) are 5 mmHg at rest and 10 mmHg with handgrip, which are normal, under 12 mmHg, with correspondingly low central aortic blood pressure (BP) of 120/70 mmHg. Her coronary arteries remain widely patent, again with obvious CSFP (Fig. 4.1).

With the pressure wire down the left anterior descending (LAD) artery, the distal-to-aorta pressure ratio, Pd/Pa, is 0.93 and rest full-cycle ratio, RFR, 0.92 (< 0.89). Continuous thermodilution is undertaken, the basal and hyperaemic indices are flow 59 and 1318 mL/min, and resistance 1318 and 261 Wood units—thus, coronary flow reserve, CFR, is 4.7 and microvascular resistance reserve, MRR, 5.1. Escalating doses of acetylcholine (ACh) are given, these are associated with a dose-dependent increase in epicardial vasospasm, but without accompanying reduction in flow, and therefore, no chest pain or ischaemic electrocardiographic changes noted (Fig. 4.2). The *respective relative indices* as proportion of basal value, in response to AC 2, 20, 100 and 200 μg, followed by verapamil 1 mg and ACh 200 μg rechallenge are

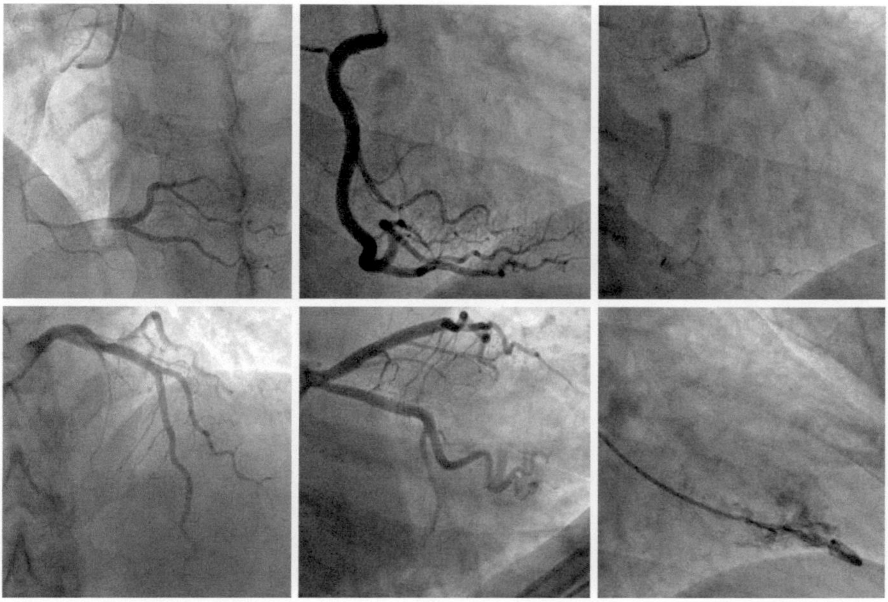

Fig. 4.1 (**Top, left to right panels**) Right coronary artery (RCA), with coronary slow flow phenomenon (CSFP) , *note* slow clearance of dye, the RCA is large, smooth, disease-free and unobstructed, and obvious contrast lingering in mid vessel. (**Bottom, left to right panels**) Left anterior descending (LAD) artery and circumflex artery with traversing contrast at 3 heartbeats, not quite opacifying the whole vessels or reaching the left ventricular apex. Left ventricular angiogram with hand injection of dye, demonstrating normal apical contractility

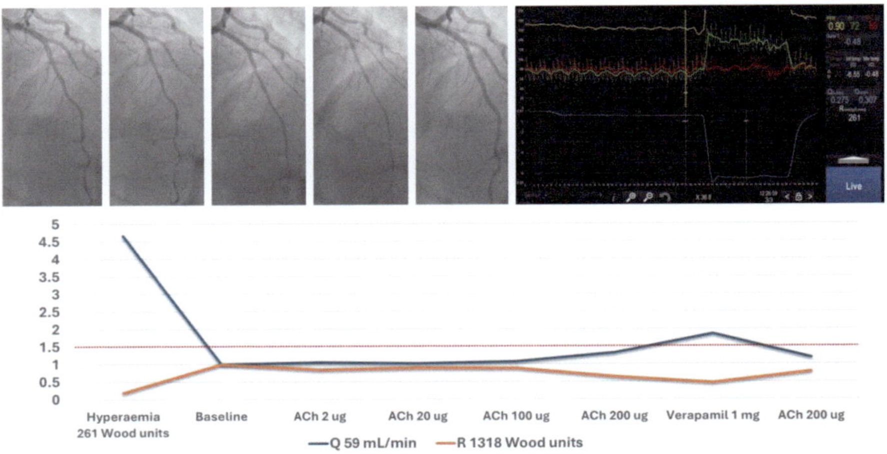

Fig. 4.2 (**Top, left to right panels**) coronary angiogram of the left anterior descending (LAD) artery following increasing intracoronary boluses of acetylcholine (ACh) sequentially from ACh 2, 20, 100 and 200 μg—causing worsening epicardial vasospasm. And ACh 200 μg after verapamil pretreatment. This time the LAD does not vasoconstrict in response to high-dose ACh. Continuous thermodilution of the LAD at hyperaemia, *note* that the steady state of mixed temperature of −0.48° Celsius is rapidly achieved with infusing saline at 20 ml/min via the Rayflow microcatheter, within 10 seconds. (**Bottom**) Haemodynamic plot of basal, hyperaemic and in response to ACh and verapamil, followed by ACh rechallenge. The vasodilatory capacity and coronary resistance are normal. Despite increasing LAD vasospasm, the flow does not fall below 1 or basal level, yet not rising by 50% in response to ACh—pathognomonic of microvascular endothelial dysfunction

flow—1.05, 1.02, 1.07, **1.32**, 1.86 and **1.18**; resistance—0.84, 0.89, 0.88, **0.64**, 0.46 and **0.78**; and Pd/Pa 0.92, 0.91, 0.91, 0.91, **0.86**, 0.92 and **0.96**—highlighted values are of ACh 200 μg before and after verapamil. Important to observe that despite increasing LAD epicardial vasospasm, the flow does not fall below the basal value, and although verapamil prevents ACh-induced epicardial vasospasm, it also at the same time "worsens" ACh-related microvascular flow increase. This verapamil-potentiated flow reduction with ACh is discussed in Chap. 3, the "Constraint heart".

Interpretation This postmenopausal woman who is a smoker turns out to have a structurally and functionally normal heart, although her stress echocardiogram in isolation was oddly abnormal. There was evident systolic and diastolic dysfunction with increased VAC, but her heart was demonstrably normal on CMR 3 months later, with VAC falling from 1.2 to 0.6. The only possible explanation in this case was that she had a fleeting episode of *takotsubo syndrome (TTS) or stress cardiomyopathy* having double-checked that she indeed had the test and it was her scan reports. She now has normal left ventricular function, unobstructed coronary arteries with preserved microvasculature. However, she has ***global endothelial dysfunction***, in response to ACh, she develops epicardial vasospasm indicating epicardial endothelial dysfunction, and her microvasculature autoregulates to maintain flow in spite of reducing coronary calibre, and the latter is not severe enough to reduce perfusion pressure gradient or Pd/Pa significantly (> 0.90). The flow nevertheless does not rise beyond 50% above baseline, which means microvascular endothelial dysfunction. Verapamil abolishes ACh-provoked epicardial vasospasm, yet it paradoxically reduces flow. In other words, the flow in response to ACh is greater with epicardial vasospasm than without it, after pretreatment with verapamil. This might explain the inconsistent efficacy of calcium channel blockers in coronary microvascular dysfunction (CMD).

Also, she fitted the bill as someone who is at risk for developing TTS, being postmenopausal and having vasoreactive coronary arteries. Finally, with further questioning, she has insomnia and poor quality sleep pattern. She describes that often at night just before falling asleep, she develops headache, chest pain, sees flashing lights and hears banging noise in her head, reminiscent of hypnagogic hallucination, due to sleep deprivation and rapid eye movement (REM) deficit. Her transient TTS could have been due to an episode of "night terror" from her dysfunctional sleep. She was advised to stop smoking, lose weight, practise healthy sleeping habits and was referred to the menopause clinic.

4.2.2 Athlete's Heart

A 56-year-old black woman started having chest pain 5 months before she was admitted to St George's Hospital. In the first month, she presented to her local emergency department three times. Her *diagnostic coronary angiogram* showed smooth and unobstructed coronary arteries, but with striking generalised *CSFP*. Her troponins were not elevated, neither was her NT-ProBNP, and her ECG showed tall QRS complexes with J-wave early repolarisation and biphasic T-wave that were static (Fig. 4.3). Standard dose oral nitrates appeared to settle her symptoms. Despite having mild asthma, in her younger days, she was into competitive powerlifting and basketball. She has continued to routinely exercise daily, but has noticed breathlessness and during recovery, experienced some chest pain. She had Covid-19 33 months prior, which she attributed her fatigue and breathlessness, not typical of her asthma to long Covid. In spite of her ECG changes, she was not hypertensive and has no coronary artery risk factors, she was postmenopausal, has a BMI of 32 kg/m^2, and not on hormone replacement therapy. She has moderate lumbar canal stenosis in L4/5, probably from her weight training. Her CMR 3 months later showed no scar, fibrosis, infarction, left atrial dilatation, no LVH, EF 62%, ESVI 31 (4–33) mL/m^2, SVI 50 (37–62) mL/m^2 and VAC 0.62 (0.6–1.0). Although her right atrium and right ventricle (EF 58%, 55–77; 93, 53–90 mL/m^2) appeared to be slightly dilated, attributed to her athletic training. Her previous D-dimer and CT pulmonary angiogram ruled out pulmonary embolism at her local hospital. She was assessed in the outpatient clinic the following year, and she has continuing symptoms both at rest and on exertion despite her oral nitrates. Hence, she was offered invasive coronary physiology which was undertaken a couple of months later.

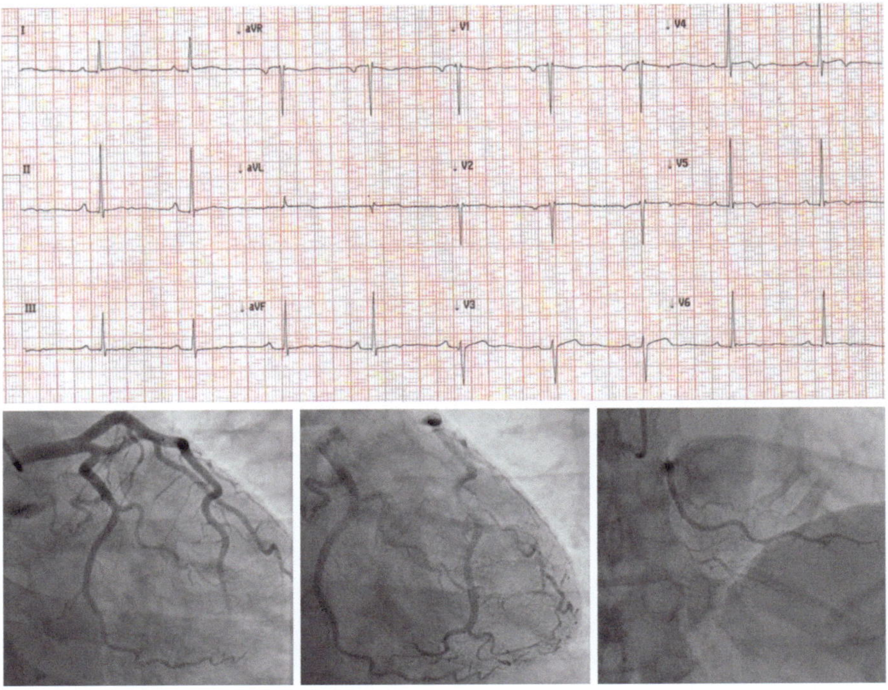

Fig. 4.3 (**Top panel**) 12-lead electrocardiogram with a heart rate of 57 beats per minute, with a J-wave post tall QRS, biphasic T-wave and normal axis—a pattern that is common in an athlete. (**Bottom, left to right panels**) First coronary angiogram undertaken about 2 years previously with generalised coronary slow flow phenomenon (CSFP) , note that at 3 heart beats, the contrast does not completely traverse to the distal vessels in the left coronary artery, and persistence of dye in distal vasculature suggesting delayed clearance. This is seen too in the right coronary artery

Procedure During her procedure, she has reactive BP, with a central aortic BP fluctuating up to 160/80 mmHg which is reflected in a raised LVEDP of 15 mmHg, without obvious LV wall motion abnormalities on LV angiogram. Her coronary arteries are disease-free and unobstructed, with less obvious CSFP compared to her coronary angiogram done nearly 2 years ago (Fig. 4.4). With the pressure wire down the LAD, Pd/Pa was 0.95 and RFR 0.93 (> 0.89), confirming unimpeded flow.

Bolus thermodilution is performed first. With IC 200 μg of adenosine, FFR is 0.92, CFR 6.5, IMR 23 and MRR 7.3; with 1000 μg adenosine—FFR is 0.90, CFR 9.3, IMR 10 and MRR 15. Although these values are supraphysiological, because the technique tends to overestimate, they do suggest that her vasodilatory capacity and coronary resistance are normal. This is confirmed with continuous thermodilution which obtained the following haemodynamic basal and hyperaemic indices; flow 69 and 374 mL/min, and resistance 1328 and 272 Wood units—CFR 5.4 and MRR 4.9.

ACh 2 μg provokes diffuse moderate epicardial vasospasm, fractional flow falls by 16% and resistance rises by 37%, but without significant reduction in Pd/Pa at 0.92, and with ACh 20 μg, there is severe epicardial vasospasm and worsening flow,

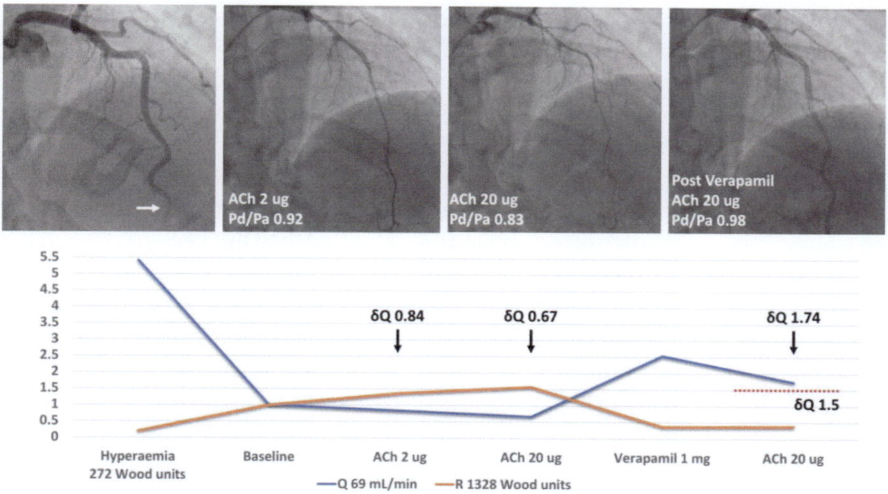

Fig. 4.4 (**Top, left to right panels**) Flow down the left anterior descending (LAD) artery is delayed, not quite reaching the apex at three heart beats—prior study about 2 years ago. Acetylcholine (ACh) 2 μg causes diffuse moderate epicardial vasospasm without a reduction in Pd/Pa. With the next dose of ACh at 20 μg, there is a dose-dependent worsening of LAD vasospasm, assiociated with chest pain and ischaemic electrocardiographic changes. The dose of ACh after verapamil pretreatment abolishes its effects. (**Bottom**) Haemodymanic indices in response to saline hyperaemia, ACh and verapamil as multiples of baseline value at 1, or unity. There is normal vasodilatory capacity and resistance, but there is also enhanced vasoreactivity to low doses of ACh, with resulting epicardial vasospasm, and flow reduction. Verapamil prevents both epicardial vasospasm. With ACh 20 μg rechallenged, flow is > 50% above baseline, and this can be interpreted as intact microvascular endothelial function, which otherwise was masked by the severe epicardial vasospasm

falling by 33%, resistance rising by 57%, and Pd/Pa falls to 0.83. This is associated with chest pain and ECG lateral ST elevation. With verapamil 1 mg, this abolishes the epicardial vasospasm, Pd/Pa 0.95, flow rises 2.5-fold and resistance falls by two-thirds. When rechallenged with ACh 20 μg, this time there is no radiographic epicardial vasospasm, Pd/Pa stays high at 0.98, flow increases by 74% (> 50%) and resistance decreases by 61%.

Interpretation This woman who is physically very active with vagal dominance has no significant coronary artery disease, normal microvascular vasodilatory capacity, and normal coronary resistance. But has both coronary and peripheral endothelial dysfunction, and the reactive BP rises during her procedure causing her LVEDP to increase, suggestive of LV diastolic dysfunction. Low doses of ACh cause diffuse epicardial vasospasm, with diminished flow. Verapamil abolishes these ACh effects, and interestingly, with verapamil on board, ACh increases flow > 50% from baseline, which fulfils the definition for preserved microvascular endothelial function. In other words, verapamil by preventing epicardial vasospasm unmasked her intact microvascular endothelial function.

This woman therefore is *highly vasoreactive epicardial coronary artery*—on top of LV diastolic dysfunction with raised LVEDP in response to increased afterload. She has normal thyroid function, haematinics and vitamin D level, but consistently elevated C-reactive protein (CRP) of 5.5 to 6 (< 5) mg/L suggesting systematic inflammation, in addition, she is on inhaled steroids which theoretically could have systemic spillover effects, although this effect is noticeable with oral steroids. She unfortunately was intolerant of oral diltiazem and verapamil, thus was maintained on a higher dose of isosorbide mononitrate at 40 mg od, and has been referred to the menopause clinic. Home monitoring of her BP shows consistent systolic BP < 130 mmHg. Her *epicardial coronary vasoreactivity* is likely to be multifactorial. Her right heart dilatation and ECG pattern are related to her athletic training, but this case exemplifies the notion that athleticism does not always preserved vascular endothelial function [12].

4.2.3 Triphasic Flow

A 61-year-old woman has been experiencing chest pain since 15 years ago, started at the time when she was perimenopausal. She has had various investigations at her local tertiary cardiac unit over the years. Her CT coronary angiogram, exercise tolerance test, echocardiogram and 24 hr Holter monitoring all had been unremarkable. She was overweight, with a *BMI of 39 kg/m2*, and has resistant hypertension on 3 antihypertensive agents; bisoprolol 2.5 mg od, ramipril 10 mg od and bendroflumethiazide 1.25 mg od. Despite these drugs, her recent office BP was high at 145/81 mmHg. She was on hormone replacement therapy—Sandrena transdermal oestradiol gel 1 mg od and Utrogestan 100 mg od nocte, in spite of which her postmenopausal symptoms continued—flushes, night sweats, urinary frequency and nocturia. She was also on vitamin D 25 μg od. She described an anginal-type pain, which was mostly exertional, rather than occurring at rest or waking her up at night. When it started, there was a lingering element of up to 30 minutes with a variable response to sublingual nitroglycerine. She has a presumptive diagnosis of coronary microvascular dysfunction (CMD) and was intolerant of verapamil. Her adenosine stress perfusion CMR 2 weeks prior to her invasive coronary physiology study was normal without LA dilatation or LVH, no gadolinium enhancement, ischaemia, scar, fibrosis or infarct—EF 59%, ESVI 30 (11–35) mL/m^2, SVI 33 mL/m^2 and VAC 0.91 (0.6–1.0).

Procedure Her coronary physiology study starts with the LV, and unexpectedly, her LVEDP is elevated > 25 mmHg with obvious *mid-cavity waisting*, with a central aortic blood pressure that is also elevated, > 160/80 mmHg (Fig. 4.5). Her coronary arteries are disease-free, the distal vessels are however tortuous with petering calibre, but the contrast as a marker of flow traverses the arteries within a single heartbeat, thus no CSFP. Continuous thermodilution is under-

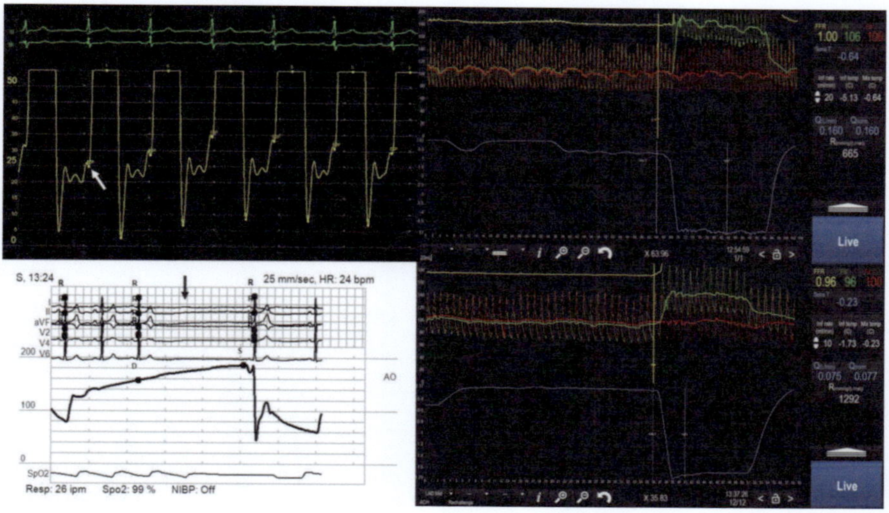

Fig. 4.5 (**Top, left to right panels**) Marked elevation in left ventricular end-diastolic pressure (LVEDP >25 mmHg, *arrow*) in response to a reactive systemic blood pressure (BP). In the absence of epicardial coronary artery disease, note the fractional flow reserve, FFR, of 1.0 and high mean distal coronary BP of 106 mmHg, in the circumflex artery. The measured hyperaemic minimal resistance is high, at 665 Wood units, if converted by a factor of 20 to index of microvascular resistance (IMR), this is 33 (< 25). (**Bottom, left to right panels**) Acetylcholine (ACh) 200 μg causes drop beats (*arrow*) peaking of T-wave in inferior leads and T-wave inversion in precordial V2 which can be due to subendocardial ischaemia. Post verapamil, ACh 200 μg causes impressive coronary slow flow phenomenon (CSFP) , in the absence of distal coronary pressure fall, or epicardial vasospasm pointing to a pure microvascular phenomenon, note failure of flow to increase, in fact slightly less than the basal flow by −7%. In other words, verapamil impairs microvascular endothelial function

taken in the circumflex artery first, the following basal and hyperaemic indices are obtained—flow 43 and 160 mL/min, and 2661 and 665 Wood units, and thus CFR is 3.7 and MRR 4. By the time the LAD is studied, the systolic BP falls < 140 mmHg, with the following corresponding results—flow 81 and 234 mL/min, and 1207 and 375 Wood units, and therefore CFR is 2.9 and MRR 3.2. Escalating doses of ACh are given (Fig. 4.6). With ACh 2 μg, obvious CSFP is observed, and it is associated flow decreases with rising resistance. Similarly with ACh 20 μg, although the measured flow is higher, it is still below baseline—this is usually interpreted as microvascular spasm. There is a clearly dose-dependent increase in mid to distal LAD vasospasm, sparing the proximal coronary arteries. Paradoxically, with ACh 100 and 200 μg, CSFP actually disappears, with increasing flow above baseline, 1.65-fold and 1.57-fold, respectively, but associated with drop beats, at the latter ACh dose, there is chest pain with ischaemic ECG changes. Verapamil 1 mg causes global vasodilatation, and ACh 200 μg rechallenge produces marked CSFP and no flow increase beyond the baseline, this being asymptomatic.

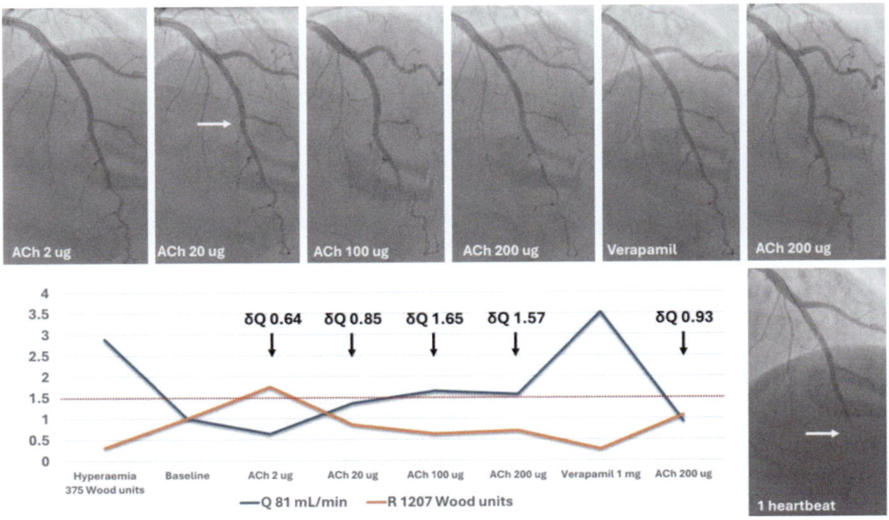

Fig. 4.6 (**Top, left to right panels**) Acetylcholine (ACh) causes a *dose-dependent epicardial vasospasm*, but it is isolated to mid to distal left anterior descending (LAD) artery. Coronary slow flow phenomenon (CSFP) is observed with ACh 2 and 20 µg, the *arrow* points to where the constrast reaches at one heartbeat. The flow improves to within one heartbeat in traversing the LAD despite worsening epicardial vasospasm with ACh 100 and 200 µg. Verapamil vasodilates the LAD. Interestingly, ACh 200 µg rechallenge does not reduce the LAD calibre, but CSFP reappears, and at one heartbeat, the contrast reaches the junction post second diagonal branch, between mid and distal LAD (**Bottom, right panel**). (**Bottom, left panel**) Haemodynamic indices at baseline, saline hyperaemia, in response to ACh and verapamil. The vasodilatory capacity is normal, coronary flow reserve, CFR, is 2.9, microvascular resistance reserve, MRR, 3.2, and minimal hyperaemic resistance 375 Wood units, which is equivalent to an index of microvascular reistance, IMR, of 19 (< 25), when divided by 20. The initial flow reduction with ACh 2 µg increases proportionally with escalating doses despite increasing epicardial vasospasm, flow increases > 50% with ACh 100 and 200 µg in the absence of CSFP, fulfilling the definition for preserved microvascular endothelial function. But ACh 200 µg provokes chest pain with electrocardigraphic ischaemic changes which implies flow diversion. Verapamil triples the flow and prevents ACh 200 µg from provoking epicardial vasospasm, but paradoxically it also abolishes ACh's ability to augment flow. Does verapamil therefore impair microvascular endothelial function?

Interpretation This woman has treated hypertension, albeit not to target with high office BP, and she exhibits procedural reactive BP initially. Her coronary arteries are unobstructed, and this allows the systemic BP to be transmitted to the microvasculature unimpeded, causing a rise in resistance with resultant low baseline flow in the Cx that is studied first. And the heart in generating flow against this rise in afterload or peripheral resistance elevated the LVEDP to a heart failure level by virtue of diastolic dysfunction.

Her contemporaneous *NT-ProBNP is* not elevated at 86 (< 125) ng/L, suggesting that she does not normally run a high LVEDP, that her BP might be better controlled outside the office or cardiac catheter laboratory, or this is an underestimate as NT-ProBNP could be inappropriately low in obesity [13, 14]. In this instance, when this hypertensive response settles, subsequent coronary physiology study in the

LAD reveals normal vasodilatory capacity and resistance. ACh causes microvascular spasm (or distal LAD spasm) and CSFP at low doses, but this is overcome at higher ACh doses, with flow that is faster and volumetrically higher, despite increasing epicardial vasospasm. Throughout the four escalating ACh doses, the Pd/Pa stays > 0.9, respectively, 0.99, 0.99, 0.98 and 0.97. *On caveat is that these figures do not cover the pressure fall in distal LAD beyond the pressure wire tip due to diffuse epicardial small vessel spasm.* She develops chest pain, and ECG changes with a flow that is 57% higher than baseline. One possible explanation is that although flow down the LAD is increased in totality, it might diversional flow, increased in the epicardium, but reduced in the subendocardium or LV apex, but the latter does not fit with transmural apical ischaemia because the left precordial leads, V3–6 are relatively unchanged.

Interesting, although verapamil dilates the LAD and increases flow, it abolishes ACh's capacity to augment flow as it did earlier at the same dose. Stated another way, verapamil curtails microvascular endothelial function in this case. She had a dobutamine stress echocardiogram (DSE) a couple of weeks later which showed a normal heart without inducible ischaemia, with an adequate heart rate response > 85%, EF 59%, without LA dilatation or LVH, but elevated E/e' 9.3 (< 8.0), ESVI 22 mL/m^2, SVi 31 mL/m^2 and VAC 0.71 (0.6–1.0). And her 24-hr ambulatory BP monitoring in the following 2 weeks, her daytime mean BP was 121/64 mmHg, with a normal nighttime dip. Her measured vitamin D level was 39 (> 50) nmol/l and oestradiol level was 214 (< 250) pmol/l on the day she had her coronary physiology study.

She was reviewed in the Menopause clinic 5 weeks after her procedure, and was advised to take vitamin D supplementation and increase the dose of oestradiol gel by 50%. Strictly, this woman has *epicardial endothelial dysfunction*. But the following observations were made: 1. Underlying hypertension and diastolic dysfunction, 2. Epicardial vasoreactivity restricted to distal vessels, 3. Preserved microvascular endothelial function, 4. Nonselective non-dihydropyridine L-type calcium channel blockers (verapamil and diltiazem) vasodilated epicardial vasculature, yet impaired blood flow. The *triphasic response to ACh*:

1. Distal LAD vasospasm with **fall in flow** and CSFP (ACh 2 and 20 μg)
2. Distal LAD vasospasm worsening with **increased flow** > 50% and resolution of CSFP (ACh 100 and 200 μg)
3. Distal LAD vasodilated with verapamil, **reduction of flow** to just below baseline level and recurrence of CSFP with ACh 200 μg rechallenge

It is not intuitive what causes the triphasic response to ACh in this woman. One possible speculative narrative is that a reduction in distal LAD calibre impedes flow and causes the CSFP in phase 1. As the microvascular endothelial function kicks into action with higher doses of ACh, the flow increases despite worsening epicardial vasospasm, with resolution of CSFP in phase 2. Verapamil resolves the epicardial vasospasm, the resulting full force of perfusion pressure coupled with ACh increases capillary permeability and the raised LVEDP increase interstitial pressure, compressing the microvasculature, reducing flow in phase 3 with reemergence of CSFP (also noted in Chap. 8—case 3).

4.2.4 Frequent Attender

This 57-year-old man was previously described in detail [15]. He first presented when he was 38, or 19 years ago when he was admitted with a troponin negative chest pain. His coronary angiogram at the time showed a moderate mid LAD lesion with generalised CSFP. He was medically treated at first but when an inpatient exercise tolerance test was performed, this turned out to be positive for ischaemia. He therefore had an intravascular ultrasound (IVIS) guided percutaneous coronary intervention (PCI) (Fig. 4.7). Although the minimal luminal area was 5 mm^2 and the lesion was in fact 50% stenotic. Because of his recurrent chest pain with a positive stress test, the mid LAD was stented with a Boston Taxus 3.5x24 mm drug-eluting stent (DES). This was nearly 2 decades ago, in current practice with better understanding of coronary physiology, this would not have happened. From then to now, he has had 14 invasive procedures involving many operators, and most were undertaken through recurrent hospitalisations. He rarely attended outpatient clinic follow-ups. Interesting to note that 13/14, or 93% were troponin negative chest pain admissions, the one time it was positive, this was a minor rise of 91 (< 14) ng/L [15]. The following arterial accesses were used—right radial x3, right femoral x9, left radial x1 and right ulnar x1—the radial arteries by now were occluded. He consistently showed CSFP and has had 2 instent restenoses (ISR) treated over the time period, including 5 IVUS and 5 pressure wiring studies. He was a nonsmoker but used cocaine, without other coronary artery disease risk factors. He was overweight

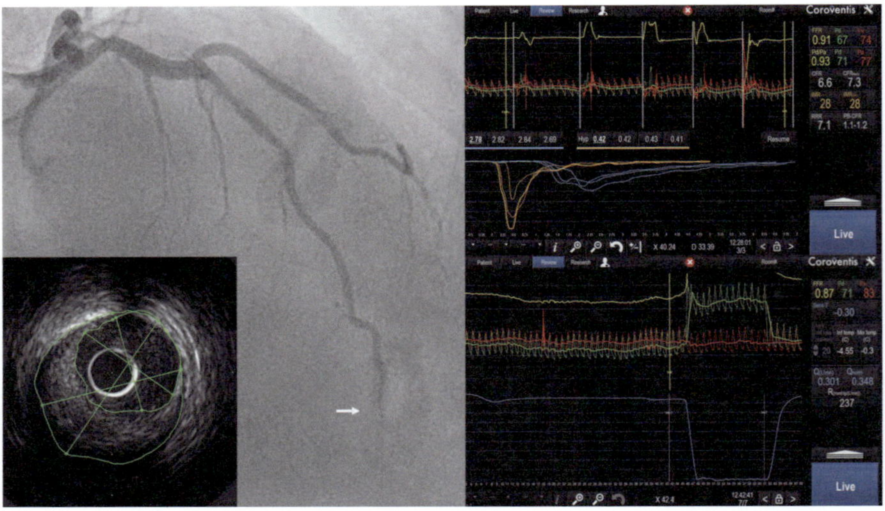

Fig. 4.7 (**Left panel**) Marked coronary slow flow phenomeon (CSFP) down the left anterior descending (LAD) artery, the *arrow* points to constrast reaching the distal LAD at 3 heart beats. The intravascular ultrasoung (*inset*) shows the original mid LAD lesion before stenting 19 years ago, with a borderline minimal luminal area (MLA) of 5 (< 4) mm^2. (**Left, top and bottom panels**) Bolus thermodiltion with discordant coronary flow reserve, CFR $\geq$ 2.5 and index of microvascular resistance, MRR $\geq$ 25, whereas continuous thermodilution finds normal microvascular function with concordant vasodilatory capacity and coronary resistance

with a BMI of 33 kg/m² and has a normal heart on echocardiogram without left atrial (LA) dilatation, or left ventricular hypertrophy (LVH), and his ECG showed right bundle branch block with left anterior fascicular block. His adenosine stress perfusion CMR when he was 44, after a pressure wire study found an FFR of 0.85 (> 0.80) in the LAD, was normal—EF 73%, LVMI 61 (56–89) g/m², without LA dilatation, ESVI 19 (13–35) mL/m², SVI 51 (39–63) mL/m² and VAC 0.37 (0.6–1.0). His coronary physiology study was undertaken after yet another troponin negative chest pain admission about 2 years ago with this update in his clinical course.

Procedure A right ulnar approach is used, as the right radial artery that was cannulated 3 times before is occluded. A 4 French sheath is used, followed by a 5 French EBU4.0 guide catheter introduced sheathlessly as was previously described [16, 17]. He has a low central aortic BP of 95/68 mmHg, and his LVEDP is 5 mmHg, which does not rise with hand gripping. The LAD has moderate ISR within the stent, with CSFP, the rest of his coronary arteries are unobstructed (Fig. 4.7).

With the pressure wire down his LAD the Pd/Pa is 0.92, RFR 0.92 (> 0.89), and bolus thermodilution is undertaken with IC adenosine 200 μg. The following haemodynamic indices are obtained—FFR 0.91, CFR 6.6, MRR 7.3 and IMR 28. Next, continuous thermodilution is carried out with these basal and hyperaemic values—flow 68 and 301 mL/min, and resistance 1226 and 237 Wood units; hence the CFR is 4.4, MRR 5.2, and the derived IMR based on minimal hyperaemic resistance of 237/20 is 12.

Escalating ACh doses are given with resultant epicardial vasospasm, but without a fall in flow, neither an increase in flow > 50% from baseline. Pd/Pa is maintained > 0.90 with ACh 2 and 20 μg, and 0.85 with ACh 100 μg. The latter dose causes severe epicardial vasospasm with intermittent drop beats, but without chest pain or ischaemic ECG changes. The LAD vasospasm is reversed by IC GTN. Verapamil 1 mg augmented flow 1.9-fold and ameliorated the effect of ACh 100 μg rechallenge, in addition to an even higher ACh dose at 200 μg. Although these higher ACh doses continue to cause intermittent drop beats (Fig. 4.8). The figures are adapted with permission from Elsevier of the published article, "Lim, PO, What causes cocaine-related coronary slow flow phenomenon? IHJ Cardiovascular Reports, 2024;8:36-39".

Interpretation This man has *premature atherosclerotic coronary artery* disease under 40 years of age due to cocaine use. He has both *epicardial and microvascular endothelial dysfunction*—ACh causes epicardial vasospasm and his coronary flow fails to rise above 50% from baseline. Nevertheless, although his CSFP gives rise to an elevated IMR, his *microvasculature is demonstrably normal* with continuous thermodilution: *normal CFR of 4.4 and hyperaemic minimal resistance of 237 Wood units.* He was advised to institute positive lifestyle changes off his drug treatment, but he has continued to present to the emergency department on a weekly basis. Unless he clearly develops ECG changes with associated troponin rise, invasive management of his coronary artery disease should be avoided, given that he already has had 14 cardiac catheterisations.

Cocaine produces intense euphoria by blocking *dopamine* reuptake in the synapses of the mesolimbic reward pathways of the brain, from midbrain ventral tegmental area (VTA) to ventral striatum (nucleus accumbens) in basal forebrain.

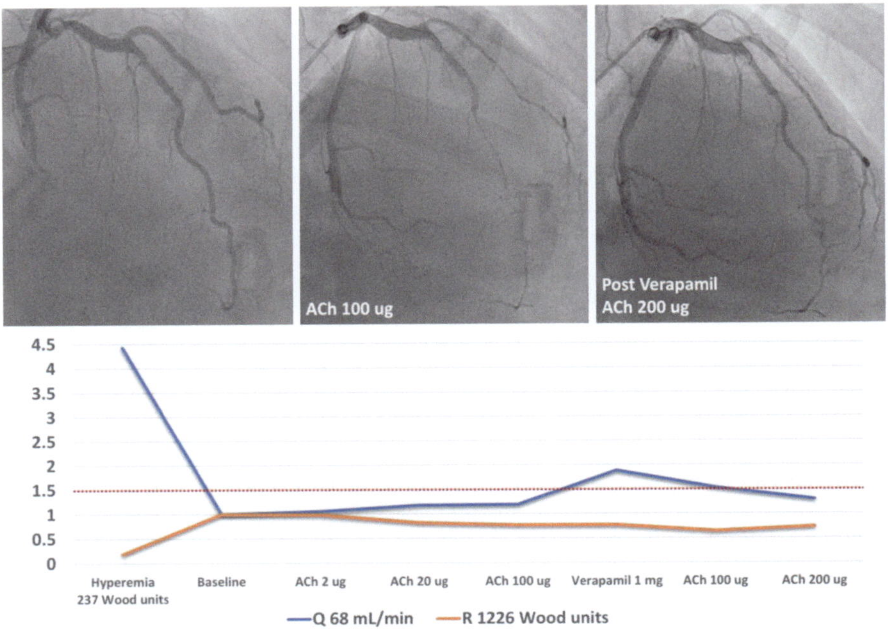

Fig. 4.8 (**Top, left to right panels**) Left anterior descending (LAD) artery at baseline with moderate diffuse instent restenosis, but non-obstructive with a fractional flow reserve, FFR of 0.87 (> 0.80) with saline hyperaemia. Acetylcholine (ACh) casuses severe epicardial vasospasm, which is ameliorated by verapamil pretreatment. (**Bottom**) Haemodynamic chart of flow and resistance from baseline, and in response to saline hyperaemia, ACh and verapamil. ACh causes epicardial vasospasm, flow does not fall, with downtrending of resistance suggesting compensatory response of the microvasculature. Yet the flow does not rise > 50%. The respective fractional flow are—4.4, 1 (basal), 1.1, 1.2, 1.2, 1.9 (verapamil), 1.5 and 1.3. The Pd/Pas are > 0.90, other then at 0.85 with ACh 100 μg before verapamil

Cocaine binds the triple monoamine transporters, acting as a serotonin–norepinephrine–dopamine reuptake inhibitor (SNDRI), reducing their synaptic clearance [18]. Elevated *norepinephrine* heightens sympathetic arousal, increasing energy and alertness, and elevated *serotonin* affects mood and confidence. Cocaine can also indirectly disinhibit dopamine neurons. For example, studies show cocaine potentiates certain γ-Aminobutyric Acid (GABA)ergic synapses in the VTA, reducing inhibitory GABA neuron firing and thereby "freeing" dopamine neurons to fire more [19]. In essence, cocaine's transport-blocking action floods the brain's reward circuitry with neurotransmitters, explaining its intense high and associated loss of inhibition. Occasional use for perceived performance enhancement has been reported among entertainers.

Cocaine's acute sympathetic stimulation apart from inducing pupillary dilatation, tachycardia and hypertension also increases epicardial coronary vasoreactivity that can be inhibited by phentolamine, an α-blocker, but made worse by beta-blockade [20, 21]. Sustained cocaine use increases endothelial endothelin-1 production, impairs endothelial nitric oxide homeostasis, promotes leucocyte migration and disrupts endothelial glycocalyx barrier, allowing low-density lipoprotein to permeate into the subintimal space [22, 23]. The cocaine-related endothelial dysfunction gives rise to early onset coronary atherosclerosis.

This man's coronary artery disease is consistent with cocaine use, the early onset atherosclerosis, and relatively high baseline coronary tone, normally functioning microvasculature that is able to generate over 4.5-fold in coronary flow with hyperaemia, but with significant endothelial dysfunction involving both the epicardial coronary and microvasculature. Verapamil doubles coronary flow yet made the CSFP worse, suggesting a disconnect between flow and CSFP as observed by others [24, 25], and it counters the epicardial reactivity to ACh rechallenge. He was advised to overcome his drug habit and implement lifestyle changes.

4.2.5 Euphoric Heart

A 65-year-old woman of mixed parentage with Jamaican heritage complained of breathlessness and angina that radiated from central chest up her neck, often at rest which usually rapidly responsive to GTN spray. She was admitted with Takostubo syndrome (TTS), requiring inotropic support in the intensive care, three and a half years ago (Fig. 4.9). Her coronary angiogram at the time revealed unobstructed

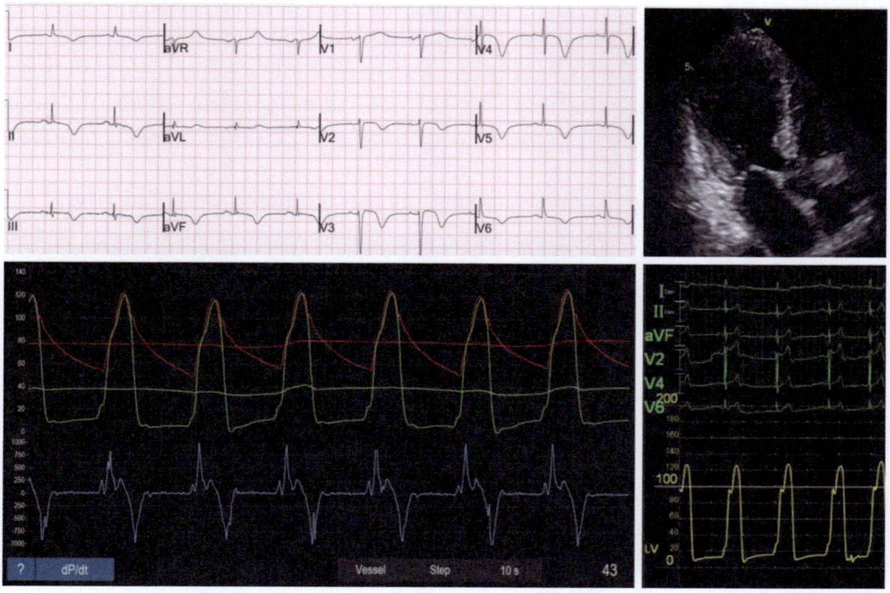

Fig. 4.9 (**Top, left to right panels**) ECG with the pathognomonic Takotsubo syndrome with the "giant" T-wave inversion and the echocardiogram in apical two-chamber long-axis view shows dykinesia in the apex and mid LV. (**Bottom, right to left panels**) The up-to-date ECG shows upright T-waves and LV pressure tracing showing elevated LVEDP, and the pressure wire in the LV confirms the high LVEDP in addition to reduced dP/dt and higher Tau

coronary arteries with a moderate lesion in the obtuse marginal branch. Her ECG was classically for TTS, with widespread deep T-wave inversion, and echocardiogram showed LV mid to apical dyskinesia with an EF of < 35%, and VAC 2.3 (0.6–1.0). Her CMR within a week revealed marked improvement in EF, at 52%, ESVI 49 (13–31) mL/m^2, SVI 51 (36–58) mL/m^2, VAC 1.0 (0.6–1.0), without LA dilatation or LVH, but mild apical hypokinesia.

She has complex and a long list of medical problems, including throat cancer in remission, thyroid dysfunction, fibromyalgia, multiple joint pain, chronic pancreatitis, aortic vasculopathy, depression, and anxiety. She had a further coronary angiogram, one and a half years ago, which found no new interval changes. Her heart has normalised in EF.

She was a lifelong *cannabis* user and was a frequent emergency department attender, nearly always unable to keep her outpatient clinic appointments and attend for investigations. Her last echocardiogram during an admission with a troponin negative chest pain showed a normal LV, EF 60–65%, with persistent mild basal RV and RA dilatation without pulmonary hypertension, average E/e' 11.9 (> 8). Unfortunate, she did not turn up for her CMR on multiple occasions. She was last admitted for an episode of inflammatory colitis one month prior to her current coronary physiology, and her last BMI was 27.5 kg/m^2.

Procedure A 4 French pigtail catheter is used to measure the LVEDP, which is 20–30 mmHg. Hence the pressure wire is advanced into the LV after upsizing to a 5 French JR4 guide catheter. This allows measurement of LV pressure-time derivatives, which indicate LV systolic and diastolic dysfunction, with raised LVEDP and central aortic systolic BP of 120 mmHg, and she runs a low pulse rate of 45 bpm; max +dP/dt (index of contractility) 966 (> 1200) mmHg/s, min -dP/dt (index of relaxation) -1035 (< −1100) mmHg/s and Weiss' Tau, τ (time constant of relaxation) 0.06 s (< 0.05).

Her coronary angiogram shows no new changes, coronary slow flow phenomenon as noted before, especially the RCA that supplies the inferobasal LV. The following hyperaemic and basal indices are obtained in duplicates; flow 348, **322**, 137 and **139** mL/min, and resistance 249, **280**, 628 and **607** Wood units, using the repeat values: CFR 2.3, MRR 2.2 and IMR 14 (280/20). These values are normal, consistent with a vasodilated resting state (Fig. 4.10).

Escalating ACh doses are given, the first dose of 2 μg is associated with 14% flow reduction and resistance increased by 26%, whereas the next three doses of 20, 100 and 200 μg are not affecting flow at all, while with 100 and 200 μg she has drop beats, and provoke a dose-response of mild-to-moderate mid LAD vasospasm. The effect of verapamil 1 mg is blunted with regard to flow but resolves the LAD vasospasm, when rechallenged with ACh 200 μg, this causes less LAD spasm, instead there is a modest rise in flow by 40% (< 50%).

Interpretation This woman has preserved vasodilatory reserve but *global endothelial dysfunction*, i.e. ACh-induced epicardial vasospasm and a blunted flow response to ACh to imply microvascular endothelial dysfunction. She has both reduced LV systolic and impaired diastolic function with low ±dP/dt and pro-

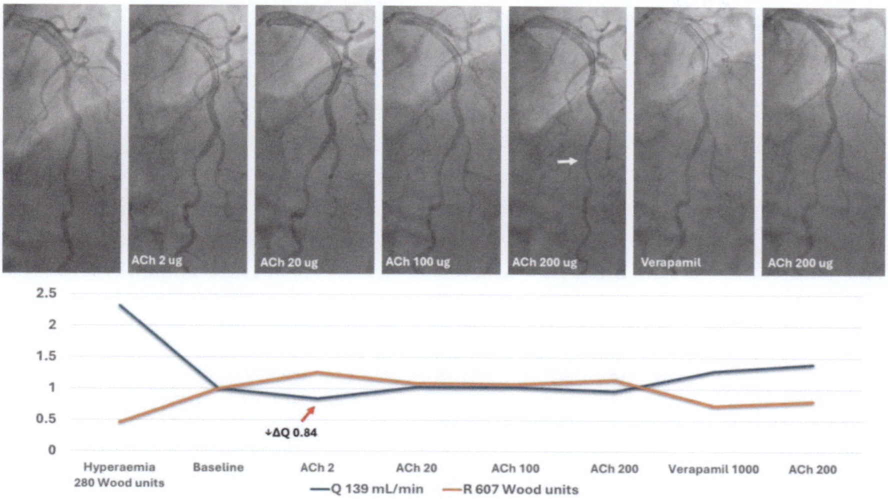

Fig. 4.10 (**Top, left to right panels**) Baseline high flow and low resistance. The LAD following acetylcholine with 2, 20, 100 and 200 μg; low-dose ACh causes flow reduction, and the last two doses of ACh cause epicardial vasospasm, but flat respnse to flow. IC verapamil abolishes the epicardial vasospasm and ameriolated rechallenge with ACh 200 μg which is potentiated with 40% increase in flow

longed Tau. Her contemporaneous NT-ProBNP is elevated at 420 (< 125) pg/L, and it was 718 the previous month proving that she has HFpEF with raised LVEDP. The reduced flow response to verapamil (flow ↑29% vs. ↑132% with hyperaemia) suggests an altered ACh signalling away from nitric oxide at the microvascular level (discussed in detail in Chap. 7).

She grew up in a community where cannabis use is part of the culture, and she smoked 1 gm divided into 3–4 rolled-up joints per day, which helped her general aches and pains, and anxiety. Cannabis is derived from the plant cannabis sativa, which is a source of fibre for fabrics, cosmetic cream, and herbal medicine to treat inflammation and provide analgesia. It has been cultivated for thousands of years, and it has different names for its different parts and derivatives; Má by the Chinese, Ganja by the Indians, kánnabis by the Greeks, Hashish by the Arabs, and it was introduced to Jamaica by indentured Indian workers in 1850s, and later adopted into the Rastafarian culture [26, 27]. In the US, it is called Marijuana from the 1930s, associating its use with Mexican immigrants, and laws were enacted to forbid it.

Hemp-derived CBD (cannabidiol) is a nonpsychoactive compound that is legal mainly for use in rare epilepsies in children. Over-the-counter CBD is consumed for attention deficit hyperactive disorder (ADHD)-related symptoms although evidence for its efficacy is lacking [28]. The psychoactive molecule is the Δ9-tetrahydrocannabinol (THC), hemp has $\leq 0.3\%$, whereas the marijuana plant has more of THC, especially the unpollinated flower bud from female plants, called sinsemilla (Spanish for without seeds), which has the highest density of trichomes, frosted tiny glands that produce the resin-like alkaloids which include THC, CBD and terpenoids [29, 30].

Cannabis is an illegal Class B drug under the Misuse of Drugs Act 1971 in the UK. In 2023–24, about 90,000 cannabis possession offences were recorded in England and Wales, and 16% led to formal charges, of that, about 2500 received custodial sentences, mostly under six months although the law allows a jail time of up to 14 years. Over the same period, 85 tonnes of herbal cannabis and 480,000 plants were confiscated [31]. On the other hand, many countries, including the US (about half the states) and Europe, have set legal limits for personal possession of cannabis in public, for example, from ≤ 5 gm in Belgium and Netherlands, to ≤ 25 gm in Germany and Portugal [32]. Therefore, recreational and habitual use of cannabis will become more common.

There is endocannabinoid system in the brain, THC-induced dopamine release in the brain's reward *mesolimbic dopamine pathway* giving a sense of euphoria, a similar effect to that of cocaine [33]. Chronic use reduces receptor sensitivity resulting in tolerance, craving and addiction. The woman in this report has cannabis dependence with her long history of moderate to heavy use.

Cannabis causes vasodilatation and reflex sympathetic tachycardia within minutes of smoking with a heart rate increasing by 20–50%, staying for 2–3 hr [34]. High doses can cause orthostatic hypotension (dizziness on standing) and palpitations. With repeated daily use, tolerance to these effects develops rapidly; chronic users tend to have lower resting heart rates and blunted blood pressure responses compared to occasional users [35]. This was observed with the woman in this case who has a heart rate in mid 40 s and BP under 120 mmHg.

Almost immediately, THC relaxes vessels by activating cannabinoid CB1 receptors on vascular smooth muscle cells (VSMC) by lowering Ca^{2+} and by opening transient receptor potential ankyrin 1 (TRPA-1) and transient receptor potential vanilloid 1 (TRPV1), which are calcium-permeable "irritant" channels found in pain-sensing nerve fibres (perivascular A δ- and C-fibres) that coil around arteries and arterioles; when they open, these nerves release neurogenic vasodilator peptides like calcitonin gene-related peptide (CGRP) and substance P. Smaller amounts of both channels also appear in the vessel wall itself, on endothelial projections that poke through the elastic lamina and on neighbouring VSMC, so they can influence tone directly, as well as via sensory nerves [36].

Minutes later THC acts like a ligand for peroxisome proliferator-activated receptor gamma (PPAR-γ), in blood vessel walls this nuclear receptor upregulates eNOS and superoxide dismutase (SOD), producing NO and converting superoxide ($O_2•^-$) to vasorelaxant H_2O_2, a mechanism that sustains dilation while damping inflammation [37]. Unfortunately the increased vascular superoxide and reactive oxygen species (ROS) react with, and scavenge NO to form peroxynitrite. So NO bioavailability collapses. In resistance vessels, THC now tips the balance in favour of α-adrenergic constriction via reduced NO-mediated VSMC vasodilatation and suppresses acetylcholine-evoked, NO-mediated dilatation, resulting in endothelial dysfunction. In addition, ROS is known to sensitise the α_1-receptor/ROCK pathway.

Because GTN donates NO extracellularly, it bypasses the damaged endothelium and acts directly on VSMC, overpowering the heightened α-tone; this explains why this lady's angina subsided so rapidly after a GTN spray. Repeated or high-dose exposure to cannabis amplifies oxidative stress, so an initially vasodilated endothelium evolves into one that is pro-spasm, pro-thrombotic and predisposed to atherosclerosis [38]. Simply, cannabis causes endothelial dysfunction via oxidative stress and NO depletion, and vasoreactivity from ROS sensitised α-adrenergic tone.

This woman's TTS could have been facilitated by cannabis-related endothelial dysfunction [39], similar cases have been reported [40, 41], and cannabis appears to increase TTS in men by nearly fivefold [42], precipitating a basal variant of TTS when combined with cocaine in a young man [43]. Importantly, she demonstrably has no CMD based on her coronary physiology which makes multivessel coronary vasospasm a potential trigger for her TTS as per Hikaru Sato's hypothesis, although it might not be that simple, and this topic is addressed in Chap. 8 [44, 45]. The chronic cannabis use has given her a brady-tolerant and hypotensive state [46, 47]. Nevertheless, her angina could be vasospastic in nature on top of her atherosclerotic coronary artery disease which is non-obstructive. Her TTS has caused a subclinical cardiomyopathy with raised LVEDP which would reduce the threshold for her angina. Although subclinical LV systolic dysfunction as seen in this lady is highly prevalent, there is increased incidence of hospitalisation with heart failure in long-term cannabis users [48–51]. She was advised to stop her drug habit.

4.3 Discussion

CSFP is simply defined as contrast taking more than three heart beats to traverse the coronary artery angiographically, TIMI ≥ 2 [6, 9, 52]. It can also be quantified by counting the angiographic frames, all vessels, as TIMI frame count (TFC) > 27, for LAD this is divided by 1.7 to correct for its length, as corrected TFC at a cine speed of 30 frames per second, each frame is 33 ms [53]. The findings of histopathological and CMR LV abnormalities [8, 54] and perfusion defects with imaging studies underpin continuing belief that CSFP is a marker of CMD [7, 55]. Mangieri et al.'s [8] 1996 endomyocardial biopsies of 10 patients (6 women) aged 38–58, with a structurally normal heart, normal LVEDP and devoid of coronary artery disease risk factors showed a whole range of patchy microscopic findings which as a whole did not point to a specific condition. Out of 28 biopsies, 8 showed arteriolar hypertrophy with interstitial expansion which was an intriguing finding, but was not specified from which of the 10 patients. This so-called "hyaline arteriolosclerosis" is commonly seen in hypertensives, 7 patients had a systolic BP of ≥ 130 mmHg and 3 of these had a systolic BP of ≥ 140 mmHg, who would be regarded as hypertensives under the updated ESC guidelines 2024 [56].

Bolus thermodilution often finds high IMR in CSFP like in *case 4* which appears to suggest CMD, but the high CFR gives a discordant result, as noted by Fineschi et al. in 2008 [57]. Harkin et al. in 2024 reported a series of patients with evidence of cardiac ischaemia on functional imagings; 104 (78.8% women), with a median age of 61.5 years, have non-obstructive coronary arteries, with high prevalence of cardiometabolic syndrome [obesity (BMI 36 vs. 28 kg/m^2), diabetes, hypertension and hyperlipidaemia: in this cohort 22% (22/104)] have CSFP, of these, 43.5% (10/23) have IMR ≥ 25, but 90% (9/10) also have CFR ≥ 2.5. This marked discordance between high IMR and high CFR in CSFP, renders CSFP a poor marker of CMD. In other words, in CSFP patients with high IMR, only 10% has CMD, and CSFP has a positive predictive value (PPV) of CMD using the generous criteria of CFR < 2.5 and/or IMR ≥ 25, of 56.6%.

However, these results are consistent with the philosophical underpinnings of bolus thermodilution as discussed in Chap. 1. In brief, its methodology is based on the central volume principle, instead of measuring the dilution within the microvasculature (an impossible task), the mean transit time of a 3 mL saline bolus is measured across a 6 cm segment of a coronary artery, and this is extrapolated to the microvasculature, the volume of distribution is cancelled off as it is assumed to become a constant under hyperaemia. Thus, IMR is a composite measure of the artery segment the saline bolus traverse, LVEDP, distal coronary pressure and intensity of hyperaemia, notwithstanding the operator and anatomical factors. These explain why IMR is high in diseased, stented and ectatic coronary arteries [44].

In contrast, continuous thermodilution allows reproducible measurement of coronary flow, and it allows changes in coronary haemodynamics in response to drugs to be precisely estimated. The cases described in this chapter are a heterogeneous group of patients (Table 4.1), but none of them has CMD as defined by a CFR of < 2, two are recreational drug users (cocaine and cannabis). Notably, all exhibit *epicardial vasoreactivity in response to ACh* and two have history of TTS. Strikingly, in *case 4*, verapamil doubles the coronary flow rate, yet CSFP becomes noticeably worse. On the other hand, *case 3* with a triphasic response to ACh: CSFP appears with a mild calibre reduction in LAD as well as a significant drop in flow with the first two ACh (2 and 20) doses; flow ≥ 50% without CSFP in response to the two higher ACh (100 and 200 μg) doses despite worsening LAD vasospasm; and with baseline LAD calibre and slightly lower than baseline flow following ACh rechallenge (200 μg) after verapamil 1 mg pretreatment, with reappearance of CSFP. With these disparate observations, without a clear pattern between CSFP, vessel calibre (with or without vasospasm) and flow physiology (high flow or low flow)—CSFP must be rheological in nature, i.e. how sticky the vessel wall is to contrast, perhaps glycocalyx degradation associated with endothelial dysfunction plays a part.

There are data to suggest that high blood osmolality is associated with CSFP [58]. Contrasts change their viscosities depending on temperature. At a body temperature of 37 °C Visipaque™ 320 (iodixanol) has a viscosity of 11.8 centipoise (cP), and Omipaque™ 300 (iohexol) has a viscosity nearly half of that at 6.3 cP; therefore the former moves down the artery twice as slow, since contrast hyperaemia is viscosity independent [59, 60]. A 80:20 dilution for Omipaque 300™ and a 70:30 dilution for Visipaque™ 320 with saline would match blood's viscosity and potentially reduce CSFP, and these dilutions do not appear to affect radiographic visibility [61]. A potential proof of concept would be to study CSFP with different contrasts of varying viscosities, if in animals, before and after endothelial stripping or denudation [62, 63]. If the hypothesis is correct, then simply switching from iodixanol to iohexol would reduce CSFP, if it is present.

Table 4.1 Coronary physiology in coronary slow flow phenomenon

Case	Age	BMI	Co-morbidities	CSFP	Vasodilatory Capacity (CFR)	Coronary Resistance (Wood units)	Vasoreactivity (ACh)	Verapamil
1	52♀	35	Smoking, asthma, irritable bowel syndrome, congenital absent of right kidney, poor sleep pattern, headache, postmenopausal and **TTS**	CSFP noted in coronary angiogram 5 months before and during study	4.7	261	**Epicardial vasospasm** and microvascular endothelial dysfunction	+++ abolished epicardial vasospasm with ACh rechallenge, yet potentiated flow reduction
2	56♀	32	Lumbar spine stenosis L4/5, asthma and previous Covid-19, postmenopausal	CSFP noted in coronary angiogram 2 years before study	5.4	272 Raised LVEDP with BP at beginning of study	**Epicardial vasospasm**	+++ abolished epicardial vasospasm with ACh rechallenge, and potentiated flow increase ≥ 50% from baseline
3	61♀	39	Resistant hypertension on 3 agents, early menopause on HRT, vitamin D deficiency. [a]Cardiac syndrome X-type angina	[b]**CSFP** (↓0.64 & ↓0.85) with low doses of ACh 2 and 20 μg, flow fell with mild epicardial vasospasm, thus "microvascular spasm" **CSFP** (↑1.65 & ↑1.57) disappeared with ACh 100 and 200 μg despite worsening epicardial vasospasm and flow increased ≥ 50% from baseline	Cx 3.7 LAD 2.9	Cx 665 (raised LVEDP and BP > 160 mmHg) LAD 375 (BP < 140 mmHg) NT-ProBNP 86 ng/L	**Epicardial vasospasm**	+++ abolished epicardial vasospasm with ACh rechallenge, yet potentiated flow reduction with reappearance of **CSFP** (↓0.93)

(continued)

Table 4.1 (continued)

Case	Age	BMI	Co-morbidities	CSFP	Vasodilatory Capacity (CFR)	Coronary Resistance (Wood units)	Vasoreactivity (ACh)	Verapamil
4	57♂	33	Cocaine	CSFP consistently noted in coronary angiograms	4.4	237	**Epicardial vasospasm** and microvascular endothelial dysfunction	+++ abolished epicardial vasospasm with ACh rechallenge, and potentiated some flow increase < 50% from baseline
5	65♀	27.5	Cannabis, throat cancer, fibromyalgia, joint pains, chronic pancreatitis, aortic vasculopathy, anxiety, depression, postmenopausal and **TTS**	CSFP consistently noted in coronary angiograms	2.3	280 [c]Raised LVEDP without raised BP, subclinical LVSD with raised NT-ProBNP 420 ng/L	**Epicardial vasospasm** and microvascular endothelial dysfunction	+++ abolished epicardial vasospasm with ACh rechallenge, and potentiated some flow increase < 50% from baseline

[a]Lingering chest pain >30 minutes with variable response to sublingual GTN, exertional
[b]Triphasic CSFP with ACh, the numbers in brackets are relative flow from baseline
[c]Evidence of left systolic dysfunction, either from or cannabis cardiomyopathy

It is possible to definitively conclude, with the support of recent data [24, 25, 64, 65], that CSFP is not a marker of CMD. But an indicator of epicardial and systemic endothelial dysfunction [66], and by extension, it is associated with high plaque burden [64]. Although it does not add to prognosis following a myocardial infarction with non-obstructive coronary arteries [67]. The exact mechanism for CSFP is yet to be defined, but appears to be more common in obese young men who smoke with metabolic syndrome, suggestively named "syndrome Y" [7, 55, 68] to complement syndrome X dominated by women, and on the flip side, young premenopausal women are not represented in any systematic CSFP series [6, 7, 9, 69, 70].

References

1. The thrombolysis in myocardial infarction (TIMI) trial. N Engl J Med. 1985;312(14):932–6. https://doi.org/10.1056/NEJM198504043121437.
2. Thiele H, Kappl MJ, Linke A, Erbs S, Boudriot E, Lembcke A, et al. Influence of time-to-treatment, TIMI-flow grades, and ST-segment resolution on infarct size and infarct transmurality as assessed by delayed enhancement magnetic resonance imaging. Eur Heart J. 2007;28(12):1433–9. https://doi.org/10.1093/eurheartj/ehm173.
3. Laster SB, O'Keefe JH, Gibbons RJ. Incidence and importance of thrombolysis in myocardial infarction grade 3 flow after primary percutaneous transluminal coronary angioplasty for acute myocardial infarction. Am J Cardiol. 1996;78(6):623–6. https://doi.org/10.1016/S0002-9149(96)00382-7.
4. Morishima I, Sone T, Mokuno S, Taga S, Shimauchi A, Oki Y, et al. Clinical significance of no-reflow phenomenon observed on angiography after successful treatment of acute myocardial infarction with percutaneous transluminal coronary angioplasty. Am Heart J. 1995;130(2):239–43. https://doi.org/10.1016/0002-8703(95)90434-4.
5. Ishihara M, Sato H, Tateishi H, Kawagoe T, Shimatani Y, Kurisu S, et al. Attenuation of the no-reflow phenomenon after coronary angioplasty for acute myocardial infarction with intracoronary papaverine. Am Heart J. 1996;132(5):959–63. https://doi.org/10.1016/S0002-8703(96)90005-8.
6. Beltrame JF, Limaye SB, Horowitz JD. The coronary slow flow phenomenon--a new coronary microvascular disorder. Cardiology. 2002;97(4):197–202. https://doi.org/10.1159/000063121.
7. Hawkins BM, Stavrakis S, Rousan TA, Abu-Fadel M, Schechter E. Coronary slow flow--prevalence and clinical correlations. Circ J. 2012;76(4):936–42. https://doi.org/10.1253/circj.cj-11-0959.
8. Mangieri E, Macchiarelli G, Ciavolella M, Barillà F, Avella A, Martinotti A, et al. Slow coronary flow: clinical and histopathological features in patients with otherwise normal epicardial coronary arteries. Catheter Cardiovasc Diagn. 1996;37(4):375–81. https://doi.org/10.1002/(sici)1097-0304(199604)37:4<375::Aid-ccd7>3.0.Co;2-8.
9. Tambe AA, Demany MA, Zimmerman HA, Mascarenhas E. Angina pectoris and slow flow velocity of dye in coronary arteries--a new angiographic finding. Am Heart J. 1972;84(1):66–71. https://doi.org/10.1016/0002-8703(72)90307-9.
10. Li J-J, Wu Y-J, Qin X-W. Should slow coronary flow be considered as a coronary syndrome? Med Hypotheses. 2006;66(5):953–6. https://doi.org/10.1016/j.mehy.2005.11.025.
11. Beltrame JF. Defining the coronary slow flow phenomenon. Circ J. 2012;76(4):818–20. https://doi.org/10.1253/circj.cj-12-0205.
12. Aagaard P, Baranowski B, Aziz P, Phelan D. Early repolarization in athletes. Circ Arrhythm Electrophysiol. 2016;9(3):e003577. https://doi.org/10.1161/CIRCEP.115.003577.
13. Wang TJ, Larson MG, Levy D, Benjamin EJ, Leip EP, Wilson PW, et al. Impact of obesity on plasma natriuretic peptide levels. Circulation. 2004;109(5):594–600. https://doi.org/10.1161/01.Cir.0000112582.16683.Ea.

14. Gabrielsen A-M, Omland T, Brokner M, Fredheim JM, Jordan J, Lehmann S, et al. The effect of surgical and non-surgical weight loss on N-terminal pro-B-type natriuretic peptide and its relation to obstructive sleep apnea and pulmonary function. BMC Res Notes. 2016;9(1):440. https://doi.org/10.1186/s13104-016-2241-x.
15. Lim PO. What causes cocaine-related coronary slow flow phenomenon? IHJ Cardiovascular Reports. 2024;8(1):36–9. https://doi.org/10.1016/j.ihjcvr.2024.04.003.
16. Ferreira-Martins J, Lim PO. Two-step distal radial artery cannulation for challenging radial anatomies. Cardiology. 2020;146(2):144–50. https://doi.org/10.1159/000510293.
17. Olaru M-M, Lim PO. Sheath tip radial artery disruption as a mechanism for forearm hematoma: insights from the distal radial artery approach. Romanian Journal of Cardiology. 2024;34(1):50–5. https://doi.org/10.2478/rjc-2024-0006.
18. Nestler EJ. The neurobiology of cocaine addiction. Sci Pract Perspect. 2005;3(1):4–10. https://doi.org/10.1151/spp05314.
19. Bocklisch C, Pascoli V, Wong JCY, House DRC, Yvon C, de Roo M, et al. Cocaine disinhibits dopamine neurons by potentiation of GABA transmission in the ventral tegmental area. Science. 2013;341(6153):1521–5. https://doi.org/10.1126/science.1237059.
20. Lange RA, Cigarroa RG, Flores ED, McBride W, Kim AS, Wells PJ, et al. Potentiation of cocaine-induced coronary vasoconstriction by beta-adrenergic blockade. Ann Intern Med. 1990;112(12):897–903. https://doi.org/10.7326/0003-4819-112-12-897.
21. Lange RA, Cigarroa RG, Yancy CW Jr, Willard JE, Popma JJ, Sills MN, et al. Cocaine-induced coronary-artery vasoconstriction. N Engl J Med. 1989;321(23):1557–62. https://doi.org/10.1056/NEJM198912073212301.
22. Pradhan L, Mondal D, Chandra S, Ali M, Agrawal KC. Molecular analysis of cocaine-induced endothelial dysfunction: role of Endothelin-1 and nitric oxide. Cardiovasc Toxicol. 2008;8(4):161–71. https://doi.org/10.1007/s12012-008-9025-z.
23. Talarico GP, Crosta ML, Giannico MB, Summaria F, Calo L, Patrizi R. Cocaine and coronary artery diseases: a systematic review of the literature. J Cardiovasc Med (Hagerstown). 2017;18(5):291–4. https://doi.org/10.2459/JCM.0000000000000511.
24. Dutta U, Sinha A, Demir OM, Ellis H, Rahman H, Perera D. Coronary slow flow is not diagnostic of microvascular dysfunction in patients with angina and unobstructed coronary arteries. J Am Heart Assoc. 2023;12(1):e027664. https://doi.org/10.1161/JAHA.122.027664.
25. Gallinoro E, Paolisso P, Bermpeis K, Tino Bertolone D, Esposito G, De Bruyne B. When "Slow Flow" Is Not "Low Flow". JACC Cardiovasc Interv. 2022;15(10):e119–e21. https://doi.org/10.1016/j.jcin.2022.02.015.
26. Rubin V, Comitas L. Ganja in Jamaica: a medical anthropological study of chronic marijuana use. The Hague: Mouton Publishers; 1975.
27. Warf B. High points: an historical geography of cannabis*. Geogr Rev. 2014;104(4):414–38. https://doi.org/10.1111/j.1931-0846.2014.12038.x.
28. Whiting PF, Wolff RF, Deshpande S, Di Nisio M, Duffy S, Hernandez AV, et al. Cannabinoids for medical use: a systematic review and meta-analysis. JAMA. 2015;313(24):2456–73. https://doi.org/10.1001/jama.2015.6358.
29. Goff NK, Guenther JF, Roberts JK, Adler M, Molle MD, Mathews G, et al. Non-invasive and confirmatory differentiation of hermaphrodite from both male and female cannabis plants using a hand-held Raman spectrometer. Molecules. 2022;27(15):4978.
30. Russo EB. Taming THC: potential cannabis synergy and phytocannabinoid-terpenoid entourage effects. Br J Pharmacol. 2011;163(7):1344–64. https://doi.org/10.1111/j.1476-5381.2011.01238.x.
31. Home O. Seizures of drugs in England and Wales, financial year ending 2024. London: Home Office; 2025.
32. European Union Drugs A. Threshold quantities for drug offences: personal possession limits in Europe. 2025.
33. Oleson EB, Cheer JF. A brain on cannabinoids: the role of dopamine release in reward seeking. Cold Spring Harb Perspect Med. 2012;2(8). https://doi.org/10.1101/cshperspect.a012229.
34. Goyal H, Awad HH, Ghali JK. Role of cannabis in cardiovascular disorders. J Thorac Dis. 2017;9(7):2079–92.

35. Colizzi M, Bhattacharyya S. Cannabis use and the development of tolerance: a systematic review of human evidence. Neurosci Biobehav Rev. 2018;93:1–25. https://doi.org/10.1016/j.neubiorev.2018.07.014.
36. Wagner JA, Járai Z, Bátkai S, Kunos G. Hemodynamic effects of cannabinoids: coronary and cerebral vasodilation mediated by cannabinoid CB1 receptors. Eur J Pharmacol. 2001;423(2):203–10. https://doi.org/10.1016/S0014-2999(01)01112-8.
37. O'Sullivan SE, Tarling EJ, Bennett AJ, Kendall DA, Randall MD. Novel time-dependent vascular actions of Δ9-tetrahydrocannabinol mediated by peroxisome proliferator-activated receptor gamma. Biochem Biophys Res Commun. 2005;337(3):824–31. https://doi.org/10.1016/j.bbrc.2005.09.121.
38. Bretón-Romero R, Lamas S. Hydrogen peroxide signaling in vascular endothelial cells. Redox Biol. 2014;2:529–34. https://doi.org/10.1016/j.redox.2014.02.005.
39. Mohammadi L, Navabzadeh M, Jiménez-Téllez N, Han DD, Reagan E, Naughton J, et al. Association of Endothelial Dysfunction with Chronic Marijuana Smoking and THC-edible use. JAMA Cardiol. 2025; https://doi.org/10.1001/jamacardio.2025.1399.
40. Haque O, Kiyani M, Husain S. Cannabis-related Takotsubo cardiomyopathy presenting with ventricular tachycardia and cardiogenic shock successfully treated with Milrinone and intra-aortic balloon pump. JACC Case Rep. 2025:104246. https://doi.org/10.1016/j.jaccas.2025.104246.
41. Grigoriadis CE, Cork DP, Dembitsky W, Jaski BE. Recurrent cardiogenic shock associated with cannabis use: report of a case and review of the literature. J Emerg Med. 2019;56(3):319–22. https://doi.org/10.1016/j.jemermed.2018.12.013.
42. Modi V, Singh A, Shirani J. Marijuana use and stress cardiomyopathy in the young. Cureus. 2021;13(10):e18575. https://doi.org/10.7759/cureus.18575.
43. Nash E, Roberts DM, Jamshidi N. Reverse Takotsubo cardiomyopathy precipitated by chronic cocaine and cannabis use. Cardiovasc Toxicol. 2021;21(12):1012–8. https://doi.org/10.1007/s12012-021-09692-9.
44. Lim PO. Is index of microvascular resistance of Sisyphean utility in Takotsubo syndrome? ESC Heart Failure. 2024;11(6):4438–40. https://doi.org/10.1002/ehf2.14943.
45. Lim PO. Is Takotsubo syndrome's 2% annual recurrence rate reducible? Am J Cardiol. 2023;209:242–3. https://doi.org/10.1016/j.amjcard.2023.09.061.
46. Sharkova J, Nickolaus T, Schaefer JR. Effects of cannabis use on the heart. Herz. 2024;49(6):420–7. https://doi.org/10.1007/s00059-024-05282-x.
47. Watanabe AH, Navaravong L, Sirilak T, Prasitwarachot R, Nathisuwan S, Page RL, et al. A systematic review and meta-analysis of randomized controlled trials of cardiovascular toxicity of medical cannabinoids. J Am Pharm Assoc. 2021;61(5):e1–e13. https://doi.org/10.1016/j.japh.2021.03.013.
48. Javed N, Sklyar E, Bella JN. Associations of cannabis use with cardiovascular and cerebrovascular diseases: a systematic review. J Card Fail 2025;31(1):327. https://doi.org/10.1016/j.cardfail.2024.10.373.
49. Kamel I, Mahmoud AK, Twayana AR, Younes AM, Horn B, Dietzius H. Myocardial infarction and cardiovascular risks associated with cannabis use. JACC: Advances. 2025;4(5):101698. https://doi.org/10.1016/j.jacadv.2025.101698.
50. Khanji MY, Jensen MT, Kenawy AA, Raisi-Estabragh Z, Paiva JM, Aung N, et al. Association between recreational cannabis use and cardiac structure and function. JACC Cardiovasc Imaging. 2020;13(3):886–8. https://doi.org/10.1016/j.jcmg.2019.10.012.
51. Storck W, Elbaz M, Vindis C, Déguilhem A, Lapeyre-Mestre M, Jouanjus E. Cardiovascular risk associated with the use of cannabis and cannabinoids: a systematic review and meta-analysis. Heart. 2025:heartjnl–2024–325429. https://doi.org/10.1136/heartjnl-2024-325429.
52. Chesebro JH, Knatterud G, Roberts R, Borer J, Cohen LS, Dalen J, et al. Thrombolysis in myocardial infarction (TIMI) trial, phase I: a comparison between intravenous tissue plasminogen activator and intravenous streptokinase. Clinical findings through hospital discharge. Circulation. 1987;76(1):142–54. https://doi.org/10.1161/01.cir.76.1.142.
53. Gibson CM, Cannon CP, Daley WL, Dodge JT, Alexander B, Marble SJ, et al. TIMI frame count. Circulation 1996;93(5):879–888. https://doi.org/10.1161/01.CIR.93.5.879.

54. Candemir M, Şahinarslan A, Yazol M, Öner YA, Boyacı B. Determination of myocardial scar tissue in coronary slow flow phenomenon and the relationship between amount of scar tissue and Nt-ProBNP. Arq Bras Cardiol. 2020;114(3):540–51. https://doi.org/10.36660/abc.2018149.
55. Aparicio A, Cuevas J, Morís C, Martin M. Slow coronary blood flow: pathogenesis and clinical implications. Eur Cardiol Rev. 2022;17:e08. https://doi.org/10.15420/ecr.2021.46.
56. McEvoy JW, McCarthy CP, Bruno RM, Brouwers S, Canavan MD, Ceconi C, et al. 2024 ESC guidelines for the management of elevated blood pressure and hypertension: developed by the task force on the management of elevated blood pressure and hypertension of the European Society of Cardiology (ESC) and endorsed by the European Society of Endocrinology (ESE) and the European stroke organisation (ESO). Eur Heart J;45(38):3912–4018. https://doi.org/10.1093/eurheartj/ehae178.
57. Fineschi M, Bravi A, Gori T. The "slow coronary flow" phenomenon: evidence of preserved coronary flow reserve despite increased resting microvascular resistances. Int J Cardiol. 2008;127(3):358–61. https://doi.org/10.1016/j.ijcard.2007.06.010.
58. Elias RR, Aziz MMN, Eweda II, Iskandar MMA. Serum osmolality as a predictor of coronary slow flow phenomenon. International Journal of Cardiovascular Academy. 2025;11(2):58–66. https://doi.org/10.4274/ijca.2025.52724.
59. Nishi T, Johnson NP, De Bruyne B, Berry C, Gould KL, Jeremias A, et al. Influence of contrast media dose and osmolality on the diagnostic performance of contrast fractional flow reserve. Circ Cardiovasc Interv. 2017;10(10). https://doi.org/10.1161/circinterventions.117.004985.
60. Rahmani R, Ramezani M, Shafiee A. The influence of low and Iso-osmolar contrast media on diagnostic performance of contrast fractional flow reserve measurement. Turk Kardiyol Dern Ars. 2022;50(4):264–9. https://doi.org/10.5543/tkda.2022.21273.
61. Im DJ, Kim Y-H, Choo KS, Kang J-W, Jung JI, Won Y, et al. Comparison of coronary computed tomography angiography image quality with high- and low-concentration contrast agents (CONCENTRATE): study protocol for a randomized controlled trial. Trials. 2016;17(1):315. https://doi.org/10.1186/s13063-016-1441-y.
62. Adjedj J, Picard F, Collet C, Bruneval P, Fournier S, Bize A, et al. Intracoronary saline-induced hyperemia during coronary Thermodilution measurements of absolute coronary blood flow: an animal mechanistic study. J Am Heart Assoc. 2020;9(15):e015793. https://doi.org/10.1161/jaha.120.015793.
63. Ohwada T, Saito T, Saitoh S, Osugi T, Ohtake A, Maehara K, et al. Specificity of vascular reactivity and remodeling after repeated endothelial injury in a swine model. Int Heart J. 2006;47(2):297–310. https://doi.org/10.1536/ihj.47.297.
64. Caiati C, Iacovelli F, Mancini G, Lepera ME. Hidden coronary atherosclerosis assessment but not coronary flow reserve helps to explain the slow coronary flow phenomenon in patients with Angiographically Normal coronary arteries. Diagnostics. 2022;12(9):2173.
65. Harkin KL, Loftspring E, Beaty W, Joa A, Serrano-Gomez C, Farid A, et al. Visual estimates of coronary slow flow are not associated with invasive wire-based diagnoses of coronary microvascular dysfunction. Circ Cardiovasc Interv. 2024;17(6):e013902. https://doi.org/10.1161/circinterventions.123.013902.
66. Wang X, Geng L-L, Nie S-P. Coronary slow flow phenomenon: a local or systemic disease? Med Hypotheses. 2010;75(3):334–7. https://doi.org/10.1016/j.mehy.2010.03.016.
67. Buller P, Kern A, Tyczyński M, Rosiak W, Figatowski W, Gil RJ, et al. Coronary slow flow is not an adverse prognostic factor in MINOCA patients in the 5-year follow-up. Medical Research Journal. 2023;0(0). https://doi.org/10.5603/MRJ.a2023.0024.
68. Leone MC, Gori T, Fineschi M. The coronary slow flow phenomenon: a new cardiac "Y" syndrome? Clin Hemorheol Microcirc. 2008;39(1–4):185–90.
69. Sen T. Coronary slow flow phenomenon leads to ST elevation myocardial infarction. Korean Circ J. 2013;43(3):196–8. https://doi.org/10.4070/kcj.2013.43.3.196.
70. Tanta Y, Ghanie A, Indrajaya T, Sukandi E, Saleh I, Maritska Z. The application of coronary contrast emptying time in diagnosing coronary slow flow phenomenon: a serial case report. Acta Med Indones. 2022;54(4):621–5.

Chapter 5
Infarcted Heart

Abstract The pathophysiology of myocardial infarction (MI) and its management continue to evolve from systemic thrombolysis in the 1980s to systematic percutaneous coronary intervention in the 2000s. The current focus is on microvascular preservation. The pain-to-balloon time remains the overwhelming factor. Microvascular obstruction assessment with the index of microvascular resistance (IMR) obtained with bolus thermodilution has limited clinical utility because during an MI, the raised left ventricular end-diastolic pressure (LVEDP) confounds it. On the other hand, aggressive medical therapy, which reduces both blood pressure and LVEDP, has potential in limiting infarct size. Continuous thermodilution post-MI even in a poor but compensated LV can demonstrate preserved microvascular function after a large MI. Further, the drug-coated balloon reduces stenting during an MI, which ameliorates stent-related embolisation, avoids side-branch occlusion, and spares long-term endothelial dysfunction, hence theoretically improving left ventricular remodelling. This undoubtedly will be evaluated in future trials, but early anecdotal experience appears to support this thesis. MI with non-obstructive coronary arteries (MINOCA), at least in men, the majority of cases are due to plaque pathology, contributed by the synergistic triad of high cholesterol, smoking and blood pressure surges from physical and mental stresses, which in the setting of a stiff vessel, can disrupt the vascular endothelium, even in the absence of a vulnerable plaque, leading to a tear that extends to the media layer, thus precipitating coronary vasospasm. This could be one underappreciated mechanism in young men who smoke presenting with a cardiac arrest. Smoking demonstrably is associated with endothelial dysfunction, provable with acetylcholine and coronary flow estimation.

5.1 Introduction

The management of myocardial infarction (MI) has evolved over the years, from a condition with high fatality to a "relatively" benign condition, albeit still a leading cause of death in industrialised nations. In the UK, there were about 100,000 MI

P. O. Lim, *Coronary Thermodilution*,
https://doi.org/10.1007/978-3-032-10734-3_5

hospital admissions per year in 2020–2023, with 4.5% 30-day mortality, but an extra 50,000 did not make it in the hospital annually [1]. It used to be treated with prolonged hospitalisation for months with strict bed rest. Hoping that this would reduce MI-related complications that often result in death.

Paul H. Wood (1907–1962), a celebrated cardiologist at National Heart Hospital at Westmoreland Street in London, in the 1950s, who famously correlated invasive haemodynamics with clinical cardiology, and lent his name to vascular resistance, "Wood unit", suffered an MI aged 54 [2]. He instructed his colleagues not to resuscitate him in the event of a cardiac arrest. He knew this would involve his chest sliced and ribs split for direct heart massage, with little prospect of survival. The external defibrillator was already invented, but it was only undergoing testings in Boston, US. He indeed suffered a cardiac arrest and as he had wished, no attempt was made to resuscitate him. Hence, he died in his prime from a thrombotic occlusion of his left anterior descending (LAD) coronary artery which has over a 90% one-year survival with today's care [3]. Incidentally, he was a heavy smoker, subsequently British doctors led an epidemiological study that linked smoking to MI, and this explains the later low prevalence of the habit amongst British doctors [4].

The next phase is percutaneous coronary intervention (PCI), which reduced in-hospital MI mortality to under 5% from 10 to 15% with thrombolysis, and cut hospital stay to between 2 and 5 days [5]. This involves mechanically unblocking the culprit coronary artery with a small balloon following heparin and the aid of dual antiplatelet therapy, under direct fluoroscopic visualisation in the cardiac catheterisation laboratory. The Controlled Abciximab and Device Investigation to Lower Late Angioplasty Complications (CADILLAC) trial [6] in 2002 launched the stent as the standard of treatment for MI, hence the present era of the coronary stent [6]. However, the balloon, now coated with an antiproliferative agent such as paclitaxel, was in fact developed in parallel with the drug-eluting stent (DES) in early 2000s, and the drug-coated balloon (DCB) is gaining ground in reducing coronary artery re-narrowing without the metal cage, which exacerbates endothelial dysfunction [7–11].

The next focus is on infarct size reduction. The bolus thermodilution's index of microvascular resistance (IMR) appears to relate to CMR infarct size, but looking at the LAD territory MI, an IMR of ≥ 40 was just a coin flip in predicting microvascular obstruction (MVO) [2, 12]. However, there is an innovative workaround [13] of measuring *absolute coronary resistance* during MI. This involves balloon occlusion of the infarct artery proximally and measures the pressure in distal vessel, which corresponds to the wedge pressure (Pw). Next, infuse room-temperature saline at a rate of 15–20 mL/min via a microcatheter. When the distal pressure rises and stabilises within 30 s (Pi), the change in pressure, $\Delta P = Pi - Pw$, divided by the infusion rate gives the resistance in Wood unit. If this is done pre- and post-angioplasty, it allows objective assessment of which revascularisation approach best preserves the microvasculature. This represents a very direct application of Ohm's law to a quasi-static, "non-contractile" microvascular bed. In this chapter, continuous thermodilution was applied to four post-MI patients treated with a variety of techniques. This is a more precise and reproducible method [14] to assess flow during hyperemia, and in response to acetylcholine to evaluate endothelial function, and coronary resistance.

5.2 Cases

5.2.1 *Hybrid Stenting of Ostial Left Anterior Descending Artery*

A 62-year-old Caucasian man with a body mass index (BMI) of 32 kg/m^2 (111 kg) was admitted with a Wellens' acute coronary syndrome. His electrocardiogram showed biphasic anteroseptal T-wave, his peak troponin T was elevated to 554 (<14) ng/L, and echocardiogram showed a normal heart without wall motion abnormalities. A diagnostic coronary angiogram was carried out, which found a critical ostial left anterior descending (LAD) artery, which was wire-cut with double buddy wire, a short 3.5/12 mm drug-eluting stent (DES) was placed as a "T-stent" covering the proximal LAD, purposefully avoiding the distal left main (LM) and ostial LAD, and the procedure was completed with a 3.5 × 40 mm drug-coated balloon (DCB) treatment across the LM into the LAD (Fig. 5.1).

Procedure He undergoes a coronary restudy with physiology 9 months later. First, his left ventricle (LV) is studied, the left ventricular end-diastolic pressure (LVEDP) is 10 mmHg at rest and 13 mmHg with handgrip, central aortic blood pressure (BP) is 133/77 mmHg, and LV angiogram reveals no wall motion abnormalities. The LM and ostial LAD plus the proximal LAD stent are widely patent, although the LAD is diffusely diseased. Continuous thermodilution is undertaken, the basal and hyperaemic indices are 61 and 257 mL/min for flow, and 1427 and 319 Wood units for resistance: Thus, coronary flow reserve, CFR, is 4.2, microvascular resistance reserve, MRR, 4.5, and derived index of microvascular resistance, IMR, 16 (319/20)—these are normal values. The distal-to-aortic pressure ratiogradient, Pd/Pa, is 0.96, full resting cycle, RFR, is 0.93 (< 0.89), and fractional flow reserve, FFR, with saline hyperaemia is 0.85 (> 0.80).

Escalating doses of acetylcholine (ACh) are given. With ACh 2 μg, the flow as proportion of basal flow falls fractionally to **0.79**, with a corresponding rise in resistance to 1.29, without evident epicardial vasospasm—Pd/Pa 0.95. With ACh 20 μg, the flow increases fractionally to 2.66 (this level is not often seen, could be spurious but the direction is consistent with the next ACh dose) with a fall in resistance to 0.45—Pd/Pa 0.93, associated with diffuse epicardial vasospasm, and with ACh 100 μg, he develops severe mid to distal occlusive LAD vasospasm, Pd/Pa 0.90, with flow at 1.85 and resistance, 0.66—he has mild angina, but is not associated with ischaemic electrocardiographic changes. Verapamil 1 mg is given, which resolves the epicardial vasospasm, Pd/Pa 0.92, flow 1.38 and resistance 0.67—which unmasks a distal LAD lesion; with the pressure wire sensor beyond it, the FFR is 0.81 with saline hyperaemia.

Interpretation This man with diffuse coronary atherosclerosis presented with a plaque rupture involving the ostial LAD treated with hybrid PCI, a combination of stent and DCB [15]. He has normal LV function, and 9 months later, he retained patency of his LM and LAD without flow limitation and *intact microvascular func-*

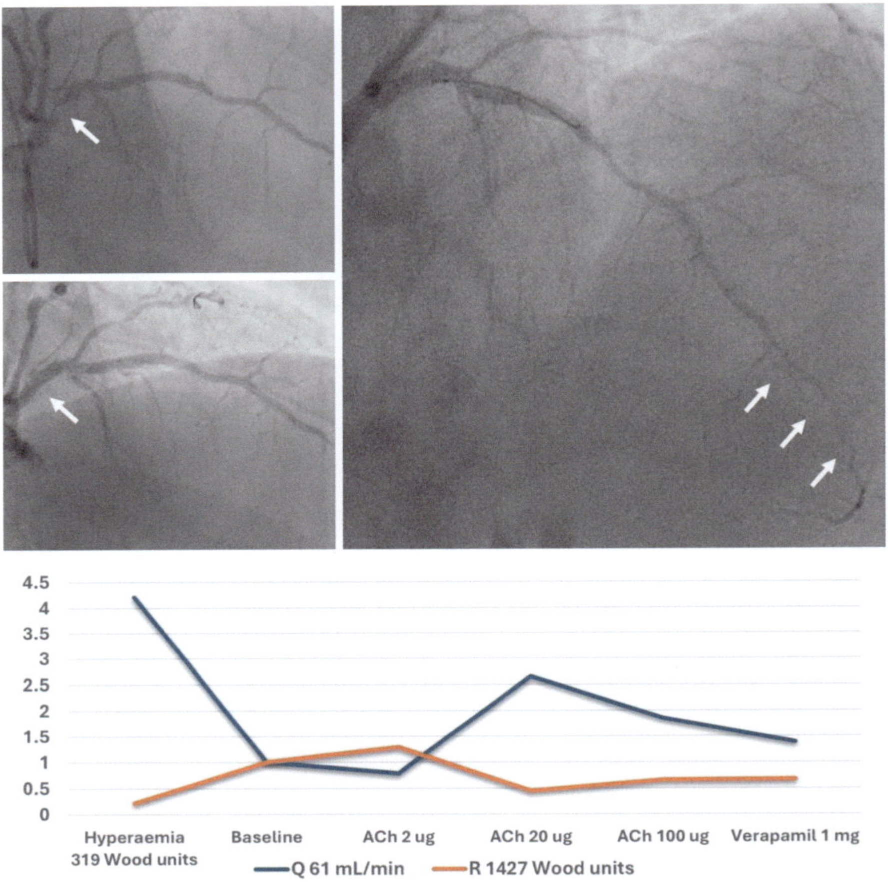

Fig. 5.1 (**Top and middle left panels**) Ostial left anterior descending (LAD) lesion (arrow), before and after coronary intervention with the hybrid stenting approach. (**Right panel**) The LAD 9 months later, with patent stent and severe distal LAD occlusive vasospasm (arrows) with acetylcholine 100 μg. (**Bottom panel**) Coronary haemodynamics, normal vasodilatory reserve without raised hyperaemic resistance, but a biphasic response to acetylcholine (ACh), flow falls with low-dose ACh, and increases ≥50% with high doses despite significant epicardial vasospasm, and verapamil, although reverses the vasospasm, does not increase flow matching with that of ACh, suggesting that its effect on the microvasculature is more limited

tion (CFR 4.2 and minimal hyperaemic resistance 319 Wood units). He has a *biphasic response to ACh*, low dose reduces flow by 21% from baseline, and medium to high doses of ACh increase flow > 50% from baseline confirming preserved microvascular endothelial function, despite epicardial vasospasm, in line with his atherosclerotic epicardial endothelial dysfunction. Calcium channel blockade although reverses the epicardial vasospasm, increases flow no more than that with ACh, which means that *its effect is predominantly epicardial and not microvascular*. This is consistent with the results of EDIT-CMD study [16]. He was switched to a vasodilating beta blocker.

5.2.2 *Thrombotic Occlusion of an Aneurysmal Left Anterior Descending Artery*

A 49-year-old Middle Eastern man woke up with an anterolateral ST-elevation Myocardial Infarction (STEMI) (Fig. 5.2). He had a cardiac arrest due to ventricular fibrillation (VF) when he arrived at the Heart Attack Centre (HAC), reversible with a single DC shock from an external defibrillator. His emergency coronary angiogram found a thrombosed aneurysmal LAD. It was wired, balloon dilated and in view the large "organised" clot, and direct full-dose weight-adjusted intracoronary thrombolysis with Tenecteplase 45 mg was delivered via a microcatheter into the aneurysm. Intracoronary vascular ultrasound (IVUS) showed a thin-walled non-atherosclerotic LAD aneurysm measuring 8.0 mm in diameter. Distal flow was noted, albeit vasoconstricted distal vessels, the pain-to-thrombectomy time was under 3 hr, at 162 min. He was heparinised for 2 days to prevent rebound thrombosis followed by long-term direct oral anti(Xa)coagulant (DOAC). His cardiovacular magnetic resonance (CMR) scan at 4 months showed extensive LAD territory infarction with an aneurysmal left ventricular apex with gadolinium enhancement,

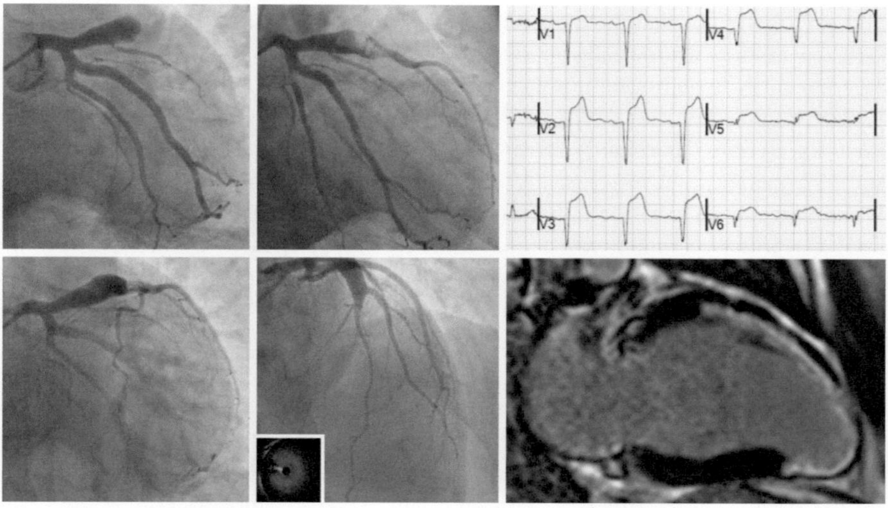

Fig. 5.2 (**Top, left to right panels**) Aneurysmal and occluded left anterior descending (LAD) artery, recanalised with balloon dilations and direct intracoronary thrombolysis delivered with a microcatheter, note the large filling defect of an "organised" thrombus. Presenting electrocardiogram with "tombstoning" anterolateral ST elevation. (**Bottom, left to right panels**) Repeat coronary angiogram at 2 years, the clot has completely resolved with long-term treatment of direct oral anticoagulant (DOAC) monotherapy, the "true" LAD is now evident, previously the visualised distal vessel was the diagonal branch, and the *inset* shows the LAD aneurysm measuring about 10 mm without evidence of atherosclerosis. Nevetheless, the microvascular function is normal with a coronary flow reserve, CFR, of 3.8 with continuous thermodilution. Finally, the negatively remodelled left ventricle with thinned and subendocardially infarcted heart in the LAD territory as shown by the gadolinium enhancement

with an ejection fraction, EF, of 40% without left atrial dilatation; the respective body surface area (BSA) indexed, end-systolic volume, ESVI, stroke volume, SVI, and ventriculo-arterial coupling, VAC (ESVI/SVI), were 68 (17–38) mL/m^2, 46 (42–66) mL/m^2, and 1.48 (0.6–1.2). His CMR was repeated about 2 years later, and the corresponding values were: 84, 39 and 2.15. His ESVI increased, SVI reduced and VAC doubled normal, with falling EF to 32% but the left atrium remained undilated. Clearly, his heart has negatively remodelled despite treatment with bisoprolol, dapagliflozin, candesartan and eplerenone, but he remained compensated for his reduced EF, with NT-ProBNP at a low level of 157 (<125) ng/L, and he was in NYHA II breathlessness, only on inclines. He was added the *fourth pillar* of heart failure therapy switching his candesartan to entresto which is a combination of valsartan, an angiotensin II Receptor blocker, and sacubitril, a neprilysin inhibitor (ARNi) [17].

Procedure He is admitted for a restudy of his coronary arteries and physiology. His left ventricle (LV) is studied, the end-diastolic filling pressure (LVEDP) is 5 mmHg, and 10 mmHg with handgrip, while the central aortic pressure is 100/65 mmHg. The LAD is widely patent without visible thrombus. In addition, it has become clear now that the previously wired artery was in fact a large diagonal branch, and the follow-up CMR (Fig. 5.2) shows subendocardial distal LAD infarction, which implies that this vessel would have been recanalised with thrombolysis after leaving the cardiac catheter laboratory 2 years ago. He goes into VF with contrast injection down his left coronary artery, converted by a single DC shock—suggesting that he is at risk of further VF with his heart failure with reduced ejection fraction, HFrEF. Continuous thermodilution is undertaken to the LAD; the basal and hyperaemic indices—flow 55 mL/min and 209 mL/min, and resistance 1267 Wood units and 274 Wood units. Therefore, CFR is 3.8, and MRR 4.7 (estimated IMR 14), with hyperaemic resistance falling by 79%. Repeat IVUS confirms a non-atherosclerotic LAD aneurysm excluding Glagov remodelling, and the maximal diameter is about 10 mm.

Interpretation It is not clear as to the aetiology of this middle-aged man's coronary aneurysm, but clearly non-atherosclerotic in nature, and the slow flow dynamics caused the vascular thrombus resulting in an MI. Acutely, intracoronary thrombolysis was the right strategy, followed by long-term DOAC. The resulting MI has led to HFrEF, which is associated with adverse remodelling overtime. His therapy has been upgraded to the four pillars of HFrEF treatment, the candesartan was converted entresto, and in view of his predilection for VF in the context of coronary ischaemia and having an EF ≤ 35%, he is considered for an automated implantable cardiac defibrillator (AICD) and will have CT coronary angiogram surveillance for his LAD aneurysm, and if this dilates further overtime, cardiac surgery might be needed, as concluded in a formal multidisciplinary meeting (MDT). Interestingly, despite the size of the MI, his microvascular function was normal (CFR 3.8, minimal hyperaemic resistance 274 Wood units), with normal LVEDP, low NT-ProBNP, and he has no angina.

5.2.3 *The Barn-Door Heart Attack*

A 62-year-old Caucasian man had an anterolateral STEMI while watching car racing on television. His echocardiogram showed severe left ventricular systolic dysfunction (LVSD) with an ejection fraction, EF < 35%. As expected, the LAD was proximally occluded (Fig. 5.3). Thrombectomy established flow, and the whole length of the LAD was wire-cut with double buddy wire followed by treatment with overlapping 3.0 × 15 mm, 3.0 × 20 mm and 2.5 × 40 mm drug-coated balloons (DCB). The flow down the vessel was TIMI III without limiting dissections on a background of diffuse post-infarct vasospasm. Adjunctive glycoprotein IIb/IIIa was given as bolus and infusion over 12 h plus dual antiplatelet therapy. The pain onset to thrombectomy time was under 4 hr, at 3 hr and 32 min. Left ventricular angiogram confirmed the echocardiographic assessment, in addition to an LVEDP of 35 mmHg. He was treated with ramipril, eplerenone, nebivolol, frusemide and colchicine. His predischarge echocardiogram a couple of days later found an apical LV thrombus with an EF of 32%; he was thus anticoagulated with warfarin in addition to clopidogrel. A CMR was performed 20 weeks later—the cardiac function has improved, EF 46%, with extensive subendocardial infarction, and the LV clot has

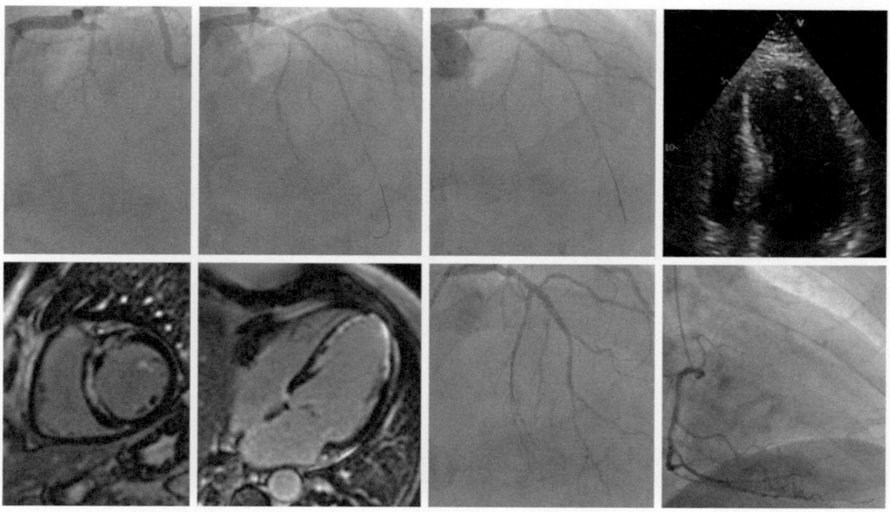

Fig. 5.3 **(Top, left to right panels)** The occluded left anterior descending (LAD) artery, recanalised following thrombectomy, and the end results after extensive wire-cut with double buddy wire and three drug-coated balloons along the whole length of the LAD—note the diffuse LAD vasospasm. Echocardiogram on day 2 that found severe left ventricular systolic dysfunction (LVSD) with an apical thrrombus. (**Bottom, left to right panels**) CMR at week 20 shows anteroseptal and apical infarction with gadolinium enhancement, mostly at the subendocardium, with improved cardiac function, resolution of apical thrombus and ventriculo-arterial coupling (VAC) at the upper range. Follow-up coronary angiogram at 5 months reveals a widely patent LAD, Pd/Pa of 0.91 and fractional flow reserve, FFR 0.86 with intracoronary adenosine 200 μg. The right coronary artery co-supplies the left ventricular apex via the posterior descending artery

resolved; the left atrium was undilated, LV slightly dilated, ESVI 57 (14–36) mL/mm², SVI 48 (40–64) mL/m², and VAC 1.2 (0.6–1.2) (Fig. 5.3). NT-ProBNP was 1739 ng/L one day following his STEMI, falling to 816 ng/L, at 5 months when he had his coronary restudy.

Procedure His ECG shows flattening of the anteroseptal ST (Fig. 5.4), and LV angiogram reveals contractility in the LV apex, LVEDP 10 mmHg and not rising

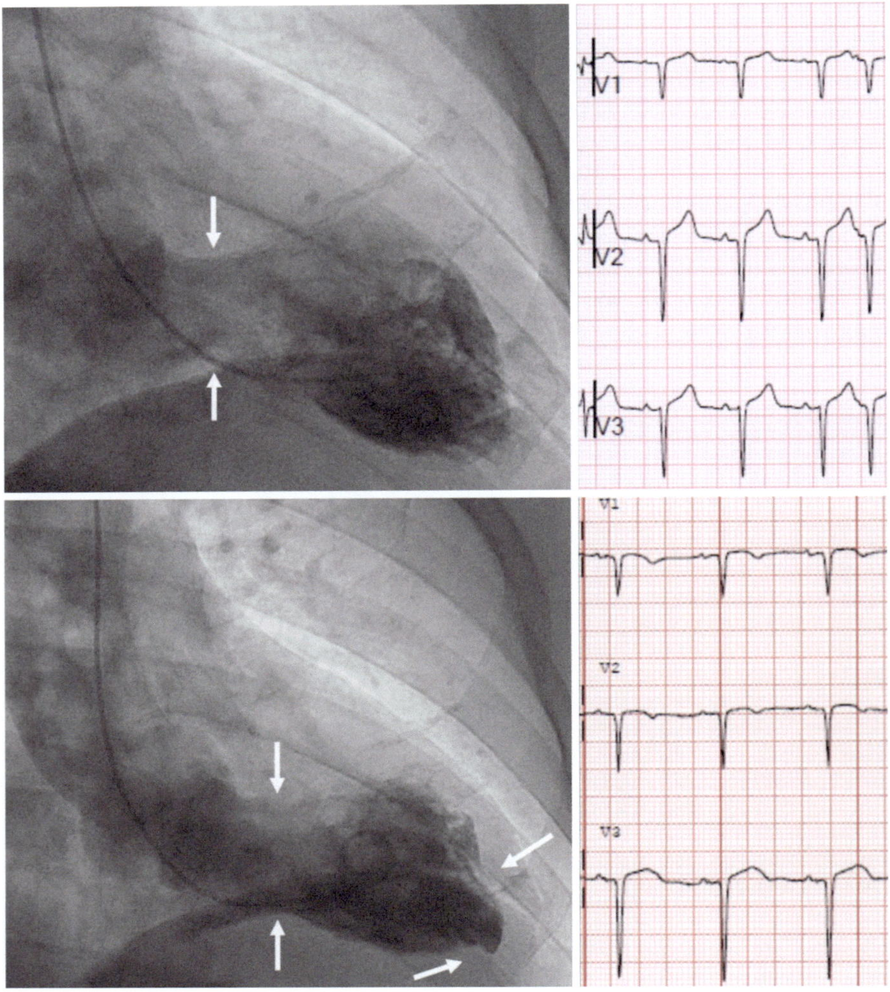

Fig. 5.4 (**Left, top and bottom panels**) Left ventricular (LV) angiogram after recanalising the left anterior descending (LAD) artery, ejection fraction (EF) < 35%—*arrows show contractile areas*, and LV end-diastolic pressure (LVEDP) is 35 mmHg. LV angiogram at 5 months, shows improvement in EF, now 45% with obvious contractility in mid anterior wall and LV apex—*more arrows of contractility*, and LVEDP is 10 mmHg. (**Right, top and bottom panels**) Electrocardiogram 18 hr post-procedure shows deep Q and persistent ST elevation consistent with the aneurysmal and akinetic antero-apical LV. At 5 months, the ST normalises

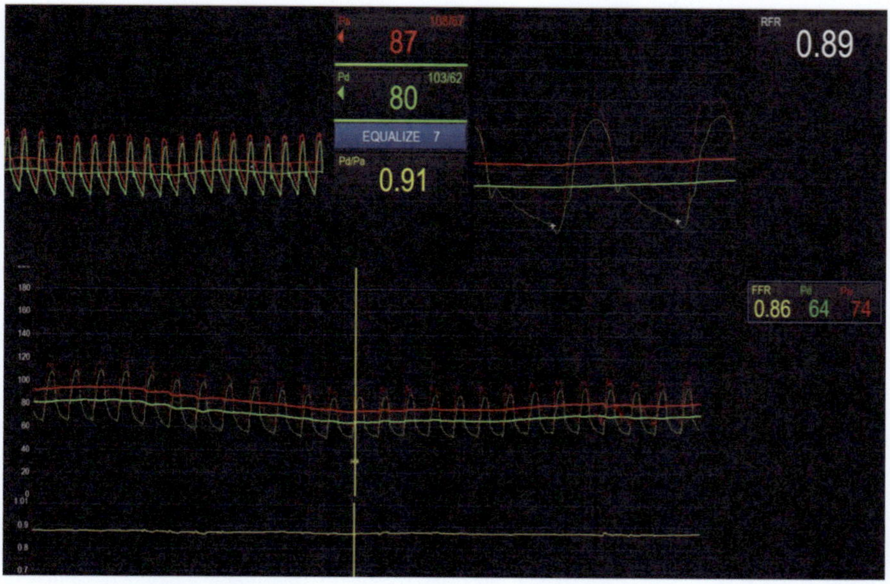

Fig. 5.5 (**Top, left to right panels**) Pd/Pa 0.91 and RFR 0.89 (< 0.89). (**Bottom panel**) Fractional flow reserve, FFR 0.86 (< 0.80), suggesting no significant flow limitation

> 15 mmHg with handgrip, with a central aortic BP of 108/67 mmHg. His LAD is widely patent (Fig. 5.3). With the pressure wire in distal LAD (Fig. 5.5), Pd/Pa is 0.91, resting full-cycle ratio, RFR 0.89 (< 0.89), and fractional flow reserve, FFR 0.86 (< 0.80) following intracoronary (IC) adenosine of 200 μg. Bolus thermodilution is undertaken to the LAD with escalating doses of IC 400, 600 and 800 μg with consistent results of increasing CFR 1.5, 2.1 and 2.3, suggesting incremental hyperaemia (Fig. 5.6). The IMR is 21, and MRR is calculated with the top adenosine dose—CFR/FFR x Rest aortic coronary pressure/Hyperaemic aortic coronary pressure = 2.30, taking into account the systemic aortic driving pressure. This is comparable to that obtained with continuous thermodilution to the same vessel; basal and hyperaemic indices—flow 89 and 170 mL/min, and resistance **915** and 402 Wood units; the MRR is therefore 2.28 (915/402), derived IMR 20 (402/20) and CFR *1.96*. Finally, the circumflex artery is studied, and the corresponding haemodynamic indices are as follow: flow 68 and 180 mL/min, and resistance **1405** and 485 Wood units; MRR 2.9, IMR 24 and CFR *2.6*.

Interpretation This man had rapid treatment of his STEMI, this might have been instrumental in his favourable clinical course, his severe LVSD improved, LV thrombus disappeared, and he was symptomatically well. The bolus thermodilution finds low CFR and IMR implying functional microvascular dysfunction. While continuous thermodilution produces concordant results, it adds more details. Counterintuitively, the LAD has low basal resistance, because of his STEMI and the associated extensive infarct, the microvascular vasodilatory reserve was partially

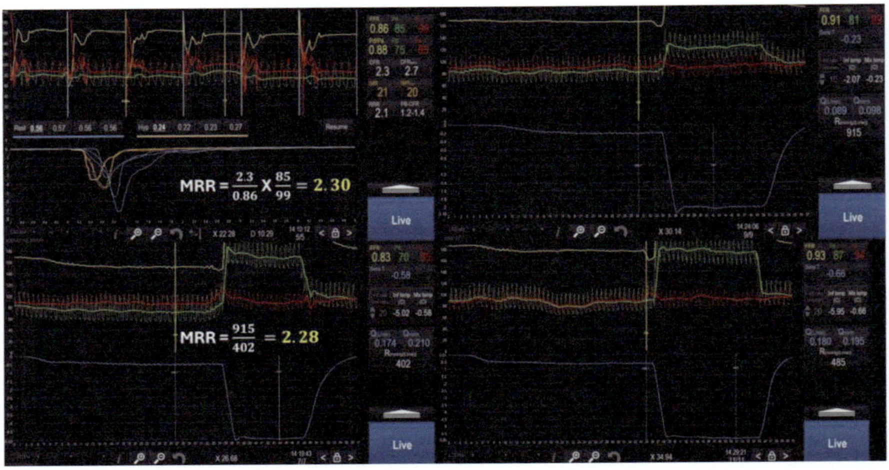

Fig. 5.6 (**Left, top and bottom**) Bolus thermodilution to the left anterior descending (LAD) artery with intracoronary adenosine 800 μg, and continuous thermodilution to the LAD with hyperaemic flow induced by 20 mL/min saline infusion through the RayFlow microcatheter. (**Right, top and bottom**) The saline flow rate was reduced to 10 mL/min to measure basal flow in the LAD, and hyperaemic flow in the circumflex (Cx) artery, which shows concordant minimal coronary resistance in LAD and Cx—402 Wood units versus 485 Wood units. Similarly, in this case, the haemodynamic indices in the LAD obtained with bolus thermodilution and continuous thermodilution are comparable; CFR 2.3 versus 1.96, IMR 21 versus 20 (402/20) and MRR 2.30 versus 2.28, diagnosing functional coronary microvascular dysfunction (CMD) due to expended vasodilatory reserve due to comparatively low basal LAD resistance—LAD 915 Wood units against Cx's 1405 Wood units

expended to maintain a normal basal flow of 89 mL/min for the LAD, this is a codominant LAD that reaches, but it does not wrap around the LV apex; the right posterior descending artery (RPDA) also reaches the LV apex. That is why the hyperaemic flow appears blunted. On the other hand, the Cx has comparatively normal microvascular function, although with a hint of borderline raised basal and hyperaemic resistance, likely related to the post-STEMI dilated LV. Nevertheless, this man has made a significant progress from the cardiac point of view.

5.2.4 Waking up with Chest Pain

A 41-year-old man of South Asian descent woke up with chest pain in the morning at 8.30 am and dialled 999 (UK emergency service number) for help within the hour. When the ambulance crew arrived and undertook an ECG, this showed inferior ST elevation. He arrived at the cardiac catheter laboratory in 40-min time. His coronary arteries turned out to be unobstructed, and the right coronary artery (RCA) was noted to be dominant with mild irregularity in the mid segment straddling an acute marginal side branch that supplied the right ventricular free wall. When his ECG was repeated post-procedure, it had normalised. His echocardiogram found a normal heart with an EF of 60%, as did his CMR—EF 61%, ESVI 30 (17–38) mL/m^2, SVi 49 (42–66) mL/m^2 and VAC 0.61 (0.5–1.0), without overt evidence of infarction, fibrosis or scar. However, his peaked troponin T was mildly elevated at 50 (<14) ng/mL but without a corresponding rise in creatine kinase 223 (<320) U/L. His only coronary risk factor was a 30 pack-year smoking (20 cigarettes a day for 30 years), without accompanying hypercholesterolaemia. He had visited his local hospital for chest pain and was prescribed aspirin although he had not been compliantly taking it. He was diagnosed with *myocardial infarction with non-obstructive coronary arteries* (MINOCA), and discharged on day 3 on standard post-MI drugs, including bisoprolol 1.25 mg od.

Five months later, he was readmitted with further chest pain associated with intermittent inferior ST elevation noted in the coronary care unit. The peak troponin was 88 (< 14) ng/mL and creatine kinase 127 (< 320) U/L (Fig. 5.7). His echocardiogram continued to show a normal heart. This time his coronary angiogram was undertaken with optical coherence tomography (OCT, Dragonfly™ OPTIS™, Abbott Laboratories, Illinois, US) to image the RCA for plaque disruption, erosion or dissection. There was a "single frame" (20 mm/s pullback, 5 frames per mm = 200 μm between frames, axial resolution 10–20 μm) showing a pinhole rupture 90° clockwise from the right ventricular side branch in the thickened intima, the green dashes around the catheter measure about 1 mm, and accordingly the rupture was 100–150 μm in diameter. This was accompanied by a limited intimomedial dissection which extended clockwise and proximally by 20 mm breaching the internal elastic lamina into the vascular media.

This was covered with a 4.0 × 38 mm drug-eluting stent (DES), and post-dilated with a 5.0 mm noncompliant balloon at 12 atmospheres. He had a body mass index (BMI) of 40 kg/m^2, and was advised to lose weight and stop smoking. His treated total cholesterol was 3.2 mmol/L and LDL cholesterol 1.7 mmol/L, well below the treatment targets of 4.0 and 2.0 mmol/L respectively. In view of his recurrent symptoms, he had a coronary physiology study in 2 months' later. He had been switched from bisoprolol to diltiazem, which was interrupted for 24 hours before his coronary function test.

Procedure The RCA is widely patent with its stent, and with the pressure wire in distal vessel, the Pd/Pa is 1.00 and RFR 0.98 (< 0.89). Continuous thermodilution is undertaken with the following basal and hyperaemic indices—flow 79 and 258 mL/min, and resistance 900 and 290 Wood units—thus, CFR is 3.3 and MRR 3.1 (Fig. 5.8). With ACh 20, 40 and 80 μg, there is initial fall in flow by one third with rising resistance with the first 2 doses, before returning to baseline with the last dose—with mild general reduction in epicardial coronary artery calibre, without ECG changes or chest pain—this would be interpreted as small vessel or microvascular spasm. The LAD is studied next, and with the pressure wire in distal vessel, the following are obtained—Pd/Pa 0.95, RFR 0.93 (< 0.89), flow 90 and 219 mL/min, and resistance 888 and 319 Wood units; therefore, CFR is 2.4 and MRR 2.8,

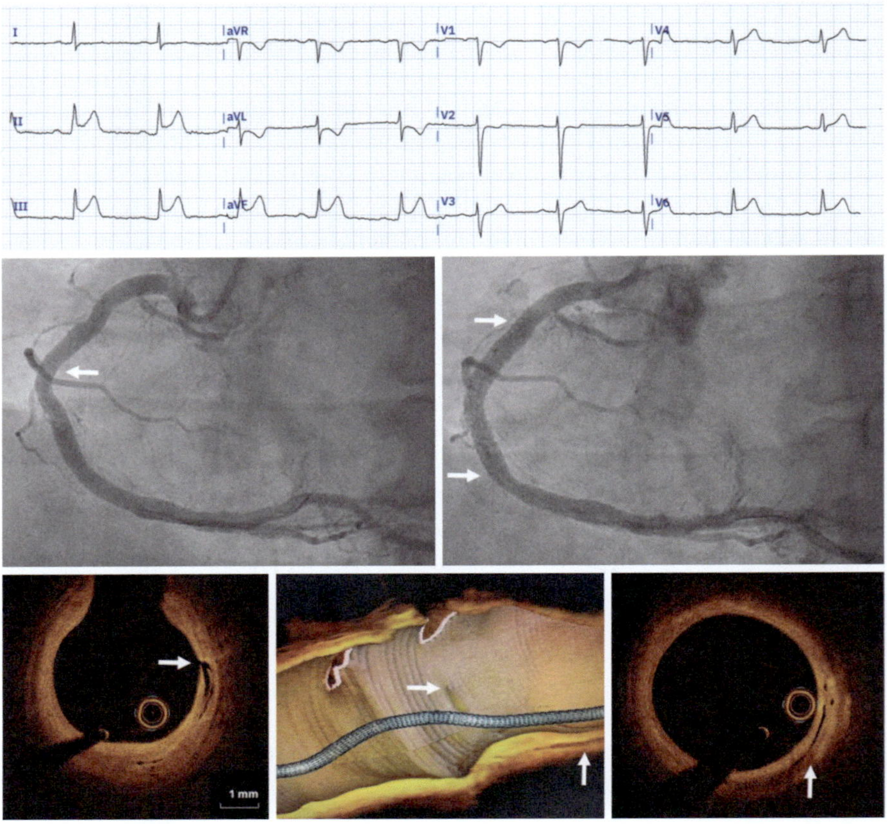

Fig. 5.7 (**Left panel**) Electrocardiogram (ECG) from the London Ambulance Service (LAS) on the second admission that shows inferolaterol ST elevation with reciprocal ST depression mostly in the aVL suggesting right posterolateral (RPL) branch territory of the right coronary artery (RCA). (**Middle, left and right panels**) The RCA at the take-off of the right ventricular (RV) branch there is a mild to moderate stenosis (**arrow**), and post-stenting, the *arrows* show the stent edges. (**Bottom, left to right panels**) Optical Coherence Tomography (OCT) shows a pinhole defect in the mid RCA at 3 o'clock from the ostium of the RV branch, corresponding to the RCA coronary angiogram as pointed in the *middle left panel* above. 3D reconstruction of the same depiction (*arrow*), in addition to intimomedial dissection, shown again in 2D cross-section

ACh 2, 20, 100 and 200 μg produced a flat haemodynamic response hovering around the baseline values without clinical sequelae, concordantly with the RCA. However, verapamil 500 μg increases flow by 30% with a matched fall in resistance.

Interpretation This young man presented recurrently with a troponin positive chest pain associated with inferolateral ST elevation on ECG. But with unobstructed coronary arteries—the most likely explanation was Prinzmetal epicardial coronary vasospasm, in his case, with a pinhole puncture with a contained intimomedial dissection. This kind of scenario is well described with plaque disruption, erosion,

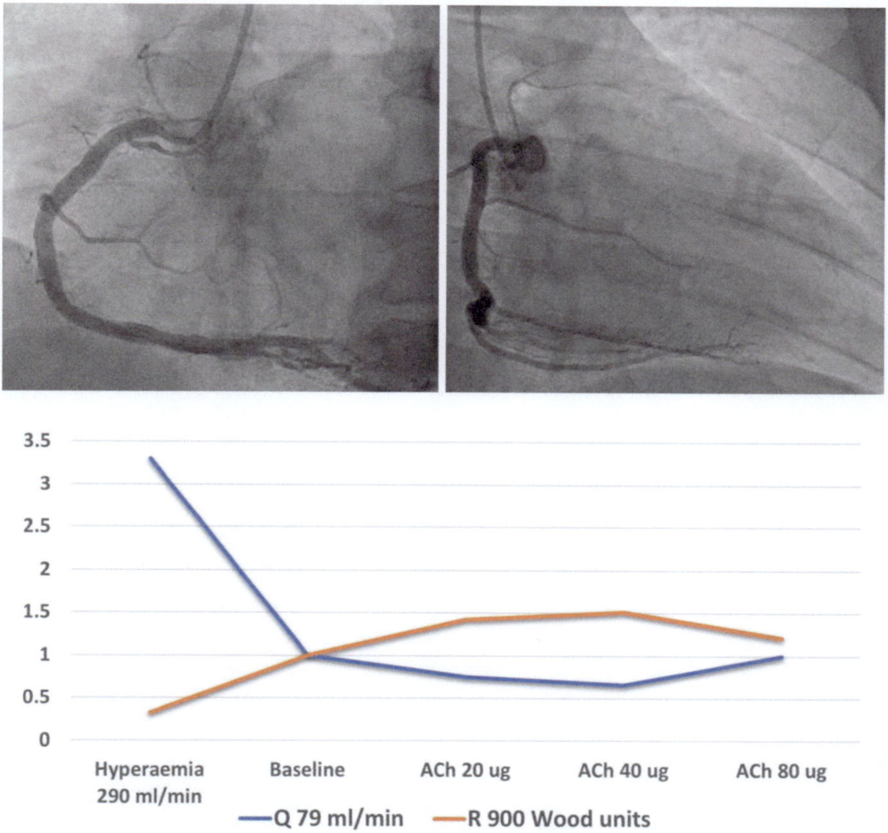

Fig. 5.8 (**Top, left and right panels**) The right coronary artery (RCA) with a widely patent stent at 2 months, and the subtended territory which is mostly the posterolateral segments of the left ventricle as confirmed in the electrocardiogram (ECG) in Fig. 5.7. (**Bottom panel**) Haemodynamic indices in response to saline and escalating doses of acetylcholine (ACh) of 20, 40 and 80 μg. The vasodilatory capacity is normal, whereas with the first 2 doses of ACh, there is a downward trend in falling flow, which rose to baseline with ACh 80 μg

dissection or haematoma [18–20]. He has normal vasodilatory capacity, a relatively low baseline coronary resistance and a muted response to ACh. Interestingly, ACh did not provoke epicardial vasospasm. He had concordant haemodynamics in the LAD, which also did not response to ACh, but vasodilated with verapamil, albeit also blunted (x2 flow usually). Therefore he has *vascular endothelial dysfunction*, and this was attributed to smoking, with mid RCA atherosclerosis and proven disruption in the endothelium on OCT. Stenting the RCA with a plaque disruption could potentially prevent segmental epicardial coronary vasospasm [21–24].

However, about 2 years following his RCA stenting, he was seen in the emergency department twice for recurrent chest pain, culminating with him being readmitted with the same presentation as before, despite his prescription of *amlodipine*

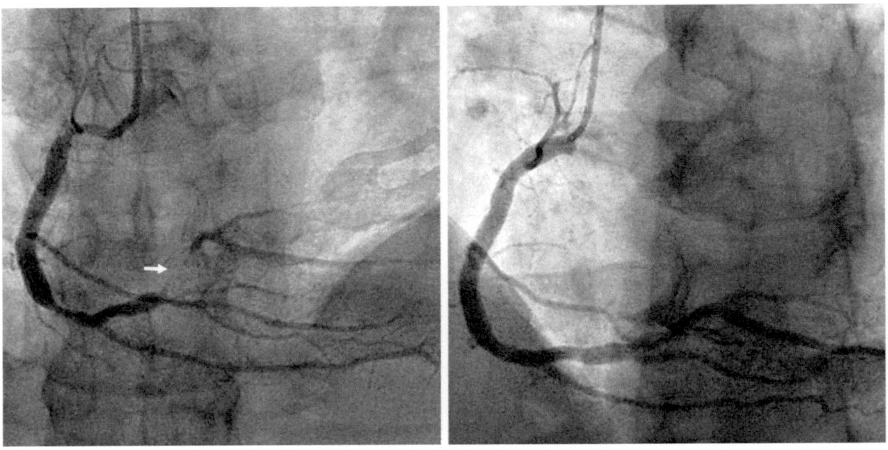

Fig. 5.9 (**Left and right panels**) The right coronary artery angiogram shows diffuse vasospasm sparing the stented segment with occlusion in the mid right posterolateral branch (*arrow*). The artery dilated following nitroglycerine, with evident atherosclerotic progression in distal vessel

5 mg od 1 month before, when his BP was noted to be 144/90 mmHg in the casualty department. Again, his echocardiogram revealed a structurally and functionally normal heart. He unfortunately had continued smoking, and his diltiazem had been discontinued following failure to elicit epicardial vasospasm with ACh in both his RCA and LAD to minimise the number of medicine he took to improve drug compliance 2 years prior. This time, on his emergency coronary angiogram, there was clear demonstration of diffuse RCA vasospasm sparing where the stent was, with occlusive vasospasm in the segment of the right posterolateral branch that had a right angle angulation (Fig. 5.9).

Intravascular ultrasound (IVUS) demonstrated no significant instent restenosis (ISR) in the RCA stent. His peak troponin T was 346 (< 14) ng/mL on this occasion. He was again strongly advised to give up smoking and was restarted on diltiazem. In addition, he has not lost any weight, with the same BMI of 40 kg/m^2 consistent with WHO's definition of clinical obesity. His abdominal ultrasound diagnosed metabolic dysfunction steatotic liver disease (MASLD), which implies a more general visceral adiposity, and his sleep study found an Epworth Sleepiness Score of 9/24 suggesting mild daytime sleepiness, apnoea-hypopnoea index (AHI) of 5 events per hour, and marked oxygen desaturation index (ODI) of 18 events per hour, with a relatively normal average oxygen saturations overnight of 96%. Nevertheless, this is suggestive of mild obstructive sleep apnoea (OSA).

In combination with smoking-related coronary vascular endothelial dysfunction and epicardial adipose tissue (EAT)-related vasoreactivity [25], the hypoxic episodes during sleep likely give rise to his epicardial coronary vasospasm, and this explains his repeated hospitalisations that usually occur in the morning, *waking up with chest pain*. The association between OSA and coronary vasospasm is well known, has been described for sudden cardiac death, and treatment with continuous positive airway pressure (CPAP) appears to alleviate the condition [26–29].

5.3 Discussion

To recap, four cases are described in this chapter. **Case 1** was a man with a BMI of 32 kg/m^2 and Wellen's acute coronary syndrome, the ostial LAD was treated with a combination of DES and DCB, he has preserved vasodilatory capacity (CFR 4.4 and Rμ 319 Wood units) and a **biphasic** response to ACh; low ACh dose (2 μg—0.79) flow reduction and high-dose ACh (20 μg—2.66 and 100 μg—1.85) flow > 50%, despite severe epicardial vasospasm. **Case 2** was a man with thrombotic occlusion of his aneurysmal LAD treated with intracoronary thrombolysis. He sustained severe LV systolic dysfunction (LVSD), but at the time of his coronary physiology study he was in compensated LVSD (LVEDP 5 mmHg) with *extensive subendocardial infarction*, nevertheless, intact vasodilatory capacity (CFR 3.8 and Rμ 274 Wood units). **Case 3** was a man with a STEMI that was revascularised with three DCB under four hours from pain onset, he had severe LVSD with apical thrombus, while in hospital, his EF improved with resolution of apical thrombus 5 months, and later, EF improved from 32% to 46%, nonetheless, with *extensive subendocardial infarction* like case 2. His LVEDP was 10 mmHg, he was relatively vasodilated at baseline with high flow and low resistance (CFR 1.96 and Rμ 402 Wood units) in the LAD, while in the Cx (CFR 2.6 and Rμ 485 Wood units). And finally **Case 4**, an overweight man with a BMI of 40 kg/m^2 with recurrent Prinzmetal-type MINOCA presentations, he was found to have a pinhole rupture with associated intimomedial tear in the mid RCA on OCT, and this was covered with a stent. He has preserved vasodilatory capacity in RCA (CFR 3.3 and Rμ 290 Wood units) and LAD (CFR 2.4 and Rμ 319 Wood units). When the RCA was challenged with ACh, low doses (20 μg—0.75 and 40 μg—0.66) were associated with a fall in flow, while non-responsive to high-dose ACh (80 μg—1.08), and for the LAD there was an initial reduction in flow with low-dose ACh (2 μg—0.74), followed by a relatively flat responses to higher doses of ACh (20 μg—1.27, 100 μg—1.03 and 200 μg—0.97). He subsequently represented 2 years later with another Prinzmetal event, this time with diffuse RCA vasospasm and subtotal occlusion of the posterolateral branch responsive to intracoronary glyceryl trinitrate (GTN). It became clear in his case, there was a link between smoking, obesity-related obstructive sleep apnoea (OSA) and RCA vasospasm.

The following are summary of three germane observations:

1. **Large infarct with extensive subendocardial scarring with moderate to severe LVSD in the absence of a raised LVEDP and central aortic hypertension—is not associated with an elevated coronary resistance, remarkably with relatively intact vasodilatory capacity** (Cases 2 and 3). Post-MI reversibility of microvascular function should thus be interpreted in the context of LVEDP and BP, and bolus thermodilution's IMR is vulnerably influenced by these factors [2, 12], even after adjusting for driving aortic pressure, by deriving the microvascular resistance reserve (MRR) [14, 30]. IMR rapidly falls within 24 hr of STEMI, while the microvascular obstruction (MVO) process progresses, and high IMR in bystander non-culprit arteries points strongly to the influence of

unaccounted LVEDP and uncorrected BP [31–33]. ACh (up to 100 μg) has been given safely in non-ischaemic dilated cardiomyopathy with severe LVSD; interestingly, those who developed multivessel epicardial vasospasm improved their LV function with calcium channel blockade [34].

2. **Flow reduction with low-dose ACh is common**; it is an early sign of endothelial dysfunction [35, 36]. it is important to escalate the ACh dose unless not tolerated. In Case 1, there was a *biphasic response* resulting in severe epicardial vasospasm, but with augmented flow with high doses of ACh, suggesting *epicardial endothelial dysfunction* yet preserved microvascular endothelial function with flow > 50%. In contrast, Case 4, his diltiazem was interrupted for 24 hours, and the drug might still be active; in both his LAD and RCA, flow reduced with low-dose ACh, yet blunted responses to higher doses of ACh, confirmative of *microvascular endothelial dysfunction* related to smoking. Continuous thermodilution allows flow to be measured even in the presence of coronary vasospasm, whereas for the doppler wire technique, apart from difficulty in obtaining a stable signal, the changing calibre of an artery introduces a squared error in cross-sectional area calculation [35].
3. **Coronary artery stenting could exacerbate epicardial endothelial dysfunction** demonstrable with increased vasoreactivity in response to ACh escalation (Case 1) [9, 10]. A smoking-related stiffer and vasoreactive epicardial coronary artery is prone to vascular injury and OSA hypoxic-driven vasospasm (Case 4). There is also emerging data to link epicardial adipose tissue (EAT) enveloping the coronary artery with vasoreactivity due to direct paracrine secretion of adipokines into the coronary vasculature [37, 38], and the heart base in the atrioventricular groove where RCA and its PL branch are, has higher fat deposition [39, 40].

5.3.1 Historical Background

Acute coronary syndrome encompasses a spectrum of unstable epicardial coronary pathologies. Ranging from the open and unobstructed artery, subtotally occluded vessel, to complete acute occlusion. The common thread is the atherosclerotic *vulnerable plaque* which either becomes inflammatorily eroded, or ruptures from haemodynamic stress, thus, exposing its lipoid core, driving a local coagulation cascade with platelets aggregating, leading to clots formation—impeding blood flow to the myocardium subtended by the culprit artery—resulting in MI [41].

This seemingly simple understanding took the better part of last century to figure out. There were two opposing camps. One side proposed that MI was primarily a cardiac necrotic phenomenon. Since at autopsy, most coronary arteries were patent, this was due to intrinsic fibrinolysis. On the other hand, the proponents of the thrombotic hypothesis argued that clots occluded the coronary artery, causing ischaemic damage to the heart muscle. This was illustrated by Klaus P. Rentrop's detailed case report of a fortuitous first primary PCI in 1978 [42, 43]. During a routine diagnostic coronary angiogram via right brachial artery cut-down in a 45-year-old truck driver, his RCA acutely occluded precipitating an inferoposterolateral STEMI, likely due to a thrombus. Nitroglycerine infusion at 3 mg/hr was tried for 30 min, assuming that it was vasospasm. As the patient became increasingly restless and his blood pressure (BP) started to fall, the occluded RCA was re-visualised, with a Sones 8 French catheter, deep-seated to the site of occlusion. The RCA occlusion was poked through with an 0.8 mm exchange wire, the Teflon coiled tip straightened by pushing the stylet forward, this has similar dimension to the current 0.035″ exchange wire, but the guidewire routinely used today measures 0.014″ which is about half the width.

Andreas Grüntzig (1939–1985) had just published on his 1.2 mm sausage-shaped balloon with a stirring wire on the balloon top used to manoeuvre the balloon into a stenosed, but non-occlusive coronary artery lesion, to balloon-dilate it as a novel treatment of coronary artery disease [44, 45]. Rentrop's patient stabilised with his ST-elevation settling, he was put on heparin infusion at 1200 U/hr, and this predated the routine use of antiplatelet agent for PCI. And he underwent 3 hr later, a coronary artery bypass grafting (CABG) surgery with two vein grafts, one to LAD and another to RCA. A coronary angiogram was repeated on day 9 post-surgery, while the graft to RCA was patent, the one to LAD had occluded, but with good flow down the native vessel, suggesting that the stenosis in LAD was not sufficiently flow-limiting. The competitive flow had shut down the graft. Indeed, he was able to complete his supine bike exercise at 50 W for 4 min, roughly similar in submaximal intensity to the Dundee step test, without angina [46, 47]. This first *chanced* Primary PCI for a catheter-induced STEMI demonstrated that early recanalisation aborts the ischaemic myocardial necrotic process. In this case, as proven by thallium-201 myocardial perfusion scan. However, it was a sobering statistic that 0.15% of diagnostic coronary angiograms resulted in death despite emergency CABG, in this pre-PCI era.

St George's Hospital at Hyde Park Corner (1733–1980) in London had three key characters in the angina story: William Heberden the Elder (1710–1801), John Hunter (1728–1793) and Edward Jenner (1749–1823); they collectively contributed to the patho-aetiology of coronary atherosclerosis, and their names are today immortalised as ward and wings in the eponymous hospital that has moved to Tooting (from 1980), in South West London. Heberden described his 20 years' experience of at least 20, mostly *short-necked fat men over the age of fifty* with chest pain, for which he coined the term, "angina pectoris" at the Royal College of Physicians, in London on July 21, 1768, as Hunter was appointed resident surgeon at St George's Hospital that year. His account was later published in 1772 in the Medical Transactions. His comprehensive description of angina with its associated features was definitive; "*Where it is felt, around the breastbone, with a sense of strangling and attendant anxiety of doom*". What he verbalised terminogically then, are well-rehearsed by medical students the world over, and readily used in eliciting angina by doctors today [48–50].

Heberden incidentally received a letter from a 52-year-old physician who after reading his paper, realised that he too suffered angina, and pledged his body upon death for autopsy. His sense of foreboding turned out to be prescient. Three weeks later, in his usual after dinner walk, he was taken ill, and leaned against a pole, begged a passerby to assist him into a neighbouring house, where he vomited, and was bled, but died in under half an hour. Bloodletting was "cure all" at the time. His will was honoured, and his post-mortem was undertaken within 48 h by Hunter, assisted by Jenner, with the following conclusions—"*there are a few specks of calcification in the aorta, the heart's vessels and valves are normal, and the left ventricle is strong and thick, but it is empty of blood, as if, it has been washed*". The coronary arteries were not specifically dissected; thus it was not immediately obvious that coronary artery disease caused angina. This was an unfortunate missed opportunity. Nevertheless, the clinical course would fit an acute MI followed by ventricular fibrillation which explains the empty left ventricle. This account was presented in 1772, and published in 1785 [51].

Jenner's subsequent clinical practice and autopsy experience in Gloucester linked angina with the calcified coronary artery in 1785. But he never published his findings, instead communicated informally with colleagues. Because, at about the same time, he noted that Hunter, whom he respected immensely as a mentor, began to suffer angina, and was keenly aware of Hunter's adverse prospect. Jenner kept his theory from him despite their voluminous correspondence over the years. In under 10 years, as expected, Hunter died suddenly, following a Governors' boardroom fracas around share of fees from trainees, and training privileges for a couple of Scottish youngsters who reminded him of his youth, who had neither done a surgical apprenticeship, nor attended medical school, who were not *bred to the profession* on 16 October 1793 [50, 52, 53]. Everard Home (1756–1832), Hunter's student and assistant, who was also married to his younger sister, Anne Hunter (1742–1821), macabrely undertook his autopsy. He confirmed to Jenner that Hunter's coronary arteries were indeed calcified and he had scars in his heart. Hunter's heart was not preserved as he had wished as an item in his museum, and Home was to publish 92 papers over the next 20 years, allegedly from Hunter's papers which he burnt on 26 July 1823 [52, 54].

It was Caleb H. Parry (1755–1822) of Bath who collated, added, and expounded on the findings of Heberden, Hunter and Jenner in 1799 [55]. He was the person Jenner communicated first with his discovery of obstructive coronary artery disease being associated with angina, and he was a proponent collapse as a major feature of angina, which he called, "syncope anginosa", it became synonymous with angina pectoris. He recorded a case of a 66-year-old priest with rest angina yet could swing lead weights a hundred times a day. His ideas illustrated with dissections of 3 angina sufferers, were published in 1800, as well as a posthumous book in 1825, which sown the seed for coronary physiology, and the concept of angina with both obstructive and non-obstructive coronary arteries (ANOCA). Thus, the centrality of blood flow to the heart muscle, from his astute observation that bradycardia and hypotension can reduce coronary perfusion giving rise angina, as has been observed by others [55–57]. The prevalence of angina was low then, Heberden only saw 20 or so cases in 20 years, whereas for the same length of time, an Interventional Cardiologist working in the same hospital albeit at a different site could see about 10,000 cases, even when divided by 13 times more population, and it is still 40-fold more common 250 years later, making coronary atherosclerosis a modern disease.

The debate about obstructive versus non-obstructive coronary artery in MI spilled over into the following century. James B. Herrick (1861–1954) reported in

1912 that coronary occlusion might not always be fatal, and highlighted the first ECG correlates of coronary ligation in canine experiments carried out in 1917 by his assistant, Fred M. Smith (1888–1946) [58–60]. However, the thrombotic hypothesis was finally settled by Marcus A. DeWood (1946–2021) in 1980 in his series of emergency coronary angiograms which showed that acute MI in 87% (110/126) of cases was associated with **thrombotic occlusion** of the coronary artery [61]. This led coronary care units (CCUs) to systemic thrombolysis, followed by rescue PCI if pain and ECG ST elevation did not settle. From the 2000s, MI has been treated with routine primary PCI with default stent implantation [5].

5.3.2 MINOCA

About 90% of patients with MI have plaque-related occlusive thrombus and the rest have MINOCA [62]. There was a distinct preponderance of women, 57.2% vs 25%, with comparable burden of angina, and similar morbidity and mortality (2.2% vs 2.1%) at 1 year post-event in the SWEDEHEART registry 2005–2022, with a cohort of 46,428 patient < 80 years of age (5281 or 11.4% MINOCA) [63, 64]. In Reynolds et al's study of women with MINOCA, 85% had identifiable causes following high resolution intravascular imaging with OCT. The majority turned out to have plaque too, but in the remaining cases, no underlying diagnosis could be established despite in-depth investigations [65]. Furthermore, people who suffered sudden cardiac death with an apparently normal heart, only 50% had an attributable aetiology, including cardiac arrhythmias [66].

With regards to **Case 4**, the finding of an RCA pinhole rupture with a tear extending into the vascular media was fortuitous. This could potentially explain his initial and repeat hospitalisation. MI is common on waking up in the morning with catecholamine surge as with this case, mirrored by blood pressure rise which incurs haemodynamic stress and injury to the vascular system. It is well documented that unaccustomed and strenuous exercises for instance shovelling snow and heavy gym workout could rupture the plaque, and sometimes the normal coronary artery with intimal thickening only (Fig. 5.10). In other words, the unstable or thin-capped fibroatheromatous plaque when subjected to haemodynamic stress erupts and exposes its thrombogenic contents, giving rise to an MI. This case implies that non-vulnerable plaque with intact luminal vessel wall is similarly liable to rupture.

The RCA at the side branch take-off is a stress area of the vessel wall as the side branch acts as an anchor for the RCA, akin to a ship's mast tied to its step becoming taut when stretched or lashed by winds. The intimal thickening is an adaptive remodelling process to deal with repetitive strain altering its elasticity, making it susceptible to rupture [67, 68]. In addition, there is a systolic component to RCA filling; hence it faces the full force of systemic blood pressure, unlike the LAD, the filling of which is mainly during diastole. Pressure-driven coronary pinhole rupture is well-recognised from barotrauma with bursting angioplasty balloon and with injecting radiographic contrast from a pressure-damped or wedged catheter tip [69].

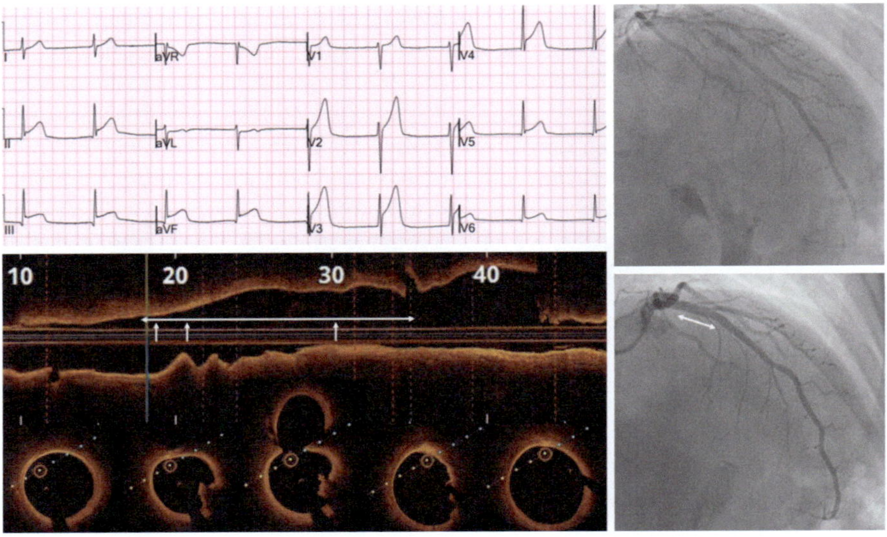

Fig. 5.10 Heart attack with gym workout. A 24-year-old man was admitted with chest pain, 2 hr after a heavy workout with weights in a Gymn. His ECG showed widespread ST elevation (**Top, left panel**). Because his echocardiogram showed a relatively well-preserved left ventricular function, EF 55% without an obvious wall motion abnormality, he was initially conservatively managed. His creatine kinase rose from 850 to 2148 (<320) U/L, troponin T 251 to 1766 (<14) ng/L and NT-ProBNP 612 (>125) pg/mL. He was a smoker since 16 and has untreated hypertension, and without hyperlipidaemia, total and LDL cholesterol were 4.5 (<5.0) and 2.7 (3.0) mmol/L respectively. He had a coronary angiogam on day 2 which found clots in the proximal LAD staddling the diagonal branch with "a cast of embolus" the distal LAD (**Top, right panel**). He was given intacoronary tenectaplase 50 mg, weight-adjusted for 98 kg, followed by daily anticoagulant dose of deltaparine until his restudy on day 7. (Bottom**, right to left panels**) The repeat coronary angiogram found a widely patent LAD and diagonal branch, and the *double-headed arrow* shows the linear dissection measuring about 18 mm on the optical coherence tomography (OCT). The OCT pullback with the *double-headed arrow* shows the longitudinal intimomedial rupture / dissection. Note the normal to normal cross-section of the artery. The *first upright arrow* points to the beginning of the luminal defect with adherrence red thrombi with complete dropout of OCT signals. The *second upright arrow* indicates the LAD at the diagonal branch take-off, and there is the normal tangential signal attenuation at both limbs. The *third upright arrrow* locates the proximal edge of the longitudinal split in the vessel wall. Bolus thermodilution was undetaken with adenosine given intravenously at 140 ug/kg/min—FFR 0.94, CFR 2.3, IMR 20 and MRR 2.4; unobstructed LAD and preserved microvascular function. This case shows that coronary artery could rupture even with normal vascular structure when there is smoking-elated endothelial dysfunction

This subtle vascular intimomedial tear has been discovered in recent years within the spectrum of aortic dissection. It is increasingly detectable with high-resolution multi-slice CT scan, accounting for at least 5% of symptomatic patients [70]. This synonymous abnormality in the aorta is applicable as well to the coronary vasculature, albeit at a microscopic scale where coronary "rupture-and-tear" is demonstrable with OCT. These OCT appearances are variously reported in the medical literature as "microchannel or laceration" and "plaque fissure or cavity" [65, 71–73]. These terminologies convey a sense of passivity, and the former is borrowed from microchannel that develops in chronic coronary occlusive segment. There is no plausible biological explanation why any connection between the vascular lumen and vessel wall should arise given that the endothelial cell membrane is permeable to allow exchanges with the circulating blood. Likewise, fissure is Latin for "split or tear", and it makes sense if this occurs in response to haemodynamic stress, as illustrated in this case by the RCA 3D reconstruction in Case 4.

The coronary pinhole rupture on OCT is smaller than a puncture by a size 12 sewing needle (410 μm) but probably would be equivalent to that made by a facial acupuncture needle (120 μm). The rupture is so small, and having a "trapdoor" opening makes it impervious to blood pressure transmission. Yet, large enough to let in red blood cells (6–8 μm) and circulating blood constituents. These include macromolecular atherogenic lipoproteins, whose mode of crossing the intact endothelium continues to be debated, passing into the subendothelial space [74]. What is notable is that OCT requires clearance of red blood cells by radiographic contrast that was injected down the RCA which then freely percolated deep within the torn intima, remote from the site of pinhole rupture, thus giving credence to the "response to injury" hypothesis of plaque pathogenesis. During acute MI presentation, blood clots usually appear on top of any coronary vascular defect like the ruptured plaque or inflammatory surface in plaque erosion or nodular calcium protrusion. This would attenuate OCT signals rendering the structures beneath invisible [75]. Nevertheless, in the EROSION III study, "microchannel and fissure" were observed in 25% of MI cases [73]. This suggests that vessel wall injury is relatively common.

In this case, the chest pain with transient ECG ST elevation coupled with a rise in troponin T suggestive of myocardial damage could only be explained by occlusive coronary vasospasm. It is conceivable that the vascular media of coronary artery which consists mostly of vascular smooth muscle cells with tightly regulated Ca^{2+} milieu, when breached and exposed directly to Ca^{2+} rich circulating blood would contract. Arterial trauma or injury, needling of a small artery or sheath insertion, could all precipitate vasospasm [76]. Myron Prinzmetal (1908–1987) in 1959 described a case series of three young men aged 42, 42 and 58 who were prone to have coronary vasospasm, those with Prinzmetal's variant or vasospastic angina. They could be readily diagnosed with acetylcholine provocation test [77]. It was prognostically important to know whether this man has predisposition for coronary vasospasm [62]. Prior to his first hospital admission, he had no angina which suggests that the intimomedial tear could be the initiator of his symptoms. In the event, acetylcholine failed to provoke coronary vasospasm in both of his stented RCA and LAD, making his case generalisable to the population at large. Instead, he has *coronary endothelial dysfunction* even with well-controlled cholesterol levels, blood pressure and ACE inhibitor treatment.

The healthy coronary artery pulsates with blood flow, and this reduces vessel wall stress. The coronary endothelial dysfunction in this man was due to his long-term and continuing smoking habit [78]. This stiffened his coronary arteries, increasing vessel wall stress and intimal thickening as seen in his RCA on OCT. Consequently, he was more at risk of stress-induced vascular injury. Plaque is basically a maladaptive healing process which could be reproduced in animals by iatrogenically inflicting vessel wall trauma [79]. Alexander Ignatowskis (1875–1955), whose work led to the cholesterol hypothesis, when his protein-rich feeding protocol was combined with hypertension in 1912, plaque formation in the rabbit's aorta accelerated, advancing the notion that haemodynamic injury, is an atherosclerotic facilitator [80]. Indeed, epidemiological studies have found, in men under 55, the triad of hypercholesterolemia, stress BP and smoking account for over 80% of the variance for cardiac events (Fig. 5.11) [81, 82].

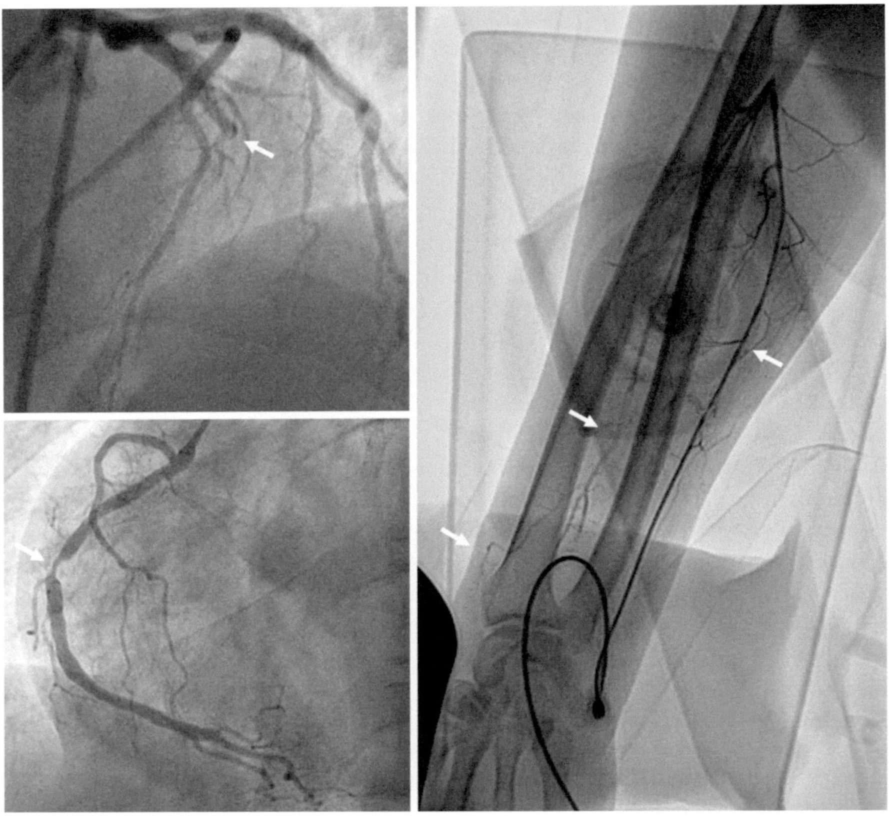

Fig. 5.11 High cholesterol. A 37-year-old man, a Gardener, was admitted for a staged procedure to his right coronary artery (RCA). He was admitted 4 months prior with an anterior ST-elevation myocardial infarction (STEMI) which precipitated an out of hospital cardiac arrest that fortunately was brief. His radial arteries were not palpable then, and hence a femoral approach was used. The occluded left anterior descending (LAD) artery was re-opened and stented, and he sustained severe left ventricular systolic dysfunction (LVSD) with LV apical thombus which improved over time, from severe to moderate. He was a 20-a-day cigarrette smoker, and his total cholesterol was 11.9 (<5.2) mmol/L and LDL cholesterol 10.16 mmol/L, which respectively reduced to 4.4 and 3.03 mmol/L with atorvastatin 80 mg od and ezetimibe 10 mg od, prior to starting a PCSK9 inhibitor, evolocumab. (**Left, top and bottom panels**) Occluded mid LAD at index presentation. Mid RCA lesion—bolus thermodilution with intracoronary adenosine 100 µg; FFR 0.88 (< 0.8, PCI to the RCA is deferred), CFR 2.3 and IMR 33 (due to epicardial disease), central aortic BP 100/60 mmHg. (**Right panel**) A right ulnar access with a 4 French sheath. Severe atherosclerotic forearm vascular disease, the ulnar atery (*top arrow*) is of small calibre, interosseous artery (*middle arrow*) that collateralises the occluded radial artery (*bottom arrow*)

It is tempting to postulate that coronary pinhole rupture is a frequent and ubiquitous occurrence. It potentially causes sudden cardiac death as coronary vasospasm could trigger fatal cardiac arrhythmias, or the break in endothelial surface would allow atherogenic lipoproteins to be seeded within the vessel wall to initiate plaque genesis. On the other hand, if the intima is neither stiff nor thickened, a tear along the dissection plane in the intimomedial layer could happen causing spontaneous coronary artery dissection (SCAD), or a localised intramural haematoma occluding the vessel lumen precipitating an MI [83]. It is equally possible that the plaque itself is subject to the same haemodynamic injury presenting as intraplaque haemorrhage. Contrary to blood extravasation via the vasa vasorum which is a low-pressure system [84]. Eventually, the coronary artery would cease to be vasospastic once the vascular tear is healed, or the vascular media is infiltrated by plaque. There is also recent understanding that transcytosis of apoprotein B LDL cholesterol across the endothelium via dedicated receptors occurs in normal vascular homeostasis. Since plaques are not uniformly distributed throughout the vascular system, but are concentrated on high- and low-stress areas, such as near bifurcations, tortuosity, etc., this would lend support to the epidemiological studies and animal experimental data that haemodynamic stress plays a major part in the atherosclerotic process [85, 86].

5.3.3 LVEDP

The central role of LV filling pressure in coronary perfusion was discussed in Chap. 1. Important to consider that, the pressure which propels blood flow down the coronary artery is the difference between mean aortic BP minus the LVEDP, as per Ohm's hydraulic analogue ($\Delta P = Q \cdot R$). Autoregulation to myocardial perfusion breaks down when this is under 50 mmHg [87] in canine experiments, which could be tolerated more with angiotensin converting enzyme (ACE) inhibition, by at least 10 mmHg lower [87, 88]. The autoregulatory range is even lower in human, closer to 40 mmHg [89, 90]. Figure 5.12 illustrates an example, BP of 140/70 = mean 93–35 = 58 mmHg, which was at the limit but it was exceeded, in the presence of LAD stenosis, if the pressure gradient was 20 mmHg, and it was subtracted, then the coronary perfusion pressure (CPP) would be 38 (< 40) mmHg, which gave rise to the LAD bidirectional "seesaw" flow phenomenon in an otherwise patent artery. When he was brought back to the cardiac catheter laboratory 10 days later after offloading with diuretics and ACE inhibition, the LAD coronary perfusion pressure (CPP) was 80–15 = 65 mmHg, which was enough to normalise his LV function.

The *seesaw flow phenomenon* that does not fill the whole artery is the **third reason** for the impeded flow, due both to ischaemic coronary microvascular dysfunction (CMD), and raised LVEDP. The other two causes are: 1. no reflow—with dye hang up, because of microvascular obstruction from spasm, or plugging with embolising clots and atherosclerotic debris exacerbated by stenting, and 2. restrictive coronary dissection, all of these causes can be differentiated with distal vessel contrast delivery via a microcatheter (Fig. 5.13). In no reflow, the contrast hangs

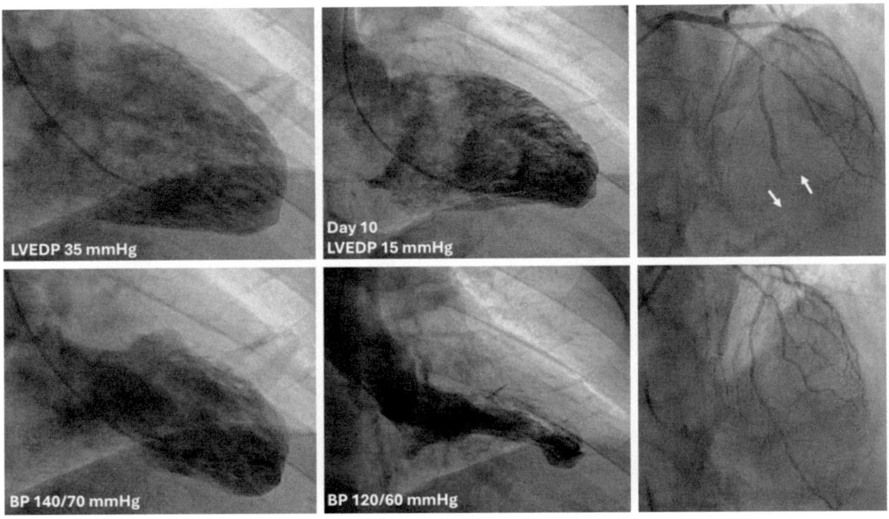

Fig. 5.12 Seesaw flow phenomenon I. A 61-year-old man was transferred for primary PCI when he developed anterolateral ST elevation following a colonic polypectomy in a local hospital. He had anaemia and was diagnosed with giant cell arteritis, started on prednisolone 60 mg od 3 days prior. (**Left, top and bottom panel**) His LV angiogram revealed severe LV systolic dysfunction (LVSD) with an EF of < 35% and a high LV filling pressure. (**Right, top panel**) Interestingly, his left anterior descending (LAD) was patent with significant bifurcation disease involving the diagonal branch—the contrast did not traverse the whole artery, but there was a "*to-and-fro*" appearance of the dye in distal vessel (*arrows*). Given that he was haemodynamically stable, his PCI was deferred, in favour of medical treatment and offloading. (**Mid, top and bottom panels**) He was brought back to the cardiac catheter laboratory 10 days later. His LV function has normalised with limited apical akinesia and the LV filling pressure has fallen. (**Right, bottom panel**) The LAD flow was now unimpeded, outlining the distal vessel. It was treated with drug-coated balloon PCI because of the length involved and the diffuse nature of the disease. His stress perfusion CMR 2 years later showed an EF of 62% with a small full thickness apical infarct, ESVI 24 (10–34) mL/m^2, SVI 39 mL/m^2 and VAC 0.62 (0.6–1.0), and without inducible ischaemia in the rest the LV

around and does not clear, in coronary *dissection*, the occlusion site can be delineated. Whereas in seesaw flow, the whole artery can be opacified with retrograde constrast injection, yet the dye clears rapidly, the mechanism is likely to be due to "systolic flow reversal and diastolic antegrade trickle" from high LVEDP causing raised microvascular resistance. Offloading the LV is key to reducing infarct size in this setting [2]. This flow pattern has been described in competitive flow in LAD due to a right ventricle fistula [91], and more generally observed as a *normal phenomenon* in a grafted coronary artery with competing flow. In practice, high LVEDP reduces CPP, and for the factional flow reserve (FFR), each rise in 1 mmHg of LVEDP beyond 15 mmHg contributes to an FFR of 0.008; when the LVEDP is 35 mmHg (Fig. 5.12), it contributes to 20 × 0.008 = 0.16, and a real FFR of 0.64 would be 0.80 [92, 93].

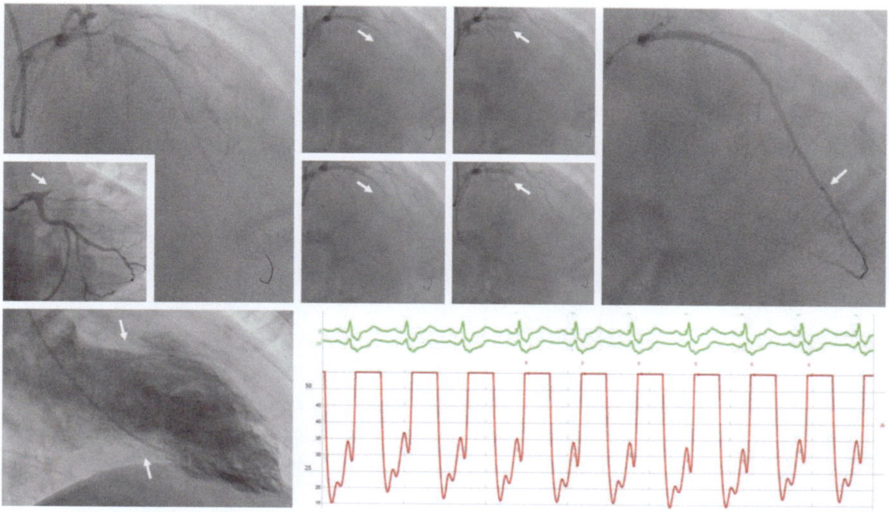

Fig. 5.13 Seesaw flow phenomenon II. A 47-year-old man with poorly controlled septaldiabetes, hyperlipidaemia, chronic kidney disease and hypertension was admitted with an anteroseptal ST elevation myocardial infarction (STEMI), and cardiogenic shock with a lactate of 2.8 (< 0.1) mmol/L, requiring metaraminol boluses and infusion at the rate of 1 mg/hr to keep his systolic blood pressure above 100 mmHg. (**Top, left panel**) His emergency coronary angiogram showed a proximally occluded left anterior descending (LAD) artery (*insert*), and following thrombectomy that revealed a critical lesion at the site of occlusion with underfilled and vasoconstricted distal LAD. The proximal and mid LAD was stented with overlapping 3.5 × 15 mm and 3.0 × 23 mm drug-eluting stents (DES), and the distal LAD was treated with overlapping 2.5 × 40 mm and 2.5 × 20 mm drug-coated balloons (DCB). (**Top, middle panel**) Despite a widely patent LAD, the flow was "*to-and-fro*" in the mid LAD, and the injected contrast did not reach the apical LAD (arrows—*left upper insert, right upper insert, left lower insert and right lower insert*). (**Top, right panel**) With retrograde dye injection using the thrombectomy catheter placed in distal LAD, the LAD was opacified forward and backward with rapid clearance of constrast. (**Bottom, left panel**) The left ventricular angiogram showed an undilated LV, with a large area of akinesia involving the LAD territory, with contractility only at the base, thus giving an EF < 35%, and LVEDP 25–30 mmHg (**Bottom, right panel**)

5.3.4 LAD Stenting

Sparing the LAD from being caged by a DES metal scaffold or limiting its stented length has become a new ideal, in particular with the complementary use of DCB [94, 95]. Comparing LAD PCI with DES against grafting with the left internal mammary artery (LIMA) in a pooled meta-analyses of 2168 patients with follow-up of 10 years, there appeared no differences in mortality of 3.9%, a target vessel revascularisation of 5.1 vs 6.4 (+1.3) % at 5 years and 13.6 vs 16.1 (2.5) % at 10 years, $p < 0.001$, showing a widening gap with time with increasing stent failure [96, 97]. A 15-year follow-up study with the first generation Cypher (sirolimus) recorded a 36.8% repeat revascularisation of the stented lesion [98]. But this was in a setting of a thick stent strut of 140 μm with durable polymer that was allergenic and caused endothelial dysfunction with increased vasoreactivity [99]. Newer generations of DES with stent stuts < 90 μm, and biodegradable polymer effectively become a bare-metal stent (BMS) in time. However, even with BMS, when challenged with spasm-inducing dosing of ACh, as used in this book, 104 patients with a BMS, two-thirds were uncovered with vasoreactivity; 49% epicardial and 16% microvascular spasm [100].

By definition, endothelial dysfunction is the prerequisite and precursor to any atherosclerotic plaque coming into being; hence it could be argued that the above findings are not surprising. However, the medical literature is replete with case reports of spontaneous coronary artery spasm associated with rest pain following stenting to imply culpability [101]. There might however be a time course, in porcine coronary artery and rabbit iliac artery stenting, the vasoreactivity appears to dissipate after 3 months following endothelisation of the stent struts, and in the case of biodegradable scaffold, the stented segment retained its vasodilatory capacity [102, 103]. This favourable effect has also been noted with DCB treatment [9, 10]. In principle, given the relentless course of stent failure against time, "caging" a segment of an artery increases wall stress and reduces pulsatility, and it impairs endothelial function. In STEMI, anecdotally, complex bifurcation PCI or PCI with long stents is associated with instent restenosis [104] and poorer LV function (Fig. 5.14). On the other hand, DCB PPCI could be associated with better LV functional recovery (Case 3) [105].

Further, LAD stenting could compromise flow down the septal branches inducing LV septal or diagonal ischaemia [106] and conduction defects (Figs. 5.15 and 5.16) [107–109]. Despite the small number of individual case reports, there have not been a published systematic series on septal ischaemia on non-invasive stress imagings. Perhaps, from a sense of inevitability that not much could be done about it, hence it is underrecognised, or because the LV septum has dual blood supply, from the LAD and RCA via the posterior descending artery. Across four large, LAD-bifurcation registries (V-RESOLVE, COBIS-II, PROGRESS-BIFURCATION and GRAND-DES) acute side-branch/diagonal occlusion occurred in roughly **1 in 10 cases**—7.4% in V-RESOLVE, 8.4% in COBIS-II, and 13% in PROGRESS-BIFURCATION, which tripled periprocedural death and MI from 5% to 15% (14.6% vs 3.5% in V-RESOLVE); by 3 years there was one-third excess events (12.3% vs 8.0% in COBIS-II), whereas proactive side-branch wiring and ballooning halved repeat revascularisation risk (6.6% vs 9.2%) in the GRAND-DES [110–114].

There are three mechanisms that stenting the LAD during STEMI increases infarct size: 1. Stent optimisation with aggressive post-dilation provokes distal embolisation of clots and atherosclerotic debris exacerbating microvascular spasm, plugging and obstruction; 2. Septal and diagonal branch occlusion due to plaque shift or thrombotic occlusion extends infarction to mid LV septum and lateral wall; and 3. Stent-induced endothelial dysfunction promotes disease progression, reduces distal vessel calibre and accelerates adverse LV remodelling. With the advent of DCB, PCI can be simplified, avoiding stenting, if possible. If not, limit stenting by

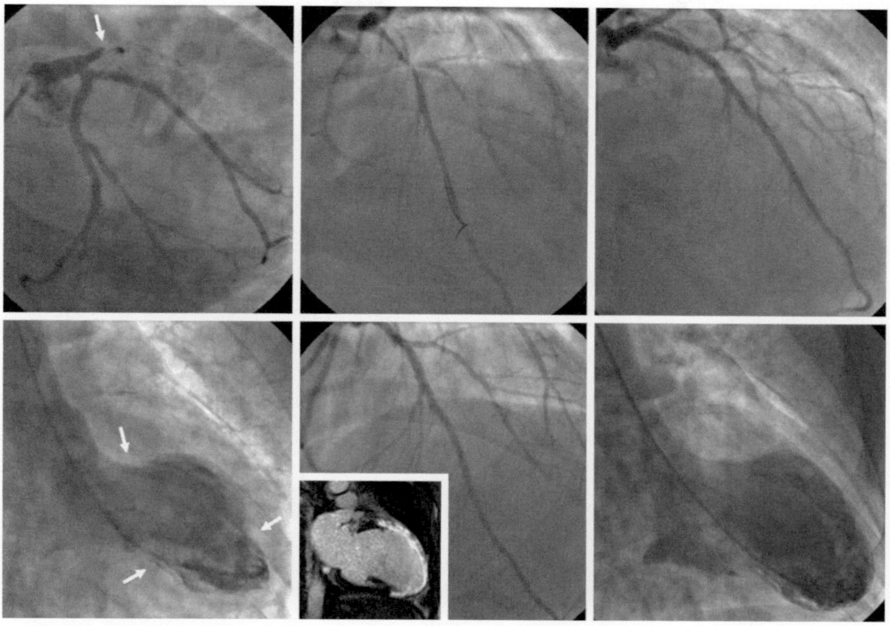

Fig. 5.14 Post-MI negative LV remodelling with Crush stenting. A 38-year-old smoker with hypertension, diabetes and hyperlipidaemia was admitted with an anterolateral ST-elevation myocardial infarction (STEMI). (**Top, left to right panels**) His coronary angiogram showed an occluded proximal LAD. Following thrombectomy, it turned out to be a bifurcation lesion involving a large diagonal branch (D). This was treated with crush stenting; 3.5 × 26 mm drug-eluting stent (DES) in LAD and 2.5 x 8 mm DES in D. In addition, the mid D was treated with a 2.0 x 14 mm drug-coated balloon (DCB). The flow was rapid, in TIMI III, and (**Bottom, left panel**) left ventricular (LV) angiogram showed "ballooning" in the mid anterior wall, but there was contractility (*arrows*) in LV apex, ejection fraction (EF) was 35–40% and LVEDP was 22 mmHg at the end of the procedure, glycoprotein IIb/IIIa was used. (**Bottom, middle panel**) At 5 months, his CMR revealed a full thickness infarct in the whole of LAD territory (*Inset*), but repeat coronary angiogram showed widely patent LAD and D with good calibre distal vessels. (**Bottom, right panel**) The corresponding LV angiogram confirmed the CMR findings, the LVEDP remained high at 20 mmHg, and EF < 35%. A CRT-D was implanted. At 2 years, he developded an instent restenosis in the proximal LAD which was treated with a DCB. His cardiac function has not changed over the last 10 years. The initial pain-to-thrombectomy time was under 4 h, yet his heart *negatively remodelled* despite excellent epicardial coronary stenting results

spot stenting using a mixture of DES and DCB, and bifurcation lesions can be simplified [15]. Further, PCI with stents, nearly a third of patients continue to require anti-anginals [115], and a similar number have demonstrable perfusion defects [116]. Hence the metaphor, "less metal, more petal"; hypothetically, in STEMI, avoiding implanting long stents and preserving side branches, along with judicious offloading the LV with proven therapy, could translate into better cardiac function [15, 105].

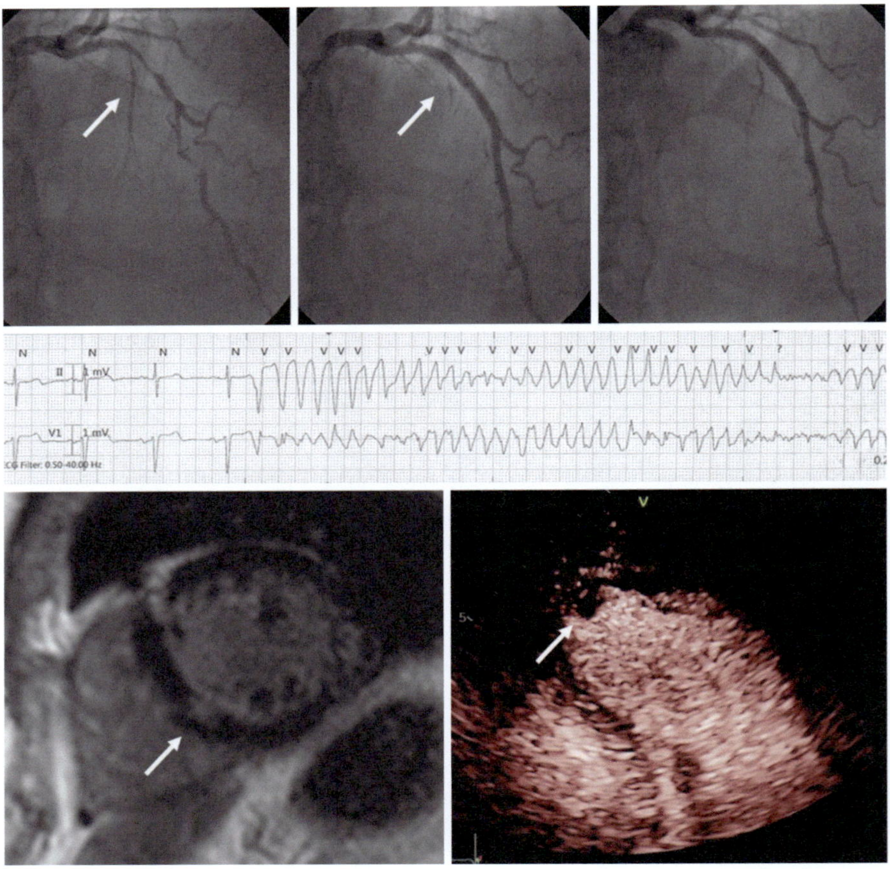

Fig. 5.15 The stented septal I. A 76-year-old man was admitted with a Wellens' acute coronary syndrome. (**Top, left to right panels**) The coronary angiogram showed a tortuous LAD with diffuse disease from proximal to mid vessel and an ostial lesion in the first septal perforator branch (S1) (*arrow*), following overlapping 4.0 × 12 mm and 3.5 × 48 drug-eluting stents (DES) trapping and subtotally occluding S1, and repeat coronary angiogram after his cardiac arrest the following day which showed patent stents and sluggish flow down S1. (**Middle panel**) The rhythm strip revealed an R on T followed by polymorphic ventricular tachycardia without QT prolongation, and he was cardioverted with a single DC shock. (**Bottom, left to right panels**) Day 4, the troponin T peaked at 844 (<14) ng/L—CMR short-axis view with late gadolinium enhancement at mid ventricular level confirming focal infarction in the posterior septum consistent with S1 occlusion, EF of 46%, and apical dyskinesia on contrast echocardiogram with an apical thrombus. He was duly anticoagulated and underwent an automated implantable cardiac defibrillator (AICD) implantation prior to hospital discharge

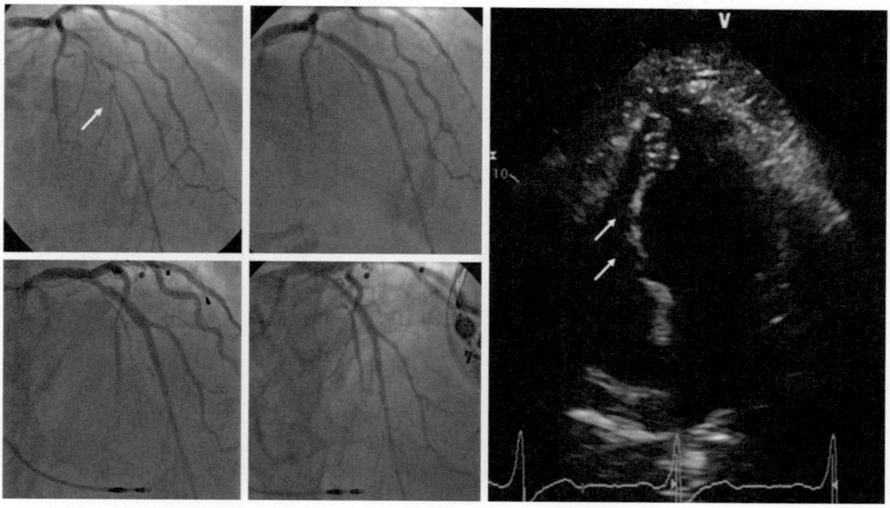

Fig. 5.16 The stented septal II. A 54-year-old man was admitted with chest pain and his ECG showed anteroseptal T inversion. His bedside echocardiogram revealed preserved cardiac function without wall motion abnormalities. (**Top, left to middle panels, bottom, left to middle panels**) His coronary angiogram showed critical LAD disease before and after the diagonal branch, and the second septal perforator branch (S2) is highlighted by the *arrow*. The LAD from the origin of the first septal perforator branch (S1) into the mid LAD was covered with overlapping 3.5 × 33 mm and 3.0 × 15 mm drug-eluting stents (DES) with resultant occlusion of S2, while the stent-trapped first diagonal branch was recrossed and treated with a 2.5 × 15 mm drug-coated balloon (DCB). The next day he collapsed with complete heart block requiring external pacing and an emergency CRT-P biventricular pacemaker was implanted. Two days later his repeat coronary angiogram showed patent stents, and as noted before, an absent S2. His left ventricular angiogram showed basal and mid anterior akinesia with moderate left ventricular systolic dysfunction and his LVEDP was raised at 15 mmHg. The creatinine kinase peaked at 1737 (<320) U/L and troponin T at 4664 (<14) ng/L. Coronary angiogram at 1 year showed progressive disease before and after the stent, with visibly reduced distal vessel calibre. Nevertheless, with the pressure wire in distal LAD, the Pd/Pa was 0.92, and with intravenous adenosine at 140 ug/kg/min, the fractional flow reserve (FFR) was 0.86 (< 0.80) and index of microvascular reserve, IMR was 22 (< 25). (**Right panel**) Echocardiogram at 8 months revealed a well-localised septal infarct

References

1. NHS Digital. Compendium – deaths within 30 days of a hospital procedures or emergency admission. Compendium – Hospital care indicators. England: NHS Digital; 2016.
2. Lim PO. Is index of microvascular resistance of Sisyphean utility in Takotsubo syndrome? ESC Heart Fail. 2024;11(6):4438–40. https://doi.org/10.1002/ehf2.14943.
3. Somerville J. Paul Wood Lecture. The master's legacy: the first Paul Wood Lecture. Heart. 1998;80(6):612–8; discussion 8–9. https://doi.org/10.1136/hrt.80.6.612.
4. Doll R, Peto R, Boreham J, Sutherland I. Mortality in relation to smoking: 50 years' observations on male British doctors. BMJ. 2004;328(7455):1519. https://doi.org/10.1136/bmj.38142.554479.AE.

5. Keeley EC, Boura JA, Grines CL. Primary angioplasty versus intravenous thrombolytic therapy for acute myocardial infarction: a quantitative review of 23 randomised trials. Lancet. 2003;361(9351):13–20. https://doi.org/10.1016/s0140-6736(03)12113-7.
6. Stone GW, Grines CL, Cox DA, Garcia E, Tcheng JE, Griffin JJ, et al. Comparison of angioplasty with stenting, with or without abciximab, in acute myocardial infarction. N Engl J Med. 2002;346(13):957–66. https://doi.org/10.1056/NEJMoa013404.
7. Akiyama Y, Matoba T, Katsuki S, Takase S, Nakashiro S, Nakano Y, et al. Comparison of endothelial dysfunction in coronary arteries with bare metal and 2(nd)-generation drug-eluting stents. J Atheroscler Thromb. 2022;29(3):379–92. https://doi.org/10.5551/jat.61366.
8. Caramori PRA, Lima VC, Seidelin PH, Newton GE, Parker JD, Adelman AG. Long-term endothelial dysfunction after coronary artery stenting. J Am Coll Cardiol. 1999;34(6):1675–9. https://doi.org/10.1016/S0735-1097(99)00411-8.
9. Lim PO. Stent, balloon and hybrid in de novo PCI: could the whole be greater than the sum of its parts? Br J Cardiol. 2023;30(4):37. https://doi.org/10.5837/bjc.2023.037.
10. Lim PO. Grüntzig's technique, relearnt. Br J Cardiol. 2024;31:123–5. https://doi.org/10.5837/bjc.2024.042.
11. Suzuki S, Kaikita K, Yamamoto E, Jinnouchi H, Tsujita K. Role of acetylcholine spasm provocation test as a pathophysiological assessment in nonobstructive coronary artery disease. Cardiovasc Interv Ther. 2021;36(1):39–51. https://doi.org/10.1007/s12928-020-00720-z.
12. Lim PO. Decoding the index of microcirculatory resistance. J Am Coll Cardiol Intv. 2024;17(1):104. https://doi.org/10.1016/j.jcin.2023.11.020.
13. van Beek KAJ, Khan S, Butt H, Demandt JPA, Eerdekens R, Dillen DMM, et al. Infarct-related myocardial resistance before reperfusion in patients with acute myocardial infarction to predict microvascular injury and clinical outcomes. Abstract. Catheter Cardiovasc Interv. 2025. https://doi.org/10.1002/ccd.70338.
14. Kern MJ. Takotsubo syndrome. J Am Coll Cardiol Intv. 2025;18(13):1657–9. https://doi.org/10.1016/j.jcin.2025.06.011.
15. Lim PO. Complete stent coverage of the coronary bifurcation is an outdated concept. Eur Heart J Case Rep. 2024;8(5) https://doi.org/10.1093/ehjcr/ytae168.
16. Jansen TPJ, Konst RE, de Vos A, Paradies V, Teerenstra S, van den Oord SCH, et al. Efficacy of diltiazem to improve coronary vasomotor dysfunction in ANOCA: the EDIT-CMD randomized clinical trial. JACC Cardiovasc Imaging. 2022;15(8):1473–84. https://doi.org/10.1016/j.jcmg.2022.03.012.
17. Evbayekha E, Idowu AB, LaRue S. Sacubitril/valsartan vs ACE inhibitors or ARBs: a systematic review and meta-analysis of randomized trials. JACC: Adv. 2025;4(3):101598. https://doi.org/10.1016/j.jacadv.2025.101598.
18. Takasaki A, Ito H, Kurita T, Dohi K. Intraplaque hemorrhage is a key finding in sudden cardiac death resulting from coronary vasospasm. JACC Case Rep. 2025;30(5):103387. https://doi.org/10.1016/j.jaccas.2025.103387.
19. Marschall A, Rivero F, Bastante T, Del Val D, Cuesta J, Alfonso F. Vasospasm associated rapid plaque progression secondary to intraplaque hemorrhage. Coron Artery Dis. 2025;36(1):84–5. https://doi.org/10.1097/mca.0000000000001384.
20. Yamamoto T, Toshimitsu I, Ishida A. Healed plaque erosion as a cause of recurrent vasospastic angina: a case report. Eur Heart J Case Rep. 2021;5(10) https://doi.org/10.1093/ehjcr/ytab349.
21. Zhang F, Xie Y, Liu H, Dang Y. The culprit of coronary artery spasm: atherosclerosis evidenced by OCT and a provocation test: a case report. Heart Surg Forum. 2024;27(12):E1375–E80. https://doi.org/10.59958/hsf.7891.
22. Ono M, Okabe T, Isomura N, Ochiai M. Successful treatment of vasospastic angina refractory to various therapies using stenting: a case report. J Cardiol Cases. 2024;30(3):97–100. https://doi.org/10.1016/j.jccase.2024.05.010.
23. Wang H, Peng G, Dong Y, Liu D. Intravascular ultrasound findings and stent implantation for a patient with coronary spastic angina at site of progressive atherosclerotic plaque

and responded poorly to medical treatment: a case report. BMC Cardiovasc Disord. 2019;19(1):300. https://doi.org/10.1186/s12872-019-01304-3.
24. Chu G, Zhang G, Zhang Z, Liu S, Wen Q, Sun B. Clinical outcome of coronary stenting in patients with variant angina refractory to medical treatment: a consecutive single-center analysis. Med Princ Pract. 2013;22(6):583–7. https://doi.org/10.1159/000354290.
25. Doukbi E, Soghomonian A, Sengenès C, Ahmed S, Ancel P, Dutour A, et al. Browning epicardial adipose tissue: friend or foe? Cells. 2022;11(6):991.
26. Loui WS, Blackshear JL, Fredrickson PA, Kaplan J. Obstructive sleep apnea manifesting as suspected angina: report of three cases. Mayo Clin Proc. 1994;69(3):244–8. https://doi.org/10.1016/s0025-6196(12)61063-5.
27. Michael F, Main A, Kumar A. Obstructive sleep apnoea as an exacerbator of vasospastic angina. EMJ Cardiol. 2023:61–5. https://doi.org/10.33590/emjcardiol/10005818.
28. Sakakibara M, Yamada S, Kamiya K, Yokota T, Oba K, Tsutsui H. Sleep-disordered breathing is an independent risk factor of aborted sudden cardiac arrest in patients with coronary artery spasm. Circ J. 2012;76(9):2204–10. https://doi.org/10.1253/circj.cj-12-0210.
29. Tamura A, Kawano Y, Ando S, Watanabe T, Kadota J. Association between coronary spastic angina pectoris and obstructive sleep apnea. J Cardiol. 2010;56(2):240–4. https://doi.org/10.1016/j.jjcc.2010.06.003.
30. Eerdekens R, El Farissi M, De Maria GL, Shetrit A, Sykes R, Ekenbäck C, et al. Prognostic value of microvascular function in takotsubo syndrome: a pooled analysis of individual patient data. JACC Cardiovasc Interv. 2025;18(13):1646–56. https://doi.org/10.1016/j.jcin.2025.05.028.
31. Cuculi F, De Maria Giovanni L, Meier P, Dall'Armellina E, de Caterina AR, Channon KM, et al. Impact of microvascular obstruction on the assessment of coronary flow reserve, index of microcirculatory resistance, and fractional flow reserve after ST-segment elevation myocardial infarction. JACC. 2014;64(18):1894–904. https://doi.org/10.1016/j.jacc.2014.07.987.
32. Rioufol G, Finet G. Invasive coronary microcirculation assessment during myocardial infarction. JACC. 2014;64(18):1905–7. https://doi.org/10.1016/j.jacc.2014.08.028.
33. Silva M, Paiva L, Teixeira R, Ferreira MJ, Gonçalves L. Microcirculation function assessment in acute myocardial infarction: a systematic review of microcirculatory resistance indices. Front Cardiovasc Med. 2022;9 https://doi.org/10.3389/fcvm.2022.1041444.
34. Inami T, Kataoka M, Shimura N, Ishiguro H, Kohshoh H, Taguchi H, et al. Left ventricular dysfunction due to diffuse multiple vessel coronary artery spasm can be concealed in dilated cardiomyopathy. Eur J Heart Fail. 2012;14(10):1130–8. https://doi.org/10.1093/eurjhf/hfs103.
35. de Jong EAM, Namba HF, Boerhout CKM, Feenstra RGT, Woudstra J, Vink CEM, et al. Assessment of coronary endothelial dysfunction using contemporary coronary function testing. Int J Cardiol. 2025;418:132640. https://doi.org/10.1016/j.ijcard.2024.132640.
36. Lee B, Francis K. Coronary endothelial dysfunction: from pathogenesis to clinical implications. Open Heart. 2022;9(2):e002200. https://doi.org/10.1136/openhrt-2022-002200.
37. Ito T, Fujita H, Ichihashi T, Ohte N. Impact of epicardial adipose tissue volume quantified by non-contrast electrocardiogram-gated computed tomography on ergonovine-induced epicardial coronary artery spasm. Int J Cardiol. 2016;221:877–80. https://doi.org/10.1016/j.ijcard.2016.07.139.
38. Kataoka T, Harada K, Tanaka A, Onishi T, Matsunaga S, Funakubo H, et al. Relationship between epicardial adipose tissue volume and coronary artery spasm. Int J Cardiol. 2021;324:8–12. https://doi.org/10.1016/j.ijcard.2020.09.074.
39. Iacobellis G, Willens HJ. Echocardiographic epicardial fat: a review of research and clinical applications. J Am Soc Echocardiogr. 2009;22(12):1311–9. https://doi.org/10.1016/j.echo.2009.10.013.
40. Trimarchi G, Carerj ML, Zito C, Bella GD, Taverna G, Cusmà Piccione M, et al. Epicardial adipose tissue: a multimodal imaging diagnostic perspective. Medicina (Kaunas). 2025;61(6):961.

41. Vergallo R, Park S-J, Stone GW, Erlinge D, Porto I, Waksman R, et al. Vulnerable or high-risk plaque. JACC Cardiovasc Imaging. 2025;18(6):709–40. https://doi.org/10.1016/j.jcmg.2024.12.004.
42. Lim PO. Angina: the ischemic triad. Am J Cardiol. 2024;223:118–9. https://doi.org/10.1016/j.amjcard.2024.05.023.
43. Rentrop P, de Vivie ER, Karsch KR, Kreuzer H. Acute coronary occlusion with impending infarction as an angiographic complication relieved by a guide-wire recanalization. Clin Cardiol. 1978;1(2):101–6. https://doi.org/10.1002/clc.4960010209.
44. Gruntzig A. Transluminal dilatation of coronary-artery stenosis. Lancet. 1978;1(8058):263. https://doi.org/10.1016/s0140-6736(78)90500-7.
45. Gruntzig A, Schneider HJ. [The percutaneous dilatation of chronic coronary stenoses--experiments and morphology]. Schweiz Med Wochenschr. 1977;107(44):1588.
46. Lim P, Shiels P, Anderson J, MacDonald T. Dundee step test: a simple method of measuring the blood pressure response to exercise. J Hum Hypertens. 1999;13(8):521–6. https://doi.org/10.1038/sj.jhh.1000869.
47. Lim PO, MacDonald TM. Step test in hypertension. QJM. 2000;93(11):703–5. https://doi.org/10.1093/qjmed/93.11.703.
48. Boden WE, Kaski JC, Berry C. Reprising Heberden's description of angina pectoris after 250 years. Eur Heart J. 2022;44(19):1684–6. https://doi.org/10.1093/eurheartj/ehac643.
49. Heberden W. Some account of a disorder of the breast. Med Trans (RCP London). 1772;2:59–67.
50. Kligfield P. John hunter, angina pectoris and medical education. Am J Cardiol. 1980;45(2):367–9. https://doi.org/10.1016/0002-9149(80)90660-8.
51. Heberden W. A letter to Dr Heberden, concerning the angina pectoris; and Dr Heberden's account of the dissection of one, who had been troubled with that disorder. Med Trans (RCP London). 1785;3:1–11.
52. Moore W. Anatomist's Heart. The knife man: blood, body snatching, and the birth of modern surgery. New York: Broadway Books; 2005. p. 524.
53. O'Brien JC. My surgical heroes. Proc (Bayl Univ Med Cent). 2013;26(1):67–75. https://doi.org/10.1080/08998280.2013.11928924.
54. Tricker J. Saints and sinner Everard home. Bull R Coll Surg England. 2012;94(9):316–8. https://doi.org/10.1308/147363512x13448516926900.
55. Parry CH. An inquiry into the symptoms and causes of the syncope anginosa, commonly called angina pectoris, illustrated by dissections. Ann Med (Edinb). 1800;5:53–78.
56. Parry CH. Elements of pathology and therapeutics: being the outlines of a work intended to ascertain the nature, causes, and Most efficacious modes of prevention and cure of the greater number of the practical disorders incident to the human frame: illustrated by numerous cases and dissections. London: Underwood; 1825.
57. Warren J. Remarks on angina pectoris. N Engl J Med Surg Collateral Branch Sci. 1812;1(1):1–11. https://doi.org/10.1056/NEJM181201010010101.
58. Herrick JB. Clinical features of sudden obstruction of the coronary arteries. JAMA J Am Med Assoc. 1912;LIX(23):2015–22. https://doi.org/10.1001/jama.1912.04270120001001.
59. Herrick JB. Thrombosis of the coronary arteries. JAMA J Am Med Assoc. 1919;72(6):387–90. https://doi.org/10.1001/jama.1919.02610060001001.
60. Smith FM. The ligation of coronary arteries with electrocardiographic study. 1918. Ann Noninvasive Electrocardiol. 2004;9(1):80–93. https://doi.org/10.1111/j.1542-474x.2004.91003.x.
61. Lim PO. Is Takotsubo syndrome's 2% annual recurrence rate reducible? Am J Cardiol. 2023; https://doi.org/10.1016/j.amjcard.2023.09.061.
62. Montone RA, Niccoli G, Fracassi F, Russo M, Gurgoglione F, Camma G, et al. Patients with acute myocardial infarction and non-obstructive coronary arteries: safety and prognostic relevance of invasive coronary provocative tests. Eur Heart J. 2018;39(2):91–8. https://doi.org/10.1093/eurheartj/ehx667.

63. Gulati M, Rodriguez-Lozano PF. A paradigm shift in myocardial infarction with nonobstructive coronary arteries care: advancing diagnostics, equity, and outcomes. J Am Heart Assoc. 2025;14(14):e040433. https://doi.org/10.1161/jaha.125.040433.
64. Welén Schef K, Tornvall P, Lindahl B, Nordenskjöld AM, Jernberg T. Angina pectoris prevalence and sick leave burden 1 year after myocardial infarction with nonobstructive coronary arteries. J Am Heart Assoc. 2025;14(14):e037264. https://doi.org/10.1161/jaha.124.037264.
65. Reynolds HR, Maehara A, Kwong RY, Sedlak T, Saw J, Smilowitz NR, et al. Coronary optical coherence tomography and cardiac magnetic resonance imaging to determine underlying causes of myocardial infarction with nonobstructive coronary arteries in women. Circulation. 2021;143(7):624–40. https://doi.org/10.1161/CIRCULATIONAHA.120.052008.
66. Chugh SS, Kelly KL, Titus JL. Sudden cardiac death with apparently normal heart. Circulation. 2000;102(6):649–54. https://doi.org/10.1161/01.cir.102.6.649.
67. Stary HC, Chandler AB, Dinsmore RE, Fuster V, Glagov S, Insull W Jr, et al. A definition of advanced types of atherosclerotic lesions and a histological classification of atherosclerosis. A report from the committee on vascular lesions of the council on arteriosclerosis, American Heart Association. Circulation. 1995;92(5):1355–74. https://doi.org/10.1161/01.cir.92.5.1355.
68. Thubrikar MJ, Robicsek F. Pressure-induced arterial wall stress and atherosclerosis. Ann Thorac Surg. 1995;59(6):1594–603. https://doi.org/10.1016/0003-4975(94)01037-d.
69. MR LM, Beanlands DS. Pinhole balloon rupture during coronary angioplasty causing rupture of the coronary artery. Catheter Cardiovasc Diagn. 1990;19(2):91–2. https://doi.org/10.1002/ccd.1810190206.
70. Chin AS, Willemink MJ, Kino A, Hinostroza V, Sailer AM, Fischbein MP, et al. Acute limited intimal tears of the thoracic aorta. J Am Coll Cardiol. 2018;71(24):2773–85. https://doi.org/10.1016/j.jacc.2018.03.531.
71. Goyal M, Kim SW, Mishra S, Sharmin S, Won H, Cho I, et al. Morphological characteristics of optical coherence tomography defined plaque fissure in patients with acute coronary syndrome. Heart Vessel. 2019;34(3):427–34. https://doi.org/10.1007/s00380-018-1271-9.
72. Ichibori Y, Ohtani T, Nakatani D, Tachibana K, Yamaguchi O, Toda K, et al. Optical coherence tomography and intravascular ultrasound evaluation of cardiac allograft vasculopathy with and without intimal neovascularization. Eur Heart J Cardiovasc Imaging. 2016;17(1):51–8. https://doi.org/10.1093/ehjci/jev110.
73. Jia H, Dai J, He L, Xu Y, Shi Y, Zhao L, et al. EROSION III: a multicenter RCT of OCT-guided reperfusion in STEMI with early infarct artery patency. JACC Cardiovasc Interv. 2022;15(8):846–56. https://doi.org/10.1016/j.jcin.2022.01.298.
74. Behbodikhah J, Ahmed S, Elyasi A, Kasselman LJ, De Leon J, Glass AD, et al. Apolipoprotein B and cardiovascular disease: biomarker and potential therapeutic target. Meta. 2021;11(10) https://doi.org/10.3390/metabo11100690.
75. Sinclair H, Bourantas C, Bagnall A, Mintz GS, Kunadian V. OCT for the identification of vulnerable plaque in acute coronary syndrome. JACC Cardiovasc Imaging. 2015;8(2):198–209. https://doi.org/10.1016/j.jcmg.2014.12.005.
76. Lindbom A. Arterial spasm caused by puncture and catheterization; an arteriographic study of patients not suffering from arterial disease. Acta Radiol. 1957;47(6):449–60. https://doi.org/10.3109/00016925709170919.
77. Ong P, Athanasiadis A, Borgulya G, Vokshi I, Bastiaenen R, Kubik S, et al. Clinical usefulness, angiographic characteristics, and safety evaluation of intracoronary acetylcholine provocation testing among 921 consecutive white patients with unobstructed coronary arteries. Circulation. 2014;129(17):1723–30. https://doi.org/10.1161/CIRCULATIONAHA.113.004096.
78. Zeiher AM, Schachinger V, Minners J. Long-term cigarette smoking impairs endothelium-dependent coronary arterial vasodilator function. Circulation. 1995;92(5):1094–100. https://doi.org/10.1161/01.cir.92.5.1094.

79. Fang SM, Zhang QH, Jiang ZX. Developing a novel rabbit model of atherosclerotic plaque rupture and thrombosis by cold-induced endothelial injury. J Biomed Sci. 2009;16:39. https://doi.org/10.1186/1423-0127-16-39.
80. Konstantinov IE, Jankovic GM, Alexander I. Ignatowski: a pioneer in the study of atherosclerosis. Tex Heart Inst J. 2013;40(3):246–9.
81. Ware WR. High cholesterol and coronary heart disease in younger men: the potential role of stress induced exaggerated blood pressure response. Med Hypotheses. 2008;70(3):543–7. https://doi.org/10.1016/j.mehy.2007.06.031.
82. Yusuf S, Hawken S, Ounpuu S, Dans T, Avezum A, Lanas F, et al. Effect of potentially modifiable risk factors associated with myocardial infarction in 52 countries (the INTERHEART study): case-control study. Lancet. 2004;364(9438):937–52. https://doi.org/10.1016/s0140-6736(04)17018-9.
83. Alfonso F, Paulo M, Gonzalo N, Dutary J, Jimenez-Quevedo P, Lennie V, et al. Diagnosis of spontaneous coronary artery dissection by optical coherence tomography. J Am Coll Cardiol. 2012;59(12):1073–9. https://doi.org/10.1016/j.jacc.2011.08.082.
84. Barger AC, Beeuwkes R 3rd, Lainey LL, Silverman KJ. Hypothesis: vasa vasorum and neovascularization of human coronary arteries. A possible role in the pathophysiology of atherosclerosis. N Engl J Med. 1984;310(3):175–7. https://doi.org/10.1056/NEJM198401193100307.
85. Zhang X, Fernández-Hernando C. The Janus-faced role of SR-BI in atherosclerosis. Nat Metab. 2019;1(6):586–7. https://doi.org/10.1038/s42255-019-0072-5.
86. Huang L, Chambliss KL, Gao X, Yuhanna IS, Behling-Kelly E, Bergaya S, et al. SR-B1 drives endothelial cell LDL transcytosis via DOCK4 to promote atherosclerosis. Nature. 2019;569(7757):565–9. https://doi.org/10.1038/s41586-019-1140-4.
87. Tani H, Saito D, Kusachi S, Nakatsu T, Hina K, Ueeda M, et al. Autoregulation by the right coronary artery in dogs with open chests; comparison with the left coronary artery. Pflugers Arch. 1990;416(4):442–7. https://doi.org/10.1007/BF00370752.
88. Rouleau JR, Simard D, Blouin A, Kingma JJG. Angiotensin inhibition and coronary autoregulation in a canine model of LV hypertrophy. Basic Res Cardiol. 2002;97(5):384–91. https://doi.org/10.1007/s003950200047.
89. Johnson NP, Gould KL, De Bruyne B. Autoregulation of coronary blood supply in response to demand: JACC review topic of the week. J Am Coll Cardiol. 2021;77(18):2335–45. https://doi.org/10.1016/j.jacc.2021.03.293.
90. Mahendiran T, Collet C, Bruyne BD. Coronary-artery autoregulation with increasing stenosis. N Engl J Med. 2024;390(21):2030–2. https://doi.org/10.1056/NEJMc2402216.
91. Yamazaki K, Kada K, Suga K, Ota T. To-and-fro coronary flow and simultaneous dual coronary artery occlusion following Fontan surgery in pulmonary atresia with intact ventricular septum. Eur Heart J Case Rep. 2025;9(5) https://doi.org/10.1093/ehjcr/ytaf208.
92. Cohoon TJ, Kern MJ. Extreme angiographic-physiologic mismatch with elevated left ventricular end-diastolic pressure. Cardiovasc Revasc Med. 2022;40:182–3. https://doi.org/10.1016/j.carrev.2021.12.031.
93. Leonardi RA, Townsend JC, Patel CA, Wolf BJ, Todoran TM, Fernandes VL, et al. Left ventricular end-diastolic pressure affects measurement of fractional flow reserve. Cardiovasc Revasc Med. 2013;14(4):218–22. https://doi.org/10.1016/j.carrev.2013.06.001.
94. Gitto M, Sticchi A, Chiarito M, Novelli L, Leone PP, Mincione G, et al. Drug-coated balloon angioplasty for de novo lesions on the left anterior descending artery. Circ Cardiovasc Interv. 2023;16(12):e013232. https://doi.org/10.1161/circinterventions.123.013232.
95. O'Callaghan D, Rai H, Giacoppo D, Coughlan JJ, Durand R, Paradies V, et al. Drug coated balloons versus drug-eluting stents in patients with de novo coronary artery disease. Catheterization and Cardiovascular Interventions.n/a(n/a). https://doi.org/10.1002/ccd.70005.
96. Gallingani A, Pampuri G, Diab N, Grassa G, Hernandez-Vaquero D, Tuttolomondo D, et al. Percutaneous coronary intervention or minimally invasive coronary bypass for isolated left anterior descending artery disease. Am J Cardiol. 2025;249:36–42. https://doi.org/10.1016/j.amjcard.2025.04.014.

97. Ndrepepa G. Minimally invasive direct coronary artery bypass or percutaneous coronary intervention with drug-eluting stents for isolated left anterior descending artery stenosis. Am J Cardiol. 2025; https://doi.org/10.1016/j.amjcard.2025.05.016.
98. Nishiura N, Kubo S, Fujii C, Shima Y, Ikuta A, Osakada K, et al. Fifteen-year clinical outcomes after sirolimus-eluting stent implantation. Circ J. 2024;88(6):938–43. https://doi.org/10.1253/circj.CJ-23-0929.
99. Minami Y, Kaneda H, Inoue M, Ikutomi M, Morita T, Nakajima T. Endothelial dysfunction following drug-eluting stent implantation: a systematic review of the literature. Int J Cardiol. 2013;165(2):222–8. https://doi.org/10.1016/j.ijcard.2012.03.084.
100. Ong P, Athanasiadis A, Perne A, Mahrholdt H, Schäufele T, Hill S, et al. Coronary vasomotor abnormalities in patients with stable angina after successful stent implantation but without in-stent restenosis. Clin Res Cardiol. 2014;103(1):11–9. https://doi.org/10.1007/s00392-013-0615-9.
101. Lim PO. Angina with coronary microvascular dysfunction and its physiological assessment: a review with cases. Br J Cardiol. 2022;29:67–72. https://doi.org/10.5837/bjc.2022.013.
102. Gogas BD, Benham JJ, Hsu S, Sheehy A, Lefer DJ, Goodchild TT, et al. Vasomotor function comparative assessment at 1 and 2 years following implantation of the Absorb everolimus-eluting bioresorbable vascular scaffold and the Xience V Everolimus-eluting metallic stent in porcine coronary arteries. JACC Cardiovasc Interv. 2016;9(7):728–41. https://doi.org/10.1016/j.jcin.2015.12.018.
103. Nakamura T, Winsor-Hines D, Yin X, Sushkova N, Chen JP, King SB, et al. Vasomotor function and re-endothelialisation after implantation of biodegradable abluminal polymer coated paclitaxel-eluting stents in rabbit iliac arteries: a time-course study. EuroIntervention. 2012;8(4):493–500. https://doi.org/10.4244/EIJV8I4A77.
104. Kong MG, Han JK, Kang JH, Zheng C, Yang HM, Park KW, et al. Clinical outcomes of long stent in the drug-eluting stent era: patient-level pooled analysis from the GRAND-DES registry. EuroIntervention. 2019; https://doi.org/10.4244/EIJ-D-19-00296.
105. Lim PO. Takayasu arteritis and stent always end in tears. Eur Heart J Case Rep. 2023;7(9) https://doi.org/10.1093/ehjcr/ytad421.
106. Xu K, Jiang Y, Yang W, Zhang W, Wang D, Zhao Y, et al. Post-procedural and long-term functional outcomes of jailed side branches in stented coronary bifurcation lesions assessed with side branch Murray law–based quantitative flow ratio. Front Cardiovasc Med. 2023;10 https://doi.org/10.3389/fcvm.2023.1217069.
107. Nojima Y, Ihara M, Adachi H, Kurimoto T, Nanto S. Rescue percutaneous coronary intervention for a lethal "jailed" septal perforator branch to resolve delayed complete atrioventricular block. Int Heart J. 2019;60(2):457–61. https://doi.org/10.1536/ihj.18-280.
108. Playán-Escribano J, Martínez-Losas P, Cobos-Gil MÁ. Electrocardiographic changes after angioplasty of the left anterior descending coronary artery. Circulation. 2019;139(12):1550–3. https://doi.org/10.1161/CIRCULATIONAHA.118.038518.
109. Sadiq MA, Azman W, Abidin IZ. Irreversible delayed complete heart block secondary to jailed first septal perforator following PCI of the left anterior descending coronary artery. J Invasive Cardiol. 2012;24(1):E13–E5.
110. Carvalho PEP, Mutlu D, Strepkos D, Alexandrou M, Ser OS, Jalli S, et al. Impact of side branch predilatation on provisional bifurcation percutaneous coronary intervention outcomes: insights from PROGRESS-BIFURCATION registry. Catheter Cardiovasc Interv. 2025;105(6):1349–55. https://doi.org/10.1002/ccd.31465.
111. Hahn JY, Chun WJ, Kim JH, Song YB, Oh JH, Koo BK, et al. Predictors and outcomes of side branch occlusion after main vessel stenting in coronary bifurcation lesions: results from the COBIS II registry (COronary BIfurcation Stenting). J Am Coll Cardiol. 2013;62(18):1654–9. https://doi.org/10.1016/j.jacc.2013.07.041.
112. Oh GC, Park KW, Kang J, Han J-K, Yang H-M, Kang H-J, et al. Association of side-branch treatment and patient factors in left anterior descending artery true bifurcation lesions: analysis from the GRAND-DES pooled registry. J Interv Cardiol. 2020;2020(1):8858642. https://doi.org/10.1155/2020/8858642.

113. Strepkos D, Alexandrou M, Mutlu D, Carvalho PEP, Ser OS, Jalli S, et al. Impact of side branch occlusion on patient outcomes after bifurcation percutaneous coronary intervention. Catheter Cardiovasc Interv. 2025;105(5):1142–8. https://doi.org/10.1002/ccd.31439.
114. Wu X, Wu M, Huang H, Liu Z, Huang H, Wang L. Risk factors and clinical consequences of side branch occlusion in left anterior descending bifurcation percutaneous coronary intervention: a validation study of the V-RESOLVE score. Front Cardiovasc Med. 2025;12 https://doi.org/10.3389/fcvm.2025.1648244.
115. Stone GW, Ellis SG, Gori T, Metzger DC, Stein B, Erickson M, et al. Blinded outcomes and angina assessment of coronary bioresorbable scaffolds: 30-day and 1-year results from the ABSORB IV randomised trial. Lancet. 2018;392(10157):1530–40. https://doi.org/10.1016/S0140-6736(18)32283-9.
116. Giedd KN, Bergmann SR. Myocardial perfusion imaging following percutaneous coronary intervention: the importance of restenosis, disease progression, and directed reintervention. J Am Coll Cardiol. 2004;43(3):328–36. https://doi.org/10.1016/j.jacc.2003.09.032.

Chapter 6
Knotted Heart

Abstract Coronary artery anomalies are encountered in at least 5% of routine catheter-based diagnostic and CT coronary angiograms. These range from the coronary artery with an anomalous aortic origin, a complex fistula and a segment of an artery that tunnels under the myocardium. The last anomaly involving the left anterior descending (LAD) artery with a myocardial bridge (MB) appears to be the commonest—up to one third of the general population. In a patient with chest pain, it might be difficult to tease out if these coronary anomalies are contributory. Nevertheless, cardiac ischaemia is dictated by blood supply and fuel demand under stress; in the cardiac catheter laboratory, adenosine or dobutamine can be used and vasoreactivity tested with acetylcholine provocation. Further, these anomalies are usually an incidental finding in patients with competing comorbidities, including hypertension, left ventricular dysfunction, and a background of atherosclerotic coronary artery disease. The pressure-derived "surrogate" flow ratios are likely to be confounded. That was the reason for using the integrated diastolic fractional flow reserve (dFFR ≤ 0.76) with dobutamine for assessing MB. Although this was introduced over 20 years ago, it has not been adopted into daily clinical practice. Alternatively, now that actual volumetric coronary flow can be accurately measured in real time with continuous thermodilution, MB can be re-evaluated, with the potential that it might become the new gold standard. In the meantime, the clinical pathophysiology of MB is better understood. According to Francisco Torrent-Guasp's helical myocardial ventricular band (HMVB) model where the heart can be origamically unfolded into a single strip of muscle, the "stray" muscle fibres running criss-cross from the right ventricle across the interventricular sulcus where the LAD is embedded to the left ventricle; when blunt-dissected with fingers the heart can be opened up like a lady's purse. The MB is relatively immuned to the atherosclerotic process which renders it highly vasoreactive. On the other hand, the pre-MB LAD is a high stress area, making it liable to develop intimal thickening with plaque formation; when subjected to haemodynamic stress it can rupture, leading to coronary thrombosis and myocardial infarction. Finally, if the MB is stented inadvertently or when it is masked by a stunned myocardium, the reappearance of MB with myocardial recovery gives rise to repetitive radial strain on the stent, causing it to restenose or even fracture.

P. O. Lim, *Coronary Thermodilution*,
https://doi.org/10.1007/978-3-032-10734-3_6

6.1 Introduction

Coronary flow restriction due to atherosclerotic plaque build-up within the vessel wall, causing a narrowing or luminal stenosis, is a relatively modern phenomenon. As discussed in the previous chapter, when William Heberden the Elder (1710–1801) described angina pectoris which it results in, just over 250 years ago, he only saw one case per year in his 20 years' practice at St George's Hospital, at the time sited in Hyde Park Corner, London [1, 2].

On the other hand, Heinrich C. Reyman (b. 1718) as part of his doctoral dissertation in Göttingen systematically dissected 6 hearts looking specifically at the coronary arteries; 35 years earlier in 1737, he found myocardial bridging (MB) instantly [3]. This high MB prevalence was confirmed in later autopsy series, but in an unselected series, it was about 15%, and in a third of cases, it was associated with other coronary artery anomalies (CAA), such as the right coronary cusp arising circumflex artery with an interarterial course between the aorta and the pulmonary artery [4]. While in a large CT coronary angiogram (CTCA) series, coronary artery anomalies (CAA) was found in 8% of cases, nearly half were MB. CTCA is four times more sensitive in detecting CAA than coronary angiogram. In a large coronary angiogram cohort of patients with chest pain, MB was found in 4% of cases [5]. Incidentally, Reyman's supervisor, Albrecht von Haller (1708–1777), gave a detailed description of the anatomical courses of the right and left coronary arteries in 1757 [6, 7], building on the French anatomist and physician Raymond de Vieussens's (c. 1633–1715) 1706 description and orientation of the two coronary arteries, who also discovered the *arterial ring* that bears his name, which links the conus branch of the right coronary artery (RCA) traversing anteriorly across the right ventricular outflow tract to the proximal segment of the left anterior descending (LAD) artery or the diagonal branch [8]. It is surprisingly rare, and in routine CTCA, it has a prevalence of 0.3% [9], but it could develop in 20% of cases if one or the other artery is occluded, providing an epicardial collateral supply [10].

As nature often exhibits bilateral symmetry, a complementary interatrial collateral vessel may arise from the atrial branch of the RCA, coursing anteriorly across the right and left atria behind the ascending aorta, towards the proximal segment of the circumflex (Cx) artery [11, 12]. Variants may also originate from the posterolateral branch of the RCA, traversing between the atria to the same destination [13]. This connecting artery was first reported by Maurice A. Kugel (1899–1946) in 1927, and it has been identified in up to 6% of patients on imaging or anatomical studies [13–15]. Thus, Vieussens' ring in front and Kugel's ring behind the aorta together form a functional coronary ring encircling the base of the heart [11, 12].

It is important to note that MB on its own does not obviously carry an adverse prognosis [16]. But it is a cause of angina with non-obstructive coronary arteries (ANOCA), and it is a diagnostic conundrum in appropriating blame, if an incidental MB causes angina. Besides MB, the plaque-free coronary artery can also be externally compressed, such as the left main coronary artery by the dilated pulmonary trunk, intramurally as it exits from the aortic root or interarterially if it has anomalous aortic origin (AAOCA) from the opposite coronary sinus [17], or blood flow that is stolen or diverted by extraneous fistulae [18–20]. In this chapter, continuous thermodilution was undertaken in four patients with various common CAA.

6.2 Cases

6.2.1 *The Tethered Left Anterior Descending Artery*

A 75-year-old Caucasian woman complained of angina, breathlessness, fatigue and dizzy spells. She has a history of depression, hypertension, hyperlipidaemia, vitamin D deficiency and a body mass index (BMI) of 34 kg/m^2. She also had human epidermal growth factor receptor 2 (HERS-2) negative left ductal breast carcinoma at 68 after local excision and sentinel lymph node biopsy—which was clear. She had 6 cycles of adjuvant chemotherapy (FEC 75) at 3 weekly intervals with intravenous fluorouracil (5FU) 600 mg/m^2, epirubicin 75 mg/m^2 and cyclophosphamide 600 mg/m^2, followed by a short course of radiotherapy, and then letrozole, an aromatase inhibitor for 4 years. As a result of her treatment, she developed static subpleural lung fibrosis. Nevertheless, her respiratory function tests were within normal limits, but she was noted to exhibit an element of dysfunctional breathing pattern at rest, despite no demonstrable oxygen desaturation. Her echocardiogram prior to her breast cancer treatment showed a normal heart. However, over the years, she developed echocardiographic left ventricular (LV) wall motion abnormalities and underwent a prior diagnostic coronary angiogram 2 years before that showed unobstructed vessels at a local hospital.

One month before her coronary physiology study, her dobutamine stress echocardiogram (DSE) at baseline showed a structurally normal heart, although there was akinesia in basal to mid inferoseptum, with an LV ejection fraction (EF) of 55–60%. She had pulmonary valvuloplasty at 11 in 1957. She has no prior history of myocardial infarction. The LV end-systolic volume index, ESVI, was 16 (13–28) m/m^2 and stroke volume index, SVI, was 18 (30–59) mL/m^2, thus a ventriculo-arterial coupling, VAC, of 0.89 (0.6–1.0). She has no left ventricular hypertrophy (LVH) nor left atrial (LA) dilatation, but elevated average E/e' of 13 (< 8), implying LV diastolic function. With dobutamine stress, her pulse rate rose from 93 to 137 bpm corresponding to 94% predicted maximal heart rate, > 85% suggesting an adequate stress test, and her BP were 140/80 and 160/90 mmHg, respectively—raised at baseline but controlled during the test. She was asymptomatic throughout, and there were no ischaemic electrocardiographic (ECG) and echocardiographic changes of note; the 2/17 akinetic segments did not improve.

Procedure Her coronary arteries are unobstructed (Fig. 6.1); the right has an anomalous aortic origin from the left coronary cusp (R-AAOCA), whereas the left anterior descending (LAD) artery has diffuse irregularity; beyond the third diagonal branch, there is an LAD segment that appears "fixed", without overt systolic coronary compression. The LV has normal systolic function with borderline raised LV end-diastolic pressure (LVEDP) which is 12 mmHg, not rising with handgrip. The basal and

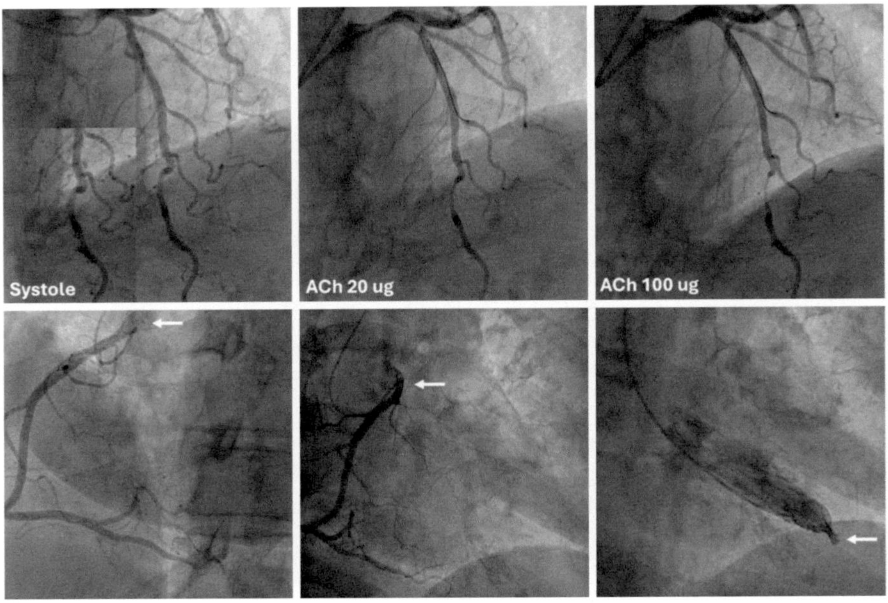

Fig. 6.1 (**Top left to right panels**) Left anterior descending (LAD) artery with a segment after the third diagonal branch that appears to be "held down", without obvious reduction in calibre during cardiac contraction in systole (*inset*). Acetylcholine (ACh) is associated with dose-dependent localised vasospasm, culminating with angina and ischaemic electrocardiographic changes. (**Bottom left to right panels**) Right Anomalous Aortic Origin of Coronary Artery (R-AAOCA) with a wide ostium (*arrows*). Left ventricular angiogram with normal contractility and a small apical pouch or diverticulum, often seen in hypertension

hyperaemic indices obtained with continuous thermodilution are; the distal-to-aortic pressure ratio (Pd/Pa) is 0.97 and fractional flow reserve (FFR), 0.97, flow 57 and 184 mL/min, and *resistance 1673 and 518 Wood units*—thus, coronary flow reserve (CFR) is 3.2 and microvascular resistance reserve (MRR), 3.2. Relative flow increases from baseline are calculated following intracoronary acetylcholine (ACh) 2, 20 and 100 μg—which are 1.1, 1.4 and 2, respectively. She develops dose-dependent LAD vasospasm, despite increased flow; the Pd/Pa is 0.83. This is associated with lateral ECG ST depression and chest pain. This is reversed with verapamil 200 μg, with a flow increase of 1.4 from baseline and relief of the LAD segmental vasospasm.

Her CTCA (Fig. 6.2) confirms that the R-AAOCA has wide ostium with a short interarterial course abutting the pulmonary truck, and in the LAD, *the mid LAD dives intramuscularly* to a depth of 3.5 mm, with a buried length of 20 mm. Looking at her echocardiogram again, she has prominent *epicardial adipose tissue* (EAT) measuring about 10 mm. As for her adenosine perfusion cardiac magnetic resonance (CMR) scan, her EF is low normal at 59%, without LVH, nor LA dilatation, but there is discordant basal to mid-septal motion, without inducible ischaemia. There is extensive *mid-wall fibrosis* in the base, involving the right ventricular insertion points. The ESVI is 28 (12–30) mL/m^2 and SVI is 40 (34–59) mL/m^2—VAC 0.7 (0.6–1.0)—these are normal values.

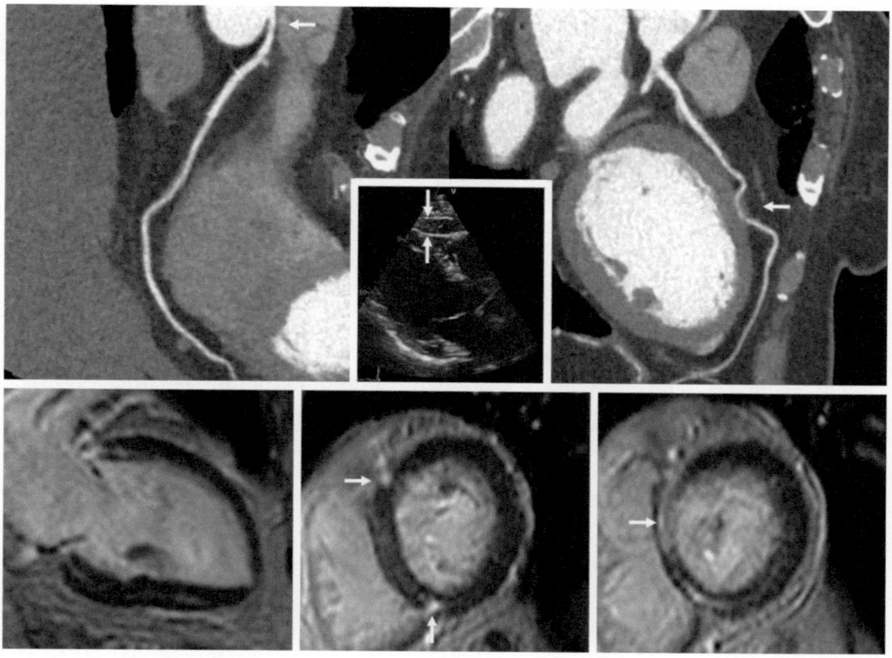

Fig. 6.2 (**Top left to right panels**) CT coronary angiogram of the Right Anomalous Aortic Origin of Coronary Artery (R-AAOCA). With a short interarterial course, the *arrow* is in the pulmonary trunk. As for the left anterior descending (LAD) artery, the mid vessel is "submerged" within the myocardium. The mid panel echocardiogram shows a prominent epicardial adipose tissue (EAT). (**Bottom left to right panels**) Cardiovascular magnetic resonance (CMR) scan shows extensive late gadolium enhancement in mid wall at the base, extending along the septum and inferiorly, and at the right ventricular insertion (*arrows*) suggestive of a cardiomyopathic process

Interpretation This woman with hypertension, which has not been treated to target, has intact vasodilatory capacity, but raised basal and hyperaemic resistance. She has preserved LV systolic function, borderline LVEDP and a small LV apical diverticulum. She has a segment of LAD within the interventricular sulcus, embedded in both muscle and EAT; this was as Erich Geiringer's (1917–1995) original description of myocardial bridging (MB) [21]. Although in this case there is no demonstrable systolic compression, yet interestingly this segment is *highly vasoreactive to ACh*. Despite this, the flow increases with ACh suggesting intact microvascular endothelial function. She also has no dobutamine-induced myocardial ischaemia implying that the *short interarterial vessel* is unlikely to be at fault [17, 18]. Further, the cardiomyopathy on her CMR is likely related to her breast cancer treatment, albeit with preserved EF and her R-AAOCA with a wide ostium together, are unlikely to be contributory, on the basis of her satisfactory dobutamine stress echocardiogram (DSE). The remaining question therefore is, if her angina is due to MB vasospasm, and her hypertension requires a tighter control as she has raised coronary resistance, which could also be contributed by her "subclinical" cardiomyopathy related to breast cancer treatment [22, 23]. EAT is separately addressed in Chap. 3.

6.2.2 *The Buried Left Anterior Descending Artery*

A 67-year-old Caucasian woman has had angina with exertion, emotion, at rest and while sleeping, over the years, and underwent 4 coronary angiograms between the ages of 47 and 58. Thus, she was diagnosed with cardiac syndrome X on ivabradine and nicorandil, despite which she was admitted to a local hospital with a troponin negative chest pain, precipitating this referral. She has asthma on long-term prednisolone 5 mg daily that adversely contributed to her diabetes, for which she took metformin and gliclazide, in addition to having hypertension and weight gain with a BMI of 44 kg/m^2. Also, she has developed adrenal insufficiency from the chronic steroid use. In an attempt to spare it, she was started on injectable omalizumab, a monoclonal antibody targeting the immunoglobulin E (IgE). She has obstructive sleep apnoea, hyperlipidaemia,was a smoker and had not needed oestrogen replacement therapy.

Procedure Her coronary angiogram shows unobstructed arteries (Fig. 6.3); the right coronary artery gives rise to a dominant posterior descending artery (RPDA) that reaches the LV apex. While the left main is short, the circumflex (Cx) artery is

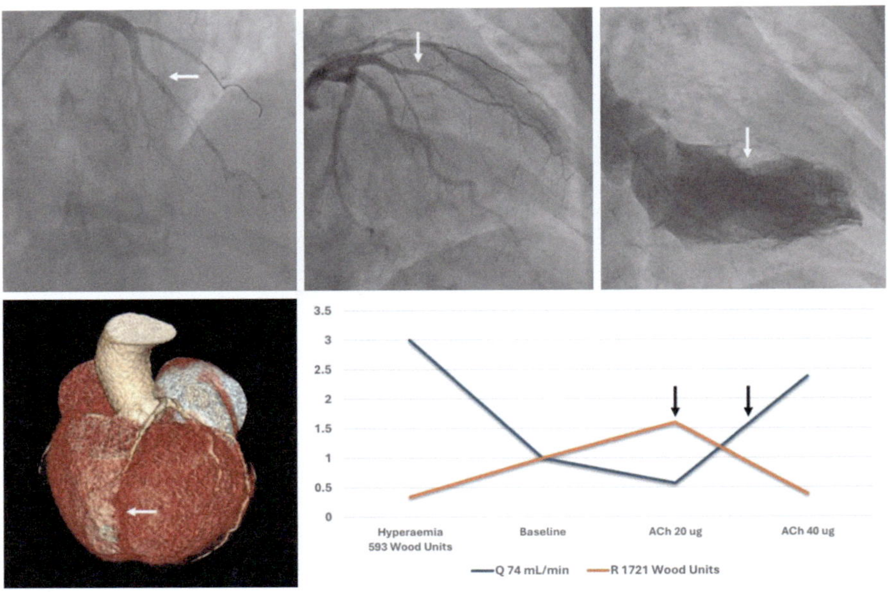

Fig. 6.3 (**Top left to right panels**) Coronary angiogram of the left anterior descending (LAD) artery; after the septal branch it dives intramuscularly along its course as pointed by the *arrows*, and left ventricular angiogram in response to a hypertensive response shows mid cavity "obstruction". (**Bottom left to right panels**) 3D CT coronary angiogram which shows that the LAD is submerged within the intraventricular groove. The haemodynamic chart plots the circumflex artery flow and resistance at baseline, hyperaemia and in response to acetylcholine (ACh). Note that ACh 20 μg raises resistance and reduces flow by half (*arrrow*) interpreted as *microvascular spasm*, yet at 40 μg, the reverse occurs (*arrrow*) which would imply that the flow reduction with ACh 20 μg is due to small vessel constriction

dominant, supplying most of inferolateral myocardium, and the left anterior descending (LAD) artery, after the septal branch, either appears to be absent, with a parallel second diagonal branch, or continues as a **small calibre and "recessive" LAD**. For this reason, continuous thermodilution is carried out in the Cx. With saline infusion rate of 20 mL/min, there is frequent heart block which may indicate that the atrioventricular (AV) nodal branch arises from the Cx; therefore the hyperaemic indices are derived with a reduced15 mL/min saline infusion rate. The basal and hyperaemic values are as follows: flow 74 and 222 mL/min, and resistance 1721 and 593 Wood units—hence, the CFR is 3.0 and MRR, 2.9. The first ACh 20 μg is associated with AV block with chest pain and a relative flow reduction to 0.56 from baseline, and a fractional rise in resistance interpreted as *microvascular spasm*. Interestingly, flow increases 2.4-fold and resistance falls 61% with doubling of ACh dose to 40 μg, despite which she develops chest pain, lateral ST depression as well as AV block. LV angiogram reveals mid-cavity obstruction, with borderline raised LVEDP of 12 mmHg, rising with handgrip to 15–20 mmHg, with a corresponding central aortic BP of 150/75 mmHg. The contemporaneous NT-ProBNP is 191 (< 125) ng/L.

Interpretation This woman has preserved vasodilatory capacity and exhibited *ACh-induced flow reduction with 20 μg,* which is overcome with higher ACh dose at 40 μg, suggesting intact microvascular endothelial function, since the flow increases by 50%, and there is no obvious radiographic vasospasm but the distal vessels are of small calibre. There could be a discordant response in the LAD, with a dose-dependent ACh-induced epicardial vasospasm, since the ACh injected down the left main dissipates down both Cx and LAD—this could have been confirmed if the flow down the LAD is measured. She has raised basal and hyperaemic resistance with high LVEDP and elevated central aortic BP.

The "confusing" orientation of the LAD is due to lifting of her heart by abdominal adiposity—making her heart appears more horizontal. She is claustrophobic; therefore a CMR could not be undertaken. Instead, she had a DSE that revealed a structurally normal heart with an EF of 60%, without LVH, but mild LA dilatation (A4C 22.9, > 20 cm^2) and average raised E/e' 14 (< 8). With dobutamine stress, her HR and BP were 58 bpm and 143/83 mmHg respectively, rising to 134 bpm and 164/90 mmHg at peak dose; thus an HR response of 88%, > 85% predicted maximal HR, suggesting adequate stress level. She did not develop chest pain, neither ischaemic ECG nor echocardiographic changes. The intramuscular course of her LAD is unlikely to be contributory with her reassuring DSE results, but potentially would be predisposed to vasospasm as in case 1. Her CTCA confirms that her LAD is buried intramuscularly throughout its course within the interventricular groove, and her ambulatory BP monitor (ABPM) reveals a daytime mean of 118/62 mmHg, with a normal nighttime dip—suggesting a well controlled BP, which is essential for her.

6.2.3 *The Anomalous Right Coronary Artery*

A 56-year-old Caucasian woman has angina with non-obstructive coronary arteries (ANOCA). About a year previously, she was admitted with an inferior myocardial infarction; she was then discovered to have a right anomalous aortic origin of coronary artery (R-AAOCA), and in the mid vessel there was haziness indicating a plaque rupture, which was directly covered with a 4.0 × 15 mm drug-eluting stent (DES). Her subsequent 12-lead ECG showed preserved R in inferior leads without a Q, and her echocardiogram on day three showed hypokinesia in basal to mid inferior wall with an EF of 52%, without LVH, or LA dilatation, ESVI 27 (13–28) mL/m^2 and SVI 29 (30–59) mL/m^2; thus VAC 0.94 (0.5–1.0). She had a DSE 3 months later; this showed no improvement in the 2/17 infarcted LV segments, and her EF remained at 52%. Undilated LA and average E/e' 7.24 (< 8), ESVI 22 (13–28) mL/m^2 and SVI 29 (30–59) mL/m^2, hence VAC 0.73 (0.6–1.0). With dobutamine stress, her HR and BP rose from 82 bpm and 144/81 mmHg to 148 bpm and 163/87 mmHg, corresponding to a maximal predicted HR of 90% (> 85%). She was asymptomatic, and there were no ischaemic ECG, nor echocardiographic findings in the viable myocardium. Despite this, she continued to have exertional angina when reviewed in the clinic 7.5 months later. The CTCA confirmed her R-AAOCA with ostial stenosis and a short interarterial course between the aorta and the pulmonary trunk (Fig. 6.4). Her BMI was 35 kg/m^2; she has hypertension and asthma, is a current smoker, 15/day, has been menopausal since 36 following her cervical cancer surgery, and has not needed oestrogen replacement therapy.

Procedure Her LV is studied first; the LVEDP is 25 mmHg without angiographic wall motion abnormalities and an EF of 55%. The LVEDP rises to 30 mmHg with handgrip, with a corresponding central aortic BP of 220/100 mmHg. Her coronary arteries are unobstructed. *An EBU3.5 5Fr guide catheter easily engaged the R-AAOCA.* Intravascular ultrasound (IVUS) is performed; this reveals an oval-shaped ostium without systolic intramural compression—area 6 mm^2, average diameter of 2.75 mm, with a reference diameter of 3.5 mm, and area of 10.3 mm^2. With the pressure wire down the vessel beyond the patent and well-apposed stent, the Pd/Pa is 0.98, rest full-cycle ratio (RFR) 0.93 (> 0.89), and FFR of 0.95 (> 0.80), following intracoronary 100 μg bolus of adenosine. Continuous thermodilution is performed, the respective basal and hyperaemic indices: flow 87 and 259 mL/min and resistance 1809 and 481 Wood units—CFR 3.0 and MRR 3.8. Escalating doses of ACh are not associated with chest pain, radiographic slow flow or vasospasm, nor ECG changes, albeit some drop beats. Instead, flow increases > 50% with a corresponding fall in resistance.

This woman's R-AAOCA is not flow limiting structurally and physiological, without ACh-induced vasoreactivity and preserved vasodilatory capacity, but raised coronary resistance and LVEDP from a hypertensive response during the procedure—for this reason, dobutamine is not used.

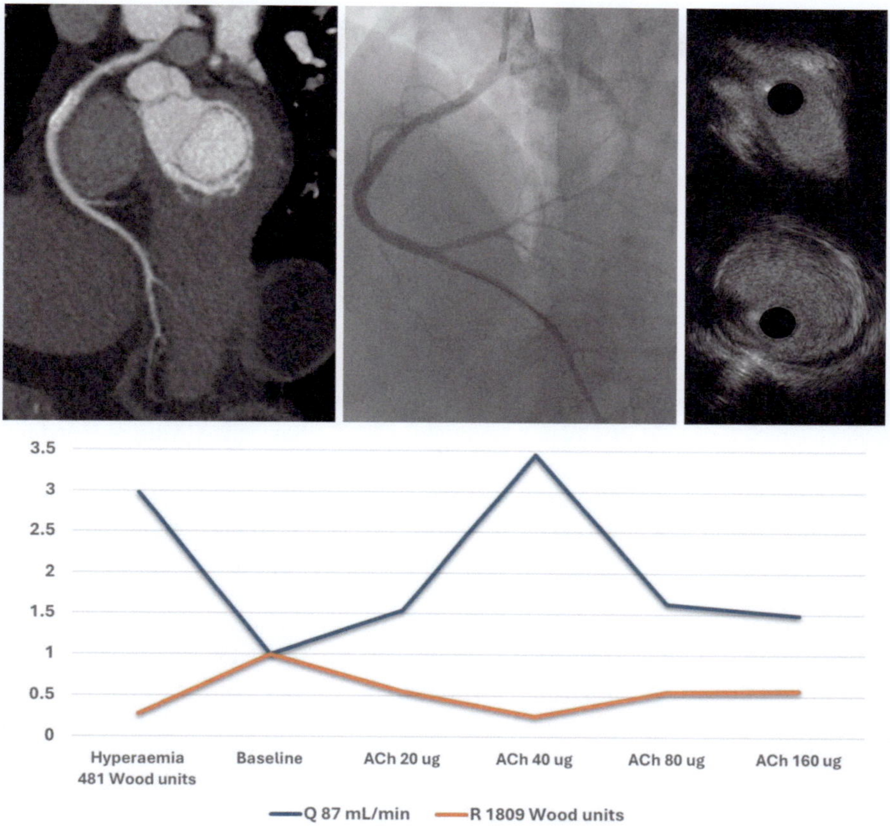

Fig. 6.4 (**Top left to right panels**) CT coronary angioram of the right anomalous aortic origin coronary artery (R-AAOCA) that shows a *pinched* ostium, and proximally it runs between the aorta as it exits against the pulmonary trunk. The corresponding coronary angiogram followed by intravascular ultrasound (IVUS) of the ostium and a reference segment. (**Bottom panel**) Haemodynamic indices derived from continuous thermodilution, from baseline and in response to hyperaemia and acetylcholine (ACh). There is elevated coronary resistance but intact vasodilatory capacity, with flow rise of > 50% in response to ACh suggesting preserved microvascular endothelial function, despite the myocardial infarction. Higher doses of ACh do not provoke epicardial vasospasm. The lack of dose dependency in increasing flow can be due to muscarinic receptor saturation and desensitisation, with nitric oxide relaxation plateau, or alternatively spill over to the media layer where the vascular smooth muscle cells are, and via nicotinic receptor coupling causing counteracting vasoconstriction in moderating flow

Interpretation Interestingly, despite early menopause and smoking, this woman has no worse coronary atherosclerotic disease than if she lacked these risk factors. She has preserved both epicardial and microvascular endothelial function. Her cardiac event was a plaque rupture likely to be related to her labile hypertension which is enough to cause cardiac stress by raising her LV filling pressure, as has she increased coronary resistance.

Her antihypertensive treatment was optimised—increasing her ramipril to 2.5 mg od and adding nebivolol 2.5 mg od, while advising her to stop smoking and lose about 10 kg in weight to bring her BMI down to < 30 kg/m^2. Her ABPM done a week later revealed a daytime mean BP of 132/77 mmHg without a nighttime dip. When reviewed in the clinic 6 weeks later, she appeared to be asymptomatic. Her NT-ProBNP is 59 (< 125) pg/mL, compared to 218 pg/mL 1 year prior.

6.2.4 The Squeezed Left Anterior Descending Artery

A 59-year old East Asian man with hypertension, diabetes and hyperlipidaemia was admitted with a troponin negative chest pain. He was previously investigated for non-specific chest pain in a local hospital, his CTCA showed LAD disease, and his DSE confirmed ischaemia in the myocardium subtended by the artery. His coronary angiogram found coronary pulmonary artery fistulae (CPAF) arising from proximal LAD, in addition to a mid-LAD MB segment. He was continued on medical treatment. His repeat CTCA at St George's Hospital confirmed that there were 2 fistulae arising from proximal LAD, inserted into the pulmonary trunk together as well as a long segment of MB in mid LAD (Fig. 6.5). His DSE undertaken 6 months later showed a structurally normal heart without overt LVH but borderline septal thickness at 1.1 cm, and no LA dilatation, average E/e' 9.74 (< 0.80), EF of 59%, ESVI 21 (11–31) mL/m^2, SVI 33 (33–47) mL/m^2, and VAC 0.62 (0.6–1.0). With dobutamine stress, the HR and BP rose from rest, 88 bpm and 137/88 mmHg to 136 bpm and 168/90 mmHg at peak dose; the HR was 85% maximal predicted suggesting an adequate stress level for the test. There was no associated chest pain nor echocardiographic inducible ischaemia, but ECG ST depression was noted in leads I and aVL. In view of his continuing angina despite high-dose beta blockade with bisoprolol 12.5 mg od, ranolazine 500 mg bd and nicorandil 10 mg bd, he was offered a coronary physiology study to understand if the CPAF or the MB was the culprit, one and a half years later. (The figures below are adapted with permission from the Hellenic Cardiological Society of the published article, "Lim PO, Is it a steal or a squeeze? HJC 2024;78:93-94.").

Procedure His coronary anatomy has not changed. Right heart catheterisation is performed with oxygen saturation samplings—right atrium (RA) 5.20 kPa, right ventricle (RV) 5.06 kPa, pulmonary artery (PA) 5.09 kPa and aorta 9.35 kPa. There is no obvious step up in oxygen content in the PA compared with RA and RV, proving that the CPAF shunt is small and the right heart pressures are normal. Continuous thermodilution is undertaken at left main (LM), mid LAD beyond the CPAF, and Cx, with the following basal and hyperaemic indices:

LM—flow 153 and 283 mL/min, and resistance 634 and 284 Wood units (CFR 1.85, MRR 2.23)

LAD—flow 86 and 173 mL/min, and resistance 1107 and 449 Wood units (CFR 2.0 MRR 2.47)

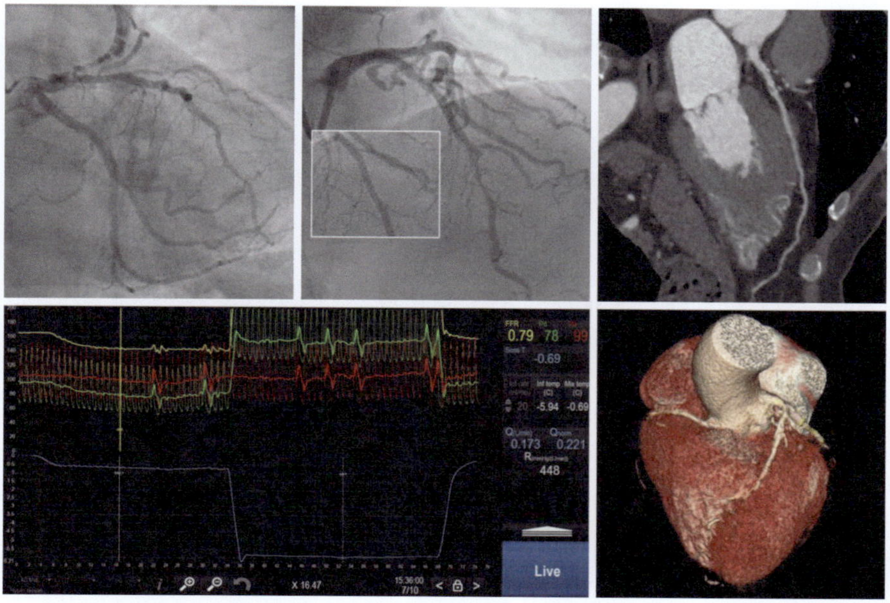

Fig. 6.5 (**Top left to right panels**) Coronary angiogram showing 2 coronary pulmonary artery fistulae (CPAF) arising from proximal left anterior descending (LAD) artery that join and attach to the pulmonary trunk as a single insertion. The mid LAD in diastole and systole (*inset*) which clearly show the myocardial bridging (MB). This is confirmed on CT coronary angiogram (CTCA); the mid LAD has an overlying myocardium. (**Bottom left to right panels**) Continuous thermodilution during dobutamine stress, exacerbating the MB with hyperaemia, resulting in an increased pressure gradient—fractional flow research (FFR) of 0.79 (< 0.8). Despite this, note the doubling of flow to 173 mL/min from a baseline of 66 mL/min with low-dose dobutamine. The 3D CT coronary angiogram shows an embedded mid LAD

Cx—flow 76 and 166 mL/min, and resistance 1156 and 533 Wood units (CFR 1.53, MRR 2.17)

Basal flow—LM 153 mL/min ~ 162 mL/min (LAD 86 mL/min + Cx 76 mL/min)—suggesting no significant flow diversion. Whereas for hyperaemic flow, LAD + Cx (339 mL/min) > LM 283 may suggest it takes a higher rate of saline infusion to produce hyperaemia in a larger subtended myocardium, and a combined LAD and Cx—CFR is 2.1.

With dobutamine infusion, at 10 μg/kg/min, Pd/Pa 0.94, flow 66 mL/min and resistance 1434 W units, at 20 μg/kg/min, Pd/Pa 0.92, flow 80 mL/min and resistance 1278 Wood units, and atropine 300 μg intravenously raises HR to 114 (72% max predicted) bpm with an hypertensive response of 210/80 mmHg. This provokes chest pain with lateral ST depression on ECG, and saline hyperaemia earlier produces an FFR of 0.79 (< 0.80).

Interpretation This man's coronary physiology is assessed in the context of hypertension, CPAF and MB. First, there is no significant step up in oxygen saturation in the PA. Second, the proximal LAD has normal calibre which suggests that there is no excess flow that would cause a compensatory aneurysmal dilatation before the CPAF. Third, the flow down the LM roughly equals to the combined flow of LAD beyond the CPAF and Cx, implying that the "steal" into the CPAF is likely to be small. For these three reasons, the CPAF in this man is unlikely to be contributory to his angina. Next, he has borderline low CFR, and high basal and hyperaemic resistance which could be concluded as CMD, but a better explanation is that this is due to hypertension. Dobutamine albeit at submaximal HR < 85% accentuates the MB leading to an increase in pressure gradient and a flat flow response with dobutamine up to 20 μg/kg/min; when atropine 300 μg is given, he becomes highly symptomatic with ECG changes and the procedure is terminated. In conclusion, this man's moderate LAD lesion at the take-offs of CPAF which on its own is not flow-limiting, but in combination with a dynamic MB causes this man's angina.

6.3 Discussion

Four cases were described (Table 6.1): (1) Hypertensive heart with mid-LAD MB (spasm) and R-AAOCA; (2) hypertensive heart with mid-distal LAD MB (likely spasm); (3) hypertensive heart and R-AAOCA; and (4) hypertensive heart with CPAF and mid-LAD MB (spasm) with positive dobutamine stress and exercise. Hypertensive LV diastolic dysfunction is associated with raised coronary resistance and elevated LVEDP, compounded by obesity in cases 1–3; these are discussed elsewhere. The focus of this chapter is on MB; CPAF was touched on earlier and R-AAOCA, if isolated, stenting is a valid option with good long-term outcome as demonstrated by Paolo Angelini (1941–2023) [18].

Erich Geiringer (1917–1995) escaped Vienna as a Jewish refugee from the Nazis to England in 1938 [24]. At 34, while he was a research fellow at the Gerontology Research Unit in the University Edinburgh, in 1951, he published a couple of papers, each with over 400 citations as sole author [21, 25]. In one he noted coronary intraplaque microchannels which only 60 years later was confirmed with intracoronary optical coherence tomography (OCT—see Chap. 5—case 4), and in a second paper he reported the definitive postmortem series of "mural", "tunnelled" or "bridging" left anterior descending (LAD) artery. He did not specify the causes of death nor gender split, but he systematically looked at the LAD of 100 subjects and concluded a bridging LAD rate of 23%. The embedded depth of 5 mm which he used is current standard reporting in CTCA which, again 60 years later, replicated his findings. In addition, he observed more intimal thickening in those without an MB, but he did not study the non-mural course of those with MB—subsequent studies revealed this to be the case in patients with MB. The mural course of LAD does confer some protection from atherosclerosis. Geringer hypothesised that in fact MB splints and protects against atherosclerosis. When the heart relaxes the MB segments suck blood along, contributing to coronary flow. He joked that as chimpanzee, and, to some extent, orangutan have embedded LAD, human perhaps descended from the wrong kind of

Table 6.1 Coronary physiology and coronary artery anomalies

Case	Age	BMI	Comorbidities	MB	Vasodilatory capacity (CFR)	Coronary resistance (Wood units)	Vasoreactivity (ACh)	Verapamil
1[a]	75 ♀	34 with EAT[a]+++	**HBP**, lipids, Vit D def, breast cancer, mid-wall LV fibrosis	Mid LAD R-AAOCA	3.2	**518** MRR 3.2 LVEDP 12	MB spasm Pd/Pa 0.84, pain and ST depression	Reversed MB spasm
2	67 ♀	44	**HBP**, asthma on steroids, diabetes, OSA, lipid, ex-smoker	Buried mid to distal LAD	3.0	**593** MRR 2.9 LVEDP 12 to 20 (NT-ProBNP 191)	Cx, biphasic— 20 µg ↓Q 44%, 40 µg ↑Q 146% (adenosine hyperaemia ↑Q 200%)	N/A
3	56 ♀	35	**HBP**, asthma, smoking and menopause at 36	R-AAOCA	3.0	**481** MRR 3.8 LVEDP 25–30, BP 220	Negative	N/A
4	59 ♀	< 30	**HBP**, diabetes and lipids	Mid LAD Coronary pulmonary artery fistula	2.0 ↓Q 23% with Dobutamine 10 µg/kg/min	**449** MRR 2.5	Dobutamine 20 µg/kg/min FFR 0.79, chest pain and ST depression LAD spasm with ACh 50 µg[b]	N/A

[a] *EAT* epicardial adipose tissue

[b] Undertaken in another unit 18 months later, RFR 0.80 (> 0.89) in LAD with bicycle exercise (intolerant of diltiazem)

primates, more akin to Gorilla and Gibbon with regard to epicardial coronary artery course [26]. He relocated to Dunedin Medical School, Otago, New Zealand in 1959. His medical activism in reproductive and population health, with his anti-establishment streak, culminated in him leading the country's nuclear disarmament movement to the international stage as a general practitioner in Wellington, in Auckland.

As observed by Geiringer the bridging segment of MB is relatively disease-free; this has been borne out by later multimodality studies; in particular, an autopsy study of 35 MB found that while the media layer varied less, the mean intimal thicknesses (IMT) across the MB were 407, 66 and 103 μm—IMT of the LAD before-MB-after [27]. The haemodynamic stress led to the pre-MB intimal thickening, increasing the likelihood of atherosclerosis and plaque rupture precipitating thrombotic occlusion and acute myocardial infarction (Fig. 6.6). As uncovered by this case, which is often underappreciated, the akinetic LV masks the MB; stenting into or across the MB could cause stent failure with recovery of myocardial contractility. In the setting of LAD chronic total occlusion (CTO) stenting, there was a 2.5-fold in stent failure rate over 2 years in a cohort of 256 patients (MB 61, 24%; 19.7 vs 8.7%, $p = 0.03$) [28]. LAD stenting does have a higher rate of stent failure compared with stenting of other coronary arteries (Cx and RCA) [29], especially if the implanted stent is > 40 mm [30], which in principle would cover an MB since MB is highly prevalent in the LAD. Thus, as discussed in the preceding chapter, LAD treatment with the drug-coated balloon (DCB) is an emerging option which potentially leads to better outcome both in LV function post-MI and in less stent failure by avoiding occult MB [31–34]. MB may not be angiographically obvious, but it is a recognised factor for repeated stent failure and fracture [35, 36], sometimes leading to stent thrombosis and MI (Fig. 6.7); therefore LAD with MB maybe better treated with a DCB [37], and percutaneous coronary intervention (PCI) guidelines discourage stenting the MB [38].

The MB is highly vasoreactive to ACh (> 90%), as can be amplified by the presence of plaque and hypertension with the presence of LVH as in cases 1, 2 and 4 [39–42], which emphasises the importance of managing coronary risk factors in these patients. And the investigation of MB remains uncertain, as it is common in the normal population; up to 1 in 7 people has MB of varying severity [16]. However, initial non-invasive testing with CTCA (depth > 2.0 mm × length > 20 mm) to define the MB [43, 44], followed by dobutamine stress echocardiogram (DSE), would help gatekeep for more invasive management. If these are negative then the focus should be on addressing vasoreactivity since isolated MB is usually benign [16]. However, in obstructive and refractory cases, surgical management might be indicated [45].

Invasive assessment of MB is on the basis of "the moderate lesion causing angina, yet has a discordant FFR of > 0.75". Abe et al. [46] in 2000 introduced the concept of *integrated* diastolic FFR ≤ 0.76; the dP or area under the curve (AUC) between *aortic dicrotic notch and the next R-wave* on gated-ECG with simultaneous aortic, LAD and LV pressure tracings; dFFR = dP-cor/dP-aor. This picked up 23/24 (95.8%) patients with functional evidence of cardiac ischaemia, whereas FFR ≤ 0.75 was seen in 20/24 (83.3%) and in a subset of patients who had CFR < 2 derived from the Doppler wire; this picked up 15/17 (88.2%). The rationale was that the coronary

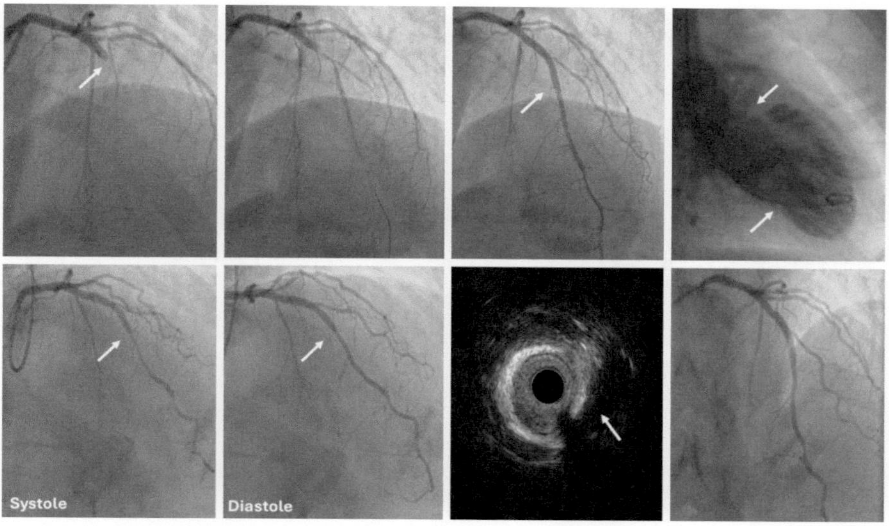

Fig. 6.6 **Inadvertent MB stenting during MI.** A 56-year-old man had an out-of-hospital cardiac arrest while cycling on a road close to St George's Hospital, a tertiary cardiac unit. He received immediate and effective bystander cardiopulmonary resuscitation (CPR) and was shocked out of ventricular fibrillation (VF) within 5 min by the London ambulance service (LAS). (**Top left to right panels**) His diagnostic coronary angiogram found an occluded mid-left anterior descending (LAD) artery (*arrow*); it was thrombectomised, which recanalised the artery, revealing an atherosclerotic plaque across the second diagonal branch. The LAD was stented with a 3.5 × 28 mm drug-eluting stent (DES) (*arrow pointing distal stent edge*). Because of persistent ST elevation despite disobliteration of the LAD, 20 mL saline hyperaemia was performed via the thrombectomy catheter placed in the mid LAD. Left ventricular angiogram demonstrated extensive dyskinesia involving the whole of the anterior wall wrapping around the apex, with an ejection fraction (EF) of < 35%, with a left ventricular end-diastolic pressure (LVEDP) of 22 mmHg at completion of procedure. His echocardiographic EF was 30%, ESVI 40 (11–31) mL/m^2, SVI 23 (33–47) mL/m^{2}and VAC 1.73 (0.6–1.0). His collapse-to-reperfusion time was 95 min which explained the normalisation of his left ventricular function within 6 weeks, on an echocardiogram that showed no wall motion abnormality—EF 51%, ESVI 24 (11–31) mL/m^2, SVI 30 (33–47) mL/m^{2}and VAC 0.82 (06–1.0). (**Bottom left to right panels**) One year later he was readmitted for a coronary restudy. The LAD stent is widely patent, and there is myocardial bridging (MB) in mid LAD preceded by a significant distal stent in-segment restenosis (*compare the LAD between systole and diastole*). Intravascular ultrasound (IVUS) demonstrates post-stent edge atheroma (*arrow*), with the pathognomonic echolucent half-moon or halo sign (*arrow*) of MB with evident systolic coronary compression. The fractional flow reserve (FFR) across the lesion is 0.80 with intracoronary adenosine 200 μg, thus the *de novo* disease is balloon-dilated and treated with a drug-coated balloon (DCB). He has remained symptom-free 15 months after his procedure

arteries, in particular LAD, fill during diastole, and the diastolic pressure gradient mapped out continuously as AUC between LAD-LV and Aorta-LV captures the full driving force for the whole diastole. Escaned et al. [47] in 2003 applied a simplified dFFR ≤ 0.76 (without LV pressure) to 12 patients with 50% systolic compression MB, out of which 9 had functional cardiac ischaemia, given dobutamine (max at 20 μg/kg/min) with 20 μg adenosine bolus.

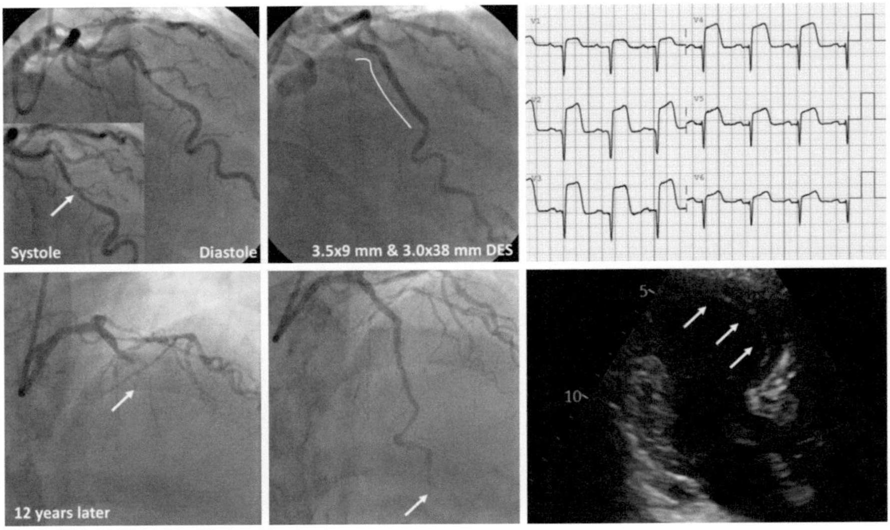

Fig. 6.7 Stenting the myocardial bridge. A 63-year-old man with diabetes was admitted 12 years ago to a local hospital with an acute coronary syndrome. His intial coronary angiogram there showed an occluded mid-right coronary artery (RCA) that was collateralised, and a long segment of left anterior descending (LAD) artery disease. He was transferred to a tertiary cardiac unit, where his RCA was recanalised and stented with a 3.0 × 38 mm drug-euting stent (DES), and the bystander LAD lesion was stented with two overlapping DES at the same sitting. (**Top left to right panels**) The mid LAD appeared "tethered" in systole (*inset*); it was stented as higlighted by the *white line*. He now presented with an anterolateral "tombsone" ST elevation myocardial infarction as shown on the electrocardiogram (ECG). (**Bottom left to right panels**) The coronary angiogram showed an occluded mid LAD with visible outline of stent struts in the occluded segment. Following balloon dilations, the flow down the artery was delayed (*arrow*) suggesting microvascular obstruction. His ECG continued to show Q and persistent ST elevation, echocardiogram in apical two-chamber view demonstrated aneurysmal and dyskinetic anterior wall. In addition, there was significant instent restenosis in the RCA which was treated separately on another day

$$\mathrm{dFFR} = \frac{\int_{\mathrm{diastole}} P_d(t)\,dt}{\int_{\mathrm{diastole}} P_a(t)\,dt}$$

Five out of the twelve developed chest pain during dobutamine infusion and only four reached the maximum dose, and MB dynamically worsened; $46.1 \pm 10.5 \rightarrow 68.7 \pm 17.9\%$ ($p < 0.0001$), and 5/12 had dFFR ≤ 0.76 vs 1/12 FFR ≤ 0.75, suggesting that dFFR unmasked more MB with flow limitation than conventional FFR. However, the sample size was too small to relate to functional ischaemia. This was taken forward by Aleksandic et al. [48] in 2021; they compared the utility of dobutamine dFFR (without adenosine) against adenosine FFR in 60 patients with symptomatic MB, and 19% or 32% had a positive exercise stress echocardiogram; dFFR had a positive predictive value (PPV) of 90% and a negative predictive value (NPV) of 98% with dobutamine while undifferentiated with adenosine. The optimal FFR ≤ 0.82 based on AUC during adenosine and dobutamine had PPV of 35.8 vs 47.6% and NPV of 71.3 vs 77% for predicting functional cardiac ischaemia. Further, FFR was observed to develop negative gradient during dobutamine when Pd > Pa with systolic overshoot. This study concluded that dobutamine was a better stressor in MB than adenosine and that FFR under-detected significant MB. Non-hyperaemic pressure ratios have been proposed as being useful in MB, but validated data are still lacking [49].

Continuous thermodilution can measure actual flow during dobutamine which may help in cases which are not clear-cut, as in case 4; the flow response was flat and the patient developed chest pain and ST depression when atropine was added to dobutamine infusion. There is a potential that this could become the new gold standard, since the basis of cardiac ischaemia is based on the definition of CFR < 2, as used by Abe et al. when they introduced dFFR ≤ 0.76 25 years ago, which appears to have been adopted at least in research but not widely used in clinical practice [46].

References

1. Heberden W. Some account of a disorder of the breast. In: Medical transactions, vol. 2. London: RCP; 1772. p. 59–67. https://archive.org/details/b24976957_0002/page/58/mode/2up.
2. Heberden W. A letter to Dr Heberden, concerning the angina pectoris; and Dr Heberden's account of the dissection of one, who had been troubled with that disorder. In: Medical Transactions, vol. 3. London: RCP; 1785. p. 1–11. https://archive.org/details/b24976957_0003/page/n21/mode/2up.
3. Reyman HC. Dissertatio de vasis cordis propriis. Bibl Anat. 1737;2:359–78.
4. Teofilovski-Parapid G, Jankovic R, Kanjuh V, et al. Myocardial bridges, neither rare nor isolated-autopsy study. Ann Anat. 2017;210:25–31. https://doi.org/10.1016/j.aanat.2016.09.007.
5. Mishra A, Jafri S, Mateen S, Jabeen F, Wani I. Myocardial bridging in patients undergoing coronary angiography for coronary artery disease. Cureus. 2024;16(5):e60087. https://doi.org/10.7759/cureus.60087.
6. Haller Av. § XXXII. Arteria coronaria dextra (inferior). In: Elementa Physiologiae Corporis Humani Tomus Primus. 1. Lausannae: Sumptibus Marci-Michaelis Bousquet & Sociorum; 1757. p. 371–4.
7. Haller Av. § XXXIII. Arteria coronaria sinistra (superior). In: Elementa Physiologiae Corporis Humani Tomus Primus. 1. Lausannae: Sumptibus Marci-Michaelis Bousquet & Sociorum; 1757. p. 375–7.
8. Christodoulou KC, Stakos D, Androutsopoulou V, et al. Vieussens' arterial ring: historical background, medical review and novel anatomical classification. Cureus. 2023;15(6):e40960. https://doi.org/10.7759/cureus.40960.
9. Doğan N, Dursun A, Özkan H. Vieussens' arterial ring: a rare coronary variant anatomy. Diagn Interv Radiol. 2019;25(2):109–13. https://doi.org/10.5152/dir.2019.17449.
10. Tsiamis E, Lazaros G, Patialiakas A, Maragiannis D, Stefanadis C. Imaging the periphery of an occluded left anterior descending coronary artery: need for selective conus artery catheterisation. Hell J Cardiol. 2008;49:357–9.
11. Varlamos C, Xenogiannis I, Mademli M, Kollias V, Rallidis L. Left main coronary artery atresia: an extremely rare albeit lethal congenital coronary anomaly. Coron Artery Dis. 2025. https://doi.org/10.1097/MCA.0000000000001518.
12. Wang J, Hu P, Yan H, Yuan H, Ma X-J. Visualising rare coronary anatomy: critical insights from multimodal imaging in RCA atresia. Acta Cardiol. 2025;80(2):195–7. https://doi.org/10.1080/00015385.2025.2450955.

13. Kugel MA. Anatomical studies on the coronary arteries and their branches: I. Arteria anastomotica auricularis magna. Am Heart J. 1928;3(3):260–70. https://doi.org/10.1016/S0002-8703(28)90324-5.
14. Angelini P. Kugel's artery: what's in a name? Questions on atrial circulation. Tex Heart Inst J. 2004;31(3):271–2.
15. Nerantzis CE, Marianou SK, Koulouris SN, et al. Kugel's artery: an anatomical and angiographic study using a new technique. Tex Heart Inst J. 2004;31(3):267–70.
16. Angelini P, Uribe C, Raghuram A. Coronary myocardial bridge updates: anatomy, pathophysiology, clinical manifestations, diagnosis, and treatment options. Tex Heart Inst J. 2025;52(1). https://doi.org/10.14503/thij-23-8300.
17. Schütze J, Stark AW, Bigler MR, Räber L, Gräni C. Misconception of 'malignant' and 'scissor-like compression' of interarterial course in anomalous aortic origin of a coronary artery: a case series. Eur Heart J Case Rep. 2024;8(8). https://doi.org/10.1093/ehjcr/ytae380.
18. Lim PO. Paolo Angelini's legacy in the study of and treatment for anomalous coronary arteries. Tex Heart Inst J. 2023;50(6). https://doi.org/10.14503/thij-23-8351.
19. Lim PO. Is it a steal or a squeeze? Hell J Cardiol. 2024;78:93–4. https://doi.org/10.1016/j.hjc.2024.03.007.
20. Lim PO. Fooled by a folded coronary artery? Cardiol Young. 2024;34(2):465–6. https://doi.org/10.1017/S1047951124000064.
21. Geiringer E. The mural coronary. Am Heart J. 1951;41(3):359–68. https://doi.org/10.1016/0002-8703(51)90036-1.
22. Mabudian L, Jordan JH, Bottinor W, Hundley WG. Cardiac MRI assessment of anthracycline-induced cardiotoxicity. Front Cardiovasc Med. 2022;9. https://doi.org/10.3389/fcvm.2022.903719.
23. Sharifkazemi M, Elahi M, Sayad M. Case report: early acute myocarditis after radiation therapy for breast cancer: a case presentation and review of literature. Front Cardiovasc Med. 2023;10. https://doi.org/10.3389/fcvm.2023.1020082.
24. Spiegl F. Obituary: Dr Erich Geiringer. The Independent. 1995, September 8, Friday.
25. Geiringer E. Intimal vascularization and atherosclerosis. J Pathol Bacteriol. 1951;63(2):201–11. https://doi.org/10.1002/path.1700630204.
26. Chase RE, de Garis CF. Arteriae coronariae (cordis) in the higher primates. Am J Phys Anthropol. 1939;24(3):427–48. https://doi.org/10.1002/ajpa.1330240323.
27. Risse M, Weiler G. Coronary muscle bridge and its relations to local coronary sclerosis, regional myocardial ischemia and coronary spasm. A morphometric study. Z Kardiol. 1985;74(12):700–5.
28. Wu X, Wu M, Huang H, et al. Impact of myocardial bridge on lesion morphology and clinical outcomes in patients undergoing IVUS-guided PCI for LAD CTO. Front Cardiovascu Med. 2025;12. https://doi.org/10.3389/fcvm.2025.1648233.
29. Calais F, Lagerqvist B, Leppert J, James SK, Fröbert O. Proximal coronary artery intervention: stent thrombosis, restenosis and death. Int J Cardiol. 2013;170(2):227–32. https://doi.org/10.1016/j.ijcard.2013.10.060.
30. Kong MG, Han J-K, Kang J, et al. Clinical outcomes of long stenting in the drug-eluting stent era: patient-level pooled analysis from the GRAND-DES registry. EuroIntervention. 2021;16(16):1318–25. https://doi.org/10.4244/eij-d-19-00296.
31. Gitto M, Sticchi A, Chiarito M, et al. Drug-coated balloon angioplasty for de novo lesions on the left anterior descending artery. Circ Cardiovasc Interv. 2023;16(12):e013232. https://doi.org/10.1161/CIRCINTERVENTIONS.123.013232.
32. Leone PP, Gitto M, Gao C, et al. Rethinking coronary artery metal implants. Prog Cardiovasc Dis. 2025. https://doi.org/10.1016/j.pcad.2025.07.005.
33. Lim PO. Grüntzig's technique, relearnt. Br J Cardiol. 2024;31:123–5. https://doi.org/10.5837/bjc.2024.042.
34. Lim PO. Gruntzig's coronary angioplasty, revisited, modified and improved. Acta Cardiol. 2024;79(7):852–3. https://doi.org/10.1080/00015385.2024.2391140.

35. Landrum EB, Schussler JM. Recurrent stent fracture due to myocardial bridging: a brief report and review of published cases. Am J Cardiol. 2023;200:75–7. https://doi.org/10.1016/j.amjcard.2023.05.016.
36. Tsujita K, Maehara A, Mintz GS, et al. Impact of myocardial bridge on clinical outcome after coronary stent placement. Am J Cardiol. 2009;103(10):1344–8. https://doi.org/10.1016/j.amjcard.2009.01.340.
37. Wu X, Wu M, Huang H, et al. Efficacy and safety of drug-coated balloon angioplasty in proximal LAD stenosis with distal myocardial bridge: a 12-month comparative study with drug-eluting stents. Front Cardiovasc Med. 2025;12. https://doi.org/10.3389/fcvm.2025.1648215.
38. 2018 ESC/EACTS guidelines on myocardial revascularization. EuroIntervention. 2019;14(14):1435–534. https://doi.org/10.4244/eijy19m01_01.
39. Bastiany A, Boivin-Proulx L-A, Allan TE, et al. Interplay between myocardial bridging, atherosclerosis, and spasm in patients with nonobstructive coronary arteries. J Soc Cardiovasc Angiogr Interventions. 2025;4(6). https://doi.org/10.1016/j.jscai.2025.103606.
40. Toya T. Coronary endothelial dysfunction and vasomotor dysregulation in myocardial bridging. J Cardiovasc Dev Dis. 2025;12(2):54. https://www.mdpi.com/2308-3425/12/2/54
41. Toya T, Naito K, Urushima T, et al. Myocardial bridging with left ventricular hypertrophy. JACC Case Rep. 2025;30(19):104047. https://doi.org/10.1016/j.jaccas.2025.104047.
42. Toya T, Yoshida S, Kuinose K, et al. Association between peripheral and coronary microvascular function and the impact of myocardial bridging. Physiol Rep. 2025;13(8):e70340. https://doi.org/10.14814/phy2.70340.
43. Rovera C, Moretti C, Bisanti F, De Zan G, Guglielmo M. Myocardial bridging: review on the role of coronary computed tomography angiography. J Clin Med. 2023;12(18):5949. https://www.mdpi.com/2077-0383/12/18/5949
44. Yu Y, Yu L, Dai X, Zhang J. CT fractional flow reserve for the diagnosis of myocardial bridging-related ischemia: a study using dynamic CT myocardial perfusion imaging as a reference standard. Korean J Radiol. 2021;22(12):1964–73. https://doi.org/10.3348/kjr.2021.0043.
45. Zhang M, Xu X, Wu Q, et al. Surgical strategies and outcomes for myocardial bridges coexisting with other cardiac conditions. Eur J Med Res. 2023;28(1):488. https://doi.org/10.1186/s40001-023-01478-9.
46. Abe M, Tomiyama H, Yoshida H, Doba N. Diastolic fractional flow reserve to assess the functional severity of moderate coronary artery stenoses: comparison with fractional flow reserve and coronary flow velocity reserve. Circulation. 2000;102(19):2365–70. https://doi.org/10.1161/01.cir.102.19.2365.
47. Escaned J, Cortés J, Flores A, et al. Importance of diastolic fractional flow reserve and dobutamine challenge in physiologic assessment of myocardial bridging. J Am Coll Cardiol. 2003;42(2):226–33. https://doi.org/10.1016/s0735-1097(03)00588-6.
48. Aleksandric SB, Djordjevic-Dikic AD, Dobric MR, et al. Functional assessment of myocardial bridging with conventional and diastolic fractional flow reserve: vasodilator versus inotropic provocation. J Am Heart Assoc. 2021;10(13):e020597. https://doi.org/10.1161/JAHA.120.020597.
49. Sternheim D, Power DA, Samtani R, et al. Myocardial bridging: diagnosis, functional assessment, and management. JACC. 2021;78(22):2196–212. https://doi.org/10.1016/j.jacc.2021.09.859.

Chapter 7
Arrested Heart

Abstract Up to half of those who suffered a myocardial infarction do not reach hospitals because of an early cardiac arrest due to ventricular fibrillation (VF). Survivors who had a coronary angiogram include a group of young men with history of smoking with patent coronary arteries. They exhibit generalised endothelial dysfunction, in response to acetylcholine; they develop epicardial vasospasm with failure of coronary flow to increase by 50% from baseline, despite preserved vasodilatory capacity to adenosine hyperaemia. This chapter presents detailed coronary physiology study of four VF cases, one woman from coronary artery thrombotic occlusion and three men with coronary artery spasm, one due to thyrotoxicosis, who had acetylcholine challenge at index admission and following treatment 1 year later. In this case, there was a biphasic, initial vasoconstrictive and blunted flow response to low-dose acetylcholine, followed by profound vasodilatation with tripling of flow rate that was slow with high-dose acetylcholine. This speculatively could be due to shifting of suppressed endothelial muscarinic nitric oxide pathway, through the same M_3 receptor to endothelial-derived hyperpolarising factor (EDHF) via Ca^{2+}-activated K^+ channel-mediated hyperpolarisation of the vascular smooth muscle cells (VSMC) across the myoendothelial gap junctions. This natural and endogenous calcium channel blockade if augmented could explain why calcium channel blockers might have less added value in some patients with coronary microvascular dysfunction, and this could potentially be tested if intracoronary verapamil's flow response is blunted with continuous thermodilution. Finally, the last two patients who had VF coincidentally shared a syndromic triad of left ventricular mid-wall fibrosis, benign early repolarisation and right coronary artery spasm, which surprisingly are pathophysiologically coherent.

7.1 Introduction

It used to be believed that selective coronary angiography would cause ventricular fibrillation (VF) which was invariably fatal, when open-chest cardiac massage was futile. That was before the invention of the direct current (DC) defibrillator. Paul

P. O. Lim, *Coronary Thermodilution*,
https://doi.org/10.1007/978-3-032-10734-3_7

H. Wood (1907–1962), whose name has become a measure of vascular resistance, as per Ohm's hydraulic analogue, pressure gradient (mmHg) = flow (L/min) × resistance (mmHg·min/L or Wood unit), was a heavy smoker and suffered an anterior myocardial infarction (MI) due to occlusion of his left anterior descending (LAD) artery at 54. He treated himself with heparin, which was forward thinking at the time during the debate whether MI was thrombotic in origin [1]. He instructed his colleagues on 13 July 1962 not to resuscitate him in the event of cardiac arrest. He did so and they respected his wish later on the day [2]. That was also the year DC defibrillator became available in the USA.

Remarkably, in the early days of non-selective coronary angiography, to avoid VF, asystolic cardiac arrest lasting 4–12 s was induced under general anaesthesia with rapid intravenous acetylcholine (ACh) 150–300 mg diluted in 5 mL saline, followed by 10 mL of saline flush and 50 mL tri-iodide contrast delivered via direct puncture of the aortic arch under the left clavicle, with a blunt needle advanced to and placed close to the coronary ostiae in July 1957 in humans—this ACh and contrast cycle could be repeated three times for cine-radiography [3, 4]. This pioneering and daring technique was developed by Georges Arnulf (1904–1994) in Lyon, France, and in one of 26 patients who had the procedure, a 59-year-old-woman developed coronary artery spasm with accompanying ECG changes, which resolved with papaverine and nicotinic acid. Thus, *the first coronary artery spasm captured on film, recognised and treated with vasodilators* in history, and Arnulf also documented pre-existing coronary artery occlusion and collaterals. He observed that in dogs, stimulation or resection of the autonomic nervous ganglia and plexus increased the calibre of the coronary artery.

It was the accidental right coronary artery (RCA) cannulation of a 26-year-old-man with rheumatic heart disease by F. Mason Sones (1918–1985) at the Cleveland Clinic, Ohio on 30 October 1958, incidentally the man went into asystole, and not VF, that launched selective coronary angiography [5]. Twenty-nine years prior in 1929, Werner Forssmann (1904–1979) at 25 and a first year surgical resident, having experimented on cadavers, then himself on 2 occasions at Auguste-Viktoria Hospital [6] in Eberswalde, near Berlin, where Richard Schneider was Chief of Surgery. There are conflicting accounts of the events, even by Forssmann, including one by his daughter, Renate [6–9]. The first attempt was aborted because his co-worker, Peter Romeis who helped him with venous access, was fearful of killing him. On his second attempt a week later, he convinced Gerda Ditzen, a scrub nurse into supplying him with sterile materials and he threaded 65 cm of a lubricated 4 French urinary catheter made of vulcanised rubber, up his left antecubital cephalic vein. He next walked down the corridor and descended with Ditzen to the basement where the X-ray department was, and the radiology nurse Eva Griessbach received him [10]. Under fluoroscopy reflected via a mirror held up by Griessbach, he repositioned the catheter tip from his axillary vein in the shoulder into his right atrium and had a chest X-ray taken despite Romeis's protestations as he burst into the room [6, 7, 9]. He further described in his seminal paper, with Schneider's permission that he inserted a catheter up the right arm into the inferior vena cava of a dying woman with septic shock, the exact diagnosis was controversial [7–9], but likely to have been infection after abortion or childbirth, since these women were ready experimental subjects in those days. He infused mixtures of glucose, adrenaline and digitalis and made some observations. He performed the autopsy 6.5 hr later and noted where the catheter tip was and that there were no vessel wall injuries or thromboses around the catheter [8]. Therefore, proving that a "central venous line" could be inserted blind, i.e. the catheter found its own way, counterflow to venous valves and avoiding side branches due to retroflex bifurcations. For his infamy, insubordination and lack of discipline, he was unable to complete his academic training in Berlin and turned to urology.

Forssmann was awarded the Nobel Prize in Physiology or Medicine 27 years later in 1956 [11]. This recognition that it was safe to instrument the heart undoubtedly inspired Sones, Jr., who had his own discovery that it was also safe to inject contrast down the coronary artery 2 years later in 1958. He published his 1000 patients' experience in 1966, which incidentally included his own mother [12]. However, he did not describe any complications although the VF rate at the time was about 1.1% [13], but ten times less in current practice [14]. In retrospect, it was fortunate that Forssmann ignored Schneider's admonishment. He later found out that the rabbit's heart went into VF when probed, and had he known this, he would have never self-experimented, thus denying us this tale of rebellion to ebullient general acceptance [10].

This chapter describes four patients who survived VF and underwent a detailed coronary physiology study.

7.2 Cases

7.2.1 Arrested Twice

A 60-year-old Caucasian woman, who was a smoker, otherwise well, developed chest pain in bed as she was about to fall asleep. She dialled 999 for emergency service after the pain persisted for 90 min. When the ambulance crew arrived 90 min later, she promptly went into VF. She was shocked out of it and taken to the heart attack centre at St George's Hospital. While in the coronary care unit awaiting the assembly of the primary coronary angioplasty team, she had another episode of VF, requiring a direct current (DC) cardioversion. Her electrocardiogram (ECG) showed hyperacute ST elevation in the anteroseptal precordial leads which corresponded to an occluded left anterior descending (LAD) artery (Fig. 7.1). The LAD was thrombectomised and clots were extracted. The flow down the LAD was restored, uncovering a long segment of non-occlusive atherosclerotic disease; this was left to be medically treated. The "door to open artery" was 57 min and call to hospital's door was 101 min—thus a total ischaemic time of just over 4 hr by 8 min. Nevertheless, the left ventricle was acutely impaired, with an ejection fraction (EF) of about 35% and a left ventricular (LV) end-diastolic filling pressure (LVEDP) of 22 (< 12) mmHg post-procedure. At 8 hr, the troponin T was 754 (< 14) ng/L, creatine kinase 625 (<200) U/L and NT-ProBNP 88 (<125) ng/L—these are modest values. Her left ventricular function rapidly improved, and her bedside echocardiogram performed

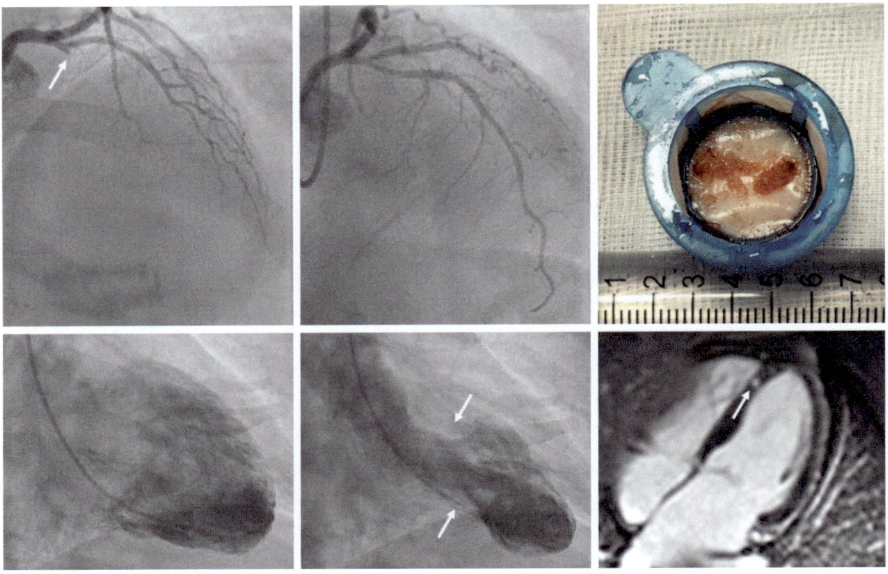

Fig. 7.1 (**Top, left to right panels**) The arrow points to the stump in the left anterior descending (LAD) artery, right after the high diagonal branch. Recanalised LAD and extracted clots—one piece measured 2.5 × 5.0 mm. (**Bottom, left to right panels**) Left ventricular angiogram in diastole and systole, demonstrating contractility mainly in the left ventricular bases. The cardiovascular magnetic resonance (CMR) scan reveals a normal heart with limited late gadolinium enhancement

at about the same time showed an EF of 55%, with hypokinesia in the LAD territory. The left atrium was not dilated, neither was there left ventricular hypertrophy, using her body mass index (BMI) of 30 kg/m^2 for calculations: end-systolic volume index, ESVI 16 (10–38) mL/m^2, stroke volume index, SVI 19 (30–56) mL/m^2 and ventriculo-arterial coupling, VAC 1.2 (0.6–1.0)—consistent with impaired contractility. She was discharged on day 3 and maintained on aspirin 75 mg od, ticagrelor 90 mg bd, lansoprazole 30 mg od, atorvastatin 80 mg od, ramipril 1.25 mg od, nebivolol 1.25 mg od and colchicine 0.5 mg od.

When assessed in the outpatient clinic 2 months later, she had no angina but was noticeably breathless with her day-to-day activities, such as climbing the stairs. Her cardiovascular magnetic resonance (CMR) scan at 10 weeks showed a normalised heart (Fig. 7.1), EF 68%, ESVI 18 (11–35) mL/m^2, SVI 38 mL/m^2 and VAC 0.5 (0.6–1.0), with scattered infarction in the LAD subtended myocardium, without inducible perfusion defects with adenosine stress.

Procedure Four months following her ST elevation myocardial infarction she is admitted to reassess her LAD and also for a formal coronary physiology to determine the cause of her exercise intolerance. She has stopped smoking and her BMI is now under 30, at 28 kg/m^2. Her LV is studied; the contractility is normal, but the LVEDP is elevated at about 20 mmHg, not rising with handgrip, and without central aortic hypertension, at 110/60 mmHg (Fig. 7.2). Her coronary arteries have not

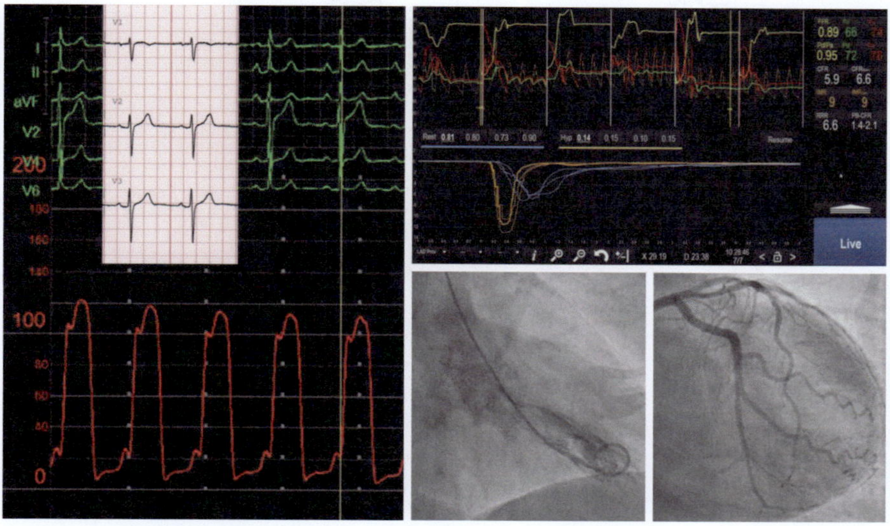

Fig. 7.2 (**Left, top to bottom panels**) Normalised electrocardiogram without evidence of Q in the anteroseptal precordial leads, but elevated left ventricular end-diastolic pressure as indicated by the *vertical yellow line* > 20 mmHg. (**Right, top to bottom panels**) Bolus thermodilution in the infarct-related left anterior descending (LAD) artery—with normal "microvascular function". Left ventricular angiogram in systole demonstrating normal systolic contraction and left coronary artery without occlusive disease

changed, and the LAD lesion remains the same. Continuous thermodilution is undertaken to the circumflex (Cx) artery with the following results at baseline and during hyperaemia: flow 39 and 97 mL/min and resistance 2132 and 866 Wood units, respectively—coronary flow reserve, CFR 2.5 and microvascular resistance reserve, MRR 2.5—low flow state with elevated resistance. The pressure wire is redirected down the LAD. The baseline distal-to-aorta pressure ratio, Pd/Pa is 0.94 and resting full-cycle ratio, RFR 0.93 (>0.89). Bolus thermodilution is performed with intracoronary adenosine bolus of 200 μg—giving a fractional flow reserve, FFR of 0.89 (> 0.80), CFR 5.9 (≥ 2.5), index of microvascular resistance, IMR 9 (< 25) and MRR 7.2—these are *barn-door* normal values. To confirm these results, continuous thermodilution is next undertaken—to obtain consistent values, as is the usual practice, duplicates are carried out, initially with hyperaemic saline infusion via the RayFlow microcatheter at 20 mL/min. However, there is a drift in the numbers, during the third study, the Pd/Pa widens, with electrographic ST depression, but without chest pain (Fig. 7.3). A coronary angiogram is taken which shows severe vasospasm where the LAD lesion is; this is relieved by intracoronary nitroglycerine and **removal of the RayFlow microcatheter.** To understand if the LAD is inherently vasoreactive, escalating doses of acetylcholine (ACh) is given with the pressure wire in situ. There is a dose-dependent fall in Pd/Pa, only with the highest dose ACh 200 μg does the Pd/Pa become borderline significant.

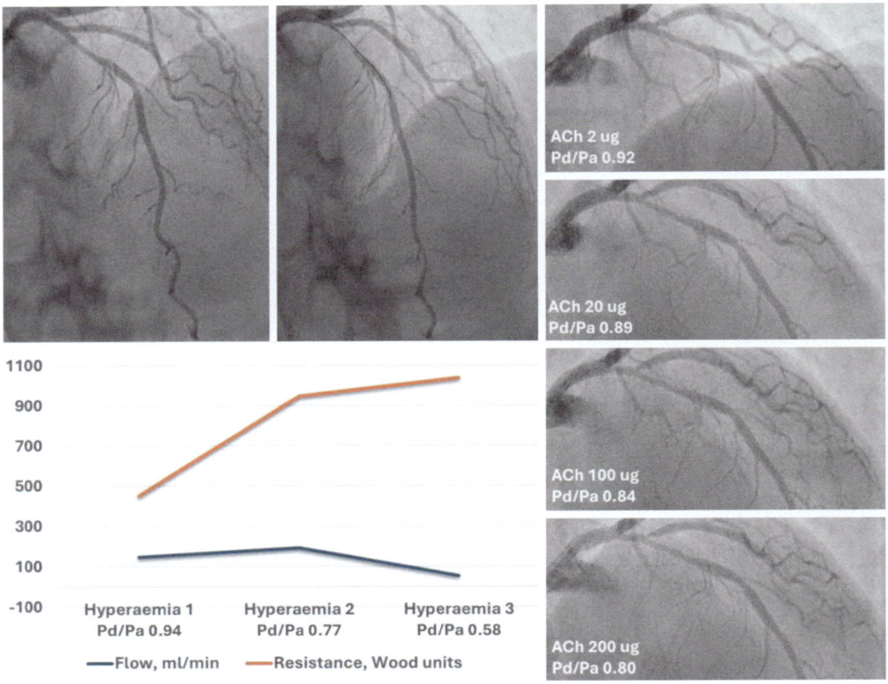

Fig. 7.3 (**Left, top to bottom panels**) The left anterior descending (LAD) artery with an eccentric moderate long segment of disease immediately after the early and high diagonal branch. In the effort to obtain reproducible readings, the hyperaemic saline infusion is repeated 3 times. And this is associated with worsening coronary haemodynamics, culminating with ischaemic electrocardiographic changes—the Pd/Pa falls with the flow and a paradoxical rise in resistance—the respective flow and resistance are 147 mL/min and 451 Wood units, 192 mL/min and 947 Wood units, and 53 mL/min and 1037 Wood units—the worsening LAD spasm is precipitated by the RayFlow saline jets. (**Right, top to bottom panels**) Acetylcholine provocation and LAD vasospasm

Interpretation This postmenopausal woman thrombotically occluded her LAD which precipitated two VF cardiac arrests, on a background of moderate atherosclerotic disease in the LAD, likely to be related to smoking, although she has moderate hyperlipidaemia, pre-treatment—LDL cholesterol 3.75 (< 2) mmol/L and total cholesterol 6.8 (< 4) mmol/L. She was rapidly revascularised at roughly 4 hr from symptomatic onset, which explains her *apparent* normalisation of ECG and cardiac function on CMR. Despite this, she continues to be breathless. She has non-obstructive coronary arteries, normal left ventricular systolic function, normotension but clearly raised LVEDP, consistent with her contemporaneously increased NT-ProBNP 133 (< 125) ng/L. While the coronary haemodynamics in the Cx are consistent and are expected with continuous thermodilution, the bolus thermodilution in the LAD returns obviously normal results. While with continuous thermodilution, the first hyperaemic minimal resistance of 451 Wood units is marginally raised and could roughly be converted with a factor of 20 to an IMR of 23 [15], and taking the maximal hyperaemic flow of 192 mL/min with the repeat study, the real CFR should be ≥ 2.0 if the basal flow is 60–90 mL/min.

Here lies the paradox, why should an area subjected to myocardial infarction with evidence of scars on CMR would have normal microvascular function as is currently defined, in contrast to the non-infarct Cx territory. The same phenomenon has been noted in the previous chapter; the coronary resistance in the infarct territory might not be raised. One possibility is that with subclinical but irreversible ischaemic damage to the interstitial tissues and capillaries, blood flow is diverted via "arteriovenous microchannels", reducing the coronary resistance. This potentially explains the *rise in microvascular resistance as the flow falls* with increasing LAD stenosis, unmasking a post-MI maladaptive microvasculature. The LAD vasospasm during continuous thermodilution is likely to be related to vessel wall stress from high rate of saline jets directed inadvertently to the atherosclerotic LAD; the proximal segment is too short to fully accommodate the saline jets away from the LAD lesion. This has previously been reported, as described in Chap. 1 [16, 17]. On the other hand, ACh although provokes epicardial vasospasm, this is non-occlusive, more an indication of *endothelial dysfunction*. In conclusion, this woman has post-infarct CMD (autoregulation failure) and heart failure with preserved ejection fraction (HFpEF, high LVEDP and raised NT-ProBNP). Her dose of nebivolol was doubled, and she was started on an SGLT2 inhibitor, dapagliflozin 10 mg od, to offload her LV.

7.2.2 Stormy Arrest

A 43-year-old Black man presented to the emergency department with neck pain which he had for a month. He was discharged with painkillers. Three months later, this time added with chest pain, nausea, breathlessness and sweating, he went back to the hospital late at night, at 8.00 pm. His vital signs were normal; he was given sublingual nitroglycerine which helped with the pain. His ECG showed sinus rhythm with tall QRS complexes and repolarisation abnormalities, mainly with inferolateral T inversion, but without overt ST depression or elevation. His troponins were mildly elevated at 33 and 54 (<14) ng/L. Eight hours later he had a witnessed VF arrest, requiring 4 DC cardioversions and 15 min of chest compressions. His immediate ECG showed lateral ST elevation and bedside echocardiogram revealed severe left ventricular systolic dysfunction.

The heart attack team assembled, and he had his diagnostic coronary angiogram a couple of hours later at 8.00 am. This demonstrated unobstructed coronary arteries, the proximal and mid LAD were irregular and appeared "beady", and LV angiogram found near normal contractility but a raised LVEDP to 20 mmHg (Fig. 7.4). His echocardiogram estimated his EF to be 40% without left atrial (LA) dilatation and borderline septal hypertrophy at 1.1 cm without left ventricular hypertrophy (LVH) with indexed LV mass at 76 (49–115) g/m^2, ESVI 40 (10–47) mL/m^2, SVI 25 (30–66) mL/m^2 and VAC 1.6 (0.6–1.0). His thyroid stimulating hormone (TSH) was undetectable, and free T4 was (9–25) 67 pmol/L. His thyroid ultrasound showed nodularity; thus he was diagnosed with thyroid storm due to Grave's thyrotoxicosis and started with propylthiouracil 200 mg tds, propranolol 40 mg tds and prednisolone 60 mg od. On day 6, he had his inpatient intravascular imaging to look for a

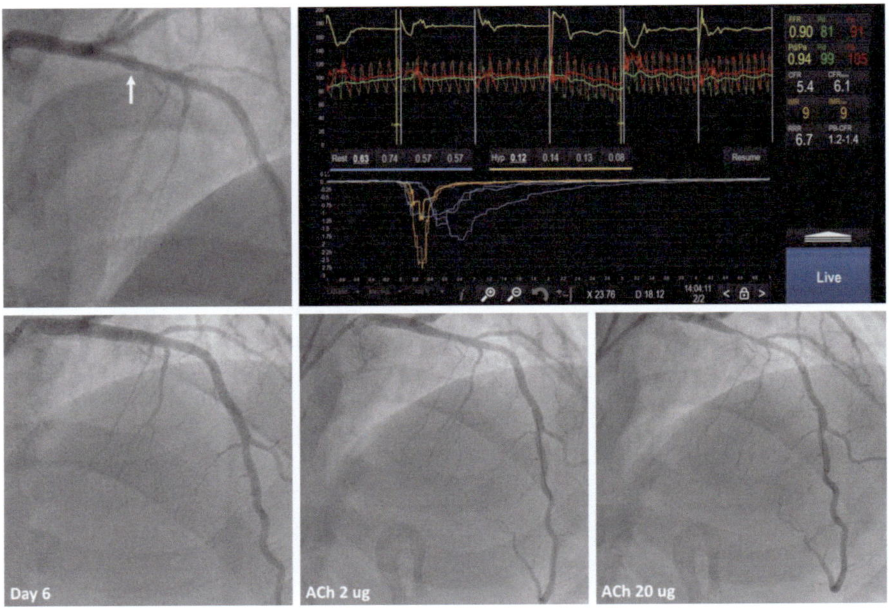

Fig. 7.4 (**Top, left to right panels**) Admission coronary angiogram following cardiac arrest shows patent coronary arteries; the proximal left anterior descending (LAD) artery appears irregular (*arrow*). On day 6, while he was still hyperthyroid, the LAD bolus thermodilution reveals normal microvascular function. (**Bottom, left to right**) On the other hand, low-dose acetylcholine (ACh) provokes a dose-dependent proximal LAD vasospasm

ruptured plaque and coronary physiology study; his free T4 had fallen to 38.2 (9–25) pmol/L.

Procedure 1 His LAD is widely patent, and the prior irregularities have disappeared. Optical coherence tomography (OCT) finds no endothelial disruption to suggest a plaque rupture, but intimal thickening in the mid LAD with a minimal luminal area (MLA) of 4.0 mm^2. Bolus thermodilution with IC adenosine 200 μg demonstrates normal haemodynamic indices—FFR 0.90, CFR 5.4, MRR 6.0 and IMR 9. He develops severe segmental proximal vasospasm LAD which resolves with IC GTN.

His CMR was undertaken on day 10—this showed a normalised heart, EF 59% with basal septal thickness of 1.1 cm, but without LVH or LA dilatation, ESVI 39 (17–38) mL/m^2, SVI 57 (42–66) mL/m^2 and VAC 0.7 (0.6–1.0). A surface automated implantable cardiac defibrillator (S-AICD) was implanted before he was discharged a week later. He was next assessed 3 months later in the outpatient clinic. A planned repeat coronary physiology study was performed when he was euthyroid, and this was *1 year* from his initial presentation. His thyroid function test was TSH < 0.02 (0.4–4.0) mU/L, Free T4 16.8 (9–25) pmol/L and T3 5.2 (1.5–3.9) pmol/L.

Procedure 2 His LV is studied first, the LVEDP is 10 mmHg, rising to 14 mmHg with handgrip; at the time his central aortic BP is 140/90 mmHg. The LAD is widely patent, as are the rest of his coronary arteries. With the pressure wire down the LAD, the Pd/Pa is 0.96 and RFR 0.95 (> 0.89). Bolus thermodilution is repeated 3 times, with the

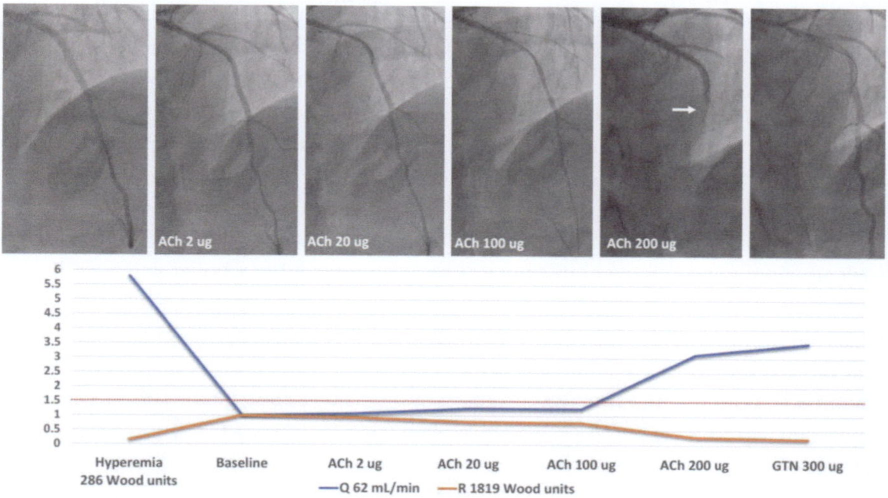

Fig. 7.5 (**Top, left to right panels**) Repeat coronary physiology study at 1 year later after his thyrotoxicosis is better treated, the left anterior descending (LAD) artery, unobstructed but escalating doses of acetylcholine (ACh) cause dose-dependent diffuse epicardial vasospasm for the first three doses. With ACh 200 μg, the LAD vasodilated with coronary slow flow phenomenon (CSFP), the arrow points to the contrast traversing the LAD at 3 heart beats; by the time the injected contrast reaches the distal vessels, it clears proximally. Curiously, CSFP is not seen with GTN at the same flow rate. (**Bottom**) Haemodynamic chart of the indices at baseline, with saline hyperaemia and in response to ACh. Both the vasodilatory capacity and microvascular resistance are normal. However, ACh flow response is blunted < 1.5, with low to medium doses, and with ACh 200 μg, the flow increases 3.1-fold, as it does with nitroglycerine, in which flow rises 3.5-fold—minus the CSFP

following values: CFR 4.1, 4.6, and 4.1; IMR 27, 24 and 23; and MRR 4.6, 5.4 and 4.4 with IC adenosine 200 μg boluses. Continuous thermodilution is next undertaken with the following basal and hyperaemic indices; flow 62 and 360 mL/min, and resistance 1819 and 286 Wood units—CFR 5.8 and MRR 6.4 (Fig. 7.5). Escalating doses of ACh are given. This time, instead of low-dose ACh inducing segmental proximal LAD vasospasm, he develops dose-dependent diffuse LAD vasospasm, the flow does not diminish, nor does it rise beyond 1.5-fold with the first three doses of 2, 20 and 100 μg—flow increases by a factor 1.08, 1.26 and 1.26 from baseline respectively, and without significant fall in Pd/Pa of 0.95, 0.94, and 0.91. Interestingly, *ACh 200 μg is associated with LAD vasodilatation and marked coronary slow flow phenomenon (CSFP), yet flow triples with a Pd/Pa of 0.95 and resistance falls by 72%.* He is asymptomatic throughout the study, without significant ECG changes.

Interpretation This man who has untreated hypertension with basal septal LVH, had thyroid overactivity related epicardial vasospasm causing VF. The fact that his cardiac enzymes were low pointed to a non-thrombotic event. His LV systolic dysfunction with a VAC of 1.6 rapidly improved, and normalised on CMR 10 days later. There was a parallel with stress cardiomyopathy, but without the ECG or the apical ballooning to go with it. There was lateral ST elevation post-resuscitation. His first coronary physiology study, albeit with reduced free T4, he exhibited ACh-induced segmental proximal LAD vasospasm, coupled with the beady appearance there seen on his emergency coronary angiogram, there was circumstantial proof that the aetiology of his presentation being epicardial vasospasm despite normal microvascular function on bolus thermodilution. It is known that thyrotoxic coronary endothelial dysfunction is an oxidative-stress–mediated loss of NO bioavailability through multiple pathways [18].

When he was clinically euthyroid with normal free T4 level, his repeat study instead found, again normal microvascular function on both bolus and continuous thermodilution. However, ACh challenge demonstrates both epicardial and microvascular endothelial dysfunction—diffuse epicardial vasospasm and coronary flow that fails to rise by 50% in the absence of epicardial flow limitation since his Pd/Pa stayed > 0.9. Interesting, the top dose ACh at 200 μg is associated with paradoxical epicardial vasodilatation and tripling of flow, this time with CSFPg. Remarkably, GTN has the same vasodilatation and flow response, but minus the CSFP.

Speculatively, at high ACh concentrations with NO synthesis inhibited, the biphasic vasodilatation shifts predominantly to an endothelium-derived hyperpolarising mechanism across myoendothelial gap junctions. ACh binds to endothelial M_3 receptors, triggering phospholipase C to generate IP_3 (inositol 1,4,5-trisphosphate), which releases Ca^{2+} from the endoplasmic reticulum and opens endothelial Ca^{2+}-activated K^+ channels, causing K^+ efflux. Through direct electrical coupling via gap junctions and the resulting rise in extracellular K^+, VSMC hyperpolarises with K^+ influx via inward-rectifier K^+ channels (Kir) and Na^+/K^+-ATPase–linked K^+ channels, which closes L-type Ca^{2+} channels, lowers VSMC $[Ca^{2+}]_i$, and induces relaxation—functionally akin to a calcium channel blocker [19–21] (Fig. 7.11). This would further support the "non-pharmacological" attenuation of ACh-induced vasodilatation with verapamil pre-treatment which directly blocks L-type Ca^{2+} channel in the VSMC, described as the Oldenburg Paradox in Chap. 1. This also offers an intriguing explanation why calcium channel blockers are not additive if natural calcium channel blockade is already augmented in the setting of endothelial dysfunction in some patients with coronary microvascular dysfunction.

7.2.3 Treadmill Emergency

A 61-year-old Caucasian man became breathless suddenly and collapsed at work. When the paramedics arrived, he was having effective chest compressions by work colleagues. He was found to be in VF, received 3 DC shocks, and was given 1 mg of adrenaline, before he returned to spontaneous circulation, within 20 min. His ECG showed aVR ST elevation with LBBB and widespread ST depression which settled into inferior ST depression with tall and peaked T-wave in the precordial V1-3, simulating de Winter sign, and his bedside echocardiogram found global LV hypokinesia. He was brought to the hospital intubated and ventilated for an emergency coronary angiogram. This found moderate disease in the mid-first diagonal branch and a tortuous mid LAD with an eccentric lesion, as well as in the mid RCA, but

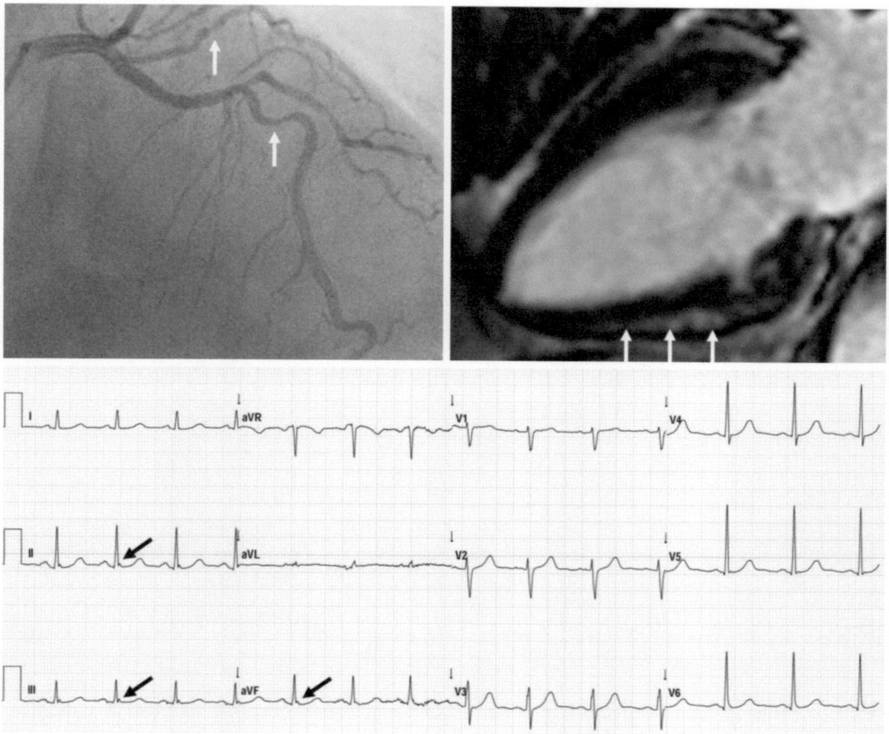

Fig. 7.6 (**Top, left to right panels**) Emergency coronary angiogram finds scattered atherosclerotic plaques, in the left anterior descending (LAD) artery, there is moderate disease in the first diagonal branch and in the tortuous mid LAD with an eccentric plaque (*arrows*). The cardiovascular magnetic resonance (CMR) scan shows inferior mid-wall fibrosis (*arrows*). (**Bottom**) A 12-lead electrocardiogram that shows a J-wave or benign early repolarisation (BER) as is pointed by the *arrows* in the inferior leads; at other times this just manifests at slurred downstroke of the QRS

with good flow throughout the vessels (Fig. 7.6). In the cardiothoracic intensive care unit (CTITU), his ECG settled, albeit with intermittent long QTc > 450 ms with a slurred QRS downstroke in the inferior limb leads as well as in precordial V4 which on occasions was visible a J-wave indicating "benign early repolarisation or BER". Although his cardiac function normalised rapidly within the next day on echocardiogram and his peak troponin T of 1252 (< 14)ng/L was modest, he needed prolonged CTITU care, partly because of his emphysema from a heavy and chronic smoking practice of 40 cigarettes per day since he was a teenager. He had Covid-19 infection 2 months prior, and suffered from sciatica, his work involved heavy lifting. On day 6 at 07:40 am he was noticed to have spontaneous inferoposterior ST elevation, associated with hypotension, and this was interpreted as he was prone to coronary vasospasm. Hence he was started on diltiazem. One day before he stepped down to the coronary care unit (CCU) after 1 month of stay in CTITU, he had his CMR. This showed an EF of 61%, undilated LA, no LVH, ESVI 24 (14–36) mL/m^2, SVI 38 (40–64) mL/m^2 and VAC 0.63 (0.6–1.0). Although there was no infarction, microvascular obstruction or oedema, there was inferobasal mid-wall late gadolinium

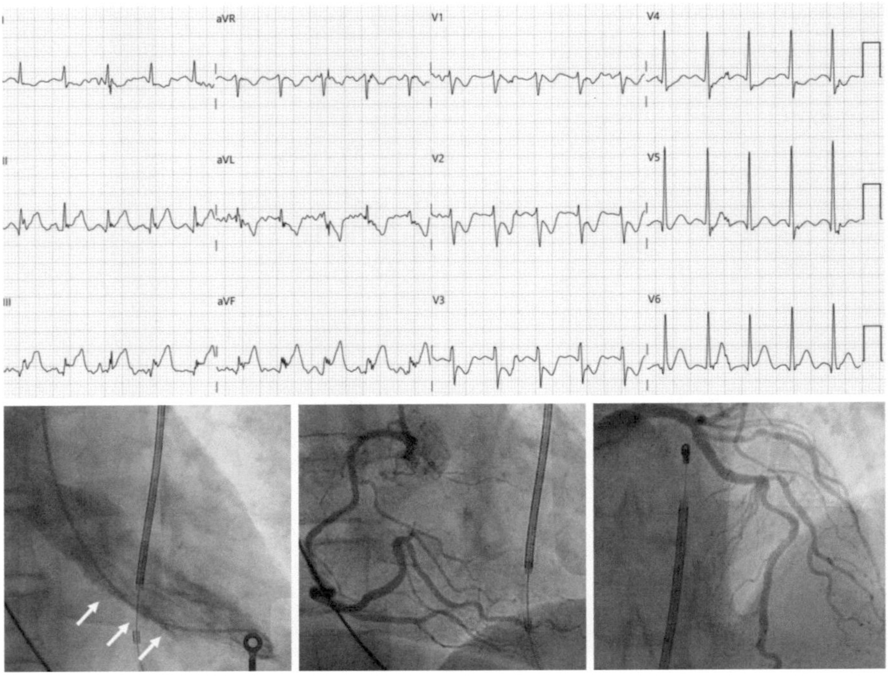

Fig. 7.7 (**Top**) 12-lead electrocardiogram that shows inferoposterolateral ST elevation with reciprocal ST depression more in aVL, more than in I—suggesting a tilt for basal inferior ischaemia. (**Bottom, left to right panels**) Repeat cardiac catheterisation during second hospital admission following the exercise tolerance test. Left ventricular (LV) angiogram depicts the LV in systole, note the hypokinetic basal inferior wall (*arrows*). Right coronary artery with moderate disease in mid vessel as is the case with the left anterior descending (LAD) artery. Note the surface automated implantable cardioverter-defibrillator (S-AICD) leads

enhancement. Following this on day 34 he had a surface automated implantable defibrillator (S-AICD) implanted before hospital discharge the next day.

When he came back for his exercise tolerance test on the treadmill 10 weeks following his VF arrest, as he was in stage 1 of Bruce protocol into 2 min and 15 s, at a heart rate of 120 bpm, he developed 2 mm inferoposterolateral ST elevation on ECG with chest pain and breathlessness, as was observed in the CTITU previously (Fig. 7.7). This was associated with intermittent alternate premature ventricular ectopics, which fortunately did not set off Torsades de Pointes (TdP). These lasted for 90 s. But the transient ST changes albeit at 1 mm recurred a minute later as his heart rate fell to 101 bpm. His pre-test heart rate was 94 bpm and BP 102/70 mmHg, and the corresponding figures were 98 and 108/68 at 7 min, at the end of the recovery period. It appeared that his ST elevation was triggered either in the morning as in CTITU during his first hospitalisation or during exercise, giving the possibility of these episodes being induced by a catecholamine surge. However, there was no evidence that he has elevated baseline catecholamines in the urine or plasma. But his 25-OH vitamin level was low at 18 (<50) ng/mL, and he had normal thyroid function. He was hospitalised again. Because of anaemia and melaena, he underwent sigmoidoscopy and was diagnosed with ulcerative colitis with systemic inflammation, raised CRP which did not completely settle; now he was treated with steroids and mesalazine. He also had influenza A. As was previously planned he underwent coronary spasm testing during this admission.

Procedure He has a BMI of 23 kg/m^2. His LV angiogram shows a subtle inferior wall hypokinesia with an LVEDP of 6 mmHg with a corresponding central aortic BP of 100/70 mmHg. The coronary artery anatomy has not changed and in view of his repeated RCA ECG changes, coronary physiology study is undertaken in that vessel. With the pressure wire in distal RCA, the Pd/Pa is 1.00 and RFR 0.97 (>0.89). Bolus thermodilution is undertaken with IC adenosine 200 μg with the following results: FFR 0.88, CFR 4.7, MRR 5.3 and IMR 23. With continuous thermodilution, the respective basal and hyperaemic indices—flow 47 and 135 mL/min and resistance 1843 Wood units and 396 Wood units—CFR 2.9, MRR 4.7 and calculated IMR 20 (Fig. 7.8). Acetylcholine (ACh) causes a dose-dependent segmental and diffuse

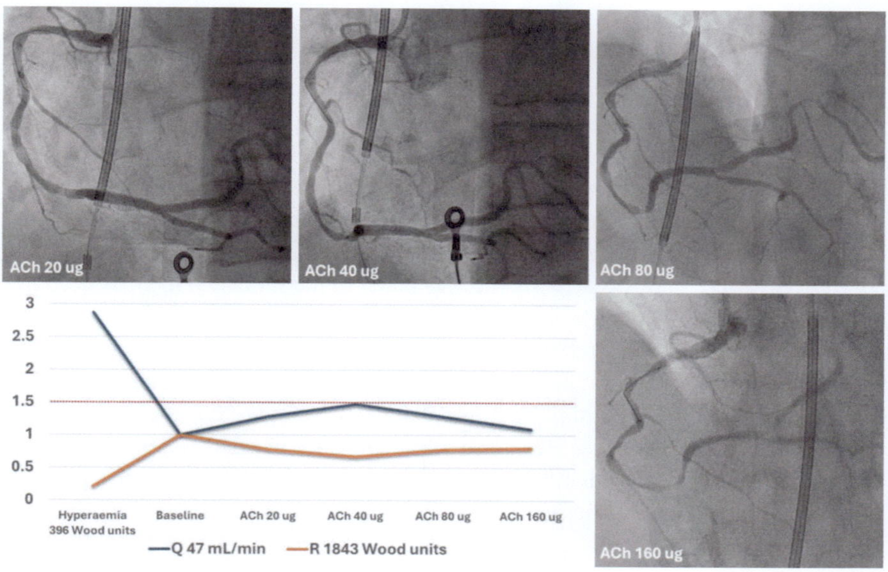

Fig. 7.8 (**Top, left to right panels and bottom, right panel**) The right coronary artery (RCA) with a dose-dependent segmental and diffuse vasospasm, with severe luminal constrictions with acetylcholine provocation. (**Bottom, left panel**) Haemodynamic indices in response to saline hyperaemia and to ACh. There is preserved microvascular vasodilatory capacity, in the setting of raised coronary resistance, relatively low basal flow for a large circulatory territory. Interestingly, flow remains above baseline and resistance starts to rise from ACh 80 μg. Since the flow does not rise by 50%, this indicates microvascular endothelial dysfunction, but the intact vasodilatory capacity allows some level of compensatory maintenance of flow despite increasing epicardial vasospasm induced by ACh. Respective flow increase with ACh 20, 40, and 160 μg is ↑Q 28, 47, 28 and 9%

epicardial vasospasm, with the last dose of ACh 160 μg, the Pd/Pa falls to 0.70, with chest pain and inferior ST depression, but without flow dipping below the baseline.

Interpretation This man has had repeated ST elevation, not quite "sharkfin as is associated with vasospasm" in RCA. In the setting of diffuse moderate coronary arteriosclerosis which he acquired from smoking-related endothelial dysfunction, that causes epicardial vasospasm, and in his case, also microvascular endothelial dysfunction, since his coronary flow does not rise > 50%, neither does it fall below the baseline, by courtesy of preserved vasodilatory capacity. There is, however, borderline increase in coronary resistance, more so at rest than during hyperaemia, which means he has high resting microvascular tone. The significance of BER in the inferior limb leads is unclear, whether it is due to myocardial fibrosis from past myocarditis, thus predisposing him to cardiac arrhythmias in the presence of myocardial ischaemia. The next question is the timing for these events. He was systemically "inflamed" from ulcerative colitis, recent Covid infection and influenza infection—a perfect storm for coronary vasoreactivity.

7.2.4 Emergency Frequenter

A 44-year-old Middle Eastern man collapsed while shopping. He received immediate bystander CPR and on arrival of London ambulance service's (LAS) crew, he was found to be in VF and was shocked 4 times, into return of spontaneous circulation (ROSC). He was intubated and ventilated at the scene and brought to the heart attack centre where he underwent his emergency cardiac catheterisation. His coronary arteries were unobstructed and he was taken to the CTITU. His bedside echocardiogram found global LV impairment with an EF of 20%. His ECG showed normal sinus rhythm with initial "peaked" T in V2-3. Two hours after admission to CTITU, he developed a short lasting "sharkfin" ST elevation in the inferoposterolateral leads which settled within 5 min into deep T wave in the corresponding leads, before normalising (Fig. 7.9). He had 2 further episodes over the next 24 hr, including one with a more traditional ST elevation in the inferolateral leads, that was also transient. His LV rapidly improved the following day with an EF of 45%. His peak troponin T was 1394 (<14) ng/L on admission, which down-trended quickly over the course of the next 2 days to 153 ng/L, as he was extubated. By the time he had his CMR on day 5, his EF was 68%; there was no evidence of infarction but late gadolinium enhancement (LGE) in mid anteroseptum and basal lateral mid to epicardial wall, in addition to isolated basal inferior crypt. There was no LA dilation or LVH, ESVI 23 (16–45) mL/m^2, SVI 54 (42–66) mL/m^2 and VAC 0.43 (0.6–1.0). An AICD was implanted on day 8 and he was discharged 4 days later on diltiazem 120 mg bd, with the diagnosis of coronary artery spasm precipitating his VF cardiac arrest. He was admitted for his coronary physiology study 10 months later, but within this period, he self-presented repeated to the emergency department 4 times,

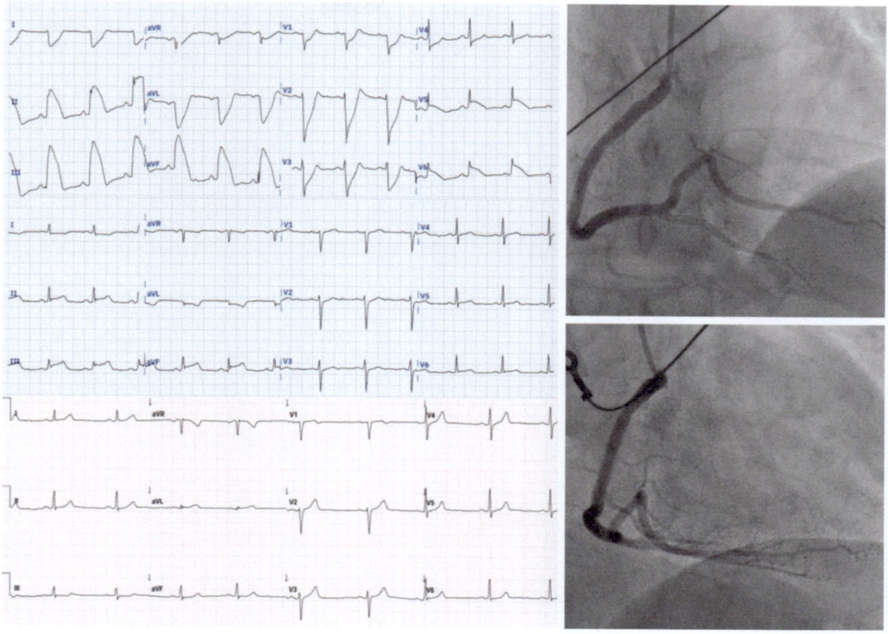

Fig. 7.9 (**Left, top to bottom panels**) 12-lead electrocardiogram (ECG) that shows "sharkfin" ST elevation in the leads corresponding to the right coronary artery (RCA)—this manifests acutely when there is a high burden of ischaemia which usually lasts for minutes and in this case, the usual matching horizontal ST elevation is also seen—as they are transitory, this suggests recurrent RCA vasospasm. The normal ECG reveals no infarctional evolution, beyond a subtle J-wave which is not consistently seen. (**Right, top to bottom panels**) The RCA angiogram shows the artery in two orthogonal views, it is a dominant vessel; there is reduction in calibre in the mid vessel that might be the site of a plaque event

and 6 more times over the next 2 years following the procedure. Most of these were for troponin negative chest pain, AICD site irritation or palpitations, without an objective diagnosis. He did however had a single shock from his AICD following chest pain 4 months after discharge when he skipped an evening dose of diltiazem. His extensive electrophysiology investigations found no predisposition for cardiac arrest. He had his mRNA Covid-19 vaccine 8 months prior to his index presentation with VF but had started having chest pain 3 months before the cardiac arrest or 5 months after his vaccination. He has been a smoker, 20 a day since he was 19, that was a 25 years smoking history.

Procedure His LVEDP is not elevated, at 13 mmHg, and not rising with handgrip, with a corresponding central aortic BP of 120/70 mmHg. His coronary arteries are unobstructed; the left anterior descending (LAD) artery is challenged with escalating doses of ACh, 2, 20, 100 and 200 μg which at higher doses produce ECG PR elongation, but without ST changes, chest pain or severe radiographic epicardial vasospasm beyond mild reduction in calibre. Since the right coronary artery is the culprit, it is studied in greater detail. It has coronary slow flow phenomenon (CSFP)

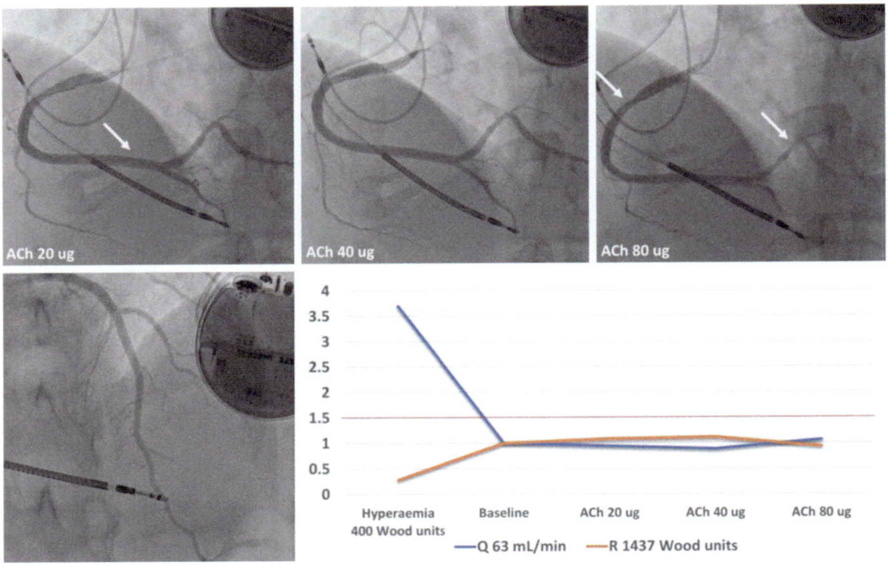

Fig. 7.10 (**Top, left to right panels**) The right coronary artery (RCA); at baseline there is coronary slow flow phenomenon (CSFP)—at three heart beats where the *arrow* is. Note the dual chamber automated implantable cardio-defibrillator (AICD) in situ. There is a dose-dependent increase in segmental vasospasm with acetylcholine (ACh) (*arrows*). (**Bottom, left to right panels**) The left anterior descending (LAD) artery which does not vasoconstrict significantly with ACh. The haemodynamic plot at baseline, with saline hyperaemia and in response to ACh. The microvascular function is normal, but there is a flat response to ACh with flow not rising by 1.5-fold implying microvascular endothelial dysfunction. The flow with respect to ACh 20, 40 and 80 μg; Q ↓6, ↓12 and ↑6%

and a mild to moderate plaque in the mid segment, without flow limitation, with the pressure wire down, the Pd/Pa is 1.01 and RFR 0.99 (> 0.89), and on optical coherence tomography (OCT) this shows intimal thickening, with a minimal diameter of 3.5 mm [5]. Continuous thermodilution is next undertaken with the following haemodynamic basal and hyperaemic indices: flow 63 and 238 mL/min and resistance 1437 and 400 Wood units; CFR 3.7 and MRR 3.6. There is a dose-dependent segmental vasospasm in the mid RCA where the plaque is also in the "kink" section of the posterolateral branch in response to acetylcholine (ACh). There is a flat response in terms of flow or resistance (Fig. 7.10).

Interpretation This young has a quintessential Prinzmetal presentation; it is likely that he has had a coronary event that set off vasospasm in his RCA. If he had OCT at the time of his presentation, this could have shown a plaque pathology such as rupture, dissection or haematoma. RCA vasoreactivity usually settles over time with plaque healing as originally described by Prinzmetal [22]. He has a normal cardiac function, whether the incidental myocardial fibrosis predisposes him to VF. Nevertheless, he has preserved vasodilatory capacity without a raised coronary resistance, but ACh induces segmental vasospasm in the RCA that is due to atherosclerotic endothelial dysfunction and the lack of rise in flow suggests microvascular endothelial dysfunction. The global endothelial dysfunction is related to his smoking habit. The cardiac event clearly has set off considerable anxiety resulting in repeated emergency contacts well beyond the natural history of his plaque pathology.

7.3 Discussion

This chapter presents four cases (Table 7.1): 1. Repeated VF in a postmenopausal woman who is a **smoker** with proximal LAD occlusion, despite normalisation of her LV function, she has diastolic heart failure or HFpEF with raised coronary resistance and a vasoreactive LAD infarct segment; 2. VF in a hypertensive man due to proximal LAD vasospasm secondary to **thyrotoxicosis**, ACh reactivity is abolished with normalised thyroxine level, but persistent vascular endothelial dysfunction, who vasodilates with ACh 200 μg with tripling of flow and CSFP, not seen with GTN; 3. VF with subsequent recurrent RCA vasospasm in a **smoker** with background LV mid-wall fibrosis and BER, and epicardial and microvascular endothelial dysfunction; and 4. VF due to RCA vasospasm in a **smoker** with background LV mid-wall fibrosis and BER, and epicardial and microvascular endothelial dysfunction.

The following themes emerged from this small sample of VF cardiac arrests:

Frequency of three:

1. More common in men
2. Smoking with its associated global endothelial dysfunction

Frequency of two:

1. LV mid-wall fibrosis
2. BER

Frequency of one:

1. Thyrotoxicosis-related vasoreactivity, which resolves the following treatment: This has been discussed elsewhere [23]
2. Biphasic paradoxical pattern: low-dose ACh flow non-responsiveness with epicardial vasospasm and high-dose ACh with marked vasodilatation with flow tripling and CSFP in treated Grave's disease (Case 2)

Cardiac arrest appears to have a gender imbalance, even when there is an arrhythmic substrate, such as Brugada syndrome; it occurs less in women [24]. They are a quarter less likely to suffer aVF during MI [25, 26] and have a third smaller infarct size than men [27]. VF in men during coronary angiography especially with the catheter tip wedged in the RCA ostium or sub-selective conus branch injection occurs on a regular basis in the cardiac catheter laboratory; this is unreported in women [24].

Table 7.1 Coronary physiology and cardiac arrests

Case	Age	BMI	Comorbidities	Aetiology	Vasodilatory Capacity (CFR)	Coronary Resistance (Wood units)	Vasoreactivity (ACh)
1*	60♀	30 to 28	**Smoking**	Proximal LAD occlusion (thrombectomy revealed a moderate underlying lesion	Cx 2.5 Q 97 LAD Q 147 Vasospasm with RayFlow 20 mL/min saline	**866** MRR 2.5 **451** LVEDP 20 BP 110/60	Proximal LAD spasm with ACh 200 μg (Pd/Pa 0.80)
2	43♂	<30	Hypertension	Thyrotoxicosis	LAD 5.8	**286** MRR 6.4 LVEDP 10 BP 140/90	1. Proximal LAD vasospasm during acute phase—20 μg 2. repeat ACh after 1 year elicited no vasospasm, but CSFP and ↑Q 213% (not seen with GTN at the same flow rate)
3	61♂	23	**Smoking**, ulcerative colitis, low Vitamin D level and inferior LV mid-wall fibrosis	RCA vasospasm BER	RCA 2.9	**396** MRR 4.7 LVEDP 6 BP 100/70	Segmental and diffuse RCA vasospasm with ACh, at 160 μg, chest pain, ST depression with relative flow preservation
4	44♂	<30	**Smoking** and anteroseptal and basal lateral LV mid-wall fibrosis	RCA vasospasm with sharkfin ST elevation BER	RCA 3.7	**400** MRR 3.6 LVEDP 13 BP 120/70	Segmental and diffuse RCA vasospasm with ACh, at 160 μg, chest pain, ST depression with relative flow preservation

ACh provocation is remarkably safe, although VF does occur rarely [28], the largest recent study published in 2024 with 556 patients (288 men), and the only VF was in a 60-year-old man who developed occlusive vasospasm in the LAD and Cx after ACh 100 μg [29]. Whether the electrophysiological resilience and ischaemic tolerance of women translate instead into more myocardial stunning resulting in apical LV ballooning, stress cardiomyopathy or Takotsubo syndrome is a matter of conjecture, which will be discussed more in the next chapter.

Smoking

The patients who present with an MI typically started smoking in their teenage years; in cases 1, 3 and 4, they had smoked cigarettes for 20–40 years. From the coronary physiology point of view they exhibit epicardial coronary reactivity and microvascular dysfunction, the inability to generate blood flow > 50% in response to ACh, i.e. generalised endothelial dysfunction, yet they have normal vasodilatory capacity when tested with adenosine. The coronary arteries become stiff, prone to tears and ruptures, from sympathetically driven haemodynamic stress, of BP rise which in itself is caused by smoking [30], and develop coronary intimal hyperplasia and atherosclerosis in conjunction with hyperlipidaemia which is also contributed by smoking. Population-attributable risk for first MI is a third with smoking, a fifth with hypertension and a half with hyperlipidaemia. While women are protected by oestrogen before menopause, men under 55 years could "abolish" their risk for MI just by addressing these three factors: smoking, stress BP and hyperlipidaemia [31, 32]. In other words, close to one-in-two MI in young men is due to smoking, each year of smoking 20/day is a loss of 3 months of life, or each cigarette puffed reduces lifespan by 20 min [33]. Staggering statistics yet smoking is immensely addictive and post-MI cessation is less than half after 1 year, and those who stopped reduced their cardiac mortality by half in 10 years [34]. Somewhat perversely, continuing smoking's risk for adverse cardiac outcome can be mitigated by statin treatment [35, 36], which means that smoking-related dyslipidaemia is one factor for endothelial dysfunction.

Smoking just one cigarette causes a rapid decrease in endothelium-dependent, flow-mediated dilation (FMD) of the brachial artery, by as much as 10% in humans, and when one cigarette worth of smoke is bubbled through buffer to make an aqueous extract and then exposed to isolated rat aortas and porcine coronary arteries, it halves the ACh-induced vasodilatation [37]. A meta-analysis of clinical studies confirms an average reduction of 3% in FMD smokers [38]; each 1% FMD reduction is 13% higher risk of future cardiovascular events in about 5 years [39]. FMD is a measure of nitric oxide (NO) bioavailability in the vascular endothelium. Cigarette smoke is a complex mixture of over 7000 chemicals; many of these drive endothelial dysfunction [40]. For example, carbon monoxide binds haemoglobin with high affinity, reducing oxygen delivery, and competes with NO for binding sites within the red blood cells which are also NO reservoir, reducing bioactive NO delivery to vascular tissues, attenuating hyperaemic vasodilatation in hypoxic tissues [41].

Nicotine

Cigarette smoking delivers a subjective sense of relaxation largely because of nicotine, which rapidly crosses into the brain, binds to *nicotinic* acetylcholine receptors, and triggers downstream release of dopamine in the mesolimbic system and other neuromodulators (serotonin, noradrenaline, ACh, glutamate, GABA and endorphins), producing transient mood modulation and relief of withdrawal-associated anxiety in dependent users [42, 43]. Because lighting up the cigarette also generates tar, carbon monoxide, and a complex cocktail of known carcinogens, it makes sense to pursue harm reduction by separating nicotine from the deadly smoke and delivering it in a controlled, non-combustion form. That logic underpins the rise of vaping or e-cigarettes, aerosolising nicotine-containing liquids so users get the pharmacologically "desirable" effects without inhaling most of the combustion by-products [44]. This has become a global industry projected to worth £20 billion in 2025 with an annual 10% growth, although still dwarfed by the tobacco market which is 40 times larger [45].

Nicotine causes endothelial dysfunction [46] in three major ways:

1. Reduces NO bioavailability via endothelial nitric oxide synthase (eNOS) uncoupling, with increased production of reactive oxygen species (ROS) such as superoxide from activation of NADPH oxidase, following nicotine's binding to endothelial nicotinic acetylcholine receptors through a series of intracellular Ca^{2+} signalling pathways including protein kinase C activation—eNOS, instead of producing NO, goes into a self-reinforcing loop making superoxide [47, 48].
2. Nicotine exacerbates pericoronary adipose tissue dysfunction with its direct activation of endothelial PI3K/Akt signalling and upregulates inflammatory cytokines increasing endothelial "stickiness" and establishing a self-reinforcing inflammatory loop [49]. This also elevates endothelin-1, promoting vasoconstriction.
3. Endothelial progenitor cells through nicotine-generated oxidative stress and inflammation plus its direct bone marrow effect impair the migration of these cells leading to failure of endothelial regeneration [50, 51]. Indeed, smokers have reduced coronary stent endothelialisation [52] and thus have a higher rate of bare-metal stent (BMS) thrombosis post-MI, 8% within 30 days despite aspirin and clopidogrel dual antiplatelet therapy (DAPT) but mitigated by stopping smoking [53], and in general, this risk is regardless of whether the newer generation of drug-eluting stent (DES) polymer coating is biodegradable or not [54].

Acetylcholine

Nicotine is a non-endogenous mimic of ACh, a xenobiotic agonist, that is why it has access to the widespread ACh receptors in humans. However, it selectively binds to nicotinic ACh receptors (nAChR) in brain, autonomic ganglia and adrenal medulla. Unlike ACh, nicotine is not broken down by acetylcholinesterase, so its action is longer-lasting and can lead to receptor desensitisation with sustained exposure. These are ionotropic, which directly open cationic channels to Na^{+} and Ca^{2+} which lead to rapid membrane depolarisation, essential for nerve transmission, e.g. neuromuscular junction to trigger muscle contraction and autonomic ganglia to propagate signals. For instance, within the parasympathetic nervous pathway, the preganglionic neuron releases ACh to nicotinic (ionotropic) receptor on the postganglionic neuron activating it quickly. Then the postganglionic neuron releases ACh onto the target organ, where muscarinic (metabotropic) receptors mediate the slower effect such as reducing heart rate in the sinoatrial or atrioventricular node. Nicotine can highjack this pathway, but the net effect is the opposite, since it also stimulates the sympathetic ganglia and the adrenal medulla, increasing catecholamine release, which tends to raise heart rate and blood pressure. Thus smokers do have higher stress BP. The two types of ACh responses were worked out by Henry H. Dale (1875–1968) that earned him the Nobel Prize in Physiology or Medicine in 1936, which he shared with Otto Loewi (1873–1961).

Rye is a sprouting grass (Fig. 7.11), since time immemorial it has been cultivated to provide grains for consumption, used for cereals, breads and beers. It can be infected by the *Claviceps purpurea* fungus, which replaces as sclerotium the flowering head of rye, a black and hard overhanging "spur". The Germans call it wulfzahn or wolf's tooth and the French *ergot* as it looks like the keratinised outgrowth midway up the back of the rooster's legs, an evolutionary dinosauric remnant used for kicking and stabbing, disposing of the occasional unwelcome territorial intruder, and climbing up the pecking order by defeating potential rivals. When replaced with metal hooks or gaffs, the trained bird is ready for cockfighting. Interestingly, this is a regulated national sport in the Philippines. Legend has it that the ancient Greeks used ergot from barley in their rituals to induce entheogenic visions [55].

One ingredient of ergot is the psychoactive lysergic acid (lys-erg-ic, etymologically, "loosened and obtained from ergot"), synthesised into lysergic acid diethylamide, LSD by Albert Hofmann (1906–2008), a Swiss Chemist with Sandoz Laboratories (Basel) in 1938 [56]. He swallowed a small amount of this derivative which crosses the blood-brain barrier easily and discovered its psychedelic effects on April 19, 1943. This led to the hippie counterculture and peace movements in the 1960s, but the drug was banned since 1968. However, illegal microdosing of LSD has come back into fashion in the Silicon Valley; purportedly it unleashes divergent thinking and produces zoning focus for creativity and problem solving, albeit with sanctioned research into treatment of mental health and chronic pain [57, 58]. Throughout recorded history, inadvertently ingesting contaminated grains cause ergotism, characterised by seizures, hallucinations, chest pains, abdominal cramps, and St Anthony's Fire—burning ischaemic legs which can turn gangrenous, due to its vasoconstrictive nitrogen-containing, often ring-shaped molecules, so-called alkaloids, isolated to ergometrine (or ergonovine) and ergotamine—with modern clinical use in childbirth and headache, respectively, at a small cost of causing coronary artery spasm [59].

Dale, while he was at the Wellcome Physiological Research Laboratories, Herne Hill, London, worked extensively with ergot. He found that certain ergot preparations powerfully slowed the heart and contracted the gut in muscarine-like parasympathomimetic fashion; both effects disappeared with atropine, which then unmasked the nicotine-like action. This persuaded him that an additional active ingredient, distinct from the known ergot alkaloids, was present; he asked his chemist colleague Arthur J. Ewins (1882–1957) to isolate it and compared it with a previously known

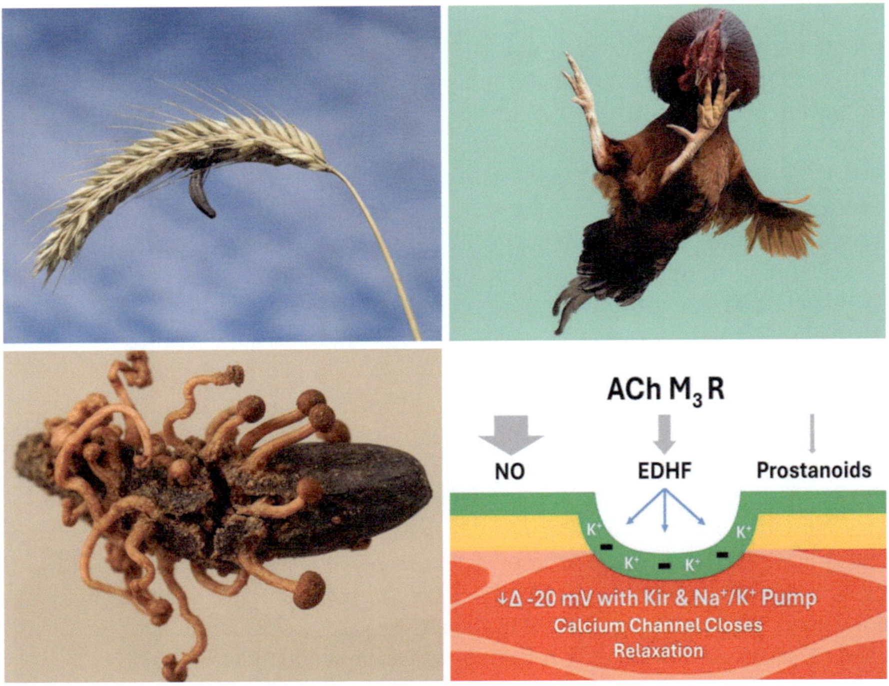

Fig. 7.11 Acetylcholine. (**Top, left to right panels**) The ergot (*Claviceps purpurea*) sclerotium of an infected rye (licensed from iStock 2099615467). An attack rooster baring its spurs, old French for ergot or cock's spur which gave the fungus its name for the likeness (Courtesy of Gregory A. Bailey from his Sculpture for a Small Planet YouTube Channel). (**Bottom, left to right panels**) Germinating ergot sclerotium with stromata bearing globose capitula (2–3 mm in diameter, AI-generated). Acetylcholine (ACh) was first naturally isolated from ergot. ACh modulates vascular tone via muscarinic type 3 receptor with three main mechanisms, nitric oxide mainly, followed by endothelium-derived hyperpolarising factor (EDHF, < 30% but could be much higher in the microvasculature, which is also activated by multiple ACh-independent agents—bradykinin, substance P, etc.) and salutarily through the prostanoids (mainly prostacyclin, PGI_2)

synthetic compound which they made in the laboratory; these molecules turned out to be one and the same. Ewins published his findings in 1914 in its current spelling, "**acetylcholine**" for the first time [60] (Fig. 7.11).

This was not the first time Dale found a synthetic molecule which turned out to be naturally occurring. Earlier in 1910, using the same methodology he discovered histamine in ergot, from the compound β-imidazolylethylamine (Greek *histos* for tissue, combined with *amine*) [61]. In the 1850s, organic chemistry preceded biochemistry, hence the formula of "make it, test it and find it". This was also how dopamine (3,4-dihydroxyphenethylamine) in 1957 [62] and GABA (γ-aminobutyric acid) in 1950 [63] were found to have a natural biological existence.

Dale found the dual effect of ACh: The muscarine-like effects could be blocked by atropine, while the nicotinic effects on the skeletal neuromuscular junctions were atropine-resistant but sensitive to curare-like agent (d-tubocurarine), as was the case with superior cervical autonomic ganglion stimulation of the cat leading to movement of the nictitating membrane (third eyelid) [64].

Separately, Loewi at the Pharmacological Institute, University of Graz, Austria in 1921 perfused an isolated frog heart, stimulated its vagus nerve to slow the rate, and then transferred the perfusate to a second heart, which also slowed, showing that the vagal stimulation had released a diffusible substance he called Vagusstoff [65]. He and Ernst Navrátil (1902–1979) showed that the effect was blocked by atropine, prolonged by eserine (physostigmine), and rapidly destroyed, pointing to Vagusstoff as a transmitter, and cycling through the known vagomimetic agents—muscarine, pilocarpine, choline, and acetylcholine; they proved that Vagusstoff was one and the same as the last agent on the list [66]. Nearly 20 years before, Loewi visited Ernest H. Starling (1866–1927) in 1902 in London and met Dale; they became lifelong friends and exchange ideas which explains the similarities of their experimental methodologies [67]. Loewi had hypothesised that nervous transmission was chemical rather than electrical, his frog heart experiment was fortuitous in two respects, he had a recurrent Easter dream about the whole experiment, and he did his experiment at 5.00 am which coincided with the frog's (Rana Esculenta) vagal inhibitory seasonal rhythm and cold spring's temperature for the acetylcholinesterase to not rapidly metabolising the ACh when he poured Ringer's solution into the second heart [67].

Choline [$HO\text{-}CH_2\text{-}CH_2\text{-}N^+(CH_3)_3$] was first isolated from pig's bile, Greek for cholé, described by the Adolph Strecker (1822–1871) in 1862, while Oskar Liebreich (1839–1908) isolated "neurine" from the brain tissue in 1865, which turned out to be a putrefied choline, trimethyl-vinyl-ammonium hydroxide [68]. Adolf von Baeyer (1835–1917) acetylated choline at very low temperature and called the compound acetyl-neurine in 1867; he won the Nobel Prize in Chemistry in 1905. Reid Hunt (1870–1948) and René de M. Taveau (1876–1950) tested this compound which they christened **acetyl-cholin** by intravenously injecting it into an anaesthetised 3 kg rabbit and found that its mean BP (152 to 36 mmHg with 200 μg) plunged, and demonstrated a dose-response with different concentrations, that it was preventable with atropine pre-treatment, and reported their findings in 1906 in the physiology section of the British Medical Journal which would not be missed by British physiologists like Dale [69]. With this prepared mind, Dale and Ewins chanced upon a compound that behaved similarly, but naturally occurring in ergot, and not a by-product that formed during ergot preparation while extracting the alkaloids for their studies. Forewarned with this knowledge from Dale, 7 years later Loewi and Navrátil found the same substance, this time as an in vivo neurotransmitter. Hence, the serendipity of synthesising a simple nitrogenous compound in 1867, which was found to be bioactive in rabbits in 1906, leading to its discovery in ergot, a rye fungus in 1914 and as a neurotransmitter in frogs' hearts in 1921, a dual action molecule in nerves and muscles. But why IV ACh 200 μg in a 3 kg rabbit causes such profound hypotension, yet the same dose IC down the LAD in healthy humans does not?

7.3.1 Endothelial Function

The European Society of Cardiology's (ESC) 2024 guidelines on functional coronary testing (*as depicted in Figure 13, page 3482 of the ESC document*) recommend a clear separation between low-dose ACh (2 and 20 µg) for testing endothelial function and high-dose ACh (100 and 200 µg) for eliciting coronary vasospasm [70]. The Stuttgart ACh dose-ladder was based on the ENCORE studies [71–75] but added ACh 200 µg to the protocol for expediency as non-selective bolus injection down the guide catheter tip engaged in the left coronary artery, instead of selective infusion into either LAD or Cx with a microcatheter. This high dose can lead to coronary vasospasm in subjects without "Prinzmetal-type" angina, which is non-exertional and has become a subject of debate whether it overdiagnoses vasospastic angina [76, 77]. To understand the nature of the concern, these three questions are addressed.

1. With intracoronary ACh, does the molecule cross unimpeded through the vascular endothelium into the subintimal space and activate the ACh Muscarinic type 3 receptor on vascular smooth muscle cell (VSMC) directly, thus causing vasoconstriction, and if low-dose ACh increases coronary flow > 50% renders clinical vasospasm impossible?
2. Is ACh-induced coronary vasospasm indicates that there is a cardiac autonomic dysfunction, or it is a general marker of vasoreactivity?
3. Has Koch's threefold postulates been satisfied with (A) ACh-provoked coronary vasospasm, and symptomatic correlation, (B) relief of symptom with treatment and (C) reduced vasoreactivity with repeat ACh challenge?

1. ***Intracoronary ACh—historical background***

ACh is a hydrophilic permanently charged quaternary ammonium ester of acetic acid and choline (2-acetoxy-N,N,N-trimethylethanaminium) with a molecular weight of 146.2 Dalton for the free base and 181.7 Dalton for the chloride salt. Because it is rapidly hydrolysed by acetylcholinesterase and related plasma cholinesterases, its action is extremely short-lived, at synapses its degradation occurs in less than a millisecond, and systemically its effective lifetime is likewise very brief, which is why in clinical settings (e.g. intracoronary testing) it must be applied locally to observe vascular effects. ACh is released from cholinergic autonomic nerve endings (primarily parasympathetic postganglionic fibres); direct cholinergic innervation of blood vessels is heterogeneous and not uniform across all vascular beds. It is not clear if ACh freely crosses the endothelial barrier when administered intravascularly.

Hunt and Taveau [69] in 1906 injected 200 µg ACh systemically into a 3 kg rabbit produced marked hypotension, but in later rabbit isolated aortic strip studies, ACh paradoxically caused contraction at a bath concentration of 19 µg [78, 79]. However, in 1961, Roger W. Jelliffe (1929–2020) reported that in serotonin-pretoned rabbit with four 2 mm aortic rings chained together, tenfold increases in acetylcholine produced three phases: an initial relaxation at total bath doses of approximately

0.2–2 μg (10^{-8}–10^{-7} g/mL), a variable contraction at 20–2000 μg (10^{-6}–10^{-4} g/mL), and a second relaxation at 2000–200,000 μg (10^{-4}–10^{-2} g/mL) [80]. In their *Nature* report in 1980, Robert F. Furchgott (1916–2009) and John V. Zawadzki (1919–1985) at the State University of New York Downstate Medical Center repeated the studies with white male New Zealand rabbits (2–3 kg). They cut transverse rings of 2.5 mm axial width, denuded the endothelium and showed that ACh produced concentration-dependent relaxation (between 0.01 and 1 μM) only when the endothelium was intact in a pre-contracted strip; removal of the endothelium abolished the relaxing response and, at higher concentrations around 1 μM, corresponding to 3.6 μg of ACh in the 20 mL bath, ACh produced contraction instead of relaxation with a maximal response at 1–2 min. They therefore postulated that ACh acting on the endothelial muscarinic receptor which could be blocked by atropine caused release of a relaxing substance, endothelium-derived relaxing factor (EDRF) [81]. This was identified to be NO. Furchgott in retrospect realised that earlier studies involved inadvertently damaged endothelium. Further, Jelliffe's 1961 study where high ACh dose caused a paradoxical vasodilatation might be relevant for case 2 but crucially proved that, with intact endothelium, ACh M_3-mediated vasodilation has an alternative pathway, later demonstrated to be due to EDHF [21].

However, the philosophy of **low-dose ACh induces vasodilatation and high-dose ACh provokes vasospasm** is firmly held. This phenomenon was studied in the swine coronary artery. Kawamura et al. [82] in 1989 injected graded doses of ACh (12.5–200 μg) into the RCA of open-chested, 5-month-old farm pigs and described a dose-dependent epicardial coronary constriction (mild at lower doses, severe at higher) with marked delay of coronary blood flow, the latter interpreted as microvascular spasm that, in some instances, occurred without severe epicardial narrowing. Histology showed no intimal thickening (rare or uncommon when present) and an intact endothelium; the relatively greater medial thickness in small coronary arteries was a normal size-dependent anatomical finding, not a pathological change, but makes spasm there more impactful. The constrictive responses were muscarinic (prevented by atropine but not by histamine 1 blockade), confirming receptor specificity. They followed up with therapeutic trials with the same findings [83, 84]. The porcine "ACh paradox" (coronary constriction despite an intact endothelium) has been replicated in other swine models: in Göttingen minipigs using carbachol (an ACh analogue), which constricts coronary arteries while dilating pre-contracted mesenteric arteries [85], and in the neonatal pig heart [86], where ACh produces coronary vasoconstriction with negative inotropy. Other porcine works, including studies of small coronary/microvascular segments, have demonstrated flow reduction or microvascular constriction in the absence of marked epicardial spasm [87, 88]. In contrast, porcine coronary arteries do dilate to other endothelium-dependent agonists such as substance P [89] (via nitric oxide) and bradykinin [90] (often via endothelium-derived hyperpolarising mechanisms), indicating preserved endothelial function. The lack of an ACh-mediated dilation reflects species/bed-specific signalling: In porcine coronary arteries endothelial muscarinic influence is minimal or functionally absent, so ACh acts directly on VSMC to evoke constriction; endothelium denudation does not alter ACh responses in pigs [91]. Finally, radioligand studies localised the ACh muscarinic receptor predominantly to the VSMC in porcine coronary arteries.

On the other hand, studies in dogs, rabbits and other animals could only demonstrate coronary flow reduction with endothelium stripping at high-dose ACh. Similarly, in humans, a flow response of > 50% with low-dose ACh precludes clinical coronary vasospasm with high-dose ACh, the triad of chest pain, ECG changes and radiographic vasospasm or slowing of flow [92].

Based on the above, the answer to question one is that, on account of the porcine studies, ACh passes unimpeded through the intact endothelium into the subintimal space and via the internal elastic lamina fenestration to activate directly the ACh M_3 receptor in the VSMC within the media layer. Thus, high-dose ACh injected down the coronary artery will spill over in a dose-dependent manner to the VSMC. However, in humans, a functional endothelium will always balance out the vasoconstrictive potential of ACh on the VSMC. In other words, a positive spasm test at high-dose ACh suggests an element endothelial dysfunction even in asymptomatic individuals.

Incidentally, Peter Ganz, a son of William Ganz (1919–2009) who made continuous thermodilution a possibility in humans, was first with his team [93] at Harvard Medical School, Boston, to demonstrate atherosclerotic coronary artery spasm with graduated 2 min ACh infusion of 0.03, 0.3, 3.0 and 30 μg into the LAD which appeared on 23 October 1986 issue of *New England Journal of Medicine.* On the other hand, a week later on 1 November 1986, *Circulation* published a Japanese group at Kumamoto City, Yasue et al.'s [94] rapid bolus of ACh within 20 s of escalating 10, 20, 30, 50, 80 and 100 μg to induce coronary artery vasospasm in patients with ANOCA with temporary pacing wire in situ. This divergent methodological differences persisted even after 40 years, the West's emphasis on coronary flow and endothelial function for research [95, 96], and the East's prominent spasm testing with temporary pacing for practice [97]. Whereas Europe has embraced both approaches in their 2024 guidelines and given coronary physiology study a Class I, Level B recommendation for ANOCA, and adopted the middle ground of giving ACh as a bolus over 1 min [70].

2. ***ACh vasoreactivity—disease or marker***

Since ACh activates the M_3 receptor in the VSMC unimpeded by a *dysfunctional endothelium*, it makes sense that a dysregulated autonomic, in particular parasympathetic nervous system overdrive, might be aetiologically responsible for vasospastic angina. When is there excess vagal activity? This is normally at night or early hours of the morning. However, it is very rare for any patient who strictly presents with only nighttime pain, while morning chest pain is more likely to be due to catecholamine surge [98]. Although high vagal tone could theoretical precede this [99] and is detectable with heart rate variability analyses [100]. On the other hand, there is recognition that obstructive sleep apnoea (OSA) with hypoxia as a trigger for vasospastic angina [101], especially with obesity, but it is also highly prevalent in those who are mildly overweight with BMI of 25–30 kg/m^2 [102]. Reflex-mediated or viscerally induced vagal surges such as carotid sinus massage [103], Bezold-Jarish reflex [104] following RCA or Cx reperfusion, either spontaneously or following PCI, retching, vomiting and coughing [105], these could be associated with profound bradycardia, peripheral vasodilatation and hypotension. Atropine is readily given in the cardiac catheter laboratory to deal with these, which are unlikely to be recurrent. Drugs such as donepezil and other acetylcholinesterase inhibitors increase vagal activity and are well-described causes of bradycardia, heart block, and related conduction issues than coronary artery spasm [106].

The fluctuation in arterial tone with flow shear stress is predominantly ACh-independent activation of endothelial nitric oxide synthase (eNOS), although non-neuronal ACh is locally produced acting in an autocrine and paracrine manner for fine-tuning. Coronary artery spasm occurs in the denervated transplanted heart [107–109] where endothelial dysfunction is inevitable [110, 111]. Except in the mesenteric circulation, where cholinergic innervation is essential for digestive function, with notable interspecies concordance including pigs, ACh via M_3 receptor signalling, whether via neuronal release or direct cellular production and activation, does not appear to be a dominant regulator of vascular nitric oxide homeostasis. Therefore, in response to question 2, intracoronary ACh-induced vasoconstriction is a sensitive indicator of endothelial dysfunction; eNOS can be activated independently of ACh through multiple mechanisms, most prominently shear stress-mediated mechanotransduction, protein kinase-dependent phosphorylation, and bradykinin signalling [47, 48].

3. ***Spasm with ACh—what does it mean?***

There is a correlation between ACh sensitivity and symptom severity. Crooijmans et al. [112] in 2025 reported data from a Dutch registry that the lower the ACh dose needed to provoke coronary spasm in ANOCA, the worse the patient's angina burden (inverse dose-response relationship, $p = 0.003$), indicating that ACh-provoked spasm mirrors the clinical severity of symptoms. Although counterintuitively, those with low ACh (< 20 μg) dose-provoked epicardial vasospasm deteriorated in angina frequency despite intensified treatment, even with calcium channel blockade (77 → 67%), but this group was small, 36, 64% women, mean age 57 ± 8, 22% with CFR < 2 and IMR ≥ 25 to suggest concomitant coronary microvascular dysfunction, and only 12 were followed up to 1 year. Notably, over half (53%) were stented, more than twice compared with other groups (ACh 100 μg 23% and ACh 200 μg 20%). Seitz et al. [113] in 2022 on the other hand reported repeat ACh challenge post-GTN 200 μg. This unmasked coexisting GTN-refractory microvascular spasm in **48%** of patients with initial epicardial spasm, while GTN fully prevented focal and 80% of diffuse epicardial spasm, but only prevented microvascular spasm in 20%, and merely attenuated it in another 49%; notably, even when spasm persisted the majority had less severe symptoms on rechallenge. However, one important message was that "microvascular spasm" defined as slow flow in the absence of epicardial constriction in the majority of cases was nitrate-resistant, which was an intriguing observation, but this *subjective criterion* was seen in **15%** in a separate study done in 2025 [114, 115]. Instead of angiographic slow flow, continuous thermodilution which allows actual flow to be measured may throw some light to this phenomenon.

There has not been a cross-over study assessing therapeutic response following a positive ACh test and repeating ACh testing. However, there is repeat ACh over time, with consistency of about one third, suggesting that there is a natural history to vasoreactivity. One prime example is following stress cardiomyopathy; the positive ACh test disappears in a matter of days suggesting that vasoreactivity is not a single disease process [116]. An early series from Canada suggested that over half the number of patients with a positive spasm test became symptom-free off treatment and turned negative on repeat spasm testing within 2 years [117], although this was about 15% in a Japanese population [118]. Even in repeatedly positive tests, the nature of epicardial spasm could shift between arteries and change between focal/segmental to diffuse spasm which would suggest altering plaque burden and endothelial dysfunction [119]. Statin for six-month appeared to reduce coronary vasoreactivity which lend support to the plaque origin of coronary artery spasm [120], and Prinzmetal's original description of variant angina were mostly of young men who smoked with coronary plaques [121]. More up-to-date series attached better prognosis and the long-term outcome is driven by age and the traditional coronary risk factors, with mortality of < 10% in 5–10 years of follow-up [122–124].

Coronary vasoreactivity is a heterogeneous condition that is overwhelmingly related to atherosclerotic coronary artery disease. The response to ACh when positive should be interpreted in a holistic manner.

7.3.2 Cardiac Arrest

Non-ischaemic cardiac fibrosis which includes LV mid-wall fibrosis has a general population prevalence of about 4–6% [125, 126], and it is associated with a 30% increase in mortality (8/54 vs 45/397) over 6 year in an Icelandic registry of people aged over 75, roughly similar to the prognostic value of ischaemic scar [125]. In a London follow-up cohort of patients with mild to moderately impaired LV, EF ≥ 40%, mid-wall fibrosis is highly prevalent in sudden cardiac death (SCD) or aborted SCD, 17.8% (18/101) vs 2.3% (7/298), ninefold higher risk over a median of 4.6 years [127]. Non-ischaemic cardiac fibrosis is a marker of ventricular arrhythmic events or SCD irrespective of cardiac function, in one aborted SCD series from Sydney, of 72 patients (48 males, aged 47.5 ± 20.5 years) two-thirds without obstructive coronary artery disease between 2012 and 2023, and a quarter has mid-wall fibrosis [128].

On the other hand, BER defined as ≥ 2 leads with J-point elevation ≥ 0.1 mV in inferior limb leads [II, III, aVF] or lateral territory [I, aVL, V4-V6] is even more common, nearly 1-in-10 of the normal population [129], and it is double in athletes with high vagal tone, which means that it could disappear with a higher heart rate [130]. BER may not be completely benign, in a 20–40 years long-term follow-up Finnish study of 10,864 middle-aged adults, those with BER > 0.2 mV in the inferior leads; there is 22.2% (8/36) vs 7.2% 736/10,234) SCD, overall for all BER: 12% vs 7.2%. Nevertheless, a small but significant risk of SCD, speculatively this risk could be compounded by the presence of structural heart disease such as cardiac fibrosis as in case 3 and 4 in this report.

BER is accentuated by vagal tone where ACh could predominate, in the presence of endothelial dysfunction as in smokers; it could be associated with coronary artery spasm. In vasospastic angina, BER has substantially higher arrhythmic risk, across 8 studies from Japan and Korea (n = 1761); BER is linked to about a fivefold increase in adverse cardiovascular events and VF, with an underlying risk of 1–3% over 2–8 years [131]. Thus, BER is a magnifier of VF in vasospastic angina but in the context of a small background risk. Therefore the combination of both should not cause any alarm, but an indication to address risk factors that contribute to endothelial dysfunction.

Mechanically, cardiac ischaemia from coronary artery spasm could augment J-wave and increase repolarisation dispersion precipitating phase 2 re-entry and VF [132], especially that there is heterogeneity in repolarisation leading to a larger epicardium to endocardium gradient, plausibly amplified by mid-wall fibrosis [133]. One common SCD scenario is related to vagal tone at night which both increases BER and causes ACh-mediated coronary vasospasm, and in the presence of mid-wall fibrosis, precipitating VF [99]. Cases 3 and 4 both share the triad of BER, mid-wall fibrosis and coronary artery spasm from endothelial dysfunction related to long-term smoking.

7.3.3 Thyrotoxicosis

Coronary endothelial dysfunction and spasm in hyperthyroidism is through a hyperadrenergic milieu (upregulated β_1 in myocardium and α-receptors in coronary VSMC), reduced nitric oxide bioavailability/oxidative stress with impaired endothelium-dependent dilation, and VSMC Ca^{2+} hyperreactivity [23]. Case 2 exhibits continuing endothelial dysfunction despite treatment although he has underlying hypertension. In this case, lower doses of ACh (2, 20 and 100 μg) are associated with blunted rise in coronary flow suggesting ineffective NO pathway, and at ACh 200 μg, there is a sudden flip with flow increasing threefold that is slow; this was previously reported in vitro by Jelliffe in 1962 [80]. Since this biphasic phenomenon is in response to ACh, it must be ACh-mediated. The most likely explanation is shifting from NO to EDHF [21]. Further, GTN increases flow to the same level implying that the endothelial dysfunction is due to reduced bioavailability of NO.

7.4 Conclusions

Smoking is a modifiable risk factor for general vascular endothelial dysfunction, which leads to early atherosclerosis and its associated coronary vasoreactivity, ischaemia and infarction. The presence of myocardial scars from past occult myocarditis might predispose to cardiac arrhythmias in the setting of ischaemia. There is also a whole host of neurohormonal mediators that could increase vasoreactivity such as thyrotoxicosis. These are generally reversible and coronary reactivity does resolve when the underlying aetiology is treated or settles on its own.

References

1. Lim PO. Is index of microvascular resistance of Sisyphean utility in Takotsubo syndrome? ESC Heart Fail. 2024;11(6):4438–40. https://doi.org/10.1002/ehf2.14943.
2. Somerville J. The master's legacy: the first Paul wood lecture. Heart. 1998;80(6):612–9. https://doi.org/10.1136/hrt.80.6.612.
3. Amplatz K. The history of coronary angiography. In: Reiber JHC, Serruys PW, editors. Quantitative coronary arteriography. Dordrecht: Kluwer Academic Publishers; 1991.
4. Arnulf G. Systematic coronary arteriography with acetylcholine cardiac arrest. Prog Cardiovasc Dis. 1959;2(3):197–206. https://doi.org/10.1016/S0033-0620(59)80001-3.
5. Cheng TO. First selective coronary arteriogram. Circulation. 2003;107(5):e42-2. https://doi.org/10.1161/01.CIR.0000053958.38681.81.
6. Heiss HW. Werner Forssmann: a German problem with the nobel prize. Clin Cardiol. 1992;15(7):547–9. https://doi.org/10.1002/clc.4960150715.
7. Braun R. Voyaging in the vein: medical experimentation with heart catheters in the twentieth century. Nuncius. 2011;26(1):132–58. https://doi.org/10.1163/182539111x569793.
8. Forssmann W. Die Sondierung des rechten Herzens. Klin Wochenschr. 1929;45:2085–7.
9. Forssmann-Falck R. Werner Forssmann: a pioneer of cardiology. Am J Cardiol. 1997;79(5):651–60. https://doi.org/10.1016/s0002-9149(96)00833-8.
10. Forrester JS. Heart healers: the misfits, mavericks, and rebels who created the greatest medical breakthrough of our lives. 1st ed. Griffin; 2016.
11. Davies MK, Hollman A. Werner Forssmann. Heart. 2002;87(5):409.
12. Proudfit WL, Shirey EK, Sones FM. Selective cine coronary arteriography. Correlation with clinical findings in 1,000 patients. Circulation. 1966;33(6):901–10. https://doi.org/10.1161/01.cir.33.6.901.
13. Shaik FA, Slotwiner DJ, Gustafson GM, Dai X. Intra-procedural arrhythmia during cardiac catheterization: a systematic review of literature. World J Cardiol. 2020;12(6):269–84. https://doi.org/10.4330/wjc.v12.i6.269.
14. Chen J, Gao LJ, Chen JL, Song HJ. Contemporary analysis of predictors and etiology of ventricular fibrillation during diagnostic coronary angiography. Clin Cardiol. 2009;32(5):283–7. https://doi.org/10.1002/clc.20394.
15. Rivero F, Gutiérrez-Barrios A, Gomez-Lara J, Fuentes-Ferrer M, Cuesta J, Keulards DCJ, et al. Coronary microvascular dysfunction assessed by continuous intracoronary thermodilution: a comparative study with index of microvascular resistance. Int J Cardiol. 2021;333:1–7. https://doi.org/10.1016/j.ijcard.2021.03.005.
16. Keulards DCJ, Van 't Veer M, Zelis JM, El Farissi M, Zimmermann FM, de Vos A, et al. Safety of absolute coronary flow and microvascular resistance measurements by thermodilution. EuroIntervention. 2021;17(3):229–32. https://doi.org/10.4244/EIJ-D-20-00074.
17. Seki R, Keulards DCJ, Gutierrez-Barrios A, Fawaz S, Mahendiran T, Bertolone DT, et al. Safety of continuous coronary thermodilution measurements. JACC Cardiovasc Interv. 2023;16(22):2794–6. https://doi.org/10.1016/j.jcin.2023.09.030.
18. Venditti P, Meo SD. Thyroid hormone-induced oxidative stress. Cell Mol Life Sci. 2006;63(4):414–34. https://doi.org/10.1007/s00018-005-5457-9.

19. Brunt VE, Fujii N, Minson CT. Endothelial-derived hyperpolarization contributes to acetylcholine-mediated vasodilation in human skin in a dose-dependent manner. J Appl Physiol (1985). 2015;119(9):1015–22. https://doi.org/10.1152/japplphysiol.00201.2015.
20. Hammarström AK, Parkington HC, Coleman HA. Release of endothelium-derived hyperpolarizing factor (EDHF) by M3 receptor stimulation in Guinea-pig coronary artery. Br J Pharmacol. 1995;115(5):717–22. https://doi.org/10.1111/j.1476-5381.1995.tb14992.x.
21. Luksha L, Agewall S, Kublickiene K. Endothelium-derived hyperpolarizing factor in vascular physiology and cardiovascular disease. Atherosclerosis. 2009;202(2):330–44. https://doi.org/10.1016/j.atherosclerosis.2008.06.008.
22. Prinzmetal M, Ekmekci A, Toyoshima H, Kwoczynski JK. Angina pectoris: III. Demonstration of a chemical origin of ST deviation in classic angina pectoris, its variant form, early myocardial infarction, and some noncardiac conditions**preliminary report. Am J Cardiol. 1959;3(3):276–93. https://doi.org/10.1016/0002-9149(59)90212-7.
23. Omar AMA, Knott K, Saba MM, Lim PO. Cardiac arrest in myocardial infarction with non-obstructive coronary artery (MINOCA) secondary to thyroid dysfunction. BMJ Case Rep. 2023;16(2). https://doi.org/10.1136/bcr-2022-253500.
24. Lim PO. Could Brugada syndrome be treated with percutaneous coronary intervention? Circ J. 2024;88(1):177. https://doi.org/10.1253/circj.CJ-23-0685.
25. Alnsasra H, Tsaban G, Weinstein JM, Nasasra M, Ovdat T, Beigel R, et al. Sex differences in ventricular arrhythmia, atrial fibrillation and atrioventricular block complicating acute myocardial infarction. Front Cardiovasc Med. 2023;10:1217525. https://doi.org/10.3389/fcvm.2023.1217525.
26. Weizman O, Marijon E, Narayanan K, Boveda S, Defaye P, Martins R, et al. Incidence, characteristics, and outcomes of ventricular fibrillation complicating acute myocardial infarction in women admitted alive in the hospital. J Am Heart Assoc. 2022;11(17):e025959. https://doi.org/10.1161/jaha.122.025959.
27. Krefting J, Graesser C, Novacek S, Voll F, Moggio A, Krueger N, et al. Sex-specific outcomes in myocardial infarction: a dual-cohort analysis using clinical and real-world data. Clin Res Cardiol. 2025; https://doi.org/10.1007/s00392-025-02627-2.
28. Takahashi T, Samuels BA, Li W, Parikh MA, Wei J, Moses JW, et al. Safety of provocative testing with intracoronary acetylcholine and implications for standard protocols. J Am Coll Cardiol. 2022;79(24):2367–78. https://doi.org/10.1016/j.jacc.2022.03.385.
29. Okuya Y, Saito Y, Kitahara H, Kobayashi Y. Omitting 50 μg of intracoronary acetylcholine injection in the left coronary artery during spasm provocation test. J Cardiol. 2024;83(1):25–9. https://doi.org/10.1016/j.jjcc.2023.07.016.
30. Haass M, Kübler W. Nicotine and sympathetic neurotransmission. Cardiovasc Drugs Ther. 1997;10(6):657–65. https://doi.org/10.1007/BF00053022.
31. Ware WR. High cholesterol and coronary heart disease in younger men: the potential role of stress induced exaggerated blood pressure response. Med Hypotheses. 2008;70(3):543–7. https://doi.org/10.1016/j.mehy.2007.06.031.
32. Yusuf S, Hawken S, Ounpuu S, Dans T, Avezum A, Lanas F, et al. Effect of potentially modifiable risk factors associated with myocardial infarction in 52 countries (the INTERHEART study): case-control study. Lancet. 2004;364(9438):937–52. https://doi.org/10.1016/s0140-6736(04)17018-9.
33. Jackson SE, Jarvis MJ, West R. The price of a cigarette: 20 minutes of life? Addiction. 2025;120(5):810–2. https://doi.org/10.1111/add.16757.
34. Biery DW, Berman AN, Singh A, Divakaran S, DeFilippis EM, Collins BL, et al. Association of smoking cessation and survival among young adults with myocardial infarction in the partners YOUNG-MI registry. JAMA Netw Open. 2020;3(7):e209649–e. https://doi.org/10.1001/jamanetworkopen.2020.9649.
35. Athyros VG, Tziomalos K, Katsiki N, Gossios TD, Giouleme O, Anagnostis P, et al. The impact of smoking on cardiovascular outcomes and comorbidities in statin-treated patients

with coronary artery disease: a post hoc analysis of the GREACE study. Curr Vasc Pharmacol. 2013;11(5):779–84. https://doi.org/10.2174/1570161111311050016.
36. Lin MJ, Lin HD, Cai CZ, Chuang MJ, Yang FC, Chiang KF, et al. Effect of statin on long-term outcomes in persistent tobacco users receiving percutaneous coronary intervention: a longitudinal, retrospective cohort study. Medicine (Baltimore). 2024;103(45):e40463. https://doi.org/10.1097/md.0000000000040463.
37. Wölkart G, Kollau A, Russwurm M, Koesling D, Schrammel A, Mayer B. Varied effects of tobacco smoke and e-cigarette vapor suggest that nicotine does not affect endothelium-dependent relaxation and nitric oxide signaling. Sci Rep. 2023;13(1):15833. https://doi.org/10.1038/s41598-023-42750-6.
38. Jia X, Zhang P, Meng L, Tang W, Peng F. The association between smoking exposure and endothelial function evaluated using flow-mediated dilation values: a meta-analysis. BMC Cardiovasc Disord. 2024;24(1):292. https://doi.org/10.1186/s12872-024-03915-x.
39. Green DJ, Jones H, Thijssen D, Cable NT, Atkinson G. Flow-mediated dilation and cardiovascular event prediction: does nitric oxide matter? Hypertension. 2011;57(3):363–9. https://doi.org/10.1161/hypertensionaha.110.167015.
40. Yugar-Toledo JC, Vilela-Martin F, Dinamarco N, Rodrigues B, Moreno H. Smoking and endothelial dysfunction: an integrated – medical and molecular review. Med Res Arch. 2022;10(9). https://doi.org/10.18103/mra.v10i9.3105.
41. Zock JP. Carbon monoxide binding in a model of hemoglobin differs between the T and the R conformation. In: Piiper J, Goldstick TK, Meyer M, editors. Oxygen transport to tissue XII. Boston, MA: Springer; 1990. p. 199–207.
42. Kim K, Picciotto MR. Nicotine addiction: more than just dopamine. Curr Opin Neurobiol. 2023;83:102797. https://doi.org/10.1016/j.conb.2023.102797.
43. Picciotto MR, Corrigall WA. Neuronal systems underlying behaviors related to nicotine addiction: neural circuits and molecular genetics. J Neurosci. 2002;22(9):3338–41. https://doi.org/10.1523/jneurosci.22-09-03338.2002.
44. College R, of P. E-cigarettes and harm reduction: an evidence review. London: Royal College of Physicians; 2024.
45. The Business Research Company.. E-Cigarettes Market Report 2025. Global: The Business Research Company; 2025.
46. Mayhan WG, Patel KP. Effect of nicotine on endothelium-dependent arteriolar dilatation in vivo. American Journal of Physiology-Heart and Circulatory Physiology. 1997;272(5):H2337–H42. https://doi.org/10.1152/ajpheart.1997.272.5.H2337.
47. Hsieh H-J, Liu C-A, Huang B, Tseng AHH, Wang DL. Shear-induced endothelial mechanotransduction: the interplay between reactive oxygen species (ROS) and nitric oxide (NO) and the pathophysiological implications. J Biomed Sci. 2014;21(1):3. https://doi.org/10.1186/1423-0127-21-3.
48. Janaszak-Jasiecka A, Płoska A, Wierońska JM, Dobrucki LW, Kalinowski L. Endothelial dysfunction due to eNOS uncoupling: molecular mechanisms as potential therapeutic targets. Cell Mol Biol Lett. 2023;28(1):21. https://doi.org/10.1186/s11658-023-00423-2.
49. Wang CN, Yang GH, Wang ZQ, Liu CW, Li TJ, Lai ZC, et al. Role of perivascular adipose tissue in nicotine-induced endothelial cell inflammatory responses. Mol Med Rep. 2016;14(6):5713–8. https://doi.org/10.3892/mmr.2016.5934.
50. Khaldoyanidi S, Sikora L, Orlovskaya I, Matrosova V, Kozlov V, Sriramarao P. Correlation between nicotine-induced inhibition of hematopoiesis and decreased CD44 expression on bone marrow stromal cells. Blood. 2001;98(2):303–12. https://doi.org/10.1182/blood.v98.2.303.
51. Li W, Du DY, Liu Y, Jiang F, Zhang P, Li YT. Long-term nicotine exposure induces dysfunction of mouse endothelial progenitor cells. Exp Ther Med. 2017;13(1):85–90. https://doi.org/10.3892/etm.2016.3916.

52. Oh S, Kim JH, Ahmad S, Jin YJ, Na MH, Kim M, et al. The effects of nicotine on re-endothelialization, inflammation, and neoatherosclerosis after drug-eluting stent implantation in a porcine model. Korean Circ J. 2025;55(1):50–64. https://doi.org/10.4070/kcj.2024.0171.
53. Honda T, Fujimoto K, Miyao Y, Koga H, Ishii M. Current cigarette smoking is an independent risk factor for subacute stent thrombosis in acute myocardial infarction patients. J Cardiol. 2014;63(5):358–64. https://doi.org/10.1016/j.jjcc.2013.10.007.
54. Kim YH, Her A-Y, Jeong MH, Kim B-K, Hong S-J, Shin D-H, et al. Impact of current smoking on 2-year clinical outcomes between durable-polymer-coated stents and biodegradable-polymer-coated stents in acute myocardial infarction after successful percutaneous coronary intervention: data from the KAMIR. PLoS One. 2018;13(10):e0205046. https://doi.org/10.1371/journal.pone.0205046.
55. Wasson RG, Hofmann A, Ruck CAP. The road to eleusis: unveiling the secret of the mysteries.. 30th anniversary ed. Berkeley, CA: North Atlantic Books; 2008.
56. Oransky I. Albert Hofmann. Lancet. 2008;371(9631):2168. https://doi.org/10.1016/S0140-6736(08)60943-5.
57. Holze F, Gasser P, Müller F, Dolder PC, Liechti ME. Lysergic acid diethylamide-assisted therapy in patients with anxiety with and without a life-threatening illness: a randomized, double-blind, placebo-controlled phase II study. Biol Psychiatry. 2023;93(3):215–23. https://doi.org/10.1016/j.biopsych.2022.08.025.
58. Ramaekers JG, Hutten N, Mason NL, Dolder P, Theunissen EL, Holze F, et al. A low dose of lysergic acid diethylamide decreases pain perception in healthy volunteers. J Psychopharmacol. 2021;35(4):398–405. https://doi.org/10.1177/0269881120940937.
59. Spencer SPE, Lowe SA. Ergometrine for postpartum hemorrhage and associated myocardial ischemia: two case reports and a review of the literature. Clin Case Rep. 2019;7(12):2433–42. https://doi.org/10.1002/ccr3.2516.
60. Ewins AJ. Acetylcholine, a new active principle of ergot. Biochem J. 1914;8(1):44–9.
61. Tiligada E, Ennis M. Histamine pharmacology: from sir Henry dale to the 21st century. Br J Pharmacol. 2020;177(3):469–89. https://doi.org/10.1111/bph.14524.
62. Ubuka T. Subchapter 131A – dopamine. In: Ando H, Ukena K, Nagata S, editors. Handbook of hormones. 2nd ed. San Diego: Academic; 2021. p. 1037–9.
63. Baxter CF. The nature of γ-aminobutyric acid. In: Lajtha A, editor. Metabolic reactions in the nervous system. Boston, MA: Springer; 1970. p. 289–353.
64. Tansey EM. Henry dale and the discovery of acetylcholine. C R Biol. 2006;329(5–6):419–25. https://doi.org/10.1016/j.crvi.2006.03.012.
65. Loewi O. Über humorale übertragbarkeit der Herznervenwirkung. Pflugers Arch Gesamte Physiol Menschen Tiere. 1921;189(1):239–42. https://doi.org/10.1007/BF01738910.
66. Loewi O, Navratil E. über das Schicksal des Vagusstoffs und des Acetylcholins im Herzen. Klin Wochenschr. 1926;5(20):894. https://doi.org/10.1007/BF01752897.
67. Heinbockel T. Introductory chapter: the neurotransmitter acetylcholine—a young centenarian. In: Heinbockel T, editor. Acetylcholine – recent advances and new perspectives. London: IntechOpen; 2023. p. 3–6.
68. Mott FW, Halliburton WD. The physiological action of choline and neurine. Philos Trans R Soc Lond B. 1899;191:211–67. https://doi.org/10.1098/rstb.1899.0007.
69. Hunt R, Taveau RM. On the physiological action of certain cholin derivatives and new methods for detecting cholin. Br Med J. 1906;2:1788–91.
70. Vrints C, Andreotti F, Koskinas KC, Rossello X, Adamo M, Ainslie J, et al. ESC guidelines for the management of chronic coronary syndromes: developed by the task force for the management of chronic coronary syndromes of the European Society of Cardiology (ESC) endorsed by the European Association for Cardio-Thoracic Surgery (EACTS). Eur Heart J. 2024;45(36):3415–537. https://doi.org/10.1093/eurheartj/ehae177.
71. Hermann M, Fischer D, Hoffmann MM, Gasser T, Quitzau K, Meinertz T, et al. CRP and CD14 polymorphisms correlate with coronary plaque volume in patients with coronary

artery disease -- IVUS substudy of the ENCORE trials. Atherosclerosis. 2012;220(1):172–6. https://doi.org/10.1016/j.atherosclerosis.2011.10.019.
72. Lüscher TF, Pieper M, Tendera M, Vrolix M, Rutsch W, van den Branden F, et al. A randomized placebo-controlled study on the effect of nifedipine on coronary endothelial function and plaque formation in patients with coronary artery disease: the ENCORE II study†. Eur Heart J. 2009;30(13):1590–7. https://doi.org/10.1093/eurheartj/ehp151.
73. Hermann M, Hellermann JP, Quitzau K, Hoffmann MM, Gasser T, Meinertz T, et al. CYP4A11 polymorphism correlates with coronary endothelial dysfunction in patients with coronary artery disease -- the ENCORE trials. Atherosclerosis. 2009;207(2):476–9. https://doi.org/10.1016/j.atherosclerosis.2009.06.009.
74. ENCORE Investigators. Effect of nifedipine and cerivastatin on coronary endothelial function in patients with coronary artery disease: the ENCORE I study (evaluation of nifedipine and cerivastatin on recovery of coronary endothelial function). Circulation. 2003;107(3):422–8. https://doi.org/10.1161/01.cir.0000046488.52939.bf.
75. Haegeli L, Quitzau K, Lüscher TF. From endothelial dysfunction to clinical events concept and update on the ENCORE trials. Eur Heart J Suppl. 2001;3(suppl_B):B12–B9. https://doi.org/10.1016/s1520-765x(01)90052-5.
76. Rehan R, Khandur C, Wong CCY, Weaver J, Jain P, Adams M, et al. Diagnostic validity of acetylcholine provocation protocols in the evaluation of coronary artery spasm in patients with ANOCA. Circ Cardiovasc Interv. 2025;0(0):e015339. https://doi.org/10.1161/CIRCINTERVENTIONS.125.015339.
77. Rahman H, Sinha A, Perera D. More is not always better: reassessing acetylcholine provocation in the diagnosis of coronary vasospasm. Circ Cardiovasc Interv. 2025;0(0):e015677. https://doi.org/10.1161/CIRCINTERVENTIONS.125.015677.
78. Furchgott RF. The pharmacology of vascular smooth muscle. Pharmacol Rev. 1955;7(2):183–265. https://doi.org/10.1016/S0031-6997(25)06984-4.
79. Furchgott RF, Bhadrakom S. Reactions of strips of rabbit aorta to epinephrine, isopropylarterenol, sodium nitrite and other drugs. J Pharmacol Exp Ther. 1953;108(2):129–43. https://doi.org/10.1016/S0022-3565(25)05163-8.
80. Jelliffe RW. Dilator and constrictor effects of acetylcholine on isolated rabbit aortic chains. J Pharmacol Exp Ther. 1962;135(3):349–53. https://doi.org/10.1016/S0022-3565(25)26242-5.
81. Furchgott RF, Zawadzki JV. The obligatory role of endothelial cells in the relaxation of arterial smooth muscle by acetylcholine. Nature. 1980;288(5789):373–6. https://doi.org/10.1038/288373a0.
82. Kawamura A, Fujiwara H, Onodera T, Wu DJ, Matsuda M, Ishida M, et al. Response of large and small coronary arteries of pigs to intracoronary injection of acetylcholine: angiographic and histologic analysis. Int J Cardiol. 1989;25(3):289–302. https://doi.org/10.1016/0167-5273(89)90219-2.
83. Kawamura A, Fujiwara H, Uegaito T, Tanaka M, Kawai C. Comparative effects of diltiazem, nifedipine, and verapamil on large and small coronary artery constriction induced by intracoronary acetylcholine in pigs. J Cardiovasc Pharmacol. 1992;19(6):915–21. https://doi.org/10.1097/00005344-199206000-00012.
84. Kawamura A, Fujiwara H, Ishida M, Takemura G, Kida M, Uegaito T, et al. Protective effects of nipradilol, isosorbide dinitrate, and bunazosin on coronary artery constriction induced by intracoronary injection of acetylcholine in pigs. Cardiovasc Res. 1990;24(12):1013–9. https://doi.org/10.1093/cvr/24.12.1013.
85. Sams A, Haanes KA, Holm A, Kazantzi S, Mikkelsen LF, Edvinsson L, et al. Heterogeneous vasomotor responses in segments from Göttingen Minipigs coronary, cerebral, and mesenteric artery: a comparative study. Vasc Pharmacol. 2023;153:107231. https://doi.org/10.1016/j.vph.2023.107231.
86. Ascuitto RJ, Ross-Ascuitto NT, Ramage D, McDonough KH, Kadowitz PJ. Acetylcholine-induced coronary vasoconstriction and negative inotropy in the neonatal pig heart. Pediatr Res. 1992;32(2):236–42. https://doi.org/10.1203/00006450-199208000-00022.

87. Cowan CL. Cholinergic regulation of resting coronary blood flow in the domestic swine. Bethesda, Maryland: Uniformed Services University of the Health Sciences, F. Edward Hebert School of Medicine; 1989.
88. Hata H, Egashira K, Fukai T, Ohara Y, Kasuya H, Takahashi T, et al. The role of endothelium-derived nitric oxide in acetylcholine-induced coronary vasoconstriction in closed-chest pigs. Coron Artery Dis. 1993;4(10):891–8.
89. Pendyala LK, Li J, Shinke T, Geva S, Yin X, Chen JP, et al. Endothelium-dependent vasomotor dysfunction in pig coronary arteries with paclitaxel-eluting stents is associated with inflammation and oxidative stress. J Am Coll Cardiol Intv. 2009;2(3):253–62. https://doi.org/10.1016/j.jcin.2008.11.009.
90. Miyata K, Shimokawa H, Yamawaki T, Kunihiro I, Zhou X, Higo T, et al. Endothelial vasodilator function is preserved at the spastic/inflammatory coronary lesions in pigs. Circulation. 1999;100(13):1432–7. https://doi.org/10.1161/01.cir.100.13.1432.
91. Gräser T, Leisner H, Tiedt N. Absence of role of endothelium in the response of isolated porcine coronary arteries to acetylcholine. Cardiovasc Res. 1986;20(4):299–302. https://doi.org/10.1093/cvr/20.4.299.
92. Feenstra RGT, Boerhout CKM, Vink CEM, Woudstra J, Wittekoek ME, de Waard GA, et al. Haemodynamic characterisation of different endotypes in coronary artery vasospasm in reaction to acetylcholine. Int J Cardiol Heart Vasc. 2022;42:101105. https://doi.org/10.1016/j.ijcha.2022.101105.
93. Ludmer PL, Selwyn AP, Shook TL, Wayne RR, Mudge GH, Alexander RW, et al. Paradoxical vasoconstriction induced by acetylcholine in atherosclerotic coronary arteries. N Engl J Med. 1986;315(17):1046–51. https://doi.org/10.1056/NEJM198610233151702.
94. Yasue H, Horio Y, Nakamura N, Fujii H, Imoto N, Sonoda R, et al. Induction of coronary artery spasm by acetylcholine in patients with variant angina: possible role of the parasympathetic nervous system in the pathogenesis of coronary artery spasm. Circulation. 1986;74(5):955–63. https://doi.org/10.1161/01.CIR.74.5.955.
95. Gulati M, Levy PD, Mukherjee D, Amsterdam E, Bhatt DL, Birtcher KK, et al. 2021 AHA/ACC/ASE/CHEST/SAEM/SCCT/SCMR guideline for the evaluation and diagnosis of chest pain: a report of the American College of Cardiology/American Heart Association Joint Committee on clinical practice guidelines. Circulation. 2021;144(22):e368–454. https://doi.org/10.1161/cir.0000000000001029.
96. Buelt A, Kennady J, Arnold M. Chest pain evaluation: updated guidelines from the AHA/ACC. Am Fam Physician. 2023;107(2):204–6.
97. Hokimoto S, Kaikita K, Yasuda S, Tsujita K, Ishihara M, Matoba T, et al. JCS/CVIT/JCC 2023 guideline focused update on diagnosis and treatment of vasospastic angina (coronary spastic angina) and coronary microvascular dysfunction. Circ J. 2023;87(6):879–936. https://doi.org/10.1253/circj.CJ-22-0779.
98. Muller JE. Circadian variation in cardiovascular events. Am J Hypertens. 1999;12(S2):35S–42S. https://doi.org/10.1016/s0895-7061(98)00278-7.
99. Yoshio H, Shimizu M, Sugihara N, Kita Y, Shimizu K, Minagawa F, et al. Assessment of autonomic nervous activity by heart rate spectral analysis in patients with variant angina. Am Heart J. 1993;125(2, Part 1):324–9. https://doi.org/10.1016/0002-8703(93)90007-V.
100. Lombardi F. Origin of heart rate variability and turbulence: an appraisal of autonomic modulation of cardiovascular function. Front Physiol. 2011;2. https://doi.org/10.3389/fphys.2011.00095.
101. Tamura A, Kawano Y, Ando S, Watanabe T, Kadota J. Association between coronary spastic angina pectoris and obstructive sleep apnea. J Cardiol. 2010;56(2):240–4. https://doi.org/10.1016/j.jjcc.2010.06.003.
102. Esmaeili N, Gell L, Imler T, Hajipour M, Taranto-Montemurro L, Messineo L, et al. The relationship between obesity and obstructive sleep apnea in four community-based cohorts: an individual participant data meta-analysis of 12,860 adults. eClinicalMedicine. 2025;83 https://doi.org/10.1016/j.eclinm.2025.103221.

103. Choi SS, Lim YJ, Bahk JH, Do SH, Ham BM. Coronary artery spasm induced by carotid sinus stimulation during neck surgery. Br J Anaesth. 2003;90(3):391–4. https://doi.org/10.1093/bja/aeg051.
104. Holland EM, Stouffer GA. Bezold-Jarisch Reflex. Catheter Cardiovasc Interv. 2022;1(2). https://doi.org/10.1016/j.jscai.2022.100029.
105. Waldmann V, Combes N, Narayanan K, Sharifzadehgan A, Bouzeman A, Beganton F, et al. Cough syncope. Am J Med. 2017;130(7):e295–e6. https://doi.org/10.1016/j.amjmed.2017.01.050.
106. Rowland JP, Rigby J, Harper AC, Rowland R. Cardiovascular monitoring with acetylcholinesterase inhibitors: a clinical protocol. Adv Psychiatr Treat. 2007;13(3):178–84. https://doi.org/10.1192/apt.bp.106.002725.
107. Bisognano JD, Lindenfeld J, Hammond E, Zisman LS. Coronary artery vasospasm causing acute myocardial infarction in a heart transplant recipient. J Heart Lung Transplant. 2005;24(3):355–8. https://doi.org/10.1016/j.healun.2003.11.405.
108. Le JN, Chang DH, Kobashigawa JA, Kittleson MM. Coronary vasospasm causing chest pain in early postoperative heart transplantation. JACC Case Rep. 2023;28:102100. https://doi.org/10.1016/j.jaccas.2023.102100.
109. Pagnoni M, Regamey J, Adjedj J, Rogati G, Muller O, Tozzi P. Case report – coronary vasospasm in transplanted heart: a puzzling phenomenon. BMC Cardiovasc Disord. 2019;19(1):305. https://doi.org/10.1186/s12872-019-01280-8.
110. Aptecar E, Benvenuti C, Loisance D, Cachera J-P, Nitenberg A. Early impairment of acetylcholine-induced endothelium-dependent coronary vasodilation is not predictive of secondary graft atherosclerosis. Chest. 1995;107(5):1266–74. https://doi.org/10.1378/chest.107.5.1266.
111. Nitenberg A, Aptecar E, Antony I, Benvenuti C, Deleuze P, Loisance D, et al. Acetylcholine-induced constriction of angiographically normal coronary arteries is not time dependent in transplant recipients: effects of stepwise infusion at 1,6,12 and more than 24 months after transplantation. J Am Coll Cardiol. 1993;22(1):151–8. https://doi.org/10.1016/0735-1097(93)90829-P.
112. Crooijmans C, Jansen TPJ, Meeder JG, Paradies V, de Vos AMJ, Woudstra P, et al. Angina severity and symptom improvement are associated with diagnostic acetylcholine provocation dose in vasospastic angina. J Am Heart Assoc. 2025;14(2):e037913. https://doi.org/10.1161/jaha.124.037913.
113. Seitz A, Feenstra R, Konst RE, Martínez Pereyra V, Beck S, Beijk M, et al. Acetylcholine rechallenge: a first step toward tailored treatment in patients with coronary artery spasm. JACC Cardiovasc Interv. 2022;15(1):65–75. https://doi.org/10.1016/j.jcin.2021.10.003.
114. Rehan R, Wong CCY, Weaver J, Jain P, Adams M, Ng MKC, et al. Impact of nitroglycerin administration on acetylcholine provocation testing in angina with nonobstructive coronary arteries. J Soc Cardiovasc Angiogr Interv. 2025:103668. https://doi.org/10.1016/j.jscai.2025.103668.
115. Vohra AS, Osborn EA. Hold the nitro: acetylcholine provocation testing for coronary vasospasm. Catheter Cardiovasc Interv. 2025:103760. https://doi.org/10.1016/j.jscai.2025.103760.
116. Angelini P, Uribe C, Tobis JM. Pathophysiology of takotsubo cardiomyopathy: reopened debate. Tex Heart Inst J. 2021;48(3). https://doi.org/10.14503/THIJ-20-7490.
117. Waters DD, Szlachcic J, Theroux P, Dauwe F, Mizgala HF. Ergonovine testing to detect spontaneous remissions of variant angina during long-term treatment with calcium antagonist drugs. Am J Cardiol. 1981;47(1):179–84. https://doi.org/10.1016/0002-9149(81)90307-6.
118. Ueda O, Kohchi K, Kishi Y, Numano F. Long lasting spasticity in controlled vasospastic angina. Heart. 1999;81(5):528–32. https://doi.org/10.1136/hrt.81.5.528.
119. Sueda S, Kurokawa K, Sakaue T, Ikeda S. What is the meaning of provoked spasm phenotypes by vasoreactivity testing? J Cardiol. 2024;83(1):1–7. https://doi.org/10.1016/j.jjcc.2023.06.013.

120. Yasue H, Mizuno Y, Harada E, Itoh T, Nakagawa H, Nakayama M, et al. Effects of a 3-hydroxy-3-methylglutaryl coenzyme a reductase inhibitor, fluvastatin, on coronary spasm after withdrawal of calcium-channel blockers. J Am Coll Cardiol. 2008;51(18):1742–8. https://doi.org/10.1016/j.jacc.2007.12.049.
121. Prinzmetal M, Kennamer R, Merliss R, Wada T, Bor N. Angina pectoris I. A variant form of angina pectoris: preliminary report. Am J Med. 1959;27(3):375–88. https://doi.org/10.1016/0002-9343(59)90003-8.
122. Bory M, Pierron F, Panagides D, Bonnet JL, Yvorra S, Desfossez L. Coronary artery spasm in patients with normal or near normal coronary arteries. Long-term follow-up of 277 patients. Eur Heart J. 1996;17(7):1015–21. https://doi.org/10.1093/oxfordjournals.eurheartj.a014996.
123. Crea F. Variant angina in patients without obstructive coronary atherosclerosis: a benign form of spasm. Eur Heart J. 1996;17(7):980–2. https://doi.org/10.1093/oxfordjournals.eurheartj.a015017.
124. Kim H-L, Kim J, Kim HJ, Lim W-H, Lee JY. Incidence and factors associated with mortality in 2,476 patients with variant angina in Korea. Sci Rep. 2017;7(1):46031. https://doi.org/10.1038/srep46031.
125. Shanbhag SM, Greve AM, Aspelund T, Schelbert EB, Cao JJ, Danielsen R, et al. Prevalence and prognosis of ischaemic and non-ischaemic myocardial fibrosis in older adults. Eur Heart J. 2018;40(6):529–38. https://doi.org/10.1093/eurheartj/ehy713.
126. Turkbey EB, Nacif MS, Guo M, McClelland RL, Teixeira PB, Bild DE, et al. Prevalence and correlates of myocardial scar in a US cohort. JAMA. 2015;314(18):1945–54. https://doi.org/10.1001/jama.2015.14849.
127. Halliday BP, Gulati A, Ali A, Guha K, Newsome S, Arzanauskaite M, et al. Association between midwall late gadolinium enhancement and sudden cardiac death in patients with dilated cardiomyopathy and mild and moderate left ventricular systolic dysfunction. Circulation. 2017;135(22):2106–15. https://doi.org/10.1161/CIRCULATIONAHA.116.026910.
128. Chandramohan S, McColl H, Hunyor I. The utility of cardiac MRI in the management of cardiac arrest survivors: a single-centre study. Heart Lung Circ. 2023;32:S258. https://doi.org/10.1016/j.hlc.2023.06.320.
129. Ji H-Y, Hu N, Liu R, Zhou H-R, Gao W-L, Quan X-Q. Worldwide prevalence of early repolarization pattern in general population and physically active individuals: a meta-analysis. Medicine. 2021;100(22):e25978. https://doi.org/10.1097/md.0000000000025978.
130. Noseworthy PA, Weiner R, Kim J, Keelara V, Wang F, Berkstresser B, et al. Early repolarization pattern in competitive athletes. Circ Arrhythm Electrophysiol. 2011;4(4):432–40. https://doi.org/10.1161/CIRCEP.111.962852.
131. Wang G, Zhao N, Zhong S, Wang H. Association of early repolarization pattern and ventricular fibrillation in patients with vasospastic angina: a systematic review and meta-analysis. Clin Cardiol. 2022;45(5):461–73. https://doi.org/10.1002/clc.23804.
132. Sato A, Tanabe Y, Chinushi M, Hayashi Y, Yoshida T, Ito E, et al. Analysis of J waves during myocardial ischaemia. Europace. 2011;14(5):715–23. https://doi.org/10.1093/europace/eur323.
133. Mercer BN, Begg GA, Page SP, Bennett CP, Tayebjee MH, Mahida S. Early repolarization syndrome; mechanistic theories and clinical correlates. Front Physiol. 2016;7. https://doi.org/10.3389/fphys.2016.00266.

Chapter 8
Flooded Heart

Abstract Stress can literally break the heart. This was called neurogenic cardiomyopathy with its distinctive widespread giant inverted T-wave on electrocardiogram (ECG) of subarachnoid haemorrhage sufferers in the 1950s. Hikaru Sato of Hiroshima set up his intracoronary thrombolysis and left ventricular angiography for acute myocardial infarction service in 1981, and two years later he found his first case, characterised by chest pain, unobstructed coronary arteries, and cardiac apical ballooning, akin to the Japanese octopus-trap pot (*Takotsubo*). Mental trigger occurs in one third of cases, about two percent recur within the year, and postmenopausal women comprise ninety percent of cases. Takotsubo syndrome (TTS) is an acute ischaemic syndrome, typically with a small and salutary troponin leak. If caught early, ECG ST elevation is evident, and coronary angiogram could show multivessel epicardial vasospasm. It is believed that catecholamine surge, causing transient microvascular spasm, with underlying coronary microvascular dysfunction (CMD) causes TTS. However, this would predict a balanced gender distribution. Since the microvasculature, unlike the epicardial coronary artery is less susceptible to atherosclerosis which infiltrates, disrupts and calcifies the vascular media, rendering epicardial vasoconstriction unlikely in older men, but their microvasculature should similarly react like in older women. However, in premenopausal women, oestrogen maintains vascular health, thus preserving compliant, patent, and vasoreactive epicardial coronary arteries. Strangely, coronary artery disease confers protection against TTS. Histologically, TTS is also a form of myocardial stunning. Cardiac abnormalities following TTS are uncommon, but cardiac imaging findings post-TTS reflect concomitant diseases' effects on the heart, and its prognosis is mainly driven by these, including hypertension, hyperlipidaemia and diabetes. This chapter describes detailed coronary physiology with continuous thermodilution in four women who have had TTS, none of whom has demonstrable CMD, but they uniformly exhibit epicardial endothelial dysfunction which is part of oestrogen-deficient normal ageing, also influenced by lifestyle-related and pre-existing vasoreactive conditions, such as smoking and migraine. One woman displays pre- and post-verapamil acetylcholine-induced coronary slow flow phenomenon (CSFP) with absolute volumetric flow increase, but associated with chest

P. O. Lim, *Coronary Thermodilution*,
https://doi.org/10.1007/978-3-032-10734-3_8

pain and ST depression on ECG. This paradoxical acetylcholine response raises the following four conjectures: 1. Acute CSFP does not equate microvascular spasm; 2. calcium channel blockade is ineffective beyond epicardial vasospasm; 3. non-nitric oxide pathways predominate in the microvasculature; and 4. unimpeded flow and microvascular vasodilatation with subendocardial postcapillary venular exudation cause angina and, if sustained, result in TTS. Cardiovascular magnetic resonance (CMR) scan pathognomonically finds scattered myocardial oedema in TTS, akin to chest X-ray and pulmonary oedema. Animal studies show that a three percent rise in myocardial interstitial water content stuns the heart.

8.1 Introduction

The first case of takotsubo syndrome (TTS) was discovered on 23 September 1983 by Hikaru Sato (1938–2021) in Hiroshima, Japan. Being an early adopter of new ideas, he set up his intracoronary thrombolysis with urokinase for ST elevation myocardial infarction (STEMI) service in 1981, after Klaus P. Rentrop's case report in Göttingen in 1979. Sato waited until he collected three TTS cases before publishing them in 1990 [1, 2]. He and his colleagues noticed that these were mostly postmenopausal women in their 60–70s with chest pain, some with ECG ST elevation and multivessel coronary artery spasm in 10% of cases, a majority with left ventricular (LV) apical ballooning, which resolved within two weeks among their cohort of thirty patients (28 women or 93%, mean age 70, 55–83 years, 1/3 with a stress trigger) they collected over the next 18 years, which they published in 2001 [3].

Inspired by Hirofumi Yasue who was the first to describe the use acetylcholine (ACh) for coronary artery spasm testing in 1986 [4], Sato performed this test in 14 patients and found that 10 or 74% had epicardial vasoreactivity, and a pre-discharge coronary angiogram in an 86-year-old woman was complicated by contrast-induced coronary slow flow phenomenon (CSFP), interpreted as microvascular vasoconstriction. CSFP, chest pain and ECG ST changes have become *sine qua non* for **microvascular spasm** in the absence of epicardial disease or vasoconstriction during coronary angiography. Sato thus hypothesised that TTS was triggered by coronary vasospasm. This was vigorously defended by Paolo Angelini (1941–2023) [5–7] who persuasively debunked catecholamine surge as a prerequisite for TTS. On the other side, John Madias successfully relegated multivessel coronary artery spasm to an epiphenomenon of TTS [8]. Nevertheless, Sato's general description of TTS remains definitive; a similar pattern has been replicated in worldwide series [9–11].

This chapter describes four women who continued to be symptomatic post-TTS, and they underwent a detailed coronary physiology study with continuous thermodilution in response to saline-induced hyperaemia, ACh and repeat ACh post-verapamil.

8.2 Cases

8.2.1 Half-hearted

A 46-year-old South Asian woman with breathlessness and angina mostly with emotional stress, which woke her up at night, was referred for a coronary physiology study. She was hospitalised 8.5 years before following a domestic discord with chest pain and a peak troponin T of 8627 (< 14) ng/L. Her ECG showed T inversion in I and aVL, coronary angiogram revealed unobstructed arteries and LV angiogram found mid-cavity "ballooning" (Fig. 8.1). Her in-hospital echocardiogram revealed her EF to be 45%, with akinetic mid-septum, anterolateral wall and average E/e' 12 (< 8). Her cardiovascular magnetic resonance (CMR) scan 7 weeks later demonstrated a normal heart: EF 57%, ESVI 28 (17–36) mL/m^2, SVI 37 (40–65) mL/m^2 and volume-derived VAC 0.76 (0.6–1.0).

She had continued to be symptomatic over the years. Nineteen months later her exercise stress echocardiogram, she did 5 min on the treadmill, stopping because of her usual symptoms, with a maximal HR of 84% predicted - 85 to 152 bpm, and BP 110/60 to 140/80 mmHg, but without significant ECG changes, nor echocardiographic ischaemia. Her CMR was repeated 5 years from the previous one found supranormal EF 84%, ESVI 8 (17–36) mL/m^2, SVI 41 (40–65) mL/m^2 and VAC 0.20 (0.6–1.0), without left ventricular hypertrophy (LVH) or left atrial (LA) dilatation. She has early menopause from her mid-thirties, with asymptomatic pituitary empty sella, primary limb lymphoedema, asthma, hypertension, coeliac disease and hyperlipidaemia.

Procedure Her coronary angiogram shows patent arteries, central aortic BP 158/86 mmHg and LVEDP 15 mmHg, which rises to 20 mmHg with handgrip (Fig. 8.2). Continuous thermodilution is performed to the left anterior descending (LAD) artery, distal-to-aortic pressure ratio (Pd/Pa) with the sensor in distal vessel is 0.98, rest full-cycle ratio (RFR), 0.95 (> 0.89), and the following basal plus hyperaemic indices are obtained: flow 62 and 154 mL/min and resistance 1636 and 627 Wood

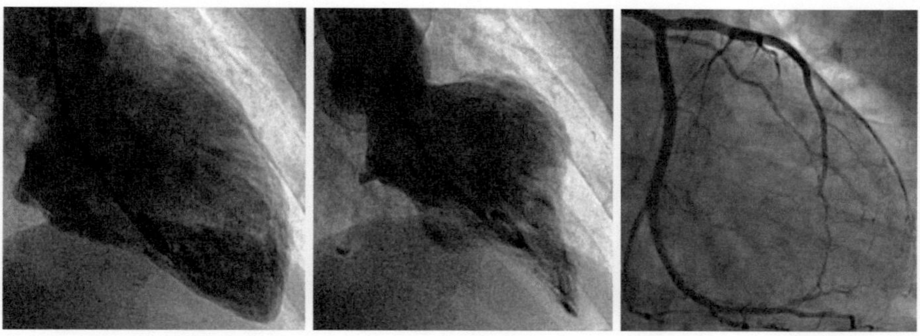

Fig. 8.1 **(Left to right panels)** Left ventricular angiogram in diastole and systole showing mid-cavity ballooning and unobstructed coronary arteries

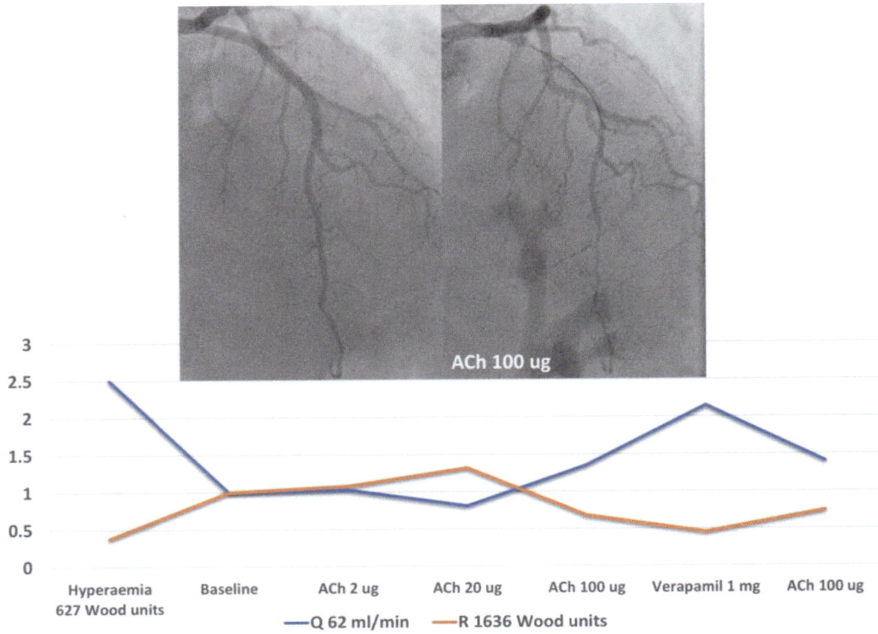

Fig. 8.2 (**Top, left to right panels**) Coronary angiogram of the left anterior descending (LAD) artery at baseline and after acetylcholine (ACh) 100 μg showing segmental and diffuse vasospasm. (**Bottom**) Flow and resistance in response to hyperaemia and drugs. Note flow reduction with ACh 20 μg and increase with ACh 100 μg, but not quite > 50%; verapamil prevents ACh-induced epicardial vasospasm but has no effect on microvascular endothelial function

units—thus, coronary flow reserve (CFR) is 2.5 and microvascular resistance reserve (MRR) 2.6. Escalating doses of ACh are given, 2 μg has no effects, 20 μg is associated with moderate proximal epicardial vasospasm with a Pd/Pa of 0.93 and a ↓19% fall in flow with ↑32% rise in resistance, and 100 μg is associated with severe proximal LAD, as well as diffuse mid to distal vasospasm, Pd/Pa 0.75, but despite this, flow actually rises by ↑35% with a ↓32% fall in resistance—she is without symptoms. She is given IC verapamil 1 mg, which doubles the flow and halves the resistance, and then rechallenged with ACh 100 μg. This time, no epicardial vasospasm is seen, with flow and resistance similar to those seen earlier during epicardial vasospasm.

Interpretation This woman has *hypertension, raised LVEDP and increased coronary resistance*, and *generalised endothelial dysfunction* as evidenced by *ACh-induced epicardial vasospasm* and *microvascular endothelial dysfunction*; the LAD flow does not rise beyond 50% in response to ACh. Her vasodilatory capacity is however preserved. In view of pre-treatment with verapamil being effective *in vivo*, she was initiated on diltiazem and then switched to lercanidipine. But these calcium channel blockers were not tolerated; hence she was converted to nebivolol instead. The priority is to control her hypertension. Her last ambulatory BP monitor (ABPM) showed a daytime mean of 111/63 mmHg with a normal night-time dip 2 years later—suggesting a well-controlled BP.

8.2.2 Apical Ballooning

A 63-year-old Caucasian woman has angina that appeared to respond to diltiazem with the presumptive diagnosis of microvascular angina. She was admitted about 3 years ago with an acute coronary syndrome characterised by deep T-wave inversion across her chest leads on 12-lead ECG, peak troponin T of 383 (< 14) ng/L, echocardiographic EF of 35%, unobstructed coronary arteries and apical ballooning on LV angiogram (Fig. 8.3). There was no apparent stressful trigger, and she woke up at 7.00 am with chest pain and a sense of foreboding and suffocation. The pain lasted for 4 hours and finally relieved by nitroglycerine given at the hospital. Her CMR performed at day 10 showed an EF of 28%, ESVI 58 (13–31) mL/m^2, SVI 23 (36–60) mL/m^2 and VAC 2.5 (0.5–1.0), confirming TTS. Two years before when she was 58, she was investigated for palpitations, chest pain and breathlessness. Her echocardiogram, CT coronary angiogram and Holter were all non-contributory, and she was reassured but was continued on her propranolol which she took for *migraine*. She stopped smoking following her hip surgery when she was 49, had gastric ulcer 5 years later requiring endoscopic treatment, and suffered disabling back and joint pains, requiring amitriptyline and buprenorphine 5 µg patches, a potent opioid. Her cardiac function improved on heart failure treatment over the next 2 years. At year

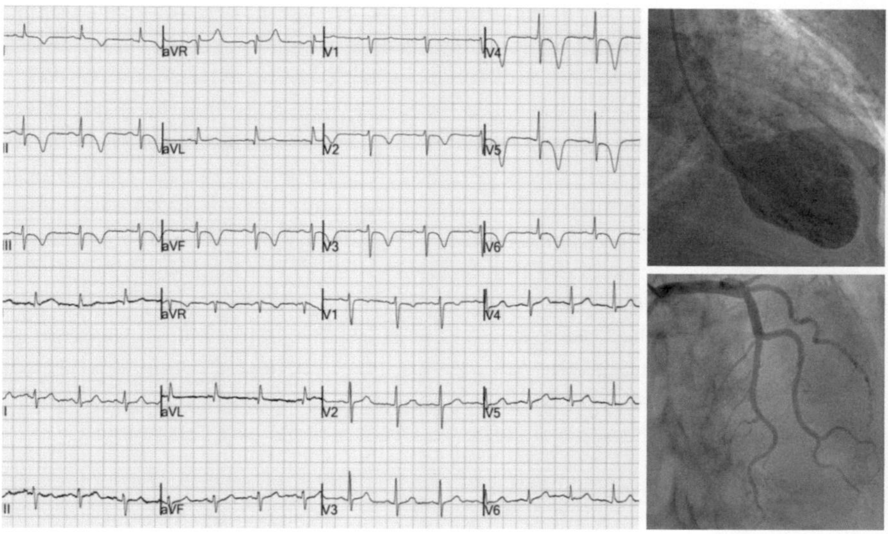

Fig. 8.3 (**Left, top and bottom panels**) Electrocardiogram (ECG) shows deep T-wave across a majority of the ECG leads, apart from aVR, aVL and V1. This is consistent with mid to apical stress cardiomyopathy, sparing the basal septum and high lateral wall. The ECG normalised at follow-up, with marked improvement in cardiac function. (**Right, top and bottom panels**) Left ventricular angiogram shows dilated apical and mid ventricle. This is done on day 3 following presentation, which explains the less impressive apical ballooning and a left ventricular end-diastolic pressure (LVEDP) of 5 mmHg, suggesting some degree of functional recovery. The coronary arteries are without significant disease, with a moderate lesion in mid-diagonal branch

4 from her TTS presentation, her echocardiographic EF was 56% with borderline dilated LA, without LVH, ESVI 22 mL/m^2, SVI 25 mL/m^2 and VAC 0.88 (2.5, 0.6-1.0), and average E/e' 6 (< 8). In contrast, her echocardiogram performed as part of her cardiac assessment 2 years before her TTS admission, and her EF was 60–65% with an undilated LA, implying that she has sustained subclinical LV systolic dysfunction.

Looking at her acute and recovery ECGs side by side (Fig. 8.3), there are a couple more interesting features beyond the widespread giant T-wave inversion: **1.** The transition chest lead, where R and S are of equal amplitude, is rotated to the left on horizontal axis in V4 during TTS presentation, and it is back in V2 at recovery; and **2.** the left ventricle facing (II, V4–6) leads' S/R amplitudes are much taller during TTS, at least doubled, and these settled later with LV recovery. This is a great example of the magnifying effect of increased blood volume within the dilated LV, as it conducts electricity well. This **Brody effect** [12] as published in 1956 is named after Daniel A. Brody (1915–1975) [13] and was elegantly confirmed by Castini et al. in 1996 [14, 15]. They demonstrated that reduced echocardiographic end-diastolic LV diameter with proximal cuff venous occlusion of the 4 limbs 10 mmHg below diastolic BP, within 5 minutes in 14 healthy men positively related to the front-facing R amplitude. This might explain the reduction in R amplitude during exercise under normal circumstances. If the opposite occurs, this can be a sign of ischaemia with exercise-induced LV dilatation.

In contrast with TTS, Ary L. Goldberger [16] in 1982 noted discordance in the R/S amplitude between the limb and chest leads in patients with idiopathic dilated cardiomyopathy (DCM). While cardiac fibrosis and thinning of myocardium reduce limb leads' R, the increased intraventricular blood volume through the Brody effect continues to magnify the R/S amplitude in chest leads—the **Goldberger triad**: **1.** *tall chest lead complexes*, SV1 or SV2 + RV5 or RV6 $\geq$ 3.5 mV; **2.** *low limb lead voltages,* total QRS amplitude $\leq$ 0.8 mV in all six limb leads (I, II, III, aVR, aVL, aVF); and **3.** *poor R progression,* R/S ratio < 1 in lead V4—with a high specificity of 99% for detecting dilated cardiomyopathy.

She was referred to the coronary physiology clinic, where she described her continuing angina which she experienced on the daily basis, at rest but not on exertion. She has no hypertension, diabetes or hyperlipidaemia, but her father who was a heavy smoker had coronary artery disease in his 40s. Her BMI was 24 kg/m2. In view of her burden of symptoms, she agreed to have the catheter-based investigation.

Procedure The LV is studied first, and the LVEDP is 15 mmHg, not rising with handgrip and central aortic BP 120/70 mmHg. As expected, her coronary arteries are unobstructed, and a pressure wire is advanced down the LAD; Pd/Pa is 0.95 and RFR 0.95 (>0.89). Continuous thermodilution is carried out with the following basal and hyperaemic values: flow 85 and 222 mL/min and resistance 1035 and 387 Wood units—CFR 2.6 and MRR 2.7 (Fig. 8.4). Increasing IC ACh doses are given—2, 20, 100 and 200 μg. With the first 2 doses, the flow falls by a third with a corresponding rise in resistance, and with reduction in epicardial calibre, but without a fall in Pd/Pa. With the 2 larger doses, the flow rises back to baseline with significant diffuse

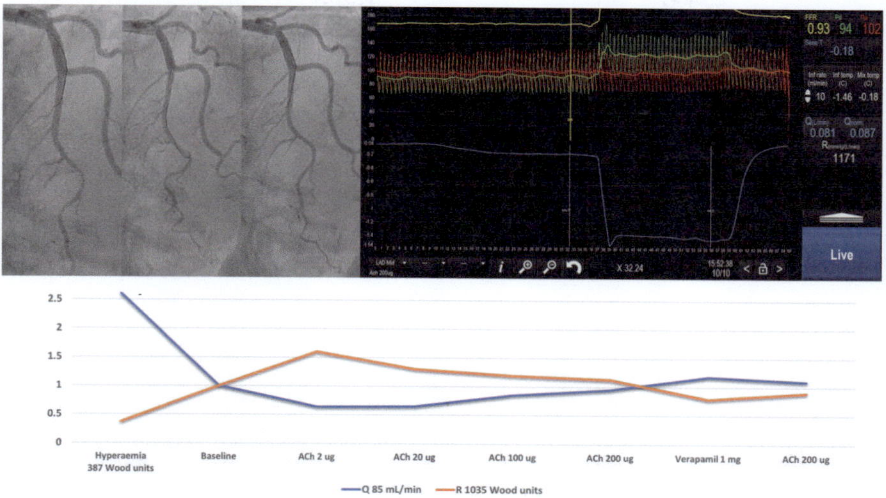

Fig. 8.4 (**Top, left and right panels**) Left anterior descending (LAD) artery showing moderate mid vessel reduction in calibre with acetylcholine (ACh) 20 µg, significantly more vasospasm with ACh 200 µg, which is ameliorated with rechallenge at the same dose following pre-treatment with verapamil 1 mg—the sequence of the LAD angiograms → ACh 20, 200 and repeat 200 µg after verapamil. Continuous thermodilution after ACh 200 µg, there is no obvious fall in Pd/Pa 0.93 and the LAD flow is roughly at the same basal level. (**Bottom**) Continuous thermodilution at baseline, hyperaemia and following ACh and verapamil. Note initial fall in flow, returning to baseline despite LAD vasospasm

mid to distal LAD vasospasm, again, without an obvious fall in Pd/Pa. Verapamil IC 1 mg increases flow by ↑18%. When rechallenged with ACh 200 µg, the epicardial vasospasm is ameliorated with a higher flow and ↑15% more compared to a prior challenge at the same ACh dose. Despite fluctuation in flow, she has no symptoms, neither does she exhibit ischaemic ECG.

Interpretation This woman has prior symptoms predating her TTS hospitalisation and continues to be symptomatic with a heart that does not fully recover her pre-TTS EF. This may explain the borderline raised LVEDP with mild LA dilatation in spite of normalisation of her VAC. She has preserved vasodilatory capacity and normal coronary resistance but exhibits a dose-dependent epicardial vasospasm with "preserved" flow but not rising > 50% suggesting concomitant *microvascular endothelial dysfunction*. Verapamil pre-treatment reduces epicardial vasospasm and marginally increases the LAD flow with high-dose ACh rechallenge. Her usual symptoms are not reproduced in vivo although she has *generalised endothelial dysfunction*. The blunted (microvascular) flow (< 1.5) in response to verapamil would be consistent with shunting to non-nitric oxide pathways within the microvasculature (discussed later and Chap. 7).

This woman had a recurrence of her TTS 22 months later, and she was bereaved of her mother passing 10 months before, after living with her as her carer for a period of time. The trigger was the stress of having to deal with the lost and resulting paperwork; this was despite being on **diltiazem 60 mg bd** which she had continued uninterrupted. She had chest pain, her troponin I peaked on admission at 517 (< 12) ng/L with widespread T-wave inversion on her ECG. Her LV improved from an EF of 31% to 55–60%, VAC 0.6 (0.6-1.0) two months later on echocardiogram, and her CMR on this second TTS admission on day 5 showed an EF of 41% and VAC 1.5 (0.6-1.0) with the characteristic increased T1/2 mapping values in mid LV suggestive of myocardial oedema. She was switched back to bisoprolol 1.25 mg od.

8.2.3 Cardiac Arrest

A 48-year-old Caucasian woman was referred for coronary vasospasm testing. Three months prior, after her bootcamp exercises, she developed left thigh pain followed by severe chest pain causing her to double up. She was admitted to a local hospital where in the emergency department she had a witnessed cardiac arrest due to ventricular fibrillation, for which she had a single DC shock, and 3 cycles of chest compressions. She was intubated and ventilated on-site. Her emergency coronary angiogram there found unobstructed coronary arteries, ECG showed widespread T-wave inversion, and her echocardiogram revealed severe LV systolic dysfunction with an EF of under 35%. She was transferred to St George's Hospital for further management. Her day 6 echocardiogram showed rapid improvement in her cardiac function, with increased EF to 52%, and CMR on day 9 found a high EF of 69%, undilated LA, no LVH, ESVI 29 (16–34) mL/m², SVI 64 (39–63) mL/m² and VAC 0.45 (0.6–1.0) (Fig. 8.5). There were diffusely increased native T1 and T2 mapping values in the absence of late gadolinium enhancement, suggesting widespread

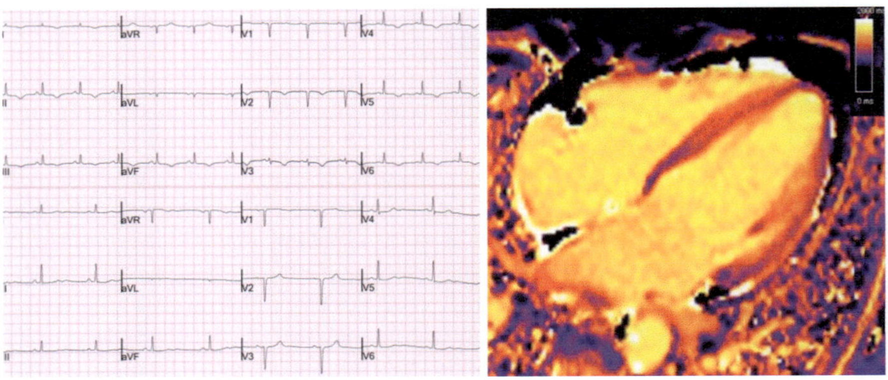

Fig. 8.5 (**Left, top and bottom panels**) The 12-lead electrocardiogram (ECG) shows widespread T inversion, apart from an upright T in aVR, which is normally inverted consistent with "whole" or mid to apical ventricular dysfunction. The repeat ECG 3 months later shows normalisation. (**Left**) Cardiovascular magnetic resonance (CMR) scan T2 colour mapping with scattered orange high readings, in the absence of late gadolinium enhancement and rapid reversal of cardiac dysfunction; these are features of Takotsubo syndrome

myocardial oedema. She in addition had aspiration pneumonia and was found to have a segmental right upper lobe pulmonary embolus and subtle bilateral small cerebellar infarctions. She was duly anticoagulated with a direct oral anticoagulant (DOAC), apixaban 5 mg twice a day, started on a beta blocker, bisoprolol 1.25 mg once a day, and had a surface AICD implanted. She had become menopausal 6 months before her cardiac arrest and had in fact been started on hormonal replacement therapy (HRT) skin patch. She has a BMI of 22 kg/m^2 and history of *migraine*. Her cardiac electrophysiological and genetic testing found no predisposition for a cardiac arrest. When she came in for her coronary physiology study, she has a low 25-hydroxyvitamin D level 42 (> 50) ng/mL, FSH 23 (> 50, FSH falls with HRT) mIU/mL and oestradiol 637 (> 92) pmol/L on a reduced HRT patch frequency, using it once every 2 days. It also transpired that prior to her cardiac event she was a heavy user of **nicotine gum** 4 mg x 30 a day—120 mg a day (well above the upper limit of 80 mg a day). Nicotine is a potent cause of endothelial dysfunction (Chaps. 3 and 7).

Procedure She has a normal LV with an LVEDP of 8 mmHg, not rising with handgrip, with a central aortic BP of 114/60 mmHg. Her coronary angiogram finds no significant coronary artery disease, but she develops catheter-induced vasospasm in her right coronary artery, responsive to IC nitroglycerine, which instead gives her a *headache* (Fig. 8.6). Initially, bolus thermodilution is performed to her LAD, Pd/Pa 0.96, RFR 0.96 (> 0.89), and following IC adenosine 200 μg, the following are obtained: FFR 0.95, CFR 6.3 and index of microvascular resistance (IMR) 11; these are normal values. Next, continuous thermodilution is undertaken with the following basal and hyperaemic haemodynamic indices: flow 55 and 145 mL/min and resistance 1502 and 434 Wood units—CFR 2.6 and MRR 3.5. Escalating doses of ACh are given, there is no significant effect with 2 μg, and with 20 μg, the flow slows to about 3 heartbeats for the dye to traverse the whole length of LAD, and with significant slowing in flow with 100 μg and 200 μg, both associated with chest pain and ST depression, *despite flow increasing over 50% that would indicate preserved microvascular endothelial function*. However there is diffuse moderate mid to distal LAD vasospasm, but without significant reduction in distal perfusion pressure. Verapamil 1 mg doubles the flow (no CSFP—one heartbeat to cross LAD), yet it does not ameliorate the effects of ACh 200 μg rechallenge despite preventing epicardial vasospasm—the CSFP reappears with similarly augmented flow, with chest pain and ST depression (Fig. 8.7)—the *paradoxical cardiac ischaemia with increased flow*.

Interpretation This woman who had TTS and her follow-up CMR at 6 months showed a completely normalised heart; she has widely patent coronary arteries, preserved vasodilatory capacity, but evident *epicardial endothelial dysfunction*, because the vessel calibre reduces in response to ACh, plus vasoreactivity as demonstrated by the RCA vasospasm due to the catheter engagement and manipulation. Also, the rise in her LAD flow > 50% with ACh implies preservation of microvascular endothelial function. The *coronary slow flow phenomenon (CSFP)* with high-dose ACh is counterintuitive, which is associated with chest pain and ST depression; ***this is quintes-***

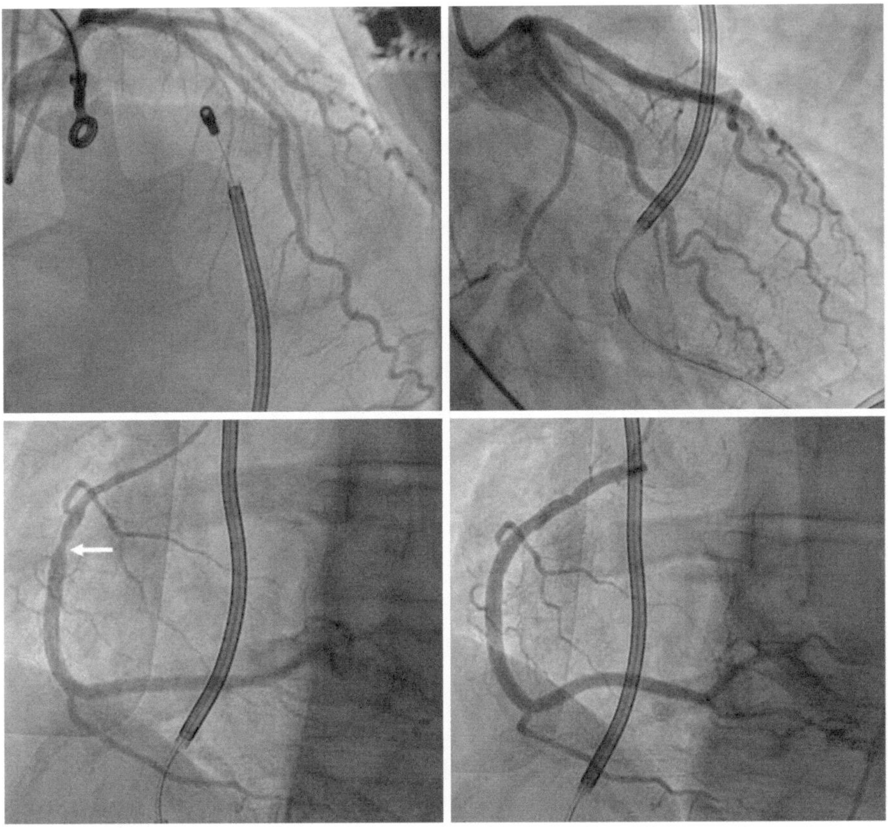

Fig. 8.6 (**Top, left and right panels**) Diagnostic coronary angiogram, which shows disease-free left coronary artery, highlighting the left anterior descending (LAD) artery on the left and the circumflex artery on the right. Note the surface automatic implantable cardioverter-defibrillator (Surface AICD) lead attached to a pad overlying the left ventricle. (**Bottom, Left and right panels**) The 4 Fr JR 4 catheter caused right coronary artery spasm and pressure-damping; it was switched to an MPA2 4Fr catheter with side holes. The *arrow* points to a discrete spasm in mid vessel, although the whole of proximal RCA is hugging the catheter. The spasm is relieved with intracoronary nitroglycerine (GTN)

sentially a "definitive" diagnosis for microvascular spasm. However, this occurred despite absolute volumetric flow increase and even following *verapamil pre-treatment, which prevented ACh-induced epicardial vasospasm and logically, would have abolished the microvascular spasm too*. This could suggest a yet "undefined vasodilatory ACh effect" on the microvasculature even when oestrogen is replete with HRT. Verapamil up to 1 mg is highly effective in relieving coronary microvascular spasm related to PCI during STEMI due clots and atherosclerotic debris embolisation [17–20]. One elaborate possibility is that *ACh has differential effects in different myocardial layers, selective subendocardial* microvascular compression from raised interstitial pressure from ACh-induced capillary leak and general microvascular vasodilatation through a different endothelium-dependent pathway, such as the

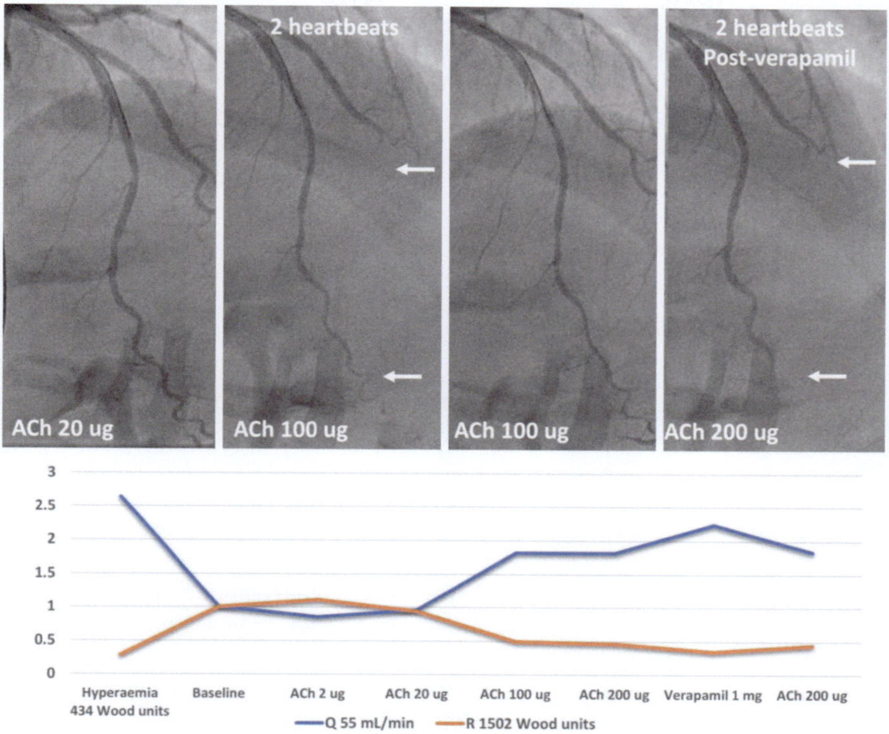

Fig. 8.7 (**Top, left to right panels**) At baseline, the contrast travels down the left anterior descending (LAD) artery under 1 heartbeat. Acetylcholine (ACh) 20 μg slows this down to 3 heartbeats, more so with ACh 100 μg, the *arrows* show the extent of the dye at 2 heartbeats and with the LAD fully opacified, the calibre is reduced, but non-occlusive. This is associated with chest pain and ST depression, similar to ACh 200 μg. Even after intracoronary verapamil 1 mg, rechallenge with ACh 200 μg *prevents epicardial vasospasm*, but not the coronary slow flow phenomenon (CSFP) or the accompanying chest pain and ST depression. (**Bottom panel**) Haemodynamic plot in response to hyperaemia and drugs. There is preserved hyperaemic vasodilatory capacity with borderline coronary resistance, ACh 20 μg reduces flow slightly, but at 100 μg and 200 μg, the flow exceeds 50% which is the definition for preserved microvascular endothelial function. Although verapamil doubles flow, it has no effect on ACh beyond preventing the reduction of epicardial calibre. This begs the question, if CSFP is due to microvascular spasm, then it is resistant to calcium channel blockade, but why does the flow markedly increase?

endothelium-dependent hyperpolarising factor (EDHF), to explain the overall increase in flow (more in the discussion and previous Chap. 7—case 2).

The trigger for TTS in this case could be a dislodged venous thrombus with exercise, embolising to the lung, causing pulmonary embolism. Her bubble echocardiogram excluded a right to left heart shunt, making systemic embolism unlikely for her cardiac event. The temporal relationship with onset of menopause and use of HRT might be contributory to the presentation. HRT is known to increase thrombotic tendency, and after her dosing was reduced, the oestradiol level was within range when she had her coronary physiology study. This could have been moderated by reducing her coronary vasoreactivity, although her migraine would imply a systemic vasoreactivity and the link between migraine and TTS is known [21]. Her vitamin D level was low at the time, which is marker of endothelial dysfunction and vasoreactivity; again it is associated with TTS [22]. She remained asymptomatic, coming off her beta blocker because of hypotension, she stopped her DOAC after 6 months and was last reviewed at her 16 months' follow-up, and she was maintained on a statin alone. In retrospect, the heavy use of nicotine gum was an important factor.

8.2.4 Train Crash

A 57-year-old Caucasian woman was admitted exactly one year previously to her local hospital and then transferred to St George's Hospital. She had intermittent chest pain for 1 week following a traumatic experience, being a passenger in a train whose driver was under the influence of cocaine, the train failed to stop, went through the buffers, and collided with the station cabin, but it remained on its tracks and no major structural damages occurred. She fortunately suffered no injuries but was badly shaken. Her ECG showed T-wave inversion in anterior chest leads, with intermittent LBBB with a QRS interval of 138 ms, without first degree heart block or left axis deviation. Her troponins were not elevated by the time she was hospitalised, and her echocardiogram showed mid to apical LV dilatation. Her coronary angiogram found non-obstructive arteries, and LV angiogram revealed apical ballooning with an LVEDP of 25 mmHg and an EF of 35%. CMR performed one month later demonstrated a normalised EF of 61%, undilated LV without LVH, but septal bounce from established LBBB. The LA was not enlarged, ESVI 30 (14–33) mL/m^2, SVI 46 (37–62) mL/m^2 and VAC 0.54 (0.6–1.0). The CMR also noted down a prominent pericardial fat pad. She was continued on ramipril but complained of angina, breathlessness, and exercise intolerance at 30 yards. Her 24-hr Holter three months later found pauses but interspersed LBBB and narrow QRS, and her treadmill exercise the following 6 months, she had chest pain during stage I with downward sloping ST depression in V5–6 and stopped exercising after completing stage II of the Bruce protocol because of breathlessness and fatigue. Baseline and peak HR and BP were 74 bpm, 114/64 mmHg and 146 bpm, 156/76 mmHg, respectively—achieving 89% predicted maximal HR, and demonstrated no chronotropic incompetence. Her chest pain resolved during recovery. She has no risk factors for coronary artery disease beyond smoking and has a BMI of 32 kg/m^2. She was on vitamin D supplementation.

Procedure Her coronary physiology study starts with the LV; there are no wall motion abnormalities, LVEDP 5 mmHg, not rising significantly with handgrip, with a central aortic BP of 130/80 mmHg. She has short left main coronary artery, as the 5Fr EBU 3.5 guiding catheter preselected her circumflex artery, and this artery is studied. As before, her coronary arteries are unobstructed. When continuous thermodilution is performed, air is inadvertently introduced via the RayFlow

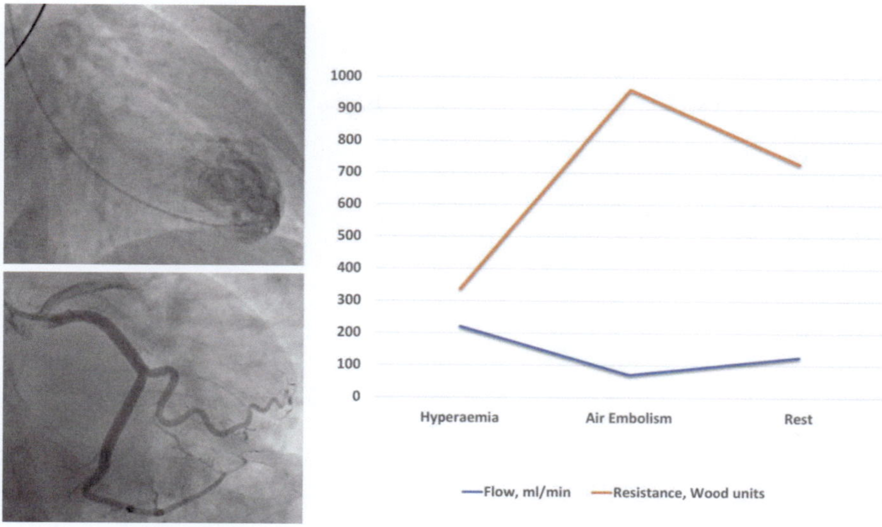

Fig. 8.8 (**Left, top and bottom panels**) Left ventricular angiogram one year previously that shows apical ballooning and unobstructed dominant circumflex artery. (**Right panel**) The coronary resistance increases by a third following an air embolus with slow flow and ST elevation and the flow halved

microcatheter down the artery, unnoticed at the time with slow flow and ST elevation (Fig. 8.8). After normal flow is established, the following basal and hyperaemic indices are obtained: flow 126 and 220 mL/min and resistance 337 and 729 Wood units—Pd/Pa 1.00, FFR 0.98, CFR 1.8 and MRR 2.2 (Fig. 8.9). ACh causes a dose-dependent segmental epicardial vasospasm with a significant fall in perfusion pressure culminating in chest pain with ACh 80 µg. With the first 2 ACh doses of 20 µg and 40 µg, the flow > 50% suggesting preserved microvascular endothelial function which failed to autoregulate or compensate when the Pd/Pa fell to 0.58. She has normal thyroid function test, and her oestradiol is < 92 pmol/L and follicular-stimulating hormone (FSH) 59.5 (> 50) mIU/mL suggesting that she is postmenopausal and oestrogen deficient despite using a hormonal coil and gel, at the time of her procedure. (The figures below are adapted with permission from Elsevier of the published article, "Lim PO, Convalescent Takotsubo Syndrome and Absolute Coronary Flow During Acetylcholine-Provoked Coronary Vasospasm, CJC Open, 2023;5:310-311".)

Interpretation This postmenopausal woman had a classical presentation of TTS, with a distinct relatable stress trigger. Her cardiac function normalised within the month, but her LBBB became established. LBBB by itself could cause exercise-related cardiac ischaemia and angina and a 10% prevalence rate of dilated cardiomyopathy every 5 years [23]. She has unobstructed coronary arteries, high basal flow which would suggest that she has preserved vasodilatory capacity, in addition to a normally functioning microvasculature, that could increase flow by > 50% in

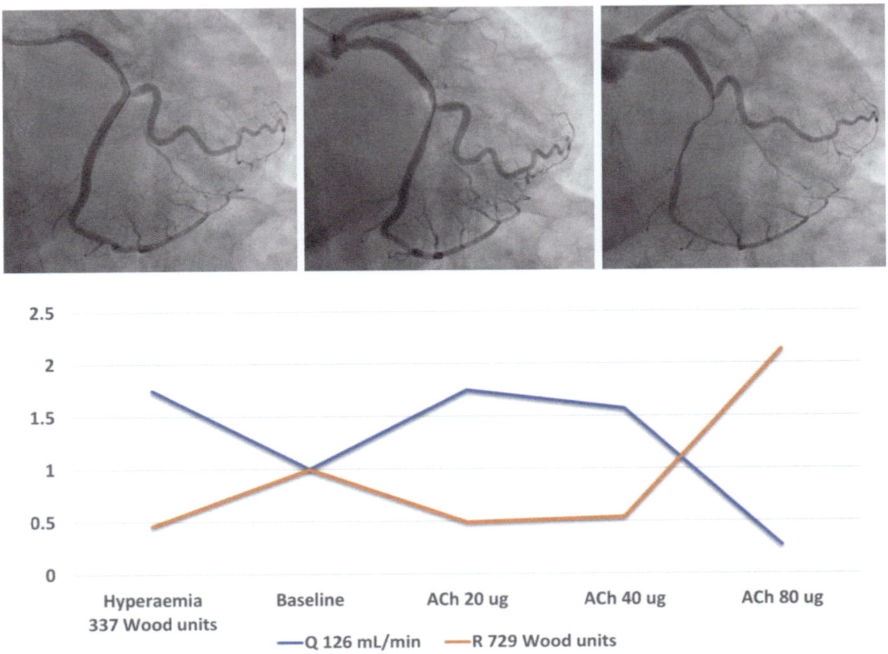

Fig. 8.9 **(Top, left to right panels)** Acetylcholine (ACh) 20 μg causes mid circumflex (Cx) artery vasospasm, associated with a Pd/Pa of 0.86, but increases flow 1.75-fold, with falling resistance by 51%; ACh 40 μg induces more mid Cx vasospasm across the obtuse marginal branch with a Pd/Pa of 0.79 (< 0.80), flow rises 1.57-fold and resistance falls by 46% and ACh 80 μg provokes severe Cx vasospasm in mid to distal vessel including the obtuse marginal branch with a Pd/Pa of 0.58 (< 0.80) with roughly halving the flow and doubling the resistance. This is associated with chest pain and electrocardiographic ST depression. (**Bottom panel**) Haemodynamic plot of flow and resistance at baseline, hyperaemia and in response to escalating doses of ACh. Note the high flow and low resistance at rest, which give the spuriously low coronary flow reserve (CFR) and microvascular resistance reserve (MRR). The first 2 doses of ACh increase flow despite worsening Cx epicardial vasospasm, and ACh 80 μg causes severe Cx vasoconstriction, precipitous rise in resistance and fall in flow causing chest pain and electrocardiographic ST depression

response to ACh which would imply intact microvascular endothelial function. The high resting flow which reduces her CFR < 2 might be due to partial hyperaemia from the 10 mL/min saline infusion rate despite her circumflex artery being codominant, and the recommendation is to reduce the saline infusion rate to 8 mL/min for a smaller vessel [24]. Also, the fact that she develops symptomatic epicardial vasospasm means that she has *isolated epicardial vasoreactivity* related to epicardial endothelial dysfunction. This would be related to smoking and oestrogen deficiency. As diltiazem SR 120 mg twice a day was not controlling her symptoms, she was switched to nebivolol, advised to stop smoking, lose weight and consider HRT. At three years follow-up she has become more breathless; this could be related to her LBBB with widening QRS to 160 ms, associated with deterioration of her EF to 45%. She has since been referred for consideration of conduction system pacing.

8.3 Discussion

8.3.1 Microvascular Angina, but Without Vasoconstriction

Of the four cases described, the common denominators are menopausal status and *epicardial vasoreactivity*, none of these woman has CMD, and of the three rechallenged with ACh following verapamil, epicardial vasospasm was abolished, yet flow was not significantly altered, in one patient, case 3—CSFP reappeared with ST depression and chest pain at the same level of augmented flow (ACh 200 μg ↑82%, Verapamil 1 mg ↑124%, and ACh 200 μg ↑84%—minus epicardial vasospasm). It is important to note that the high-dose ACh-provoked epicardial vasospasm in cases 1–3 was not associated with flow reduction, in cases 1 and 3, the flow actually increased, while in case 2, it was flat and case 4 the flow fell with segmental circumflex artery vasospasm—this was likely to be related to smoking-induced endothelial dysfunction (Table 8.1). In other words, although L-type calcium channel blockade is the first choice therapy in ACh-elicited coronary vasospasm, it is either poorly tolerated or its effect on the microvascular level is less obvious as discussed in the previous chapter.

Case 3's biphasic response has not previously been described in the medical literature with absolute flow estimation, and ACh-induced CSFP due to microvascular spasm which was refractory to IC verapamil is an unlikely explanation for two reasons:

1. IC verapamil increased absolute volumetric flow after the first ACh 200 μg challenge which meant that if there was microvascular spasm this was abolished with a ↑124% flow increase from baseline.
2. If there was microvascular spasm with ACh 200 μg pre- and post-verapamil, the flow should fall, not increased by ↑82% and ↑84%, respectively. Interestingly, the CSFP was not seen with verapamil, but with ACh, it was dissociated from flow, and this was discussed in Chap. 4.

The phenomenon of increased flow due to microvascular vasodilatation, yet causing cardiac ischaemia is the ***Oldenburg Paradox***, as discussed in Chap. 1. Briefly, the presumptive explanation is that in the setting of endothelial dysfunction, where nitric oxide bioavailability is compromised and its pathway suppressed, alternate vasodilatory mechanisms are recruited, which are also endothelium-dependent, such as the hyperpolarising factors and prostanoids, coupled with ACh-induced postcapillary venular leakiness [25], raising capillary-blood filtration, which momentarily overcomes lymphatic drainage, and thus interstitial pressure rises, and this compresses the subendocardial venules exacerbated by a raised LVEDP, with resultant flow diversion to the epicardium, and reduced flow to the endocardium. Further, nitrates via venodilatation reduce the venular pressure exacerbate the situation, firstly by making the venules compressible from *without* in the context of a raised interstitial pressure and secondly by increasing arteriolar-venular gradient collapsing the venules from *within* as per Starling's resistor/collapsible-tube model, the so-called waterfall effect. On positron emission tomography (PET) or CMR this would appear as subendocardial hypoperfusion. Since this is a mechanical compression due to

Table 8.1 Coronary physiology and Takotsubo syndrome

Case	Age	BMI	Comorbidities	Vasodilatory capacity (CFR)	Coronary resistance (Wood units)	Vasoreactivity (ACh)
1	46♀	25	**Mid LV TTS 8.5 years**, pituitary empty Sella, primary limb lymphoedema, asthma, hypertension, coeliac disease, hyperlipidaemia and menopause at mid-30 s CMR EF 84%, VAC 0.20	LAD 2.5 LAD wraps around LV apex but small calibre distally, large Cx, and RCA/RPDA supplies the LV base (LAD - left anterior descending artery, Cx - circumflex artery, RCA - right coronary artery and RPDA - right posterior descending artery)	**627** MRR 2.6 LVEDP 15 → 20 handgrip BP 158/86	Dose-dependent epicardial vasospasm with ACh 2 (↑3%), 20 (↓19%) and 100 (↑35%) μg (Pd/Pa 0.98 → 0.96 → 0.93 → 0.75) but without flow reduction Verapamil (↑115%) abolished the epicardial vasospasm ACh 100 ug (↑40% - **Δ↑5%**)
2	63♀	24	**Apical and mid TTS 3 years**, with subclinical LV systolic dysfunction, ex-smoker, ***migraine***, gastric ulcer and joints pain Recurrent TTS 22 months later, on diltiazem 60 mg bd	LAD 2.6 LAD and RCA/RPDA both reach the LV apex, and small Cx	387 MRR 2.7 LVEDP 15 → 15 handgrip BP 120/70	Diffuse distal spasm with flow reduction ACh 2 (↓36%), 20 (↓35%), 100 (↓15%), 200 μg (↓5%) Verapamil 1 mg (↑18%) abolished the epicardial vasospasm ACh 200 μg (↑10% - **Δ↑15%**)

3	48♀	22	**Global TTS with VF 3 months**, ***migraine***, **vitamin D deficiency**, early menopause on HRT and heavy nicotine gum use	LAD Bolus thermodilution 6.3 Continuous thermodilution 2.6 LAD wraps around LV apex, RCA and Cx are equal size	IMR 11 **434** MRR 3.5 LVEDP 8 → 8 handgrip BP 114/60	Flow reduction ACh 2 (↓15%, Pd/Pa 0.92), 20 (↓4%, Pd/pa 0.96, CSFP), 100 (↑82%, Pd/Pa 0.92, CSFP) and 200 μg (↑82%, Pd/pa 0.88, CSFP)—dose-dependent epicardial vasospasm and CSFP Verapamil 1 mg (↑124%, Pd/Pa 0.96) with fast flow and abolished the epicardial vasospasm ACh 20 μg (↑84 **Δ↑2%**, Pd/Pa 0.96, CSFP)
4	57♀	32	**Apical TTS 1 year**, LBBB QRS 135 ms, smoking, **vitamin D deficiency** and menopause Pericardial fat pad on CMR	Cx 1.8 **126** → 220 Raised baseline flow (the 10 mL/min saline infusion rate could have caused partial hyperaemia despite the Cx being a codominant vessel) LAD wraps around LV apex, modest-sized Cx, and RCA/RPDA reaches mid LV	729 → 337 MRR 2.2 LVEDP 5 → 5 handgrip BP 130/80	Dose-dependent epicardial vasospasm with ACh 20 (↑75%), 40 (↑57%) and 80 (↓73%) μg (Pd/Pa 1.00 → 0.86 → 0.79 → 0.58)

microvascular vasodilatation and not vasoconstriction, calcium channel blockade will not work, as increasingly acknowledged in recent studies, such as the EDIT-CMD (Efficacy of Diltiazem to Improve Coronary Microvascular Dysfunction) [26–29] and CorCTA (Coronary Microvascular Function and CT Coronary Angiogram) [30–33].

8.3.2 TTS Triggers

TTS occurs predominantly in postmenopausal women, mostly of the apical LV variant, less commonly involving the mid ventricle, and rarely the basal subtype which has been reported with higher prevalence in pheochromocytoma [34, 35], and subarachnoid haemorrhage [36, 37]. TTS is thought to be triggered by catecholamine surge with underlying CMD, among many other hypotheses [38–42]. Sato was familiar with the ECG pattern following subarachnoid haemorrhage, a hyperadrenergic event which would indicate associated TTS, noted since the 1950s [2]. Although the *fleeting* CMD hypothesis is increasingly overstated since acute features of CMD are short-lived, and patients with *pre-existing* CMD are not predisposed to developing TTS [43, 44]. Most TTS patients are asymptomatic prior to TTS, their acute haemodynamic features of CMD are artefactual mimics from low BP and high LVEDP [43], and in the majority of cases, their heart normalised within days to weeks.

Nevertheless, there is roughly a 2% recurrence rate per annum [45, 46], yet not preventable by beta blockade suggesting that catecholamine surge is not a universal requirement for TTS as challenged by Angelini earlier, or idiomatically put, “it is a spark, but not the only matchstick in the box” [45, 47]. Neither do calcium channel blockers prevent TTS recurrence as seen in case 2 (diltiazem 60 mg bd), which goes against epicardial or microvascular spasm as a necessary trigger [8, 48]. Abu-Fanne et al. reported a 76-year-old woman with recurrent TTS; the second TTS episode was related to an asthmatic exacerbation while taking verapamil 360 mg in three divided doses [48]. However, the long-term prognosis of TTS is driven more by age [49] and comorbidities than by persistent LV dysfunction as a result of TTS [9, 10].

As demonstrated in the four cases in this chapter, the marker for TTS appears to be epicardial endothelial dysfunction which means that their coronary arteries are vasoreactive. None of the women has CMD. TTS occurs in heart transplant patients: a 75-year-old woman 13 years post-transplant precipitated by a family argument [50]; a 44-year-old woman 15 months post-transplant, with a status epilepticus trigger [51]; and in a 67-year-old man 10 years post-transplant from work-related stress [52], which suggests cardiac innervation is not essential for TTS [50, 51]. The transplanted hearts are upregulated with β_2-adrenergic receptors in the LV, especially the apex and α_1-adrenergic receptors in the microvasculature, yet TTS is rare in cardiac transplant patients. The adrenergic receptor density hypothesis does not easily explain the non-apical variants of TTS. There is as yet no translatable animal models of TTS [6, 53–55]. TTS cannot be induced in animals at physiological doses of adrenaline seen in humans [54], and TTS is relatively uncommon in pheochromocytoma, 8–11%, yet nearly a third are at LV base, a quarter global LV, and still with a female preponderance [34, 56–58].

8.3.3 Oestrogen

TTS predominantly affects women, so does spontaneous coronary artery dissection (SCAD) (Fig. 8.10). It is possible that these two cardiac conditions are 2 sides of the same coin, the latter is associated with too much and the former too little oestrogen. However, large TTS registries do not collect data on HRT use [59]; hence "efficacy by omission", but combining TTS from two small studies where HRT use was documented, it was 15/70 or 21%, in accord with the 4 patients described here, ¼ or 25% [21, 60]. It makes logical sense that HRT is protective if initiated early, but unclear in what formulation, at which dose, and if oestrogen works in synergy with other hormones [55, 61, 62].

When case 3 was studied, this woman developed epicardial vasospasm despite an oestradiol level 637 (> 92) pmol/L, well above 250 pmol/L recommended for bone protection [63]. This could be related to her general vasoreactivity given that she suffered from migraine and importantly, with her judicious use of nicotine gum. Interestingly, migraine has been flagged up as being more common in TTS, with a prevalence of 44% (11/25) in a small case series linking systemic vasoreactivity with TTS [21]. Case 2 also has migraine, making this cohort of four TTS patients with 50% migraine prevalence.

Oestrogen is a potent vasodilator, acting on multiple fronts: endothelial NO synthase (eNOS) gene transcription in the endothelium, it inhibits endothelial production of endothelin-1, it amplifies the endothelium-dependent hyperpolarising factor (EDHF) pathway which reduces Ca^{2+} influx into the vascular smooth muscle cell (VSMC), it increases prostacyclin (PGI_2), which is a vasodilator, and it directly modulates VSMC contractile signalling pathways [64–67]. Previous SCAD is a contraindication for *systemic* HRT, but not topical or transdermal preparations, because of the potential link with recurrent cardiac events [68–70]. The stress of pregnancy and labour with hormonal excess account for a third of SCAD cases in women under 40 [71]. Hypertension and pre-eclampsia are cumulative risk factors [69]. Taken together, the intima of a maximally dilated artery is more likely to split, especially if there is a large fluctuation of BP. Without atherosclerotic tethering, the coronary dissection spreads in piecemeal along the intimal plane, akin to a balloon or football that is hyperinflated, which makes it liable to rupture.

The flipside is having too little oestrogen which predisposes to endothelial dysfunction and coronary vasoreactivity, particularly when there are concomitant adverse coronary risk factors present such as smoking, diabetes, hypertension and hyperlipidaemia. This is illustrated by a transgender young man of 31, who 6 years previously underwent gender reassignment surgery which included bilateral salpingo-oophorectomy and testosterone hormonal therapy. His oestrogen level dropped precipitously to postmenopausal level. He developed vascular endothelial dysfunction and inducible epicardial coronary vasospasm with ACh 100 μg, although it was likely contributed by smoking too [72].

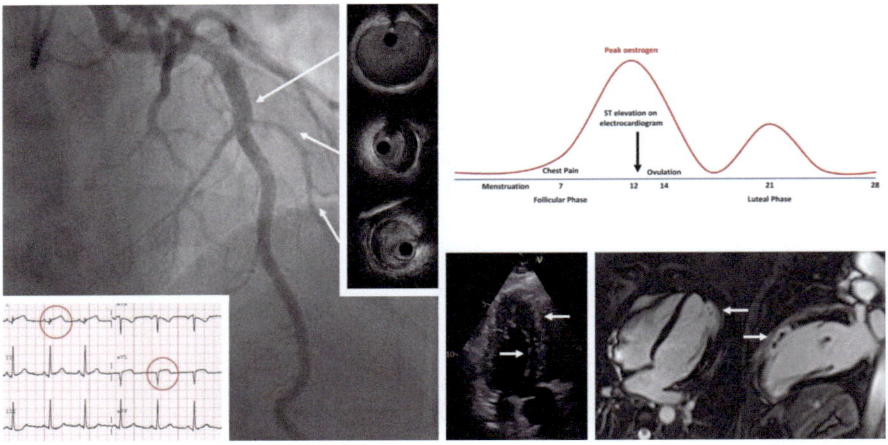

Fig. 8.10 Spontaneous coronary artery dissection and menstrual cycle. A 32-year-old woman was admitted to a local hospital with chest pain and elevated troponins. Initially without ECG changes and preserved cardiac function on echocardiogram, thus she had a diagnosis of myopericarditis. While she was an inpatient for a week, she had more chest pain with ST elevation in I and aVL, with reciprocal ST depression in aVF. She was transferred to St George's Hospital and had an urgent coronary procedure. She has no cardiac risk factors, has a BMI of 32 kg/m^2 and used a copper intrauterine device (IUD) for contraception which caused menorrhagia, plus being a regular blood donor, she donated blood a week before her hospitalisation. Her haemoglobin was 9.9 (12-15.5) g/dL and ferritin 9 (24-307) ng/L. **(Left panel)** Her ECG shows as red-circled ST elevation in the high lateral leads (*inset*), and her left anterior descending (LAD) artery changes in calibre after the diagonal branch with proximal haziness. Intravascular ultrasound (IVUS) of the diagonal branch as depicted confirms a double lumen with subintimal dissection, extending distally (*inset*). Since the diagnosis of spontaneous coronary artery dissection (SCAD) was not in doubt, IVUS was not repeated down the distal LAD to avoid exacerbating the SCAD. Her peak troponin T was 1,346 (< 14) ng/L, creatine kinase 1,491 (< 200) U/L and NT-ProBNP 1,037 (< 125) pg/mL. **(Right, top to bottom panels)** Taking a detailed menstrual history, there was a suggestion that her chest pain started on day 7 of her period, culminating with her ST elevation myocardial infarction at the presumptive peak oestrogen level during the follicular phase, before ovulation. Her echocardiogram shows dyskinetic mid anterior wall with apical left ventricular contractility (*arrows*), and cardiovascular magnetic resonance (CMR) scan shows a well circumscribed transmural infarction with microvascular obstruction (MVO) in the diagonal territory (*arrows*). It could be that her oestradiol level rose to exert maximal endothelium-dependent vasodilatation. This, coupled with the blood pressure fluctuation associated with haemodynamic stress of anaemia, speculatively caused vascular wall strain at the diagonal bifurcation, which acted like a windsock on a sailboat, thus breaking the endothelial continuity giving rise to SCAD in her case

8.3.4 Cardiac Migraine

Attilio Maseri (1935–2021) who systematically demonstrated the use of nitrates and coronary vasoreactivity, pioneered use of positron emission tomography (PET) in angina with non-obstructive coronary arteries (ANOCA), hypothesised that **pockets of microvascular ischaemia** are responsible for the angina and ECG changes. PET is the gold standard non-invasive ischaemic testing technique, but it is not widely available because it is costly to set up, expensive to maintain and upkeep, and the radioisotope tracer used could impart a radiation dosing up to 10 times that of a diagnostic coronary angiogram, at 20 mSv, or 10 years of natural ground radiation exposure. However, one unique feature of PET is its ability to measure *absolute tissue perfusion* across the myocardial layers or thickness, thus allowing *subendocardial ischaemia* (SEI) to be detected. Since normal coronary vasodilatory capacity is defined as ≥ 2.0, which is a ratio of stress versus basal flow, a high baseline flow due to expended hyperaemic reserve such as in diffuse small vessel disease, or stress and tachycardia, which increase basal flow by as much as 30%, would erroneously give a low CFR (Case 4) [73]. Further, dipyridamole used as a stressor works by increasing interstitial adenosine, a by-product from the myocytes by blocking its uptake into the red blood and endothelial cells, its excess in the surrounding of VSMC through A_2A adenosine receptor activation causes vasodilatation, and it has a short half-life of < 10 seconds. Caffeine, which is a competitive agonist of adenosine receptors, confounds PET's hyperaemic flow, giving a spuriously low CFR.

Taking all of the above into account, Johnson and Gould [74] refined and enriched their series of patients with ANOCA who had PET in Houston, Texas, over 17 years to July 2024. They looked in detail at 7,416 out of 14,008 patients without significant regional perfusion defects; of these, 314 patients had **angina and/or ST changes** during testing, and they could be split into 3 groups. The majority or 79% (248) had **SEI** with normal CFR but many of these had *structural heart disease*, 11 patients or 3.5% had low CFR, these were the "pure blood" CMD group and the rest **17.5% or 55 patients were "non-ischaemic", without demonstrable flow reduction.** In other words, in this state-of-the-art PET series, CMD was only found in 0.07% of patients over the 17 years—1 patient every 18 months. Of note, the **non-ischaemic group**, 89% (49/55) had ST depression, and 6/55 had angina, of which 7% had both angina and ST depression. Most were women, 80% (44/55) with a mean age of 64, whereas women represented 34% of the total cohort of 14,008 scans. The idea of non-ischaemic angina with or without ST depression is an interesting one. This is akin to headache due to cerebral vasodilation; hyperaemic stretching of the coronary microvasculature can activate mechanoreceptors as well as sympathetic activation with release of substance P and calcitonin gene-related peptide (CGRP), causing both chest pain and ECG changes. This is exemplified by lingering chest pain following stenting of a coronary artery. This phenomenon can perhaps aptly be called "cardiac migraine". This profound insight is consistent with the esteemed authors' [74] *non-recommendation* of a more general use of calcium channel blockers in ANOCA, without a doubt their large series encompassed many patients with reactive coronary arteries if they were tested with ACh. Further, recent RCTs such as the EDIT-CMD [26, 27, 29, 75] and CorCTA [30–33] found these drugs to lack efficacy. In other words, cardiac ischaemia with hyperaemic flow comprised 16% of the Texas PET ANOCA cohort. If the angina is due to vasodilatation, then drugs that cause vasodilatation will not be useful. Gould incidentally was the cardiologist who ushered in the coronary physiology era with his seminal work on coronary flow reserve in 1974; CFR < 2 as the working definition for cardiac ischaemia which has been adopted into routine clinical practice for both invasive and non-invasive assessments of coronary artery disease (Chap. 1) [76].

8.3.5 Flash Myocardial Oedema

As demonstrated in this chapter, the four TTS women all showed epicardial endothelial dysfunction with vasoreactivity due to multiple factors; chief among them was oestrogen deficiency, but smoking, migraine, hypertension, nicotine gum, etc. also contributed. However, case 3 woman was replete with the hormone from HRT suggesting that the postmenopausal state may be more complex with regard to vascular health. However, restoration of endothelial function with HRT is time sensitive and is not immediate. It takes at least six months to happen, and her TTS occurred three months into starting treatment [77]. Further, her high-dose nicotine gum exposure would have negated her HRT.

Sato's original hypothesis of multivessel coronary vasospasm turned out to be an epiphenomenon for TTS after all [8]. The Oldenburg Paradox through "subendocardial interstitial exudation" akin to pulmonary oedema might be the actual trigger for TTS, as a spectrum of women with ANOCA. CMR finding of increased T1/2 mapping signals as in case 3 indicates scattered oedema is a pathognomonic TTS sign [78–80].

The potential microvascular endothelial shunt from NO to EDHF pathway could prime the heart towards ischaemic myocardial stunning, as both share the "K^+-hyperpolarising and Ca^{2+}-limiting" strategy. Histologically, but with a bias towards the catecholamine-trigger, TTS myocardial tissue shares all features within the continuum of post-ischaemically stunned and infarcted myocardium: *interstitial oedema* (stunning and "vasospastic" TTS [81]), myofibrillar disruption (stunning), contraction band necrosis (infarction) and *early* mononuclear cell infiltration (TTS) [82–85]. The last histological feature would favour a rapid tissue repair, appears unique in TTS, also a sign of systemic inflammation, as seen in coronavirus 2019 (COVID-19) infection with its cytokine storm which incidentally makes the capillaries leakier and is associated with a less skewed TTS gender distribution [86, 87]. Capillary filtration is a balance of hydrostatic and oncotic pressures with intact endothelial glycocalyx plus efficient lymphatic drainage to prevent interstitial pressure rise [88]. The lymphatic capacity to drain excess fluid declines with age [89, 90]. Where there is inflammation, there is increased postcapillary venular permeability in favour of net filtration [91], so do hypoosmolality, hypoalbuminemia and hyponatraemia—they are all associated with TTS [92–94]. Importantly, canine experimental studies show that increasing the interstitial myocardial water content by three percent is enough to stun the heart [95].

The Oldenburg Paradox requires a large enough flow to increase the capillary hydrostatic pressure; this potentially explains why TTS is rare in older men because of their near universal atherosclerosis, where hyperaemic flow surge cannot be generated, but in older women, their coronary arteries are relatively unobstructed. This could also account for the TTS variants, where flow increases most during stress, for example in case 1, this woman has smaller calibre distal LAD and a dominant circumflex artery which would encourage capillary exudation in mid LV. This mid LV TTS variant has variously been called Greek vase, ace of spade and hawk's beak, and it accounts for about 15% of caseload [96, 97]. There is an indication that in these cases the LAD appears as lesser calibre, not wrapping around the LV apex

[98–101] or has disease [102]. Extrapolating this to women with ANOCA, their limited myocardial interstitial oedema causes lingering chest pain well described in cardiac syndrome x beyond thirty minutes and *unresponsive to nitrates* [103]—that is, until lymphatic clearance takes over. Smooth muscle spasm in general cannot usually be sustained before fatigue sets in, and this pain should be "colicky" in waves instead of being constant. All the above conjures up a crime scene of an impossible reach; *the clue is in the large puddle of cold water.*

References

1. Ishihara M. Takotsubo cardiomyopathy and left ventricular outflow tract obstruction. Circ J. 2015;79(4):758–60. https://doi.org/10.1253/circj.CJ-15-0089.
2. Nagai M, Dote K, Ishihara M, Kurisu S, In memoriam—Dr. Hikaru Sato: the discoverer of Takotsubo syndrome. European Heart J. 2022;43(18):1693–6. https://doi.org/10.1093/eurheartj/ehac146.
3. Kurisu S, Sato H, Kawagoe T, Ishihara M, Shimatani Y, Nishioka K, et al. Tako-tsubo-like left ventricular dysfunction with ST-segment elevation: a novel cardiac syndrome mimicking acute myocardial infarction. American Heart J. 2002;143(3):448–55. https://doi.org/10.1067/mhj.2002.120403.
4. Yasue H, Horio Y, Nakamura N, Fujii H, Imoto N, Sonoda R, et al. Induction of coronary artery spasm by acetylcholine in patients with variant angina: possible role of the parasympathetic nervous system in the pathogenesis of coronary artery spasm. Circulation. 1986;74(5):955–63. https://doi.org/10.1161/01.CIR.74.5.955.
5. Angelini P. Transient takotsubo syndrome and its recurrence: why does it happen, why does it end, and why does it rarely reappear? Int J Cardiol. 2021;330:142–4. https://doi.org/10.1016/j.ijcard.2021.02.033.
6. Angelini P, Gamero MT. Opportunities and limitations in the study of transient takotsubo syndrome in animal models. 2020.
7. Angelini P, Uribe C, Tobis JM. Pathophysiology of Takotsubo cardiomyopathy: reopened debate. Tex Heart Inst J. 2021;48(3) https://doi.org/10.14503/thij-20-7490.
8. Madias JE. Coronary vasospasm is an unlikely cause of Takotsubo syndrome, although we should keep an open mind. Int J Cardiol. 2014;176(1):1–5. https://doi.org/10.1016/j.ijcard.2014.06.069.
9. Movahed MR, Javanmardi E, Hashemzadeh M. High mortality and complications in patients admitted with Takotsubo cardiomyopathy with more than double mortality in men without improvement in outcome over the years. J Am Heart Assoc. 2025;14(10):e037219. https://doi.org/10.1161/JAHA.124.037219.
10. Schweiger V, Cammann VL, Crisci G, Gilhofer T, Schlenker R, Niederseer D, et al. Temporal trends in Takotsubo syndrome. JACC. 2024;84(13):1178–89. https://doi.org/10.1016/j.jacc.2024.05.076.
11. Templin C, Ghadri JR, Diekmann J, Napp LC, Bataiosu DR, Jaguszewski M, et al. Clinical features and outcomes of Takotsubo (stress) cardiomyopathy. N Engl J Med. 2015;373(10):929–38. https://doi.org/10.1056/NEJMoa1406761.
12. Feng L, Lin Z, Ji Y, Lim PO. Post-infarct lateral extension—Brody effect or stent thrombosis? J Electrocardiol. 2025;91:154014. https://doi.org/10.1016/j.jelectrocard.2025.154014.
13. Brody DA. A theoretical analysis of intracavitary blood mass influence on the heart-lead relationship. Circ Res. 1956;4(6):731–8. https://doi.org/10.1161/01.res.4.6.731.
14. Castini D, Vitolo E, Ornaghi M, Gentile F. Demonstration of the relationship between heart dimensions and QRS voltage amplitude. J Electrocardiol. 1996;29(3):169–73. https://doi.org/10.1016/s0022-0736(96)80078-1.

15. Mirvis DM. Physiology and biophysics in electrocardiography. J Electrocardiol. 1996;29(3):175–7. https://doi.org/10.1016/s0022-0736(96)80079-3.
16. Goldberger AL. A specific ECG triad associated with congestive heart failure. Pacing Clin Electrophysiol. 1982;5(4):593–9. https://doi.org/10.1111/j.1540-8159.1982.tb02285.x.
17. Fu Q, Lu W, Huang Y-j, Wu Q, Wang L-g, Wang H-b, et al. Verapamil reverses myocardial no-reflow after primary percutaneous coronary intervention in patients with acute myocardial infarction. Cell Biochem Biophys. 2013;67(3):911–4. https://doi.org/10.1007/s12013-013-9581-0.
18. Su Q, Li L, Liu Y. Short-term effect of verapamil on coronary no-reflow associated with percutaneous coronary intervention in patients with acute coronary syndrome: a systematic review and meta-analysis of randomized controlled trials. Clin Cardiol. 2013;36(8):E11–6. https://doi.org/10.1002/clc.22143.
19. Taniyama Y, Ito H, Iwakura K, Masuyama T, Hori M, Takiuchi S, et al. Beneficial effect of intracoronary verapamil on microvascular and myocardial salvage in patients with acute myocardial infarction. JACC. 1997;30(5):1193–9. https://doi.org/10.1016/S0735-1097(97)00277-5.
20. Vijayalakshmi K, Whittaker VJ, Kunadian B, Graham J, Wright RA, Hall JA, et al. Prospective, randomised, controlled trial to study the effect of intracoronary injection of verapamil and adenosine on coronary blood flow during percutaneous coronary intervention in patients with acute coronary syndromes. Heart. 2006;92(9):1278–84. https://doi.org/10.1136/hrt.2005.075077.
21. Scantlebury DC, Prasad A, Rabinstein AA, Best PJM. Prevalence of migraine and Raynaud phenomenon in women with apical ballooning syndrome (Takotsubo or stress cardiomyopathy). Am J Cardiol. 2013;111(9):1284–8. https://doi.org/10.1016/j.amjcard.2013.01.269.
22. Dande AS, Sena SF, Wasserman HS, Warshofsky MK, Belsky JL. Prevalence and consequences of vitamin D insufficiency in women with Takotsubo cardiomyopathy. J Clin Endocrinol Metabol. 2013;98(5):E872–E6. https://doi.org/10.1210/jc.2013-1082.
23. Thein A-S, Dixit S, Soliman EZ, Heckbert SR, Psaty BM, Gottdiener J, et al. Left bundle branch block as a risk factor for heart failure. JAMA Netw Open. 2025;8(8):e2525801–e. https://doi.org/10.1001/jamanetworkopen.2025.25801.
24. Gallinoro E, Candreva A, Colaiori I, Kodeboina M, Fournier S, Nelis O, Di Gioia G, Sonck J, van 't Veer M, Pijls NHJ, Collet C, De Bruyne B. Thermodilution-derived volumetric resting coronary blood flow measurement in humans. EuroIntervention. 2021;17(8): e672–e679. https://doi.org/10.4244/EIJ-D-20-01092
25. Claesson-Welsh L, Dejana E, McDonald DM. Permeability of the endothelial barrier: identifying and reconciling controversies. Trends Mol Med. 2021;27(4):314–31. https://doi.org/10.1016/j.molmed.2020.11.006.
26. Beneduce A, Leone Antonio M, Berry C, Chieffo A. Coronary vasomotor disorders. JACC Cardiovasc Imaging. 2022;15(9):1677–8. https://doi.org/10.1016/j.jcmg.2022.06.019.
27. Jansen Tijn PJ, Konst Regina E, de Vos A, Paradies V, Teerenstra S, van den Oord Stijn CH, et al. Efficacy of diltiazem to improve coronary vasomotor dysfunction in ANOCA. JACC Cardiovasc Imaging. 2022;15(8):1473–84. https://doi.org/10.1016/j.jcmg.2022.03.012.
28. Rahman H, Sinha A, Demir OM, Perera D. EDIT-CMD: are we comparing apples with oranges? JACC Cardiovasc Imaging. 2022;15(9):1674–6. https://doi.org/10.1016/j.jcmg.2022.04.027.
29. Stone PH. Progressive understanding of coronary microvascular disease and vasomotor dysfunction. JACC Cardiovasc Imaging. 2022;15(8):1485–7. https://doi.org/10.1016/j.jcmg.2022.04.020.
30. Berry C, Sidik NP, McEntegart MB. Response by Berry et al to letter regarding article, "invasive Endotyping in patients with angina and no obstructive coronary artery disease: a randomized controlled trial". Circulation. 2024;150(1):e5–6. https://doi.org/10.1161/circulationaha.124.069708.
31. Nishi T, Saito Y, Kobayashi Y. Letter by Nishi et al regarding article, “invasive Endotyping in patients with angina and no obstructive coronary artery disease: a randomized controlled trial”. Circulation. 2024;150(1):e3–4. https://doi.org/10.1161/CIRCULATIONAHA.124.068798.

32. Sidik NP, Stanley B, Sykes R, Morrow AJ, Bradley CP, McDermott M, et al. Invasive Endotyping in patients with angina and no obstructive coronary artery disease: a randomized controlled trial. Circulation. 2024;149(1):7–23. https://doi.org/10.1161/CIRCULATIONAHA.123.064751.
33. Taqueti VR. Prevalence of abnormal coronary function in patients with angina and no obstructive coronary artery disease on coronary computed tomography angiography: insights from the CorCTA trial. Circulation. 2024;149(1):24–7. https://doi.org/10.1161/CIRCULATIONAHA.123.066571.
34. Y-Hassan S, Falhammar H. Clinical features, complications, and outcomes of exogenous and endogenous catecholamine-triggered Takotsubo syndrome: a systematic review and meta-analysis of 156 published cases. Clin Cardiol. 2020;43(5):459–67. https://doi.org/10.1002/clc.23352.
35. Rashidghamat E, Gregory SM, Lim P. An unusual cause of myocardial infarction. BMJ. 2010;340:c1038. https://doi.org/10.1136/bmj.c1038.
36. Kumai T, Inamasu J, Watanabe E, Sugimoto K, Hirose Y. Differences between Takotsubo cardiomyopathy and reverse Takotsubo cardiomyopathy associated with subarachnoid hemorrhage. IJC Heart Vasc. 2016;11:99–103. https://doi.org/10.1016/j.ijcha.2016.05.010.
37. Shoukat S, Awad A, Nam DK, Hoskins MH, Samuels O, Higginson J, et al. Cardiomyopathy with inverted Tako-Tsubo pattern in the setting of subarachnoid hemorrhage: a series of four cases. Neurocrit Care. 2013;18(2):257–60. https://doi.org/10.1007/s12028-011-9658-9.
38. Crea F, Iannaccone G, La Vecchia G, Montone RA. An update on the mechanisms of Takotsubo syndrome: "at the end an acute coronary syndrome". J Mol Cell Cardiol. 2024;191:1–6. https://doi.org/10.1016/j.yjmcc.2024.04.009.
39. Ghadri J-R, Wittstein IS, Prasad A, Sharkey S, Dote K, Akashi YJ, et al. International expert consensus document on Takotsubo syndrome (part II): diagnostic workup, outcome, and management. Eur Heart J. 2018;39(22):2047–62. https://doi.org/10.1093/eurheartj/ehy077.
40. Ghadri J-R, Wittstein IS, Prasad A, Sharkey S, Dote K, Akashi YJ, et al. International expert consensus document on Takotsubo syndrome (part I): clinical characteristics, diagnostic criteria, and pathophysiology. Eur Heart J. 2018;39(22):2032–46. https://doi.org/10.1093/eurheartj/ehy076.
41. Pelliccia F, Kaski JC, Crea F, Camici PG. Pathophysiology of Takotsubo syndrome. Circulation. 2017;135(24):2426–41. https://doi.org/10.1161/CIRCULATIONAHA.116.027121.
42. Shetrit A, Freund O, Banai A, Amar Shamir R, Avivi I, Zornitzki L, et al. Coronary microvascular dysfunction in patients with Takotsubo syndrome. Heart Lung. 2024;68:46–51. https://doi.org/10.1016/j.hrtlng.2024.06.007.
43. Lim PO. Is index of microvascular resistance of Sisyphean utility in Takotsubo syndrome? ESC Heart Failure. 2024;11(6):4438–40. https://doi.org/10.1002/ehf2.14943.
44. Caglioni S, Mele D, Milzi A, Bergamaschi L, Pavon AG, Landi A. Impact of coronary microvascular dysfunction in Takotsubo syndrome: cause, consequence or both? Rev Cardiovasc Med. 2024;25(5):163. https://doi.org/10.31083/j.rcm2505163.
45. Raposeiras-Roubin S, Santoro F, Arcari L, Vazirani R, Novo G, Uribarri A, et al. Beta-blockers and long-term mortality in Takotsubo syndrome. JACC: Heart Failure. 2025;13(5):815–825. doi:https://doi.org/10.1016/j.jchf.2024.11.015.
46. Lim PO. Is Takotsubo syndrome's 2% annual recurrence rate reducible? Am J Cardiol. 2023;209:242–3. https://doi.org/10.1016/j.amjcard.2023.09.061.
47. Ducharme A. A critical appraisal of Beta-blocker therapy in Takotsubo syndrome. JACC: Heart Failure. 2025;13(5):826–828. doi:https://doi.org/10.1016/j.jchf.2025.02.012.
48. Abu-Fanne R, Rott D, Klein M, Leitersdorf E, Pollak A. Recurrent apical ballooning despite treatment with verapamil. Cardiology. 2007;108(3):210–3. https://doi.org/10.1159/000096779.
49. Lim PO. Complete stent coverage of the coronary bifurcation is an outdated concept. European Heart J Case Rep. 2024;8(5) https://doi.org/10.1093/ehjcr/ytae168.
50. Covino S, Marotta L, Delle Femine FC, D'Arienzo D, Liccardo B, Natale F, et al. The conundrum of biventricular Takotsubo syndrome after heart transplantation: a case report. Transplant Proc. 2025; https://doi.org/10.1016/j.transproceed.2025.03.019.

51. Shikama T, Shikama M, Hayase N, Doi K. Takotsubo syndrome following status epilepticus in a heart transplant recipient: a case report. Clin Pract Cases Emerg Med. 2025;9(1):17–20. https://doi.org/10.5811/cpcem.41970.
52. Miyake R, Ohtani K, Hashimoto T, Yada R, Sato T, Shojima Y, et al. Takotsubo syndrome in a heart transplant recipient with poor cardiac sympathetic reinnervation. ESC Heart Failure. 2020;7(3):1145–9. https://doi.org/10.1002/ehf2.12632.
53. Dong F, Yin L, Sisakian H, Hakobyan T, Jeong LS, Joshi H, et al. Takotsubo syndrome is a coronary microvascular disease: experimental evidence. Eur Heart J. 2023;44(24):2244–53. https://doi.org/10.1093/eurheartj/ehad274.
54. Izumi Y, Okatani H, Shiota M, Nakao T, Ise R, Kito G, et al. Effects of metoprolol on epinephrine-induced takotsubo-like left ventricular dysfunction in non-human primates. Hypertens Res. 2009;32(5):339–46. https://doi.org/10.1038/hr.2009.28.
55. Madias JE. Estrogens for protection from an index and recurrent episodes of takotsubo syndrome? J Endocrinol. 2021;250(3):L1–2. https://doi.org/10.1530/joe-21-0147.
56. Zmaili M. When a rare manifestation of a rare disease has an atypical form: Pheochromocytoma-associated Takotsubo cardiomyopathy. Int J Cardiol. 2023;371:295–6. https://doi.org/10.1016/j.ijcard.2022.09.018.
57. Szatko A, Glinicki P, Gietka-Czernel M. Pheochromocytoma/paraganglioma-associated cardiomyopathy. Front Endocrinol. 2023;14 https://doi.org/10.3389/fendo.2023.1204851.
58. Aw A, de Jong MC, Varghese S, Lee J, Foo R, Parameswaran R. A systematic cohort review of pheochromocytoma-induced typical versus atypical Takotsubo cardiomyopathy. Int J Cardiol. 2023;371:287–92. https://doi.org/10.1016/j.ijcard.2022.08.053.
59. Kato K, Di Vece D, Kitagawa M, Yamamoto K, Miyakoda K, Aoki S, et al. Clinical characteristics and outcomes in takotsubo syndrome—review of insights from the InterTAK registry. J Cardiol. 2025;85(4):263–7. https://doi.org/10.1016/j.jjcc.2025.01.009.
60. Salmoirago-Blotcher E, Dunsiger S, Swales HH, Aurigemma GP, Ockene I, Rosman L, et al. Reproductive history of women with Takotsubo cardiomyopathy. Am J Cardiol. 2016;118(12):1922–8. https://doi.org/10.1016/j.amjcard.2016.08.083.
61. Fu L, Liu Y, Wang J, Sun Y, Zhang L, Wu T, et al. Cardioprotection by low-dose of estrogen and testosterone at the physiological ratio on Ovariectomized rats during ischemia/reperfusion injury. J Cardiovasc Pharmacol. 2017;70(2):87–93. https://doi.org/10.1097/fjc.0000000000000497.
62. Fu L, Zhang H, Machuki JO, Zhang T, Han L, Sang L, et al. Reply to: estrogens for protection from an index and recurrent episodes of takotsubo syndrome? J Endocrinol. 2021;250(3):L3–L. https://doi.org/10.1530/joe-21-0227.
63. Zhu Z, Zhao J, Fang Y, Hua R. Association between serum estradiol level, sex hormone binding globulin level, and bone mineral density in middle-aged postmenopausal women. J Orthop Surg Res. 2021;16(1):648. https://doi.org/10.1186/s13018-021-02799-3.
64. Ganz P. Vasomotor and vascular effects of hormone replacement therapy. Am J Cardiol. 2002;90(1a):11f–6f. https://doi.org/10.1016/s0002-9149(01)02218-4.
65. Miller VM, Duckles SP. Vascular actions of estrogens: functional implications. Pharmacol Rev. 2008;60(2):210–41. https://doi.org/10.1124/pr.107.08002.
66. Pinto S, Virdis A, Ghiadoni L, Bernini G, Lombardo M, Petraglia F, et al. Endogenous estrogen and acetylcholine-induced vasodilation in normotensive women. Hypertension. 1997;29(1):268–73. https://doi.org/10.1161/01.HYP.29.1.268.
67. Visniauskas B, Kilanowski-Doroh I, Ogola BO, McNally AB, Horton AC, Imulinde Sugi A, et al. Estrogen-mediated mechanisms in hypertension and other cardiovascular diseases. J Hum Hypertens. 2023;37(8):609–18. https://doi.org/10.1038/s41371-022-00771-0.
68. Pan AL, Fergusson D, Hong R, Badawi RA. Spontaneous coronary artery dissection following topical hormone replacement therapy. Case Rep Cardiol. 2012;2012:524508. https://doi.org/10.1155/2012/524508.
69. Hayes SN, Kim ESH, Saw J, Adlam D, Arslanian-Engoren C, Economy KE, et al. Spontaneous coronary artery dissection: current state of the science: a scientific statement from the American Heart Association. Circulation. 2018;137(19):e523–e57. https://doi.org/10.1161/CIR.0000000000000564.

70. Mori R, Macaya F, Giacobbe F, Moreno V, Quadri G, Chipayo D, et al. Association between hormone therapy and short-term cardiovascular events in women with spontaneous coronary artery dissection. Revista Española de Cardiología (English Edition). 2023;76(3):140–216. https://doi.org/10.1016/j.rec.2022.07.004.
71. Nebeski D, Basic C, Svanvik T, Schaufelberger M, Ostgard Thunstrom E, SWED-PREG. Incidence of spontaneous coronary artery dissection during pregnancy in Swedish women between 1997 to 2019, a retrospective observational cohort study based on national Swedish health-registers. Eur Heart J. 2022:43(Supplement_2). https://doi.org/10.1093/eurheartj/ehac544.1172.
72. Eguchi M, Watanabe Y, Uemastu M, Sato A. Vasospastic angina in a young female-to-male transsexual. European Heart J Case Rep. 2025; https://doi.org/10.1093/ehjcr/ytaf026.
73. Mahendiran T, Wilgenhof A, De Bruyne B. The elusiveness of "rest": the challenges of assessing resting coronary physiology. Circulation. 2025;152(3):147–9. https://doi.org/10.1161/CIRCULATIONAHA.125.074343.
74. Johnson NP, Gould KL. Subendocardial ischemia: does CMD really exist? Cardiovasc Revasc Med. 2025; https://doi.org/10.1016/j.carrev.2025.01.008.
75. Jansen Tijn PJ, Damman P, van Royen N. Elias-Smale Suzette E. Reply JACC: Cardiovas Imag. 2022;15(9):1678–9. https://doi.org/10.1016/j.jcmg.2022.07.005.
76. Gould KL, Lipscomb K, Hamilton GW. Physiologic basis for assessing critical coronary stenosis: instantaneous flow response and regional distribution during coronary hyperemia as measures of coronary flow reserve. Am J Cardiol. 1974;33(1):87–94. https://doi.org/10.1016/0002-9149(74)90743-7.
77. Saitta A, Altavilla D, Cucinotta D, Morabito N, Frisina N, Corrado F, et al. Randomized, double-blind, placebo-controlled study on effects of raloxifene and hormone replacement therapy on plasma no concentrations, endothelin-1 levels, and endothelium-dependent vasodilation in postmenopausal women. Arterioscler Thromb Vasc Biol. 2001;21(9):1512–9. https://doi.org/10.1161/hq0901.095565.
78. Arcari L, Camastra G, Ciolina F, Limite LR, Danti M, Sclafani M, et al. Myocardial oedema contributes to interstitial expansion and associates with mechanical and electrocardiographic changes in takotsubo syndrome: a CMR T1 and T2 mapping study. European Heart J Cardiovasc Imag. 2023;24(8):1082–91. https://doi.org/10.1093/ehjci/jead035.
79. Kato K, Daimon M, Ishibashi I, Kobayashi Y. Myocardial edema in Takotsubo syndrome — serial cardiovascular magnetic resonance imaging of the natural course —. Circ J. 2017;81(9):1368–9. https://doi.org/10.1253/circj.CJ-17-0065.
80. Sykes R, Ang DTY, Berry C. Takotsubo is an acute myocardial ischaemic syndrome. Eur Heart J. 2025;46(17):1582–5. https://doi.org/10.1093/eurheartj/ehaf020.
81. Tokunou T, Sadamatsu K. Recurrence of Takotsubo cardiomyopathy with coronary slow flow phenomenon. J Cardiol Cases. 2012;5(2):e100–e6. https://doi.org/10.1016/j.jccase.2011.10.003.
82. Wittstein IS, Thiemann DR, Lima JA, Baughman KL, Schulman SP, Gerstenblith G, et al. Neurohumoral features of myocardial stunning due to sudden emotional stress. N Engl J Med. 2005;352(6):539–48. https://doi.org/10.1056/NEJMoa043046.
83. Nef HM, Möllmann H, Kostin S, Troidl C, Voss S, Weber M, et al. Tako-Tsubo cardiomyopathy: intraindividual structural analysis in the acute phase and after functional recovery. Eur Heart J. 2007;28(20):2456–64. https://doi.org/10.1093/eurheartj/ehl570.
84. Grassi S, Campuzano O, Cazzato F, Coll M, Puggioni A, Zedda M, et al. Postmortem diagnosis of Takotsubo syndrome on autoptic findings: is it reliable? Sys Rev Cardiovasc Pathol. 2023;65:107543. https://doi.org/10.1016/j.carpath.2023.107543.
85. Duncker DJ, Schulz R, Ferrari R, Garcia-Dorado D, Guarnieri C, Heusch G, et al. "Myocardial stunning": remaining questions1. Cardiovasc Res. 1998;38(3):549–58. https://doi.org/10.1016/s0008-6363(98)00061-3.
86. Ghasemi H, Kazemian S, Nejadghaderi SA, Shafie M. Takotsubo syndrome and COVID-19: a systematic review. Health Sci Rep. 2023;6(1):e972. https://doi.org/10.1002/hsr2.972.

87. Sharma K, Desai HD, Patoliya JV, Jadeja DM, Gadhiya D. Takotsubo syndrome a rare entity in COVID-19: a systemic review-focus on biomarkers, imaging, treatment, and outcome. SN Compr Clin Med. 2021;3(1):62–72. https://doi.org/10.1007/s42399-021-00743-4.
88. Pillinger NL, Kam P. Endothelial glycocalyx: basic science and clinical implications. Anaesth Intensive Care. 2017;45(3):295–307. https://doi.org/10.1177/0310057x1704500305.
89. Harris NR, Bálint L, Dy DM, Nielsen NR, Méndez HG, Aghajanian A, et al. The ebb and flow of cardiac lymphatics: a tidal wave of new discoveries. Physiol Rev. 2023;103(1):391–432. https://doi.org/10.1152/physrev.00052.2021.
90. Ji R-C. The emerging importance of lymphangiogenesis in aging and aging-associated diseases. Mech Ageing Dev. 2024;221:111975. https://doi.org/10.1016/j.mad.2024.111975.
91. Juchem G, Weiss DR, Knott M, Senftl A, Förch S, Fischlein T, et al. Regulation of coronary venular barrier function by blood borne inflammatory mediators and pharmacological tools: insights from novel microvascular wall models. Am J Physiol Heart Circ Physiol. 2012;302(3):H567–81. https://doi.org/10.1152/ajpheart.00360.2011.
92. López-Trejo FI, Cedillo-Urbina MR, Maldonado-Tenesaca AP, Rivera-Guerrero JC, Andrade-Cuellar EN. Hyponatraemia-induced Takotsubo syndrome secondary to idiopathic syndrome of inappropriate antidiuretic hormone: a case report. European Heart J Case Rep. 2025;9(2) https://doi.org/10.1093/ehjcr/ytaf006.
93. Patnaik S, Punjabi C, Nathan R, Khurram I, Witzke C, Lai YK. Bland and broken hearted: a case of hyponatremia induced Tako-tsubo cardiomyopathy. Int J Cardiol. 2015;187:267–71. https://doi.org/10.1016/j.ijcard.2015.03.272.
94. Watanabe Y, Yoshikawa T, Isogai T, Sakata K, Yamaguchi T, Arao K, et al. Impact of hypoalbuminemia on in-hospital mortality in patients with takotsubo syndrome: a multicenter registry of the Tokyo cardiovascular care unit network. J Cardiol. 2023;82(5):356–62. https://doi.org/10.1016/j.jjcc.2023.06.006.
95. Dongaonkar RM, Stewart RH, Geissler HJ, Laine GA. Myocardial microvascular permeability, interstitial oedema, and compromised cardiac function. Cardiovasc Res. 2010;87(2):331–9. https://doi.org/10.1093/cvr/cvq145.
96. Sheppard MN. Takotsubo syndrome-stress-induced heart failure syndrome. Eur Cardiol. 2015;10(2):83–8. https://doi.org/10.15420/ecr.2015.10.2.83.
97. Cammann VL, Würdinger M, Ghadri JR, Templin C. Takotsubo syndrome: uncovering myths and misconceptions. Curr Atheroscler Rep. 2021;23(9):53. https://doi.org/10.1007/s11883-021-00946-z.
98. Roncalli J, Carrie D, Fauvel J-M, Losordo D. A "hawk's beak" to identify the new transient midventricular Tako-Tsubo syndrome. Int J Cardiol. 2008;127:e179–80. https://doi.org/10.1016/j.ijcard.2007.04.140.
99. Peters S. Mid-ventricular ballooning in atherosclerotic and non-atherosclerotic abnormalities of the left anterior descending coronary artery. J Cardiol Cardiovasc Med. 2016;1:009–10. https://doi.org/10.29328/journal.jccm.1001002.
100. Medina YAC, López Blanco PF, González Niño RA. Hawk's beak form in Midventricular Takotsubo syndrome: two case reports from Latin America. Open Cardiovasc Med J. 2021;15:52–5. https://doi.org/10.2174/1874192402115010052.
101. Lima G, Trejo-Paredes MC, Cardoso E. A mid-ventricular variant of Takotsubo cardiomyopathy: a case study and review of literature. Cureus. 2020;12(7):e9403. https://doi.org/10.7759/cureus.9403.
102. Matta A, Roncalli J, Elbaz M, Lhermusier T, Campelo-Parada F, Bouisset F, et al. Midventricular Takotsubo cardiomyopathy with hawk's beak appearance: a case report. Am J Case Rep. 2020;21:e919563. https://doi.org/10.12659/ajcr.919563.
103. Kunadian V, Chieffo A, Camici PG, Berry C, Escaned J, Maas AHEM, et al. An EAPCI expert consensus document on Ischaemia with non-obstructive coronary arteries in collaboration with European Society of Cardiology Working Group on Coronary Pathophysiology & Microcirculation Endorsed by coronary vasomotor disorders international study group. EuroIntervention. 2021;16(13):1049–69. https://doi.org/10.4244/eijy20m07_01.

Chapter 9
Stiff Heart

Abstract Over a third of patients with angina have non-obstructive coronary arteries (ANOCA) on diagnostic coronary angiogram. There is a group of these individuals, comprising predominantly of women with angina, where the defining features include the phenomenon of lingering symptoms after a trigger has long passed, and variable responsiveness to glyceryl trinitrate spray. Many but not all have objective evidence of cardiac ischaemia with non-invasive tests, and in some, pacing stress can cause lactate spillover in the coronary sinus. Excluding obvious vasoreactivity with spasm testing, they were previously labelled as cardiac syndrome X, but are now reclassified as coronary microvascular dysfunction (CMD). Diagnosed as reduced coronary flow reserve (CFR), or the inability of the heart to double the hyperaemic coronary flow, that is, a CFR < 2.0. This chapter describes 3 selective cases of CMD diagnosed with coronary bolus and continuous thermodilution and postulates on their varied mechanisms which include both extra- and intracardiac constraints on the myocardial microvasculature.

9.1 Introduction

The resting coronary flow is not affected until an epicardial stenosis is over 85% in severity. But hyperaemic flow starts to decline beyond a moderate 30–45% narrowing. With a pressure gradient across a lesion of over 40 mmHg, the heart is unable to double its flow to meet any increase in metabolic demand, despite normal microvascular function in the dog's circumflex artery, using the perivascular electromagnetic flow transducer, and contrast-induced hyperaemia [1, 2]. This is hyperaemic flow as proportion of baseline flow or the coronary flow reserve (CFR) < 2. The same principle has been applied to humans, but non-invasively, utilising the positron emission tomography (PET) with Oxygen-15 labelled water ($H_2{}^{15}O$), that, when a coronary stenosis is > 80% the hyperaemic flow equals basal flow, negating the microvascular vasodilatory reserve [3].

Although in an elegant and precise study with continuous thermodilution, involving graduated balloon occlusion of a stented proximal left anterior descending

P. O. Lim, *Coronary Thermodilution*,
https://doi.org/10.1007/978-3-032-10734-3_9

(LAD) artery in a 63-year-man, a distal coronary pressure fall of 70%, or a fractional flow reserve, FFR of 0.30 is when CFR starts to fall below 2.0. This level of perfusion pressure is often encountered in well-collateralised distal vessels subtended by an epicardial chronic total occlusion (CTO), or a coronary wedge pressure of 30 mmHg implies adequate collateral recruitment—suggesting the resilience of a competent microvasculature in humans [4]. This explains why so many patients with CTO are relatively symptom-free. However, when the microvasculature is dysfunctional, a low CFR measured non-invasively and invasively, quadruples mortality over a mean period of 3 years, in patients with non-obstructive coronary arteries. The proviso is that most of these patients are much older with a mean age of 65 and have multiple comorbid conditions replete with traditional risk factors—hypertension, diabetes and smoking [5, 6]. It is likely that coronary microvascular dysfunction, CMD as defined by CFR < 2 is a prognostic marker in this group of high risk individuals with advanced multi-organ vasculopathy. Conceivably, in the event of an acute coronary syndrome, they are less able to autoregulate flow to their myocardium, resulting in a larger infarct or initiating a catastrophic cardiac arrhythmic event.

However, the above scenario does not apply to the "cardiac syndrome X" patients with a more benign prognosis, comparable to that of the general population, who are mostly women in their fifties with high symptomatic burden and angina that persists beyond half an hour, outwith the triggers, resulting in repeated hospital admissions and multiple invasive investigations [7]. Who continue to pose a clinical conundrum today, after the label was first coined by Harvey G. Kemp Jr. (1935–2010) in 1973, over half a century ago [8]. These are patients with a triad of **angina** with **non-obstructive coronary arteries** (ANOCA) and evidence of **myocardial ischaemia**. Although the latter may not be objectively demonstrable. Philip MacCarthy's tour de force review of the subject in 2008 questions whether flow limitation in diffuse non-obstructive coronary atherosclerosis is underestimated, the so-called diminishing gradual pressure gradient, especially in smaller distal vessels, as discussed in Chap. 1. As per Hagen-Poiseuille's law, resistance in the smaller vessel rises $\propto 1/r^4$; disproportionately with a small change in calibre, not picked up by the distal pressure sensor of a pressure wire—potentially invalidating the assumption that any flow reduction must be microvascular in nature if the epicardial coronary artery is non-obstructive.

MacCarthy also reflects on the heterogeneity of findings with invasive techniques available then, in estimating coronary flow, including coronary sinus thermodilution, against which the "gold standard" PET is validated, and the pitfalls of the coronary doppler wire—where precise measure of changing coronary calibre is needed, plus often inconsistent signals in practice. He prophesises that when it is possible to measure *absolute coronary flow* with artery-specific thermodilution, coupled with evaluation of endothelial function, is when further progress can be had in this patient population [9]. Three such case studies are now presented in this chapter.

9.2 Cases

9.2.1 A Structurally Supranormal Heart

A 59-year-old woman who was treated for hypothyroidism (on thyroxine 50/75 μg on alternate day), because of regular attendances at the emergency department with both angina and breathlessness—four times over the past year, underwent a one-stop coronary physiology study. She has right bundle branch block (RBBB) on her ECG. Her heart was normal on echocardiogram and her CT coronary angiogram showed a mild plaque in the proximal left anterior descending (LAD) artery. A stress perfusion cardiovascular magnetic resonance (CMR) scan with intravenous adenosine was obtained beforehand. Her BMI was 28 kg/m^2. She has no cardiac abnormalities—ischaemia, infarction, scar or fibrosis; left ventricular ejection fraction (EF) 68 (59–77) % without left ventricular hypertrophy, end-systolic volume index (ESVI) 17 (14–33) ml/m^2, and stroke volume index (SVI) 36 (37–62) ml/m^2, thus her volume-derived ventriculo-arterial coupling (VAC) was 0.47 (0.6–1.0)—the heart worked harder and emptied more blood, with less left in it—suggesting undercoupling either from a stress-related sympathetic hyperactivity, a low preload or a high afterload state. Her NT-proBNP was mildly elevated at 149 (< 125) ng/L. Two years before, she was started on Evorel Conti® (oestradiol 50 μg and norethisterone Acetate 170 ug) x2 patch twice a week.

Procedure Her left ventricle is studied first (Fig. 9.1); her blood pressure is highly labile, rising to a peak left ventricular systolic pressure of 160 mmHg from a normal baseline cuff blood pressure (BP) despite sedation with midazolam 1 mg, to as high as 180 mmHg during the rest of her procedure. The left ventricular end-diastolic pressure (LVEDP) is elevated at 20 mmHg with hyperdynamic contractility, and an early, or reversed dicrotic notch appearance—since the second peak (post-aortic valve opening) is taller, this is likely to be an extraventricular phenomenon such as a reactively high afterload than left ventricular outflow tract obstruction as seen in the aortic waveform in hypertrophic cardiomyopathy.

The coronary arteries are unobstructed, the right coronary artery is dominant with the posterior descending artery supplying the left ventricular apex, thus the LAD is of relatively small calibre distally. Continuous thermodilution is undertaken in the LAD. The basal flow is estimated 4 times until consistency is obtained; 84, 47, 53 and **57** mL/min, with corresponding resistance of 1610, 2893, 2158 and **2321** Wood units; whereas the hyperaemic flow is repeated 3 times; 129, 142 and **115** mL/min, respective resistance of 848, 739 and **890** Wood units. Using the last consistent values, the coronary flow reserve, CFR is 2.0, microvascular resistance reserve, MRR 2.6 and an estimated index of microvascular resistance, IMR from a minimal hyperaemic resistance of 890/20 = 45 [10]. These numbers are consistent with the diagnosis of CMD. The hyperaemic resistance is also estimated once from the circumflex artery and this is concordantly elevated at 1109 Wood units, or an estimated IMR of 55.

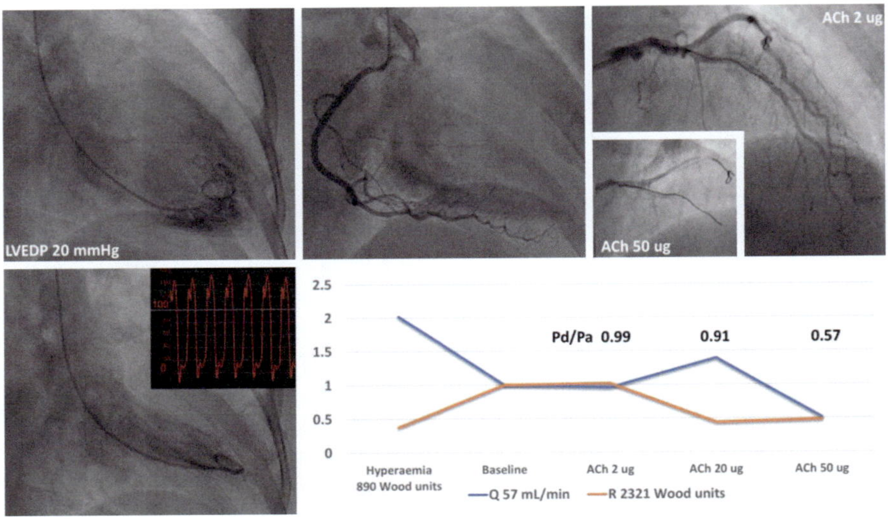

Fig. 9.1 **(Left panels)** Left ventriculogram demonstrates a hypercontractile ventricle with supranormal ejection fraction, an apparent reversed dicrotic notch and raised left ventricular end-diastolic pressure. (**Top middle and right panels**) Dominant right coronary artery that supplies the left ventricular apex and left anterior descending (LAD) artery following intracoronary acetylcholine (ACh) 2 µg; the *inset* shows occlusive vasospasm with ACh 50 µg. (**Lower right panel**) Continuous thermodilution is undertaken in the LAD; note the high basal and hyperaemic resistance with restricted vasodilatory capacity. ACh is not associated with flow higher than 1.5-fold from baseline and at 50 µg; the flow plummeted with a fall in distal-to-aortic pressure ratio (Pd/Pa) and without corresponding rise in resistance, which means that this is purely an epicardial vasospastic phenomenon in the context of generalised endothelial dysfunction

Finally, acetylcholine (ACh) is given intracoronarily in escalating doses. ACh 2 µg produces no appreciable effect from baseline, whereas ACh 20 µg increases flow, albeit less than 50% and with associated vagal response of bradycardia and dropped beats. The next dose of ACh 100 µg can only be half-given (effective dose of 50 µg), she develops chest pain, anterior electrocardiographic ST elevation, the flow falls, as with the distal-to-aortic pressure ratio, Pd/Pa, and her coronary angiogram demonstrates severe generalised epicardial vasospasm with hypotension—which is reversible with intracoronary nitroglycerine and intravenous metaraminol.

Interpretation This woman has neither full house of traditional coronary disease risk factors beyond taking atorvastatin 40 mg od for hyperlipidaemia nor demonstrable heart disease functionally and structurally on non-invasive tests. Interestingly, she has labile haemodynamics which could be stress-related, with a systemic hypertensive response associated with diastolic dysfunction and a high EF. In principle this could mimic CMD, with the high reactive coronary resistance, but the low basal flow could be consistent with a non-dominant LAD. However, it has been reported that when indexed to myocardial mass subtended [11], the hyperaemic flow remains comparatively low which would support a hypertensive response imitating CMD in this woman, with concordance in the circumflex territory.

On the other hand, her response to ACh suggested generalised endothelial dysfunction with a clinically significant epicardial vasospasm at a relatively small dose of ACh at 50 μg. This could be expected as she has atherosclerosis; the low Pd/Pa without an accompanying rise in coronary resistance pointed to her not having microvascular spasm, but endothelial dysfunction. She was titrated up on a vasodilating beta blocker, nebivolol, to 5 mg od. While this was being done, over the past one year, she has presented to the emergency department three more times, illustrating the high morbidity of ANOCA which is indistinguishable from those with obstructive coronary artery disease [12–15]. She was next referred to a specialist menopause clinic to assess the adequacy of her hormone replacement therapy (HRT).

9.2.2 *Subtle Cardiac Abnormalities and Normotension*

A 47-year-old premenopausal woman was seen in the emergency department with angina two years prior. Her CT coronary angiogram showed unobstructed coronary arteries; echocardiogram revealed a normal heart with a small rim of pericardial effusion, and her 24-hour Holter picked up no significant rhythm disturbances. She was slightly overweight with a BMI of 28, has no hypertension but had gestational diabetes and her recent HbA1c was 43 (< 43) mmol/mol suggesting that she was pre-diabetic. She has mild asthma, vitamin D deficiency and labile calcium level swinging between hypercalcaemia and hypocalcaemia with consistent hypophosphatemia, but without hyperparathyroidism. She has no history of connective tissue disease or family history of hypertrophic cardiomyopathy. Her CMR found a normal and undilated heart without hypertrophy, fibrosis or infarction, with an EF of 68%. A couple of inferior basal myocardial crypts were noted, the significance of which was unclear, plus trace gadolinium enhancement observed in the right ventricular insertion which could imply remodelling of the right ventricle. The ESVI was 16 (16–34) ml/m^2 and SVI 33 (39–63) ml/m^2—VAC, 16/33 = 0.48 (0.6–1.0), a small left ventricular cavity with low stroke volume and resulting undercoupling. Her left atrium was not dilated, neither has she right ventricular dilatation or pulmonary hypertension. As was known, she has a persistent albeit a small rim of global pericardial effusion. Her NT-ProBNP was slightly elevated at 154 (< 125) ng/mL.

Procedure In view of her symptomatic burden, she is admitted for a coronary physiology study. Her left ventricle (LV) is studied first, the LV angiogram reveals no wall motion abnormalities, but her LVEDP is elevated between 25 and 30 mmHg with normal central aortic BP of 120/60 mmHg without a systolic gradient between her LV and aorta (Fig. 9.2). During the course of her procedure, her systolic BP has been running at 90-100 mmHg. Her coronary arteries are unobstructed—LAD has tortuosity and petering calibre as it reaches the apex. Bolus thermodilution is undertaken to the LAD, because the left main is short; there is a tendency for the 5 French EBU3.5 guide-catheter tip to point to the roof, and it is stabilised with a pressure wire in the LAD and a second guidewire in the circumflex artery. As there

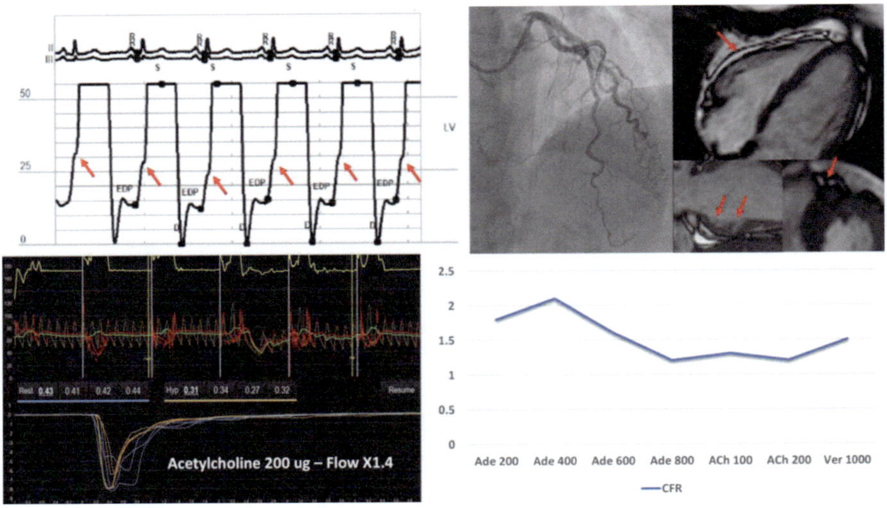

Fig. 9.2 **(Top panels, left to right)** Left ventricular pressure tracing with diastolic upstroke inflexion indicating a raised left ventricular end-diastolic pressure, LVEDP; coronary angiogram shows left anterior descending (LAD) artery that is unobstructed which is tortuous with tapering calibre; and CMR with 3 features of unknown significance—1. pericardial effusion, 2. inferobasal myocardial crypts, and 3. gadolinium enhancement in the right ventricular insertion. (**Bottom panels, right to left**) Bolus thermodilution is performed in the LAD, and the resulting increase in flow in response to escalating intracoronary doses of adenosine, acetylcholine and verapamil; Acetylcholine 200 μg does not provoke epicardial vasospasm, nor heart block; instead the flow bluntedly rises by 1.4 fractionally to suggest microvascular endothelial dysfunction, but in the context of "functional" coronary microvascular dysfunction, CMD with increased basal flow, whether this is a spurious finding

is a concern that the guide-catheter tip may not be coaxial, the bolus thermodilution is repeated four times with escalating intracoronary adenosine doses from 200, 400, 600 to 800 ug, with concordantly low CFR values; 1.8, 2.1, 1.6 and 1.2, and IMR of 18, 14, 13 and 17, and MRR of 1.89, 2.43, 2.16 and 1.63. With ACh, 100 and 200 μg, the flow increases are 1.3- and 1.40-fold without provoking epicardial vasospasm or any vagal phenomenon, and with verapamil 1 mg, the flow rises 1.5-fold.

To understand the above findings in actual values, the indices obtained with bolus thermodilution can be converted using Ohm's equation, *Pressure pushes Flow against Resistance*, using a conversion of IMRx20 = hyperaemic resistance, Rμ, – 360, 280, 260 and 340 Wood units; hyperaemic flow = distal coronary pressure / Rμ: with escalating doses of adenosine; 181, 221, 196 and 156 mL/min; divided by the respective CFR give basal flow of 101, 105, 123, and 130 mL/min. Averaging the values—Rμ **310** Wood units, basal and hyperaemic flow; **115** and **189** mL/min—CFR 1.6. From departmental data of continuous thermodilution in the LAD, the mean basal flow is about 70 ± 18 mL/min. Therefore, her basal flow is 2/3 higher, if not, her CFR would have been normal at 2.7 (189/70), with a low hyperaemic resistance or IMR.

Interpretation This lady has minor cardiac abnormalities yet high burden of symptoms. Her LV has elevated filling pressure without systemic hypertension, and she has restricted vasodilatory capacity without raised coronary resistance or increased vasoreactivity. Nevertheless, she has endothelial dysfunction as ACh does not increase the LAD flow by 50%. She therefore fulfills the diagnosis of "functional" CMD due to high resting or basal flow, and she expended or used up part of her vasodilatory reserve. It is not immediately clear what is the pathophysiology for this phenomenon, whether the high LVEDP causes subendocardial ischaemia, and the increased flow is an attempt to compensate for this. What could cause the high LVEDP, despite the persistent pericardial effusion with organisation; the pericardium itself is not thickened on CMR, but to show pericardial constraint, simultaneous LV/RV pressure measurement is required.

In the absence of left atrial dilatation, the high LVEDP is unlikely to be sustained although the NT-ProBNP is mildly elevated in support of this finding. The only possibility would be *primary diastolic dysfunction* which in isolation is unusual without evident myocardial abnormalities on CMR, but could explain the *discordance between a raise LVEDP without elevated coronary resistance.* The other possibility is the haemodynamic indices obtained are inexact, as explained in Chap. 1; bolus thermodilution is confounded by many factors that cannot be easily accounted for. In this case, the IMR could be spuriously low; if the 25–30 mmHg from the LVEDP is added, the IMR indeed would be raised. IMR correlates poorly with LVEDP, not because they are unrelated, because physiologically microvascular flow is critically affected by LVEDP (through extravascular compression even when the intrinsic microvasculature is normal), but because of the inaccuracy in measuring IMR which has a within-subject coefficient of variation of about 25% [16], and wide grey zone between 19 and 31 [17]. After all, the fractional flow reserve (FFR) is correctable by 0.008 for every 1 mmHg rise in LVEDP > 15 mmHg [18–20]. Further, the concept of *functional* CMD is debatable and has no biological plausibility or basis [21]. On the other hand, if her coronary resistance is indeed high, this would be consistent with extracardiac constraint; the rim of pericardial effusion is in fact effusive-constrictive, contributing to her symptomatology.

Nevertheless, she was symptomatically improved with nebivolol, ranolazine and dapagliflozin, but has continued to be severely restricted by breathless at one year. This prompted a repeat coronary physiology study; this time with continuous thermodilution it revealed a concordantly low CFR of 1.4 (basal flow 64 mL/min) and MRR 1.5, but elevated hyperaemic minimal resistance of 873 Wood units (normal IMR of < 25 with bolus thermodilution 1 year prior); ACh 2, 20 and 100 μg did not provoke epicardial vasospasm as before, but with 100 μg, flow fell by 30% below baseline precipitating retching but without ischaemic ECG changes. Her LVEDP was still elevated 25-30 mmHg with aortic systolic BP of 110-120 mmHg. There was early LV diastolic "dip" and pressure equalisation with simultaneous LV and RV pressure measurement, and a hint of systolic BP discordance with respiration. Her LV pressure-time derivatives, the maximal and minimal ±dP/dt; +1870 (> 1200) and -1756 (< -1100) mmHg/s were normal, while Weis's Tau (τ) was mildly prolonged at 0.05 (< 0.05) s. In canine experiments done in the 1990s,

normal peak ±dP/dt with discordantly lengthened Tau is the hallmark of pericardial constraint [22], and invasive features of pericardial constraint occur late with intrapericardial pressure over 15 mmHg, whereas clinical constraint is measurable with echocardiogram when it is just above 4 mmHg [23]. Her previous year's study with bolus thermodilution suggested *functional* CMD; yet, the repeat study with continuous thermodilution revealed genuinely *restricted vasodilatory capacity with raised coronary resistance*, likely due to extracardiac constriction. Her follow-up echocardiogram with better images measured her epicardial adipose tissue to be 1 cm thick. Thus, raised LVEDP in the absence of structural or functional cardiac abnormalities and without hypertension *point toward* extracardiac factors.

9.2.3 Right Ventricular Dilatation

A 73-year-old man with arrhythmogenic right ventricular cardiomyopathy (ARVC) first identified 30 years ago and plakophilin-2 (PKP2) gene mutation has become breathless with exercise and he desaturated when he was upright, termed "Platypnea-Orthodeoxia Syndrome" (POS). He was admitted repeatedly to his local hospital with right heart failure and fluid retention, requiring intravenous diuretic treatment. His deterioration coincided with echocardiographic left ventricular septal flattening from dilating right ventricle, increased tricuspid regurgitation plus left-to-right shunt via a patent foramen ovale (PFO), and electrocardiographic PR and QRS prolongations (Fig. 9.3). He had spontaneous coronary artery dissection (SCAD) in his distal circumflex artery 5 years previously and has an automated implantable cardioverter defibrillator (AICD) in situ. The atrial pacing with ventricular sensing mode was converted to DDDR to reduce PR length. To further investigate his symptom, a one-stop coronary work-up was undertaken. His BMI was 24 kg/m^2.

Procedure His coronary arteries are unobstructed but with generalised coronary slow flow phenomenon (CSFP). The underfilled left ventricle has a borderline filling pressure of 12 mmHg, whereas his central aortic pressure is on the low side, at 100/70 mmHg. The right coronary artery (RCA) is studied with continuous thermodilution; hyperaemic flow 66 mL/min and resistance, **1291** Wood units; corresponding basal values are 37 and *2165* respectively: giving a coronary flow reserve, CFR of 1.78, and microvascular resistance reserve, MRR of 1.67 (< 2.1) [24]. Escalating doses of ACh induce no changes in coronary haemodynamics nor vasospasm, but with the highest dose, coronary flow increases. The respective coronary indices for left anterior descending (LAD) artery: 82, **1160**; 98, *913*; CFR 0.84, MRR 0.79, and for circumflex (Cx) artery: 79**, 1219**; 86, *1157*; CFR 0.92, MRR 0.95.

Interpretation Advanced ARVC is associated with volume-overloaded right heart without pulmonary hypertension and a low cardiac output state because of right-to-left direct ventricular interaction (DVI) with pericardial constraint. These appear to have selectively affected RCA in abolishing systolic flow component as is known, by **doubling its basal coronary resistance** from right ventricular stretch, compared

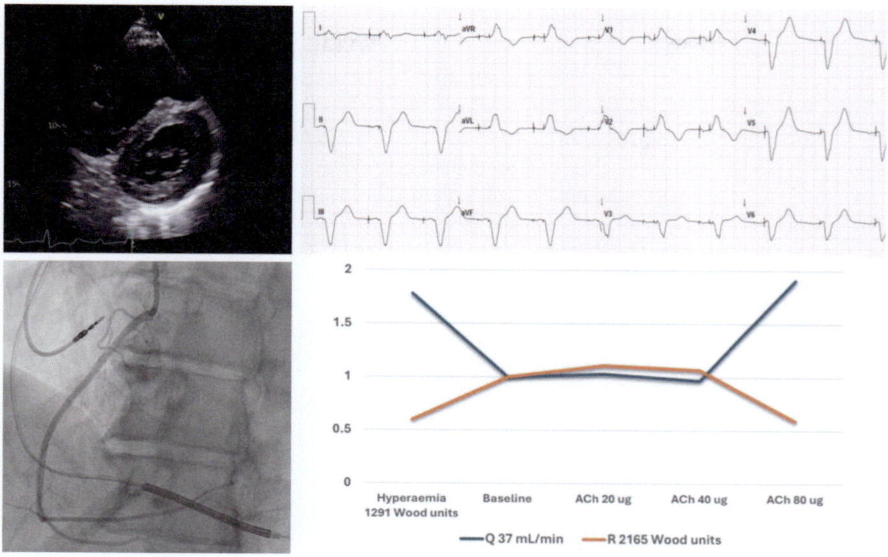

Fig. 9.3 Dilated right ventricle with a "D-shaped" left ventricle in diastole on echocardiogram (**left upper panel**), DDDR-paced rhythm on 12-lead electrocardiogram with PR set at 208 ms and prolonged QRS duration, 189 ms (**right upper panel**), disease-free codominant right coronary artery with atrial and defibrillator leads in situ (**left lower panel**), and coronary haemodynamics; raised basal and hyperaemic resistance [Rμ 1291 Wood units, equivalent to an index of microvascular resistance, IMR of 65 (< 25)] with a coronary flow reserve, CFR of 1.78; suggesting *impaired vasodilatory capacity with increased minimal resistance during hyperaemia*, consistent with the diagnosis of coronary microvascular dysfunction (CMD), and acetylcholine 20 μg and 40 μg did not alter coronary flow, but at 80 ug, the flow increased 1.9-fold, with a 41% fall in resistance indicating intact endothelial function or shunting to EDHF pathway (Chap. 7) (**right lower panel**)

to LAD and Cx, and restricting flow in all three coronary arteries with concordantly elevated hyperaemic resistance, thus diagnosing CMD. But blunted flow in response to lower doses of ACh and increased flow ≥ 50% with ACh 80 μg suggesting preserved endothelial function, and fascinatingly, no angina in this case despite the CFR < 2.0. The main symptom was exercise intolerance, closing the PFO has not altered his breathlessness despite increasing his oxygen saturation.

9.3 Discussion

In the absence of obstructive epicardial coronary arteries, failure of coronary flow to at least double under stress or hyperaemia, **CFR < 2.0 defines CMD**. However, this seemingly simple definition belies the heterogeneity and complexity of CMD as illustrated by the case studies presented (Table 9.1). Case 1 and 2 fulfilled the diagnosis of heart failure with supranormal ejection fraction, HFsnEF [25]. Both were middle-aged women, with EF ≥ 65% and low SV with equally low ESV resulting

Table 9.1 Coronary physiology and CFR < 2.0

Case	Age	BMI	Comorbidities	Vasodilatory Capacity (CFR)	Coronary Resistance (Wood units)	Vasoreactivity (ACh)
1	59♀	28	Hypothyroidism and hyperlipidaemia HRT CMR EF 68%, VAC 0.47	LAD 2.0 Flow did not rise >50% with ACh 2 and 20 ug	**LAD 890** MRR 2.6 **Cx 1109** LVEDP 20 BP 180/110 NT-ProBNP 149	Generalised epicardial vasospasm with ACh 50 (Pd/Pa 0.96 → 0.51)
2	47♀	28	Gestational diabetes and pre-diabetes, asthma and vitamin D deficiency CMR EF 68%, VAC 0.53. Inferobasal crypts and RV insertion LGE enhancement, rim of pericardial effusion	LAD bolus thermodilution 1.67 (average of 4 studies) Flow (derived) baseline and hyperaemic—115 (raised) and 189 mL/min (*see text for the repeat study with continuous thermodilution 1 year later*)	**310 (derived from IMR × 20)** LVEDP >25 BP 120/60 NT-ProBNP 154	No epicardial vasospasm or flow reduction with bolus thermodilution, but when flow was measured with continuous thermodilution 1 year later, it failed to rise by x1.5 suggesting microvascular endothelial dysfunction
3	73♂	24	ARVC	RCA 1.78 LAD 0.84 Cx 0.92	RCA 1291 vs **2165 (x2 in LAD and Cx)** LAD 1160 vs **913** Cx 1219 vs **1157** LVEDP 12 (underfilled LV from diastolic ventricular interaction (DVI) due to RV dilatation shifting the septal to the LV during diastole) BP 100/70	No epicardial vasospasm and flow increased x1.9 with ACh 80 μg

in ventriculo-arterial undercoupling, raised LVEDP, microvascular endothelial dysfunction, and nominally raised NT-ProBNP. Whether HFsnEF is systematically associated with CMD merits further exploration. However, the similarities diverted when it came to detailed coronary physiology; case 1 exhibited labile hypertension, whereas case 2 veering on the side of hypotension. And case 1, an older postmenopausal woman with evident proximal LAD atherosclerosis, responded with occlusive epicardial vasospasm with a relatively low ACh dose of 50 ug, which was not replicated in case 2, a perimenopausal woman, even with the highest ACh dose at 200 ug. Although ACh did not increase flow by 50% in both cases suggesting microvascular endothelial dysfunction. Case 1 had continuous thermodilution, whereas case 2 initially had bolus thermodilution, but repeated measures were obtained regardless of techniques to ensure consistency of data. While continuous thermodilution is highly reproducible without operator dependency, bolus thermodilution is *reassuring* with a negative test result, i.e. concordant CFR ≥ 2.5 and IMR < 25 [26]. The European Society of Cardiology has in 2024 codified blanket CMD as CFR < 2.5 and/or IMR ≥ 25 [27], which might be overly inclusive, since there is increasing uncertainty if a raised coronary resistance per se, and by implication, IMR, in isolation has any practical clinical value, since flow augmentation is demonstrably not compromised [28]. Further, IMR is a *composite index* encompassing epicardial disease rheology and high LV filling pressure, where it derived its prognostic value from, and with more precise measurement of resistance with the Doppler technique, high hyperaemic resistance in the presence of a normal CFR ≥ 2.5 represents microvascular adaptation that does not impact on long-term outcome, neither does it when assessed in parallel to CFR (see Chap. 1.4.4 on the challenges of defining resistance) [29]. When the bolus thermodilution indices are abnormal, the methodology adopted here is to repeat measurements with escalating intracoronary adenosine dosing. In the LAD, incremental hyperaemia can be maximised with 200 μg of adenosine, all the way up to 800 ug, and in practice, 1000 μg could be safely given as a rapid bolus [30]. Converting IMR by a factor of twenty to hyperaemic resistance allowed for absolute baseline flow to be estimated. To differentiate, if the low CFR was due to high basal flow, i.e. expended vasodilatory reserve, or from restricted vasodilatory capacity, in which case the resting flow would be low; in case 2, the former turned out to be the case [10]. However, as alluded to earlier, the notion of *functional* CMD (↓CFR and ↓IMR) is pathophysiological incoherent, due to wandering resting indices and/or unadjusted LVEDP or coronary wedge pressure [21], and its significance disappears when indexed to the subtented myocardial mass [11]. Indeed, case 2's repeat coronary physiology study with continuous thermodilution a year later though replicated the low CFR, but this was due to restricted hyperaemic and not expanded basal flow, i.e. expended vasodilatory reserve, in addition to a raised coronary resistance, overturning the "functional" CMD label. This serves as a cautionary tale the clinical fallacy of CMD dichotomy of structural and functional classifications based on an IMR threshold. Further, in practice LVEDP and coronary resistance ***always*** rise together [31, 32], even when LVEDP is "spuriously" raised by extracardiac factors (transmural LV preload pressure = LVEDP - right atrial pressure (RAP) as surrogate, LVEDP ≥ 15 mmHg → ↓subendocardial blood flow).

The common link between case 1 and case 2 is likely to be oestrogen, in the former, the lack of, and the latter, its continuing effects. Oestrogen protects against atherosclerosis and oxidative stress—it contributes to women as much as a decade's additional lifespan [33, 34]. There is ample experimental data to support oestrogen having endothelial-dependent vasodilating and direct calcium channel antagonistic properties in negating ACh-induced coronary vasoreactivity, reducing both coronary and peripheral vascular resistance, thus promoting myocardial perfusion and enhancing cardiac output by increasing stroke volume [35–39]. In addition, oestrogen modulates the autonomic nervous system, and its deficiency leads to sympathetic overactivity [40]. In other words, case 1 can reasonably be relabelled as cardiac syndrome "oestrogen"; it is the "X" factor, or minus it. The stiffened vasculature and reduced LV lusitropy cause a labile and heightened BP response to stress, as well as increased LVEDP with reduced stroke volume. These changes are seen in all postmenopausal women, why then only a small proportion are symptomatic? The key answer could be diet, lifestyle, healthcare access and burden of concomitant diseases, interacting adversely, leading to myocardial and microvascular maladaptation [41].

Studies in populations, or countries such as Japan where plant-based polyphenolic diet rich in phyto-oestrogens and antioxidants are consumed, appear to have better cardiac prognosis, reduced comorbid risk profile and less CMD (CFR < 2.0) [42–44]. In up-to-date clinical practice, and with better understanding of the risk benefits of oestrogen replacement in postmenopausal women, which is time sensitive, it is now more judiciously recommended in women under 60, but should be started early, as the arteries stiffen almost immediately after the last period; endothelial dysfunction becomes irreversible in due course, and before the atherosclerotic process sets in [45–49]. The recently published guidelines by UK's National Institute for Health and Care Excellence reflect these sentiments (NICE, GID-NG10241, November 7, 2024). It makes logical sense to offer postmenopausal women with ANOCA under 60, without contraindications, oestrogen replacement therapy—this is clearly an area that demands further studies, as we better understand the strengths and weaknesses of different formulations, and their associations with thromboembolic events and cancers. Specialist-led complex menopause clinics are now available in the UK.

Case 2 was a perimenopausal woman, who has tendency for hypotension, thus without systemic or coronary hypertension. Yet, on the basis of her initial bolus thermodilution, she has increased basal coronary flow which has been described before—using up part of her vasodilatory capacity giving a low CFR, and has reduced SV and cardiac output [50]. She has mild cardiac abnormalities without epicardial vasoreactivity despite her microvascular endothelial dysfunction, by extension, LV diastolic dysfunction and a raised LVEDP. She has "functional" CMD. Trying to make sense of this phenomenon if it exists, in which, *Angina in spite of heightened coronary flow* could mean—regional, as in the subendocardium, or pockets of ischaemia due to prearteriolar constriction with arteriolar steal and lingering adenosine within extracellular or interstitial space, as proposed by Maseri [51]. The adenosine-induced vasodilatation may account for the raised basal coronary flow, and its reduced clearance causes persistent angina via its algogenic activation of A_1 adenosine receptor, long after a physical or emotional trigger has resolved [52, 53]. Although conceivably, primary or secondary cardiac interstitial hypertension from high flow capillary leak overwhelming lymphatic drainage can compress the the postcapillary venules explaining all the above features (Chap. 1). There is no rational explanation why there should be selective prearteriolar vasospasm, unless there is localised inflammation which should be self-limiting, and this is not gender specific. In this case, the diabetes and accompanying insulin resistance can potentially contribute to cardiac lymphatic dysfunction. She appeared to respond to the triple therapy of nebivolol, ranolazine and dapagliflozin for her angina but not breathlessness and exercise intolerance. As discussed earlier, her repeat coronary physiology study found a low CFR due to restricted vasodilatory range, in addition to an element of extracardiac constraint which might be the dominant feature in her case.

Raised LVEDP can impact coronary perfusion, as can increased intrapericardial pressure. The dilated right ventricle in case 3 with ARVC caused pericardial constraint, increasing coronary resistance and reducing hyperaemic coronary flow and thus CFR. This has been observed in constrictive pericarditis and cardiac tamponade [54, 55]. Surgical right ventricular disarticulation, pericardiectomy and biventricular pacing have been tested in the past as a treatment strategy for ARVC with intractable ventricular tachyarrhythmias [56]. However, with advances in ablation and AICD, the arrhythmic issue has been settled, although only 7% of ARVC patients live beyond the seventh decade because of relentless right heart failure [57]. Percutaneous approach to pericardiectomy is being tested for removing pericardial constraint in HFpEF; perhaps in the future, cases such as this with lengthening QRS interval and dilating right ventricular can be managed with this approach plus cardiac resynchronisation therapy (CRT-D) [58].

In conclusion, as MacCarthy suspected, current availability of flow measurement techniques allows CFR < 2.0 to be defined more robustly, but this may not equate CMD automatically as there are complex interacting factors at play, in particular raised LVEDP in the first two cases and pericardial constraint in the second case, while the third case was due to a dilating right ventricle. These make the heart stiff, reducing its vasodilatory capacity. Finally, predicting the future in the guise of McCarthy, three innovations will likely happen soon: 1. **Beat-to-beat absolute coronary flow** by simply updating the software, keep the RayFlow microcatheter saline infusion rate at 10 mL/min (or can be determined individually to exclude partial hyperaemia, if Pd/Pa falls, in which case reduce the saline infusion rate to 8 mL/min [59]), measure the infusate temperature (T_i) at catheter tip proximally, then advance the wire down the coronary artery. Keep the wire in the same position throughout the study, measuring the continuous mixed temperature (T_m) in response to adenosine given either intravenously or intracoronarily, escalating the dose until maximal hyperaemic flow is achieved, and assess flow following ACh, verapamil and other drugs. This may be better than predicting the T_i which will introduce systematic errors [60]; 2. **N-of-1 approach** [61] or personalised evaluation, instead of the current reverse validation of haemodynamic indices based on population averages. Individualise assessment for targeted drug therapy in the cardiac catheter laboratory, moving away from empirical polypharmacy and prolonged therapeutic dose escalation; and 3. **Smartphone App-based AI-powered symptoms' diary** to examine treatment response [62], with an inbuilt standardised exercise tolerance indicator, such as the metronomic Dundee step test [63].

References

1. Gould KL, Lipscomb K. Effects of coronary stenoses on coronary flow reserve and resistance. Am J Cardiol. 1974;34(1):48–55. https://doi.org/10.1016/0002-9149(74)90092-7.
2. Gould KL, Lipscomb K, Hamilton GW. Physiologic basis for assessing critical coronary stenosis: instantaneous flow response and regional distribution during coronary hyperemia as measures of coronary flow reserve. Am J Cardiol. 1974;33(1):87–94. https://doi.org/10.1016/0002-9149(74)90743-7.
3. Uren NG, Melin JA, De Bruyne B, et al. Relation between myocardial blood flow and the severity of coronary-artery stenosis. N Engl J Med. 1994;330(25):1782–8. https://doi.org/10.1056/NEJM199406233302503.
4. Mahendiran T, Collet C, Bruyne BD. Coronary-artery autoregulation with increasing stenosis. N Engl J Med. 2024;390(21):2030–2. https://doi.org/10.1056/NEJMc2402216.
5. Taqueti VR. Coronary flow reserve: a versatile tool for interrogating pathophysiology, and a reliable marker of cardiovascular outcomes and mortality. Eur Heart J. 2022;43(16):1594–6. https://doi.org/10.1093/eurheartj/ehac001.
6. Kelshiker MA, Seligman H, Howard JP, et al. Coronary flow reserve and cardiovascular outcomes: a systematic review and meta-analysis. Eur Heart J. 2021;43(16):1582–93. https://doi.org/10.1093/eurheartj/ehab775.
7. Kemp HG Jr, Vokonas PS, Cohn PF, Gorlin R. The anginal syndrome associated with normal coronary arteriograms: report of a six year experience. Am J Med. 1973;54(6):735–42. https://doi.org/10.1016/0002-9343(73)90060-0.
8. Kemp HG Jr. Left ventricular function in patients with the anginal syndrome and normal coronary arteriograms. Am J Cardiol. 1973;32(3):375–6. https://doi.org/10.1016/S0002-9149(73)80150-X.
9. Melikian N, De Bruyne B, Fearon WF, MacCarthy PA. The pathophysiology and clinical course of the normal coronary angina syndrome (cardiac syndrome X). Prog Cardiovasc Dis. 2008;50(4):294–3. https://doi.org/10.1016/j.pcad.2007.01.003.
10. Rivero F, Gutiérrez-Barrios A, Gomez-Lara J, et al. Coronary microvascular dysfunction assessed by continuous intracoronary thermodilution: a comparative study with index of microvascular resistance. Int J Cardiol. 2021;333:1–7. https://doi.org/10.1016/j.ijcard.2021.03.005.
11. Mahendiran T, Stalikas N, Gallinoro E, Keulards D, Sakai K, Bouisset F, Viscusi MM, Corradetti S, Sonck J, van 't Veer M, Wilgenhof A, Pijls NHJ, Collet C, De Bruyne B. Coronary flow and resistance patterns indexed by subtended myocardial mass in coronary microvascular dysfunction. EuroIntervention. 2025;21(16):921–32. https://doi.org/10.4244/EIJ-D-25-00229.
12. Flanagan L. My journey with ischemia and nonobstructed coronary arteries. Circ Cardiovasc Qual Outcomes. 2022;15(7):e008745. https://doi.org/10.1161/circoutcomes.121.008745.
13. Helen H, Danielle P, Sarah B, et al. Living with myocardial ischaemia and no obstructive coronary arteries: a qualitative study. Open Heart. 2024;11(1):e002569. https://doi.org/10.1136/openhrt-2023-002569.
14. La S, Tavella R, Wu J, et al. The patient journey in chronic coronary syndromes with/without obstructive coronary arteries. European Heart J Qual Care Clin Outcome. 2025; https://doi.org/10.1093/ehjqcco/qcaf012.
15. Théberge ET, Burden E, Leung K, et al. Unveiling the longitudinal journey: 3-year follow-up of women with MINOCA and INOCA in a specialized heart Centre. CJC Open. 2024;6(12):1462–75. https://doi.org/10.1016/j.cjco.2024.08.013.

16. Emanuele GDT, Bertolone E, Fernandez-Peregrina P, Paolisso K, Bermpeis G, Esposito A, Gomez-Lopez A, Candreva N, Mileva M, Belmonte T, Mizukami S, Fournier M, Vanderheyden E, Wyffels J, Bartunek J, Sonck E, Barbato C, Collet B, De Bruyne. Reproducibility of bolus versus continuous thermodilution for assessment of coronary microvascular function in patients with ANOCA. EuroIntervention. 2023;19(2):e155–66. https://doi.org/10.4244/EIJ-D-22-00772.
17. Jason G, Aziz M, Samit S, Olga T, Yuhei K, Fahed AC, Evan S, Alok S, op den Buijs J, Joia S, Richard R, Brian B, Hayder H. Predictors of variability in coronary flow reserve and microvascular resistance measurement using the bolus Thermodilution technique ABSTRACT. Catheter Cardiovasc Interv. 2025; https://doi.org/10.1002/ccd.70301.
18. Cohoon TJ, Kern MJ. Extreme angiographic-physiologic mismatch with elevated left ventricular end-diastolic pressure. Cardiovasc Revasc Med. 2022;40s:182–3. https://doi.org/10.1016/j.carrev.2021.12.031.
19. Leonardi RA, Townsend JC, Patel CA, et al. Left ventricular end-diastolic pressure affects measurement of fractional flow reserve. Cardiovasc Revasc Med. 2013;14(4):218–22. https://doi.org/10.1016/j.carrev.2013.06.001.
20. Lim PO. Is index of microvascular resistance of Sisyphean utility in Takotsubo syndrome? ESC Heart Failure. 2024;11(6):4438–40. https://doi.org/10.1002/ehf2.14943.
21. Mahendiran T, Wilgenhof A, De Bruyne B. The elusiveness of "rest": the challenges of assessing resting coronary physiology. Circulation. 2025;152(3):147–9. https://doi.org/10.1161/CIRCULATIONAHA.125.074343.
22. Frais MA, Bergman DW, Kingma I, Smiseth OA, Smith ER, Tyberg JV. The dependence of the time constant of left ventricular isovolumic relaxation (tau) on pericardial pressure. Circulation. 1990;81(3):1071–80. https://doi.org/10.1161/01.CIR.81.3.1071.
23. Gonzalez MS, Basnight MA, Appleton CP. Experimental pericardial effusion: relation of abnormal respiratory variation in mitral flow velocity to hemodynamics and diastolic right heart collapse. J Am Coll Cardiol. 1991;17(1):239–48. https://doi.org/10.1016/0735-1097(91)90733-P.
24. Vos A, Jansen TPJ, Veer M, et al. Microvascular resistance reserve to assess microvascular dysfunction in ANOCA patients. J Am Coll Cardiol Intv. 2023;16(4):470–81. https://doi.org/10.1016/j.jcin.2022.12.012.
25. Ono R, Falcão LM. Supra-Normal Left Ventricular Function. Am J Cardiol. 2023;207:84–92. https://doi.org/10.1016/j.amjcard.2023.08.169.
26. Ford TJ, Stanley B, Sidik N, et al. 1-year outcomes of angina management guided by invasive coronary function testing (CorMicA). JACC Cardiovasc Interv. 2020;13(1):33–45. https://doi.org/10.1016/j.jcin.2019.11.001.
27. Vrints C, Andreotti F, Koskinas KC, Rossello X, Adamo M, Ainslie J, Banning AP, Budaj A, Buechel RR, Chiariello GA, Chieffo A, Christodorescu RM, Deaton C, Doenst T, Jones HW, Kunadian V, Mehilli J, Milojevic M, Piek JJ, Pugliese F, Rubboli A, Semb AG, Senior R, ten Berg JM, Van Belle E, Van Craenenbroeck EM, Vidal-Perez R, Winthe S, Borger M, Gudmundsdóttir IJ, Knuuti J, Ahrens I, Böhm M, Buccheri S, Capodanno D, Christiansen EH, Collet J-P, Dickstein K, Eek C, Falk V, Henriksen PA, Ibanez B, James S, Kedev S, Køber L, Kyriakou M, Magavern EF, McInerney A, William J, Caius ME, Mersha O, Mihaylova B, Mindham R, Neubeck L, Neumann F-J, Nielsen JC, Paolisso P, Paradies V, Pasquet AA, Piepoli M, Prescott E, Rakisheva A, Rocca B, Ruel M, Sandner S, Saraste A, Szummer K, Vaartjes I, Wijns W, Windecker S, Witkowsky A, Zdrakovic M, Zeppenfeld K, Shuka N, Bouraghda MA, Hayrapetyan HG, Reinstadler SJ, Musayev O, De Pauw M, Kušljugić Z, Valeri G, Bosko S, Maria K, Tomas K, Nielsen LH, Abdel-Aziz IS, Pekka TA, Benamer PH, Nadaraia K, Richardt G, Papafaklis MI, Dávid B, Gudmundsdóttir IJ, Arik W, Carmine RB, Kulzhanovich Z, Shpend E, Saamay A, Iveta M, Bachir A, Jolita B, Bruno P, Philip D, Valeriu R, Nebojsa BEG, Mohamed B, Admir D, Irena M, Kristin AK, Miguel BA, Coimbra LB, Alexandru P, Luca BB, Dušan B, Martin H, Zlatko F, Román F-P, Anna H, Raban JMY, Bani M, Rania H, Vedat AE, Nesukay G, Neil SA, Borisovich S. ESC guidelines for the management of chronic coronary syndromes. Eur Heart J. 2024;45(36):3415–537. https://doi.org/10.1093/eurheartj/ehae177.

28. Ahmet T, Yaren A, Ilke KT, Sabahattin U, Parker KH, van de Hoef TP, Sezer M, Piek JJ. The impact of high microvascular resistance on coronary wave energetics depends on coronary microvascular functionality Abstract. Eur Heart J Open. 2025;5(3). https://doi.org/10.1093/ehjopen/oeaf050.
29. Tas A, Alan Y, Damman P, van de Hoef TP, Tas IK, Türkmenoğlu EG, van Royen N, Perera D, Umman S, Parker KH, Piek JJ, Sezer M. Differential interaction of high microvascular resistance with coronary flow reserve across coronary microvascular dysfunction Endotypes. JACC Adv. 2025;4(12):102353. https://doi.org/10.1016/j.jacadv.2025.102353.
30. Jong C-B, Lu T-S, Yan-Tyng Liu P, et al. High dose escalation of intracoronary adenosine in the assessment of fractional flow reserve: a retrospective cohort study. PLoS One. 2020;15(10):e0240699. https://doi.org/10.1371/journal.pone.0240699.
31. Bernd WW, Schaper J, Baan AC, Arntzenius EL, Yellin. Cardiac dynamics quantification of extravascular coronary resistance. Springer Netherlands Dordrecht; 1980. p. 249–59.
32. Raff WK, Kosche F, Lochner W. Extravasale Komponente des Coronarwiderstandes und Coronardurchblutung bei steigendem enddiastolischen Druck. Coronary extravascular resistance and coronary blood flow at increasing enddiastolic pressure. Pflugers Arch Eur J Physiol. 1971;327(3):225–33. https://doi.org/10.1007/BF00586860.
33. Horstman AM, Dillon EL, Urban RJ, Sheffield-Moore M. The role of androgens and estrogens on healthy aging and longevity. J Gerontol A Biol Sci Med Sci. 2012;67(11):1140–52. https://doi.org/10.1093/gerona/gls068.
34. Lim PO. Could Brugada syndrome be treated with percutaneous coronary intervention? Circ J. 2023;88(1):177. https://doi.org/10.1253/circj.CJ-23-0685.
35. Collins P, Rosano GM, Sarrel PM, et al. 17 beta-estradiol attenuates acetylcholine-induced coronary arterial constriction in women but not men with coronary heart disease. Circulation. 1995;92(1):24–30. https://doi.org/10.1161/01.cir.92.1.24.
36. Gilligan DM, Quyyumi AA, Cannon RO 3rd. Effects of physiological levels of estrogen on coronary vasomotor function in postmenopausal women. Circulation. 1994;89(6):2545–51. https://doi.org/10.1161/01.cir.89.6.2545.
37. Leonardo F, Medeirus C, Rosano GM, et al. Effect of acute administration of estradiol 17 beta on aortic blood flow in menopausal women. Am J Cardiol. 1997;80(6):791–3. https://doi.org/10.1016/s0002-9149(97)00520-1.
38. Reis SE, Gloth ST, Blumenthal RS, et al. Ethinyl estradiol acutely attenuates abnormal coronary vasomotor responses to acetylcholine in postmenopausal women. Circulation. 1994;89(1):52–60. https://doi.org/10.1161/01.cir.89.1.52.
39. Volterrani M, Rosano G, Coats A, Beale C, Collins P. Estrogen acutely increases peripheral blood flow in postmenopausal women. Am J Med. 1995;99(2):119–22. https://doi.org/10.1016/s0002-9343(99)80130-2.
40. Vongpatanasin W, Tuncel M, Mansour Y, Arbique D, Victor RG. Transdermal estrogen replacement therapy decreases sympathetic activity in postmenopausal women. Circulation. 2001;103(24):2903–8. https://doi.org/10.1161/01.CIR.103.24.2903.
41. Sorop O, Zandbergen L, van Drie R, Merkus D, Duncker DJ. Coronary microvascular dysfunction in postmenopausal minipigs with multiple risk factors. Physiology. 2024;39(S1):2552. https://doi.org/10.1152/physiol.2024.39.S1.2552.
42. Ma L, Liu G, Ding M, et al. Isoflavone intake and the risk of coronary heart disease in US men and women. Circulation. 2020;141(14):1127–37. https://doi.org/10.1161/CIRCULATIONAHA.119.041306.
43. Shimazu T, Kuriyama S, Hozawa A, et al. Dietary patterns and cardiovascular disease mortality in Japan: a prospective cohort study. Int J Epidemiol. 2007;36(3):600–9. https://doi.org/10.1093/ije/dym005.
44. Shimokawa H, Suda A, Takahashi J, et al. Clinical characteristics and prognosis of patients with microvascular angina: an international and prospective cohort study by the coronary vasomotor disorders international study (COVADIS) group. Eur Heart J. 2021;42(44):4592–600. https://doi.org/10.1093/eurheartj/ehab282.

45. Cho L, Kaunitz AM, Faubion SS, et al. Rethinking menopausal hormone therapy: for whom, what, when, and how long? Circulation. 2023;147(7):597–6. https://doi.org/10.1161/circulationaha.122.061559.
46. Gu Y, Han F, Xue M, Wang M, Huang Y. The benefits and risks of menopause hormone therapy for the cardiovascular system in postmenopausal women: a systematic review and meta-analysis. BMC Womens Health. 2024;24(1):60. https://doi.org/10.1186/s12905-023-02788-0.
47. Liu Y, Li C. Hormone therapy and biological aging in postmenopausal women. JAMA Netw Open. 2024;7(8):e2430839. https://doi.org/10.1001/jamanetworkopen.2024.30839.
48. Samargandy S, Matthews KA, Brooks MM, et al. Arterial stiffness accelerates within 1 year of the final menstrual period: the SWAN heart study. Arterioscler Thromb Vasc Biol. 2020;40(4):1001–8. https://doi.org/10.1161/atvbaha.119.313622.
49. Vitale C, Mercuro G, Cerquetani E, et al. Time since menopause influences the acute and chronic effect of estrogens on endothelial function. Arterioscler Thromb Vasc Biol. 2008;28(2):348–52. https://doi.org/10.1161/ATVBAHA.107.158634.
50. Rosen SD, Uren NG, Kaski JC, et al. Coronary vasodilator reserve, pain perception, and sex in patients with syndrome X. Circulation. 1994;90(1):50–60. https://doi.org/10.1161/01.CIR.90.1.50.
51. Maseri A, Crea F, Kaski JC, Crake T. Mechanisms of angina pectoris in syndrome X. J Am Coll Cardiol. 1991;17(2):499–506. https://doi.org/10.1016/S0735-1097(10)80122-6.
52. Crea F, Pupita G, Galassi AR, et al. Role of adenosine in pathogenesis of anginal pain. Circulation. 1990;81(1):164–72. https://doi.org/10.1161/01.cir.81.1.164.
53. Sylvén C, Beermann B, Jonzon B, Brandt R. Angina pectoris-like pain provoked by intravenous adenosine in healthy volunteers. Br Med J (Clin Res Ed). 1986;293(6541):227–30. https://doi.org/10.1136/bmj.293.6541.227.
54. Akasaka T, Yoshida K, Yamamuro A, et al. Phasic coronary flow characteristics in patients with constrictive pericarditis. Circulation. 1997;96(6):1874–81. https://doi.org/10.1161/01.CIR.96.6.1874.
55. Jarmakani JMM, Mchale PA, Greenfield JC Jr. The effect of cardiac tamponade on coronary haemodynamics in the awake dog1. Cardiovasc Res. 1975;9(1):112–7. https://doi.org/10.1093/cvr/9.1.112.
56. Zacharias J, Forty J, Doig JC, Bourke JP, Hilton CJ. Right ventricular disarticulation. An 18-year single Centre experience☆. Eur J Cardiothorac Surg. 2005;27(6):1000–4. https://doi.org/10.1016/j.ejcts.2005.02.020.
57. Groeneweg JA, Bhonsale A, James CA, et al. Clinical presentation, long-term follow-up, and outcomes of 1001 Arrhythmogenic Right ventricular dysplasia/cardiomyopathy patients and family members. Circ Cardiovasc Genet. 2015;8(3):437–46. https://doi.org/10.1161/circgenetics.114.001003.
58. Borlaug BA, Carter RE, Melenovsky V, et al. Percutaneous pericardial resection. Circ Heart Fail. 2017;10(4):e003612. https://doi.org/10.1161/CIRCHEARTFAILURE.116.003612.
59. Gallinoro E, Candreva A, Colaiori I, Kodeboina M, Fournier S, Nelis O, Di Gioia G, Sonck J, van 't Veer M, Pijls NHJ, Collet C, De Bruyne B. Thermodilution-derived volumetric resting coronary blood flow measurement in humans. EuroIntervention. 2021;17(8):e672–9. https://doi.org/10.4244/EIJ-D-20-01092.
60. Mahendiran T, Fawaz S, Viscusi M, Keulards D, Crooijmans C, Jansen TPJ, Everaars H, Gallinoro E, Candreva A, Bouisset F, Mizukami T, Bertolone D, Belmonte M, Seki R, Svanerud J, Sonck J, Wilgenhof A, Keeble TR, Damman P, Knaapen P, Collet C, Pijls NHJ, De Bruyne B. Simplification of continuous intracoronary thermodilution. EuroIntervention. 2024;20(19):e1217–26. https://doi.org/10.4244/EIJ-D-24-00215.
61. Christopher A, Rajkumar Michael J, Foley F, Ahmed-Jushuf S, Chotai FA, Simader M, Mohsin A, Salih S, Ganesananthan N, Bual R, Petraco SS, Nijjer S, Sen J, Sehmi N, Ruparelia JN, Dungu A, Kabir K, Tang R, Gamma JR, Davies T, Kotecha GD, Cole JP, Howard TR, Keeble GJ, Clesham PD, O'Kane FE, Harrell JDP, Francis MJ, Shun-Shin RK, Al-Lamee. The role

of the collateral circulation in stable angina: an invasive placebo-controlled study. Circulation. 2025; https://doi.org/10.1161/CIRCULATIONAHA.125.074687.
62. Nowbar AN, Howard JP, Shun-Shin MJ, Rajkumar C, Foley M, Basu A, Goel A, Patel S, Adnan A, Beattie CJ, Keeble TR, Sohaib A, Collier D, McVeigh P, Harrell FE Jr, Francis DP, Al-Lamee RK. Daily angina documentation versus subsequent recall: development of a symptom smartphone app Abstract. European Heart Journal - Digital Health. 2022;3(2):276–83. https://doi.org/10.1093/ehjdh/ztac015.
63. Lim PO. Step test in hypertension. QJM. 93(11):703–5. https://doi.org/10.1093/qjmed/93.11.703.

Chapter 10
Hypertensive Heart

Abstract Hypertension is a risk factor for cardiac mortality, and it is associated with angina. For the latter, the mechanisms can be diverse. In the absence of obstructive coronary artery disease, these can range from endothelial dysfunction predisposing to coronary vasospasm, as well as vascular and left ventricular remodelling giving rise to coronary microvascular dysfunction and left ventricular hypertrophy respectively, and collectively they produce structural and electrical abnormalities in the hypertensive heart. This chapter presents three illustrative cases within hypertension's natural history, involving coronary thermodilution and acetylcholine provocation. Left ventricular diastolic dysfunction and raised coronary microvascular resistance are early common denominators responsible for exercise intolerance, leading to heart failure with preserved ejection fraction.

10.1 Introduction

Hypertension is a multifaceted conundrum. Although the strongest predictor is age, but given that rural people on a subsistence diet who are physically active, and nuns on prayerful monastic lives do not become hypertensive as they grow old suggest that it is largely a lifestyle manifestation, unless there is a clear-cut identifiable secondary cause [1, 2]. Excess mortality associated with hypertension does not "trough" until a systolic blood pressure (BP) of under 100 mmHg has led the European Society of Cardiology (ESC) to recommend a tighter treatment target to under 130 mmHg in 2024 [3]. Nevertheless, BP begins to rise when the systemic vasculature becomes stiff—with endothelial dysfunction which appears to be reversible, but there is a tipping point when hypertension becomes "essential", through neurohormonal adaptation and end-organ damage [4, 5].

Increased awareness of hypertension being a potent cardiac risk factor, also a multiplier in conjunction with diabetes and smoking for premature death, makes population screening mandatory. The archetypical feature of hypertension is a raised systemic vascular resistance, from non-compliant conductant vasculature and constricted microvasculature. To overcome this afterload, inter alia, the heart

P. O. Lim, *Coronary Thermodilution*,
https://doi.org/10.1007/978-3-032-10734-3_10

generates pressure through the Frank-Starling mechanism: higher outflow resistance reduces cardiac stroke volume leading to a raised residual end-systolic volume (ESV) increasing left ventricular stretch following renewed diastolic filling; this is how alpha-1 receptor agonists such as metaraminol work as an immediate treatment for hypotension, by increasing resistance to flow, also known as the Anrep effect [6]. However, when this results in a higher left ventricular filling pressure (LVEDP), it suggests reduced left ventricular compliance, or diastolic dysfunction. The high LVEDP in turn reduces coronary perfusion pressure via extravascular compression of the subendocardial microvasculature, and this is transmitted to the pulmonary vasculature via the left atrium, hence the twin siblings of angina and breathlessness, which are interchangeable. A dilated left atrium that occurs late from this constant back pressure is a reliable advanced marker of this phenomenon. This is why exercise intolerance occurs in hypertension from diastolic dysfunction or heart failure with preserved ejection fraction (HFpEF) [7].

10.2 Cases

10.2.1 Epicardial Vasospasm and Endothelial Dysfunction

A 61-year-old Black woman complained of breathlessness. She has secondary hypertension due to ACTH-dependent Cushing's syndrome treated with right adrenalectomy 2 years ago, in addition to type 2 diabetes, hyperlipidaemia, past smoking and coronary angioplasty to her right coronary artery 3 years prior. She was also overweight and has obstructive sleep apnoea.

Procedure She undergoes a one-stop diagnostic coronary angiogram, proceeding to a physiology study if her arteries are patent. Her coronary arteries are unobstructed and she has elevated central aortic BP of 140/67 mmHg. Her left ventricular angiogram shows no wall motion abnormalities, LVEDP at rest is 8 mmHg, but it rises to 20 mmHg with handgrip. Continuous thermodilution is undertaken to the left anterior descending (LAD) artery—this artery is tortuous with diminishing calibre towards the apex. The basal and hyperaemic indices are as follows: 61 to 161 mL/min and 1481 to 509 Wood units; thus coronary flow reserve, CFR, is 2.6 and microvascular resistance reserve, MRR 2.9. Acetylcholine (ACh 2, 20 and 100 μg) provokes a dose-dependent epicardial vasospasm with falling distal-to-aortic pressure ratio, Pd/Pa: baseline 0.92, 0.92, 0.84 and 0.73—she experiences angina at the last ACh dose, intracoronary glyceryl trinitrate (GTN) 200 μg returns the Pd/Pa to 0.91, and flow back to baseline. However, despite the epicardial vasospasm, she increases her flow with ACh > 1.5-fold.

Interpretation This lady has *intact vasodilatory capacity*, and as expected from her long-standing hypertension, ***raised coronary resistance*** with ***reduced left ventricular diastolic compliance***. She has *isolated epicardial endothelial dysfunction* as ACh provokes flow-limiting vasospasm but interestingly this did not extend to her microvasculature as it increases flow in response to ACh, suggesting *preserved microvascular endothelial function*. As the main issue is epicardial vasoreactivity, the mainstay treatment would be calcium channel blockade, and her beta blocker could be discontinued. ACh 100 μg increases flow by 90% while verapamil 200 μg raises flow by 85%, at a similar level and abolishing the ACh-induced epicardial vasospasm. Her follow-up cardiovacular magnetic resonance (CMR) scan reveals mild LV septal hypertrophy (1.1 cm); otherwise she has a normal heart (Fig. 10.1).

10.2.2 Left Ventricular Diastolic Dysfunction

A 48-year-old Caucasian woman has a three-year history of angina associated with breathlessness and palpitations, triggered both by physical exertion and emotion. Her symptoms were reproduced on a Bruce protocol treadmill test in which she managed 6 min and 42 s. Her heart rate (HR) peaked at 157 bpm from 98 bpm; 91% (> 85%, 220—age) maximal HR predicted, and corresponding BP; 164/99 and 126/79 mmHg. However, there were no objective ischaemic electrocardiographic, nor echocardiographic changes, despite her symptoms and adequacy of exercise stress level. Her CT coronary angiogram could not be completed because of tachycardia, but she has zero coronary calcium score. Her transthoracic echocardiogram showed a normal heart without LVH in spite of her hypertension; she was managed

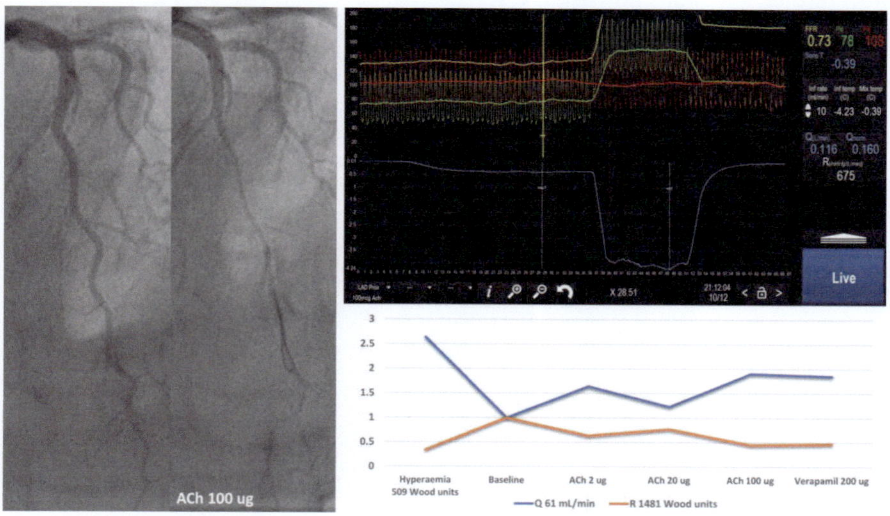

Fig. 10.1 **(Left panels)** Left anterior descending (LAD) artery at baseline and severe epicardial vasospasm in response to acetylcholine (ACh) 100 μg. Continuous thermodilution undertaken to the LAD after ACh 100 μg (**top right panel**); note the fall in perfusion pressure to a Pd/Pa of 0.73, but flow is increased 1.9-fold (**bottom right panel**), which also shows preserved vasodilatory capacity on a background of raised coronary resistance and intact microvascular endothelial function. Intracoronary verapamil abolishes the epicardial vasopasm, without augmenting flow beyond that which is induced by ACh

on ramipril and bisoprolol. She takes atorvastatin for her hyperlipidaemia which is yet to target, has been a smoker for 26 years, smoking 10 per day, and is perimenopausal with rising follicular stimulating hormone (FSH) at 55 (< 30) IU/L, with normal thyroid function and Vitamin D level.

Procedure Her coronary angiogram as expected shows unobstructed coronary arteries (Fig. 10.2). Her BP is labile during her procedure, with a central aortic systolic BP rising from 125 to 162 mmHg, > 150 mmHg when her LVEDP is measured; this is raised to 18 mmHg, rising to 20 mmHg with handgrip. Bolus thermodilution is undertaken to the LAD, initially with intracoronary adenosine 200 μg which gives the following results; fractional flow reserve, FFR 0.92, CFR 4.2, index of microvascular resistance, IMR 13 and MRR 5.4. These are reproducibly repeated with 1 mg of adenosine; FFR 0.92, CFR 4.1, IMR 14 and MRR 5.2 (Fig. 10.3). The higher dose of adenosine is well tolerated and appears to amplify the saline bolus signal.

Continuous thermodilution is next performed in the LAD (Fig. 10.2). The basal and hyperaemic flow are 62 and 197 mL/min, respectively, with paired resistance of 1767 and 475 Wood units; therefore, CFR 3.2, MRR 3.7 and estimated IMR 24 (475/20). Increasing doses of intracoronary acetylcholine (ACh) are given. Low doses of ACh are associated with a flow reduction > 10%, from the baseline without overt epicardial vasospasm. Higher doses are associated with a flow increase over 1.5-fold in the absence of any reduction in epicardial calibre suggesting preserved endothelial function. Interestingly, intracoronary verapamil 1 mg does not increase flow further, but blunts flow with ACh rechallenge. Also, escalating ACh is not associated with bradyarrhythmias in this woman.

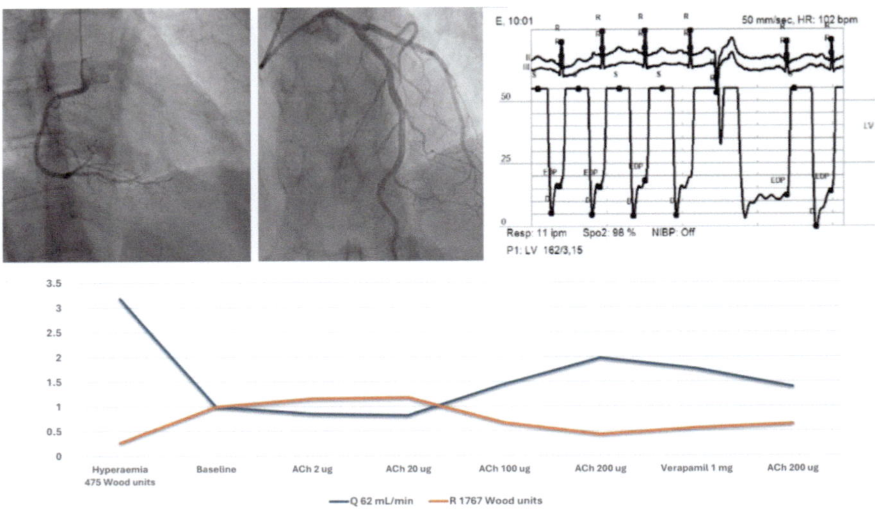

Fig. 10.2 **(Upper panel)** Right and left coronary arteries are without significant disease. Labile blood pressure (BP) during the procedure, with high systolic BP reflected in a raised left ventricular end-diastolic pressure (LVEDP) and coronary resistance. **(Lower panel)** Coronary haemodynamics during hyperaemia and in response to acetylcholine and verapamil

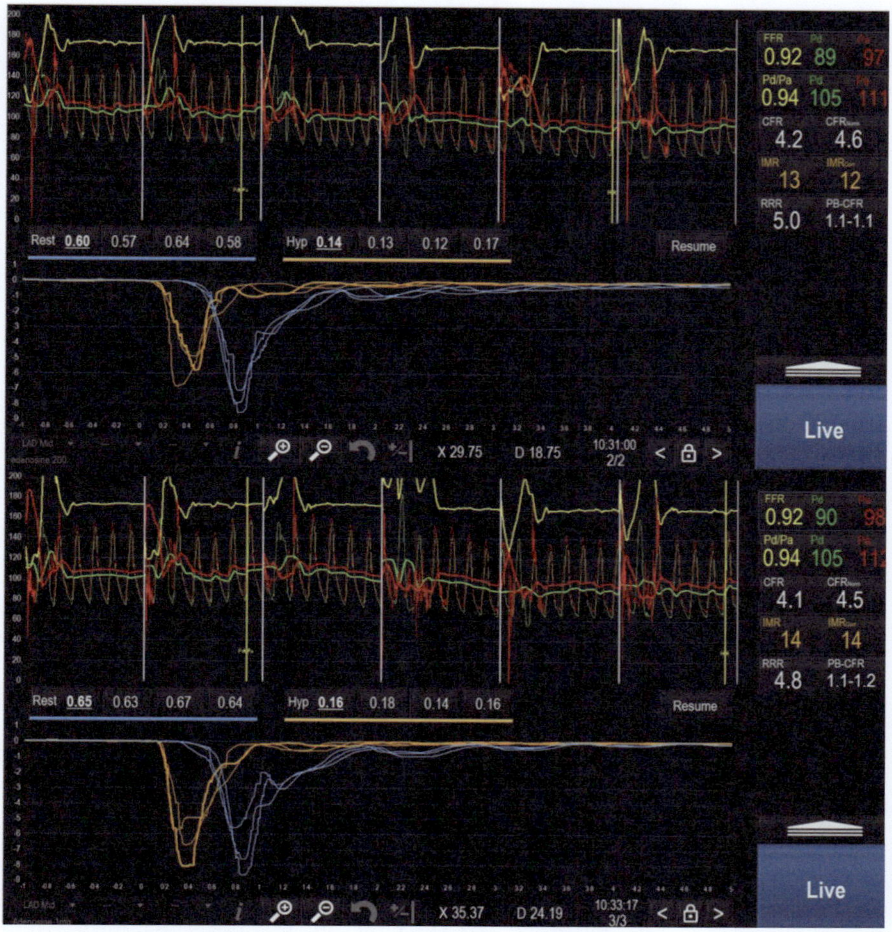

Fig. 10.3 Bolus thermodilution on the left anterior descending (LAD) artery with intracoronary adenosine, initially with 200 µg (**upper panel**) followed by 1 mg (**lower panel**). With the higher adenosine dose, the signal appears to be magnified but with concordant results

Interpretation This lady has raised rest and hyperaemic coronary resistance secondary to systemic hypertension, with corresponding rise in LVEDP suggestive of diastolic dysfunction, but preserved microvascular function and without overt vasoreactivity with ACh challenge. The initial flow reduction would traditionally be interpreted as an early "microvascular spasm in the absence of epicardial vasospasm", but it could also be due to an element of epicardial vasospasm from *first-pass* ACh as discussed in Chap. 1. This case also illustrates two further points, the limitation of bolus themodilution in detecting raised coronary resistance, and the Oldenburg Paradox, verapamil-potentiated flow reduction with ACh rechallenge (Chap. 1). The focus in this case would be beta blockade, strict control of BP and risk factor management.

At 1 year follow-up her BP was well controlled on ramipril 1.25 mg od and nebivolol 2.5 mg od, and her ambulatory daytime mean BP was 101/68 mmHg. Her breathlessness resolved, had less angina, and converted from smoking to vaping—nicotine is a potent disruptor of endothelial function and causes coronary artery spasm.

10.2.3 Left Ventricular Mid-cavity Obstruction

A 75-year-old South Asian woman complained of angina and breathlessness. She has labile hypertension and hyperlipidaemia. Her recent clinic BP was reproducibly elevated at 145–147/87-89 mmHg off treatment. When she was 61, she had a dobutamine stress echocardiogram (DSE). Even though there was no inducible cardiac ischaemia, she exhibited left ventricular mid-cavity obstructive (MCO), with a gradient of 95 mmHg in the context of mild concentric LVH, at peak dose of dobutamine 30 μg/kg/min achieving 90% (> 85%) of her maximal predicted HR (Fig. 10.4). This was associated with angina and a fall in BP to 94/58 mmHg. Her diagnostic coronary angiogram then showed unobstructed coronary arteries—she was reassured and discharged from clinic. As she was planning to have a right hip revision surgery, she underwent cardiac fitness assessment in view of her continuing symptoms and regular use of nitroglycerine spray. A repeat DSE was undertaken. Her HR response was 89% (> 85%) predicted, with a baseline BP of 161/78 mmHg, falling to 131/77 mmHg at peak dobutamine dose of 30 μg/kg/min. However, she reported no symptoms during the test, neither was there ischaemic electrocardiographic or echocardiographic changes. Her NT-ProBNP was mildly raised at 198 (<125) pg/mL.

Procedure She undergoes a coronary physiology study. She has a demonstrable MCO gradient of 25–30 mmHg (Fig. 10.5). The resting LVEDP is 16 mmHg, rising rapidly to over 20 mmHg with handgrip. Her coronary arteries remain unobstructed. Continuous thermodilution is undertaken to LAD; it appears meandering and of small calibre distally. The following are obtained; basal and hyperaemic indices—flow 63 to 86 mL/min, and resistance 1632 to 976 Wood units respectively: CFR 1.4 and MRR 1.7. Low-dose 2 μg and 20 μg acetylcholine provoke a dose-dependent epicardial vasospasm with a minor fall in flow < 10% and Pd/Pa of 0.92, culminating with a run of atrial fibrillation. Verapamil pre-treatment although alleviates acetylcholine's effect; there is continuing fall in flow by 11%. Instead, the mid-LAD myocardial bridging becomes more apparent, but non-obstructive, Pd/Pa 0.94. The circumflex (Cx) artery is also studied; flow 86 mL/min to 145 mL/min and resistance 1519 Wood units to 581 Wood units: CFR 2.1 and MRR 2.6—with transient atrioventricular block during saline hyperaemia.

Interpretation This woman has a low coronary flow state with restrictive vasodilatory capacity, associated with raised basal and hyperaemic resistance. In other words, she has quintessential coronary microvascular dysfunction (CMD). In addi-

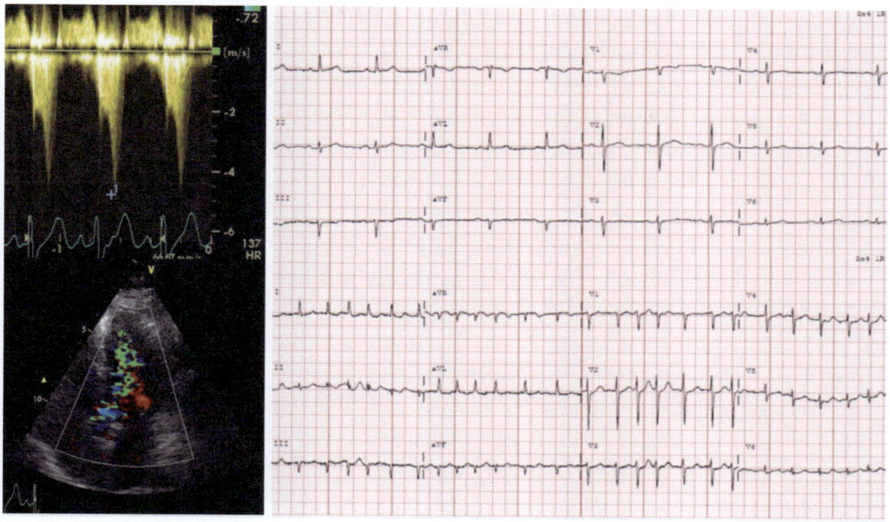

Fig. 10.4 Left panels—(**top**) Dynamic "sharkfin" doppler gradient, and (**bottom**) turbulent flow across the mid-left ventricle on dobutamine stress echocardiogram undertaken 14 years ago. **Right panels**—(**top**) Electrocardiograms show left axis deviation with transition chest lead at V2 suggestive of left ventricular hypertrophy (LVH), and (**bottom**) acetylcholine or vagal-mediated self-limiting atrial fibrillation

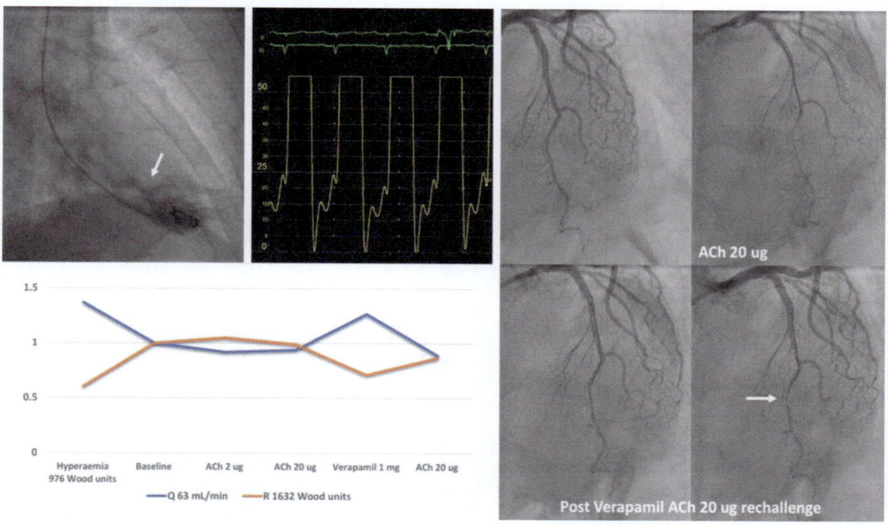

Fig. 10.5 Top panels (left to right)—Left ventricular angiogram with early contraction in mid-left ventricle causing an obstruction to flow (arrow), thus a gradient, resistant exercise with hand-grip raises left ventricular diastolic filling pressure, baseline angiogram of left anterior descending artery and vasospasm of the artery following acetylcholine. **Bottom panels (left to right)** Continuous thermodilution chart showing high basal and hyperaemic resistance with impaired vasodilatory capacity, failure of flow to increase with acetylcholine, instead epicardial vasospasm occurs, ameliorated by verapamil without flow increase which unmasks underlying myocardial bridging (*arrow*)

tion, she has generalised or both epicardial and microvascular endothelial dysfunction. Although the ACh-induced epicardial vasospasm was angiographically severe with incidental mid-LAD myocardial bridging, the distal coronary pressure was maintained, i.e. no fall in perfusion pressure and she was asymptomatic.

Although verapamil pre-treatment prevented ACh-provoked epicardial vasospasm, it paradoxically reduced flow at the microvascular level; this was described as "unmasking" microvascular spasm (resistant to GTN [8–11]), but in this case, it was a demonstration of the *Oldenburg Paradox*; verapamil-potentiated microvascular endothelial dysfunction—**ACh flow ↓, Verapamil flow ↑ and ACh rechallenge flow ↓↓**. If it was unmasking of microvascular spasm the flow should not fall further, but should stay the same at the pre-verapamil level; this phenomenon has been reproduced often as described elsewhere in the book.

In addition, she has clear MCO associated with diastolic dysfunction—a form of HFpEF. The novel finding was that the degree of CMD was segmental in the presence of MCO, *LAD was affected more than Cx*, although both arteries have concordantly high resistance.

This case potentially provided an explanation for her labile hypertension; when her MCO is accentuated, even if her systemic BP is low, she actually has intraventricular hypertension, and when the MCO is "relieved", her intracardiac hypertension is transmitted peripherally. MCO during dobutamine stress echocardiography as with this woman 14 years before is usually disregarded as artefactual in practice; hence it may not be reported routinely [12].

The question is, whether vasodilators such as calcium channel blockers or diuretics that deplete volume, which can increase MCO, should be avoided—there is clinical evidence that these should be avoided in highly symptomatic patients [13]. In the first instance, she is cautiously treated with a vasodilating beta blocker in view of her CMD, MCO and vasoreactivity.

Her cardiovascular magnetic resonance (CMR) scan on nebivolol 2.5 mg od 3 weeks later shows a functionally normal heart with an EF of 57% and volume-derived VAC 0.75 (0.6-1.0), without LA dilatation or LVH—which suggests that MCO is preload-dependent in hypertensives and can occur in a structurally normal heart.

10.3 Discussion

High coronary resistance, whether at baseline or at hyperaemia, is a signature finding of transmitted hypertension to the coronary circulation, especially if the coronaries are unobstructed. Reduced left ventricular compliance is another key feature, when the LVEDP is raised and it rises early with physical or emotional stress. These however can be masked or modified by drug therapy and procedural anxiety. Vasodilators such as long-acting oral nitrates and calcium channel blockers are routinely withheld for at least 24–48 h prior to coronary physiology study, to facilitate spasm testing with acetylcholine. Thus, uninterrupted antihypertensive agents or concomitant drugs may influence coronary haemodynamics in ways that are not yet well delineated. Pragmatically, if clinic BP is uncontrolled (> 180 mmHg systolic), it is advisable to defer the procedure. In other words, continuing symptoms despite drug treatment while uncovering abnormal coronary physiology will better guide further management. Although BP can be labile during the stressful invasive procedure (Chap. 1).

The conclusions of the three cases presented herein are (Table 10.1): (1) epicardial vasoreactivity, (2) left ventricular diastolic dysfunction, and (3) CMD with LV MCO. These cases are representative of the natural history of hypertension—from initial endothelial dysfunction with increased afterload, leading to hypertensive heart adaptation, and finally CMD. The varying pathophysiological mechanism can be targeted by lifestyle modification or drug treatment. In the early phase, salt and stress may synergistically initiate, promote and maintain hypertension, later vasodilators and drugs targeting the renin angiotensin aldosterone axis will be essential, and finally diuretics and beta blockers, when HFpEF sets in [4]. Hypertension in isolation, coronary flow is not usually compromised until heart failure occurs but in practice, comorbid habits or conditions usually cluster, perpetuating and magnifying each other's influence, such as sedentary lifestyle, excessive salt intake, smoking, diabetes, hyperlipidaemia and kidney dysfunction—through common pathways of stiffening of outflow vasculature, resulting in adverse ventriculo-arterial coupling (VAC) [14]. This is defined by the ratio (0.6–1.0) between residual volume of blood in LV following contraction (end-systolic volume, ESV) and volume of blood ejected by LV (stroke volume, SV) at each cardiac cycle. These volume-derived indices can be estimated easily with echocardiography. The higher this ratio is, the harder the heart works via myocardial stretch to generate the pressure needed to push blood down the non-compliant vasculature; this negatively impacts coronary haemodynamics, and raised ESV indexed to body surface area is a powerful predictor of HFpEF [15]. Mechanistically, a lower ESV suggests more "stored" potential energy, that, when the heart recoils compliantly into diastole, this aids rapid filling of left ventricle with higher myocardial stretch at lower end-diastolic pressure, i.e. a more efficient heart, the exception is, if the low ESV is secondary to hypertrophic cardiomyopathy.

The degree of afterload can be summed up as arterial elastance—how much pressure the heart needs to generate to push 1 mL of blood out into the aorta—the ratio between LV end-systolic pressure (ESP) over SV; while the SV can be obtained with echocardiography, not so for ESP, but for all intents and purposes, it is the same as central "aortic" BP, unless there is valvular heart disease—and it can be reconstructed non-invasively with validated devices such as SphygmoCor®. Nevertheless, there is discrepancy between central BP (ESP) and brachial (cuff, peripheral) BP [16]. The central BP is what the heart sees and it is more prognostic—drug treatment can spuriously normalise cuff BP, yet central BP remains uncontrolled; this is fairly common with beta blockade [17]. Another more practical indicator of afterload is pulse wave velocity (PWV). This is a pulse wave generated by the heart, travelling between two fixed points within the vasculature, in particular between carotid and femoral arteries, detectable as time delay over that distance, with applanation tonometry. The faster the pulse wave, the stiffer the artery is. Within the

Table 10.1 Coronary physiology and hypertension

Case	Age	BMI	Comorbidities	Vasodilatory Capacity (CFR)	Coronary Resistance (Wood units)	Vasoreactivity (ACh)
1	61♀	31	Cushing syndrome related hypertension, diabetes, hyperlipidaemia, obstructive sleep apnoea, previous right coronary artery angioplasty and past smoking CMR EF 61%, VAC 0.67, septal LVH 1.1 cm	LAD 2.6	**509** MRR 2.9 LVEDP 8 → 20 handgrip BP 140/67	Dose-dependent epicardial vasospasm with ACh 2 (ΔQ ↑64%), 20 (↑23%) and 100 (↑90%) µg (Pd/Pa 0.92 → 0.92 → 0.84 → 0.73) but without flow (Q) reduction, in fact > 50% from baseline, and verapamil (↑85%) abolished the epicardial vasospasm and increased flow at the same magnitude implying intact microvascular endothelial function
2	48♀	25	Hypertension, hyperlipidaemia, perimenopause	LAD Bolus Thermodilution IC adenosine 200 µg 4.2 adenosine 1 mg 4.1 Continuous Thermodilution 3.2	**IMR** **Adenosine 200 µg 13** **Adenosine 1 mg 14** **(underestimated coronary microvascular resistance)** **475** LVEDP 18 → 20 handgrip BP 125 → 162	Early flow (Q) reduction ACh 2 (ΔQ ↓15%), 20 (↓18%), 100 (↑45%), 200 µg (↑98%) Verapamil 1 mg (↑76%) Rechallenge ACh 200 µg (↑38%—**Δ↓60%**) *Oldenburg Paradox*
3	75♀	23	Hypertension, hyperlipidaemia	LAD 1.4 63 → 86 mL/min Genuinely reduced vasodilatory capacity, resting flow was not raised Cx 2.1 86 → 145 mL/min	LAD 1632 vs **976** Cx 1519 vs **581** LVEDP 16 → 20 handgrip BP 126 → 145 NT-ProBNP 198	Flow reduction with escalating ACh: 2 µg (ΔQ ↓8%, Pd/Pa 0.95), and 20 µg (↓6%, Pd/Pa 0.92)—dose-dependent epicardial vasospasm Verapamil 1 mg (↑27%) ACh 20 µg (↓11%)—**Δ↓5%**) *Oldenburg Paradox*—vasospasm resolved yet flow fell with obvious myocardial bridging but Pd/Pa 0.94 suggesting that the reduced flow was at the microvascular level

Framingham population, it strongly relates to hypertension and diabetes and is an independent predictor of cardiovascular events, as much as 50% for those outlying within one standard deviation from a normalised age-adjusted value [14, 18]. It is believed that a stiff artery allows "undampened and non-peristaltic" pressure to be transmitted full force distally into any end-organ's microvasculature; for example, in the kidney, it causes pre-glomerular arteriolar constriction, leading to compensatory post-glomerular arteriolar contraction, resulting in glomerular hypertension and hence kidney dysfunction. The same occurs within the cardiac microvasculature, and it induces the remodelling triad, especially in the presence of myocardial hypertrophy; (1) inward eutropic media hyperplasia of the arterioles without increasing its diameter, hence luminal constriction, (2) perivascular fibrosis or collagen deposition restricting vasodilatation, and (3) rarefaction or reduction in capillary density, reducing tissue perfusion. These structural changes *increase microvascular resistance* shifting the autoregulatory range upward and to the right and lower the vasodilatory reserve. Increased baseline metabolic demand is met by enhanced myocardial oxygen extraction, rather than by basal flow increase. Thus, predisposing to earlier autoregulatory failure at lower perfusion pressure leading to doubling of mortality in ST elevation myocardial infarction (STEMI), and progressing to HFpEF which is characterised by LVH, left atrial enlargement and raised NT-ProBNP where CMD is highly prevalent [19, 20]. Since increased afterload causing cardiac pressure overload is one of the root causes of hypertension, it is not surprising that PWV is a sensitive early marker of CMD in hypertensives with non-obstructive coronary arteries [21].

Another hallmark of hypertension is LVH, with an increase in cardiac mass; the process becomes maladaptive [22]. It is an adverse prognostic factor with doubling of cardiac mortality for every 100 g/m^2 increase in the weight of the heart, but this is modifiable by drug treatment [23]. It relates more to ambulatory BP than clinic BP, but even better predicted by submaximal exercise BP, which can be obtained using a simple 3-min step test [24–26]. The morphology of LVH is usually concentric, i.e. similar thickening of the septal and posterior wall, but can be asymmetric, affecting the basal septum more, and this gives rise to LV outflow tract obstruction (LVOTO), phenotypically simulating hypertrophic cardiomyopathy, especially in the elderly [27]. On the other hand, MCO is underappreciated, often detected during dobutamine stress echocardiography and discounted as artefactual, but it is modifiable with beta blockade [28, 29]. Unlike LVOTO, MCO is loading dependent, seen more in patients who are fluid depleted [30]. In other words, when MCO is relieved, the high end-systolic pressure (ESP) is transmitted peripherally; when it is prominent, the obstruction to flow reduces BP transmission, to the extent of causing collapses [31], which can cause angina with diffuse ST-segment elevation or breathlessness with spuriously low BP. The behaviour of MCO has parallels with use of cardiac-specific myosin inhibitor in relieving LVOTO in hypertrophic cardiomyopathy; the high ESP is then transmitted unimpeded, precipitating malignant hypertension [32]. LVH has differential histological remodelling across the myocardium, concentrated more on the subendocardium rendering it more susceptible ischaemia, identifiable electrocardiographically as "anterior tall R complex with lateral ST strain pattern" [33]. This also explains the phenomenon of angina with lactate rise despite preservation of coronary flow, and coronary sinus reducer (CSR) appears to ameriolate this by redistributing blood supply to the subendocardium [34–36].

In conclusion, the hypertensive heart from the coronary physiology point of view is characterised by LV diastolic dysfunction with raised LVEDP and increased coronary microvascular resistance. IMR from bolus themodilution is not sufficiently sensitive to detect the latter compared with hyperaemic resistance obtained with continuous themodilution. Epicardial endothelial dysfunction as expressed by ACh-provoked spasm or vasoreactivity is not inevitable, but is highly prevalent and CMD could be due to MCO or LVOTO and LVH.

References

1. Timio M, Verdecchia P, Venanzi S, Gentili S, Ronconi M, Francucci B, et al. Age and blood pressure changes. A 20-year follow-up study in nuns in a secluded order. Hypertension. 1988;12(4):457–61. https://doi.org/10.1161/01.hyp.12.4.457.
2. He J, Tell GS, Tang YC, Mo PS, He GQ. Effect of migration on blood pressure: the Yi People Study. Epidemiology. 1991;2(2):88–97. https://doi.org/10.1097/00001648-199103000-00002.
3. McEvoy JW, McCarthy CP, Bruno RM, Brouwers S, Canavan MD, Ceconi C, et al. 2024 ESC guidelines for the management of elevated blood pressure and hypertension. Eur Heart J. 2024;45(38):3912–4018. https://doi.org/10.1093/eurheartj/ehae178.
4. Lim PO, Struthers AD, MacDonald TM. The neurohormonal natural history of essential hypertension: towards primary or tertiary aldosteronism? J Hypertens. 2002;20(1):11–5. https://doi.org/10.1097/00004872-200201000-00003.
5. Lim PO, Tzemos N, Farquharson CA, Anderson JE, Deegan P, MacWalter RS, et al. Reversible hypertension following coeliac disease treatment: the role of moderate hyperhomocysteinaemia and vascular endothelial dysfunction. J Hum Hypertens. 2002;16(6):411–5. https://doi.org/10.1038/sj.jhh.1001404.
6. Lim HS. Law of the Heart. In: Hemodynamic physiology in advanced heart failure and cardiogenic shock. Cham: Springer Nature; 2024. p. 3–23.
7. Lim PO, MacFadyen RJ, Clarkson PB, MacDonald TM. Impaired exercise tolerance in hypertensive patients. Ann Intern Med. 1996;124(1 Pt 1):41–55. https://doi.org/10.7326/0003-4819-124-1_part_1-199601010-00008.
8. Ford TJ, Mikhail P. Acetylcholine (re)challenge: from diagnosis to targeted therapy. J Am Coll Cardiol Intv. 2022;15(1):76–9. https://doi.org/10.1016/j.jcin.2021.11.022.
9. Rehan R, Wong CCY, Weaver J, Jain P, Adams M, Ng MKC, et al. Impact of nitroglycerin administration on acetylcholine provocation testing in angina with nonobstructive coronary arteries. J Soc Cardiovasc Angiogr Interv. 2025:103668. https://doi.org/10.1016/j.jscai.2025.103668.
10. Seitz A, Feenstra R, Konst RE, Martinez Pereyra V, Beck S, Beijk M, et al. Acetylcholine rechallenge: a first step toward tailored treatment in patients with coronary artery spasm. JACC Cardiovasc Interv. 2022;15(1):65–75. https://doi.org/10.1016/j.jcin.2021.10.003.
11. Vohra AS, Osborn EA. Hold the nitro: acetylcholine provocation testing for coronary vasospasm. J Soc Cardiovasc Angiogr Interv. 2025. https://doi.org/10.1016/j.jscai.2025.103760.
12. Jhawar MB, Balla S, Alpert MA, Chockalingam A. Left ventricular outflow tract and midcavity obstruction may cause false-positive dobutamine stress echocardiograms. Eur J Echocardiogr. 2011;12(3):E14. https://doi.org/10.1093/ejechocard/jeq158.

13. Harrison MR, Grigsby CG, Souther SK, Smith MD, DeMaria AN. Midventricular obstruction associated with chronic systemic hypertension and severe left ventricular hypertrophy. Am J Cardiol. 1991;68(8):761–5. https://doi.org/10.1016/0002-9149(91)90650-a.
14. Vasan RS, Pan S, Xanthakis V, Beiser A, Larson MG, Seshadri S, et al. Arterial stiffness and long-term risk of health outcomes: the Framingham Heart Study. Hypertension. 2022;79(5):1045–56. https://doi.org/10.1161/HYPERTENSIONAHA.121.18776.
15. Kato M, Kitada S, Kawada Y, Nakasuka K, Kikuchi S, Seo Y, et al. Left ventricular end-systolic volume is a reliable predictor of new-onset heart failure with preserved left ventricular ejection fraction. Cardiol Res Pract. 2020;2020:3106012. https://doi.org/10.1155/2020/3106012.
16. McEniery CM, McDonnell B, Munnery M, Wallace SM, Rowe CV, Cockcroft JR, et al. Central pressure: variability and impact of cardiovascular risk factors. Hypertension. 2008;51(6):1476–82. https://doi.org/10.1161/HYPERTENSIONAHA.107.105445.
17. Baba BA, Johan PT, Mohan JC. Comparision of central aortic pressure to brachial artery pressure in hypertensive patients on drug treatment: an observational study. Indian Heart J. 2018;70 Suppl 3(Suppl 3):S208–12. https://doi.org/10.1016/j.ihj.2018.10.418.
18. Mitchell GF, Hwang S-J, Vasan RS, Larson MG, Pencina MJ, Hamburg NM, et al. Arterial stiffness and cardiovascular events. Circulation. 2010;121(4):505–11. https://doi.org/10.1161/CIRCULATIONAHA.109.886655.
19. Shah SJ, Lam CSP, Svedlund S, Saraste A, Hage C, Tan R-S, et al. Prevalence and correlates of coronary microvascular dysfunction in heart failure with preserved ejection fraction: PROMIS-HFpEF. Eur Heart J. 2018;39(37):3439–50. https://doi.org/10.1093/eurheartj/ehy531.
20. De Luca G, Nardin M, Algowhary M, Uguz B, Oliveira DC, Ganyukov V, et al. Impact of hypertension on mortality in patients with ST-elevation myocardial infarction undergoing primary angioplasty: insights from the international multicenter ISACS-STEMI registry. J Hypertens. 9900. https://doi.org/10.1097/hjh.0000000000003890.
21. Rezaeian P, Shufelt CL, Wei J, Pacheco C, Cook-Wiens G, Berman D, et al. Arterial stiffness assessment in coronary microvascular dysfunction and heart failure with preserved ejection fraction: an initial report from the WISE-CVD continuation study. Am Heart J Plus. 2024;41:100390. https://doi.org/10.1016/j.ahjo.2024.100390.
22. Zhou W, Brown JM, Bajaj NS, Chandra A, Divakaran S, Weber B, et al. Hypertensive coronary microvascular dysfunction: a subclinical marker of end organ damage and heart failure. Eur Heart J. 2020;41(25):2366–75. https://doi.org/10.1093/eurheartj/ehaa191.
23. Cooper RS, Simmons BE, Castaner A, Santhanam V, Ghali J, Mar M. Left ventricular hypertrophy is associated with worse survival independent of ventricular function and number of coronary arteries severely narrowed. Am J Cardiol. 1990;65(7):441–5. https://doi.org/10.1016/0002-9149(90)90807-d.
24. Lim PO, Donnan PT, MacDonald TM. How well do office and exercise blood pressures predict sustained hypertension? A Dundee Step Test Study. J Hum Hypertens. 2000;14(7):429–33. https://doi.org/10.1038/sj.jhh.1001041.
25. Lim PO, MacDonald TM. Step test in hypertension. QJM. 2000;93(11):703–5. https://doi.org/10.1093/qjmed/93.11.703.
26. Lim PO, Donnan PT, MacDonald TM. Blood pressure determinants of left ventricular wall thickness and mass index in hypertension: comparing office, ambulatory and exercise blood pressures. J Hum Hypertens. 2001;15(9):627–33. https://doi.org/10.1038/sj.jhh.1001229.
27. Topol EJ, Traill TA, Fortuin NJ. Hypertensive hypertrophic cardiomyopathy of the elderly. N Engl J Med. 1985;312(5):277–83. https://doi.org/10.1056/NEJM198501313120504.
28. Christiaens L, Duplantier C, Allal J, Donal E, Nanadoumgar H, Barraine R, et al. Normal coronary angiogram and dobutamine-induced left ventricular obstruction during stress echocardiography: a higher hemodynamic responsiveness to dobutamine. Echocardiography. 2001;18(4):285–90. https://doi.org/10.1046/j.1540-8175.2001.00285.x.
29. Madaric J, Bartunek J, Verhamme K, Penicka M, Van Schuerbeeck E, Nellens P, et al. Hyperdynamic myocardial response to beta-adrenergic stimulation in patients with chest pain

and normal coronary arteries. J Am Coll Cardiol. 2005;46(7):1270–5. https://doi.org/10.1016/j.jacc.2005.06.052.
30. Harrison MR, Grigsby CG, Souther SK, Smith MD, DeMaria AN. Midventricular obstruction associated with chronic systemic hypertension and severe left ventricular hypertrophy. Am J Cardiol. 1991;68(8):761–5. https://doi.org/10.1016/0002-9149(91)90650-A.
31. Ordine L, Losi MA, Canciello G, Borrelli F, Esposito G. Symptomatic orthostatic hypotension due to standing mid-left ventricular obstruction: a case report. Eur Heart J Case Rep. 2024. https://doi.org/10.1093/ehjcr/ytae566.
32. Maurizi N, Antiochos P, Muller O, Wuerzner G, Monney P. Accelerated hypertension following mavacamten introduction in severe obstructive hypertrophic cardiomyopathy with hypertension: a case report. Eur Heart J Case Rep. 2024;8(9). https://doi.org/10.1093/ehjcr/ytae450.
33. Escaned J, Lerman LO. Coronary microcirculation and hypertensive heart failure. Eur Heart J. 2020;41(25):2376–8. https://doi.org/10.1093/eurheartj/ehaa437.
34. Sheridan DJ, Kingsbury MP. Mechanisms of reduced coronary reserve in cardiac hypertrophy. In: Sheridan DJ, editor. Left ventricular hypertrophy. 1st ed. London: Churchill Livingstone; 1998. p. 135–43.
35. Foley MJ, Rajkumar CA, Ahmed-Jushuf F, Simader FA, Chotai S, Pathimagaraj RH, et al. Coronary sinus reducer for the treatment of refractory angina (ORBITA-COSMIC): a randomised, placebo-controlled trial. Lancet. 2024;403(10436):1543–53. https://doi.org/10.1016/S0140-6736(24)00256-3.
36. Wlodarczak S, Rola P, Jastrzebski A, Barycki M, Kedzierska M, Korda A, et al. Implantation of a coronary sinus reducer for refractory angina due to coronary microvascular dysfunction. Kardiol Pol. 2024;82(1):103–4. https://doi.org/10.33963/v.kp.98104.

Part III

Chapter 11
Selfish Heart

Abstract The heart metaphorically is the mother of organs. It feeds others first, pumping blood systemically during systole, receiving its own supply later during diastole through left ventricular suction, via peripheral pulse wave reflection, and it extracts every ounce of oxygen akin to feeding on leftovers, hence the altruistic heart. It works hard at generating ever more blood pressure culminating with hypertension, in order to maintain flow for other organs to fulfil their metabolic needs, as they age with rising resistance. The reflected hypertension to the coronary circulation causes hypertensive adaptations and raised microvascular resistance, giving rise to the latter's dysfunction compounded by cardiac hypertrophy and diastolic dysfunction. Now the heart turns selfish; in order to perfuse itself it generates even more blood pressure to the extent of accelerating end-organ damage elsewhere. This vicious cycle ends with heart failure with preserved ejection fraction. In women, as oestrogen wanes with its cardiovascular protection in menopause, their coronary arteries are unobstructed from delayed atherosclerosis; they become rigid with increased vasoreactivity from endothelial dysfunction, giving rise to transmitted coronary hypertension precipitating angina and predispose to Takotsubo syndrome. Thus, this purported natural history of the women's heart; selfless and resilient until it stiffens and breaks.

11.1 Introduction

This is a short chapter to consolidate materials from the last 10 chapters and explore the potential link between transmitted coronary hypertension and cardiac symptomology. Angina with non-obstructive coronary arteries (ANOCA), more often than not, is paired with breathlessness, its twin sibling. "Coronary hypertension" and cardiac ischaemia cause angina and left ventricular (LV) diastolic dysfunction; the latter raises left ventricular end-diastolic pressure (LVEDP) that is conducted through the left atrium (LA) to the pulmonary vasculature, and the stretch of these vessels is felt as breathlessness. LA dilatation is a late feature; hence ANOCA

P. O. Lim, *Coronary Thermodilution*,
https://doi.org/10.1007/978-3-032-10734-3_11

patients usually have a functionally and structurally normal heart, but there is recent interest in LA strain [1].

Diastolic heart failure expresses itself as exercise intolerance, the gold standard used to be a rise in pulmonary wedge pressure during exercise, but this is too invasive for routine practice [2]. Thus, preserved LV ejection fraction ($\geq$ 50%) with cardiac imaging studies coupled with a raised brain natriuretic peptide (BNP) is the current definition for heart failure with preserved ejection fraction (HFpEF) [3, 4]. It makes sense therefore coronary physiology study ideally includes LV study, as illustrated by the case examples below. Table 11.1 charts the key pioneers discussed in previous chapters summarising the milestones.

11.2 Coronary Hypertension

US President Franklin D. Roosevelt died of cerebral haemorrhage from hypertension in 1945, although at the time it was thought to be "essential" for tissue perfusion [5]. It was the Framingham study started in 1948 which identified it as a predictor of mortality [6].

$$\text{Blood pressure} = \text{Cardiac output}\left(\text{Stroke Volume} \times \text{Heart Rate}\right) \\ \times \text{Systemic Vascular Resistance}$$

With rising resistance, pressure needs to also rise to maintain the same flow which could spiral into malignant hypertension as happened to Roosevelt. To break this cycle, resistance needs to be reduced with vasodilators. Hypertension's quintessential haemodynamic footprint is that of a raised systemic vascular resistance. But in a closed system, circulatory volume could be factored in as stroke volume, increasing flow or cardiac output thence BP. It is evident that in experimental and clinical studies that volume loading increases BP, and diuretics reduce BP. Hence volume expansion from dietary salt and its retention from kidney dysfunction or hormonal inhibition causes hypertension in salt-sensitive individuals. In addition, vascular endothelial dysfunction is a precursor of hypertension, by raising resistance [7]. Left untreated, hypertension begets hypertension via increasingly irreversible and elevated resistance [8, 9].

The coronary circulation is part of the systemic vasculature although the arteries predominantly fill during diastole following the dicrotic notch, mostly by suction during the rapid left ventricular filling phase [10]. Further coronary filling is via pulsed wave reflection from the periphery; that is how intra-aortic balloon pump or drug-induced rise in systemic vascular resistance (e.g. metaraminol, noradrenaline, etc) partly works in increasing coronary flow [11]. Therefore, it is shielded from the full force of systolic BP unlike the kidney or the brain. Nevertheless, it is logical to surmise that hypertension transmitted down the coronary artery causes cardiac end-organ damage too, albeit with some gender-specific differences.

Table 11.1 Coronary physiology and pioneers

	Pioneers	Contributions	Implications
1	Andreas Vesalius (1514–1564)	First detailed human anatomy and gave coronary artery its name	Foundation of scientific anatomy
2	Isaac Newton (1643–1727)	Three laws of motion and calculus	Foundation of fluid dynamics and quantitative coronary physiology
3	Stephen Hales (1677–1761)	Applied plant physiology to animals. First to measure invasive arterial BP, calculated cardiac output and demonstrated microvascular resistance. Conformist clergyman (from ages of 32 to 83) of St Mary (with St Alban) church where he is buried, at ferry road in Teddington, TW11 9NN. St George's hospital is a bird's flight of 6.7 miles due east	Inspired **Werner Forssmann** (1904–1979) to self-catheterise his right heart, this won him the Nobel Prize in Medicine or Physiology in 1956. This motivated **F. Mason Sones** (1918–1985) who two years later carried out the first selective coronary angiogram followed by his 1000 patients' series which included his own mother, published in 1966 **Paul H. Wood** (1907–1962) in 1945 started invasive right heart physiology in the UK and lent his name to vascular resistance, R "Wood unit" as per Ohm's hydraulic analogue—mmHg/L/min or P/Q. This has been adapted to coronary physiology, where Q is in mL, thus the coronary Wood unit is 1000 times more than systemic or pulmonary Wood unit, which means coronary resistance is normally x30 times systemic resistance; this is offset by the heart maximally extracting oxygen at rest; thus when there is demand, flow needs to increase
4	Ernest Starling (1866–1927)	Described the preload stretch-contractility principle of the heart, introduced dynamic flow resistance and capillary filtration equation	Foundation of cardiovascular physiology The major principle of heart failure management is to reduce cardiac overstretch—restoring left ventricular pressure-volume dynamics to the left; from plateau to ascending limb of the Frank-Starling curve to the left; that is why end-systolic left ventricular volume is a powerful prognostic sign—a marker of systolic left ventricular filling reserve

(continued)

Table 11.1 (continued)

	Pioneers	Contributions	Implications
5	William Ganz (1919–2009)	Measurement of blood flow with continuous thermodilution in the coronary sinus in 1964. Escaped from the Nazis followed by communist-administered Prague in 1969 with his wife and two sons, one of them, Peter, described endothelial dysfunction with acetylcholine in humans in 1986	This was adapted to coronary thermodilution in 2007 by **Nico H. J. Pijls** and **Bernard de Bruyne**, who in turn were instructed by **K. Lance Gould's** seminal work on the definition of coronary ischaemia in 1974
6	Olaf Oldenburg	**Cardiac ischaemia with vasodilatation in the presence of endothelial dysfunction** In 2001 described the paradox of coronary vasodilatation in 52 patients (37% women, mean age 52, 25–79) with non-obstructive left anterior descending (LAD) artery with IC verapamil 1 mg increasing flow by a mean of 132% (x2.3), associated with a mean negative lactate extraction ratio (LER) of −14.7% across the aorta and coronary sinus—interpreted as *washout* of pre-existing cardiac ischaemic metabolites, but did acknowledge the possibility vasodilatory ischaemia and coronary steal (14 patients had Circumflex artery > 50% stenosis) [63]. In 1996, **Masaaki Takeuchi** using IC papaverine 10 mg in 28 patients (32% women, mean age 52, 29–71), flow in the LAD increased by a mean of 303% (x4.0) and LER –82.2% [64]. Three years before, **Kensuke Egashira** found that in 9 patients (33% women, mean age 50, 32–57) with ANOCA and *endothelial dysfunction* defined by blunted flow response to ACh, IC papaverine 10 mg was associated with mean LER −13.4% vs +14.0% in control; with the same flow increase 366% (x4.7) vs 411% (x5.1), $p = 0.47$ [65]—*normal hyperaemic flow with cardiac ischaemia in the presence of endothelial dysfunction* There is evidence that endothelial dysfunction is associated with increased capillary permeability through disruption of inter-endothelial gap function and glycocalyx degradation [66–69]. Capillary filtration is cleared primarily by lymphatics; interstitial fluid builds up when these are overwhelmed [70–73]	The paradox of increased coronary flow causing cardiac ischaemia can only be explained by microvascular transcapillary fluid dynamics. This **Oldenburg Paradox** gives rise to a framework that *supports current standard practice* with emerging therapies: Improving endothelial function is key, with positive lifestyle changes (diet, obstructive sleep apnoea, smoking and vaping), manage coronary risk factors and drug with pleiotropic effects—statin and renin-angiotensin-aldosterone system inhibitors It predicts lack of efficacy for nitrates and calcium channel blockers, these drugs should be trialled as per guidelines but avoid prolonged drug therapy or excessive dose escalation if angina is not reduced over a set period. Manage diabetes, and hypertension to systolic BP < 130 mmHg as per European Society of Cardiology 2024 guidelines Treat obesity—epicardial adipose tissue causes pericardial constraint and impacts on cardiac lymphatic function [74–78] Sodium–glucose cotransporter 2 inhibitor (SGLT2i). Early evidence that this drug group reduces interstitial oedema [79, 80] Coronary sinus reducer (CSR) which increases venous back pressure to keep the postcapillary venules from collapsing in the subendocardium during diastole [59–61]

Premenopausal women are less likely to develop atherosclerotic coronary artery disease, less prone to arrhythmic sudden cardiac death, but are liable to have spontaneous coronary artery dissection (SCAD) [12–14]. Postmenopausal women on the other hand are predisposed to and predominate in Takotsubo syndrome (TTS), ANOCA and HFpEF [13, 15–18]. All in all, women are less likely to suffer cardiac death until older age compared to men [19]. The common denominator appears to be the direct or pleiotropic effects of oestrogen on the coronary circulation and elsewhere, especially that early or postmenopausal women are inclined to develop vascular endothelial dysfunction [7, 20], as discussed in Chap. 8. Coupled with the resulting stiff vessels and postmenopausal salt sensitivity, the rate of hypertension accelerates with age, and even a small amount of salt loading could precipitate extreme BP rise [21]. Further, the fact that hormone replacement therapy albeit started early delays cardiac events fulfils Koch's postulates regarding the culpability of oestrogen deficiency [22]. Additionally, Eastern countries where diet rich in phyto-oestrogen is consumed appear to have less cardiac death [12].

In older women, an unobstructed artery allows full-force transmission of BP causing coronary hypertension. This leads to increased coronary resistance culminating in coronary microvascular dysfunction (CMD) [23]. Then a vicious cycle is created with the heart raising the BP to perfuse itself spiralling into HFpEF which is highly prevalent in older women. The cardiac origin of hypertension to perfuse itself comes mostly in sympathetic and neurohormonal overdrive with peripheral vasoconstriction and volume retention—through increase in heart rate, stroke volume and contractility [24].

11.3 Definition of Coronary Hypertension

> A pathophysiological state where raised systemic arterial pressure is transmitted as elevated distal coronary pressure into the microvasculature, producing vascular remodelling, and impairing diastolic myocardial function—especially in the absence of epicardial stenosis.

In hypertension, the autoregulatory curve shifts upward and rightward; thus low BP is not well tolerated and coronary flow reduces, and this is demonstrated by animal models of coronary hypertension [25]. This is the reason for cardiogenic shock during an acute myocardial infarction; hypertension is both a risk and a prognostic factor [26]. Aortic banding increases afterload [27], this causes left ventricular hypertrophy (LVH); the reflected BP to the coronary microvasculature induces end-organ damage in the form of interstitial and perivascular fibrosis and inflammation, arteriolar wall thickening and capillary rarefaction [28]—leading to vascular endothelial dysfunction, rise in intrinsic microvascular resistance and LV diastolic dysfunction, and pressure-overload HFpEF [29]. In humans, hypertensive crisis is associated with myocardial interstitial oedema, likely through increased capillary hydrostatic pressure [30].

Surgical correction of coarctation of aorta is time-sensitive; a gradient of 20 mmHg is regarded as significant, and if left untreated, such patients have an average lifespan of 35 years [31]. According to a Mayo Clinic series with a mean follow-up of 17 years, hypertension resolution depended on at what age surgical correction was undertaken; ≤ 5, 60% → 40%, 5–15, 70% → 60%, 15–25, 80% → 75%, and ≥ 25, 90% → 80% [32]. This illustrates the selfish heart principle, even after removal of the aortic obstruction, reducing the afterload; the heart with its "irreversible" end-organ damage with higher intrinsic resistance generates BP at the expense of other organs to perfuse itself, despite its vasodilatory range not being tapped. Resetting the BP with drugs forces the heart to compensate by expending its vasodilatory reserve—hence, normal baseline flow in the setting of elevated coronary resistance is a suggestion that this is happening. Akin to hypercalcaemia with normal parathyroid hormone level which diagnoses primary hyperparathyroidism [33]. Yet, lowering BP in hypertension translates into improved outcome in kidney failure, stroke and even myocardial infarction and heart failure—and the heart simply adapts without increased symptoms. Another example is the hypertensive response during myocardial infarction; the heart's distress call to augment its coronary perfusion via the cardiac afferent sympathetic nerves lead to an immediate neurohormonal activation. The increased cardiac workload is counterproductive, potentially increasing and extending infarction, leading to cardiogenic shock [34–36]. Thus, inadvertently the heart is acting like a self-saboteur.

There are no experimental data of creating isolated coronary hypertension until end-organ damage sets in, and if this would result in the cardiac origin of hypertension. In humans, there is compelling and emerging evidence that the unobstructed coronary arteries in women in later lives with loss of oestrogen buffer predisposes to systemic hypertension. The full force of BP transmission to the coronary microvasculature causes end-organ damage that begets further hypertension. Epidemiological data from the US suggest that half of women become hypertensive by 50 and three quarters are hypertensive over the age of 60, catching up with the men, but premenopausal women are about half as likely as the men to be hypertensive [37]. BP is generated by the heart; it is its "choice" to generate more pressure than is needed by other organs to the extent of causing damage to them. Synonymously, a "primary" cardiomyopathy without systolic dysfunction, but with high prevalence of CMD such as hypertrophic cardiomyopathy (HCM, Chap. 1—Fig. 1.2), is associated with hypertension which accelerates microvascular remodelling, compounds morbidity, and confers adverse prognosis at a younger age [81]. This merits further investigation, although by definition BP control does not reduce left ventricular hypertrophy, if the level of BP control improves outcome in those under the age of 50. Below are two illustrative cases of women with ANOCA and hypertension.

11.4 Cases

11.4.1 Why Does Verapamil Attenuate Flow Increase with Acetylcholine?

A 67-year-old Caucasian woman was referred to the Coronary Physiology Clinic for a ten year history of chest pain that caused her to retire early. She has had extensive gastrointestinal and cardiac investigations, settling with the diagnosis of "microvascular angina" on a background of hypertension, and was recently diagnosed with Sjogren's dry eyes. Her perfusion CMR 2.5 years ago revealed a normal heart without LA dilatation, LVH, scar, infarct or fibrosis, with adenosine stress in which her heart rate rose from 60 to 90 bpm and associated splenic "switch off" to signify hyperaemia; she had chest pain and was found to have a *subtle mid-circumferential subendocardial perfusion defect*, thus reinforcing her cardiac cause for her symptom. Her BMI then was 29 kg/m^2, volume-derived ventriculo-arterial coupling (VAC) of 0.46 (0.6–1.0), and EF 68%. However, despite good control of her BP with candesartan 8 mg od, indapamide 1.5 mg od and a combination of adizem XL 300 mg and SR 90 mg daily, in addition to deponit (GTN) 5 mg per day transdermal patch, phyllocontin 200 mg bd, simvastatin 20 mg and estradot patches 25 μg x2/week, she continued to be symptomatic. Dropping her diltiazem SR 90 mg evening dose did not exacerbate her chest pain. She also has *migraine with aura* and GTN-induced headaches; thus she avoided using it, although response to GTN for her chest pain was variable.

Her perfusion CMR seven years before and another twelve years earlier were normal, but hinted at a dilated LA 23 (< 20) cm^2 and corrected 13 (< 10) cm^2/m^2) in the middle scan, VAC 0.62. Her echocardiogram eight years ago was normal, another performed ten years ago found a mildly dilated LA with incomplete systolic anterior movement of the mitral leaflet.

Procedure The LV is studied (Fig. 11.1); LV angiogram shows normal contractility, EF > 65%, central aortic BP 155/78 mmHg and LVEDP 20–25 mmHg. With the pressure wire in the LV, she is given dobutamine (ug/kg/min) at an escalating dose; rest, 5, 10, 20, and **20 plus atropine** 300 μg; the corresponding LVEDP (mmHg): 15, 13, 11, 10 and **15**; dP/dt, max (> 1200 mmHg/s): 2014, ↑3%, ↑23%, ↑140%, and **↑165%**; min (< −1100 mmHg/s): −1899, ↓−7%, ↓−21%, ↓−34% and **↓− 54%;** and Weiss Tau, τ (< 0.05 s) are: 0.04, 0.04, 0.04, 0.03 and **0.03**. At peak dose, HR 92 to 128 (84% of maximal age-predicted HR) bpm and BP 158 to177 mmHg. Pullback of the pressure wire from the LV apex, through the LV outflow and into the aorta, shows no intra LV gradient.

Her diagnostic coronary angiogram reveals no significant epicardial coronary artery disease (Fig. 11.2). The pressure wire is advanced down the left anterior descending (LAD) artery; the distal-to-aortic pressure ratio (Pd/Pa) is 0.95, and resting full-cycle ratio (RFR), 0.92 (> 0.89). Basal and hyperaemic indices with saline flow rate of 10 and 20 mL/min with the RayFlow microcatheter; flow, Q 92, **94**, 220 and **229** mL/min and resistance, R 1248, **1400**, 501 and **494** Wood units. Using the

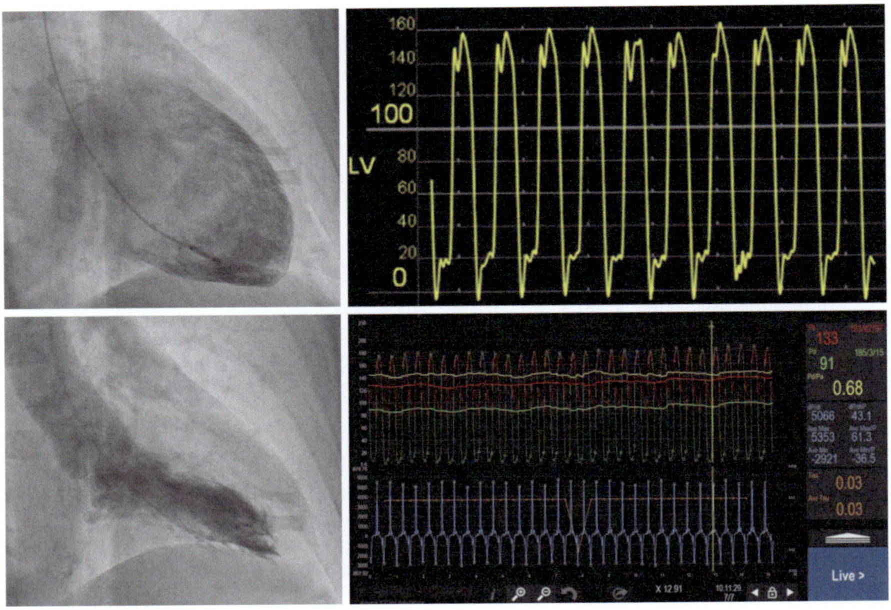

Fig. 11.1 (**Left, top and bottom panels**) The LV angiogram shows normal LV hypercontractility, EF > 65%. (**Right, top and bottom panels**) LV pressure tracing shows raised LVEDP and a systolic impulse gradient or "first" peak, followed by a slow systolic rise reaching 160 mmHg suggesting increased systemic vascular resistance, consistent with chronic hypertension, which through the Anrep effect opposes LV emptying and increases LVEDP, leveraging the "fibre-stretch" end-systolic" LV reserve, the reserve of preload-dependent Frank-Starling mechanism. Dobutamine stress is tolerated with increased systolic contractility and diastolic relaxation, without rising Weiss Tau, τ (< 0.05)

duplicates; coronary flow reserve (CFR) is 2.4, microvascular resistance reserve (MRR), 2.8 and estimated index of microvascular resistance (IMR), 25 (494/20).

Coronary haemodynamics are obtained with acetylcholine (ACh) 2, 20, 100 and 200 μg with increasing doses, as change from baseline: Q 0.83, 1.03, 0.98, and 1.43; and R 0.99, 0.80, 0.81 and 0.58. Initial fall with ACh 2 μg, flat response to ACh 20 and 100 μg, followed by ↑43 (< 50) % increase. There are no ECG changes, nor chest pain provoked, but dose-dependent moderate diffuse distal angiographic epicardial vasospasm. Verapamil 1 mg increases Q by ↑48%, and R falls by ↓54%. When rechallenged with ACh 200 μg the flow is unchanged from baseline; Q 4% and R 24%.

Her contemporaneous NT-ProBNP is elevated at 149 (< 125) pg/mL.

Interpretation This woman has unobstructed coronary arteries, preserved microvascular vasodilatory capacity, but *central aortic hypertension* with *raised LVEDP* and increased *coronary resistance*. Thus, HFpEF. In addition, she exhibited reduced flow with low-dose ACh, reducing distal vessel calibre, and flat response to high ACh doses quintessential of *generalised endothelial dysfunction*, verapamil modestly increased flow but negated the raised flow with high ACh dose. In other words,

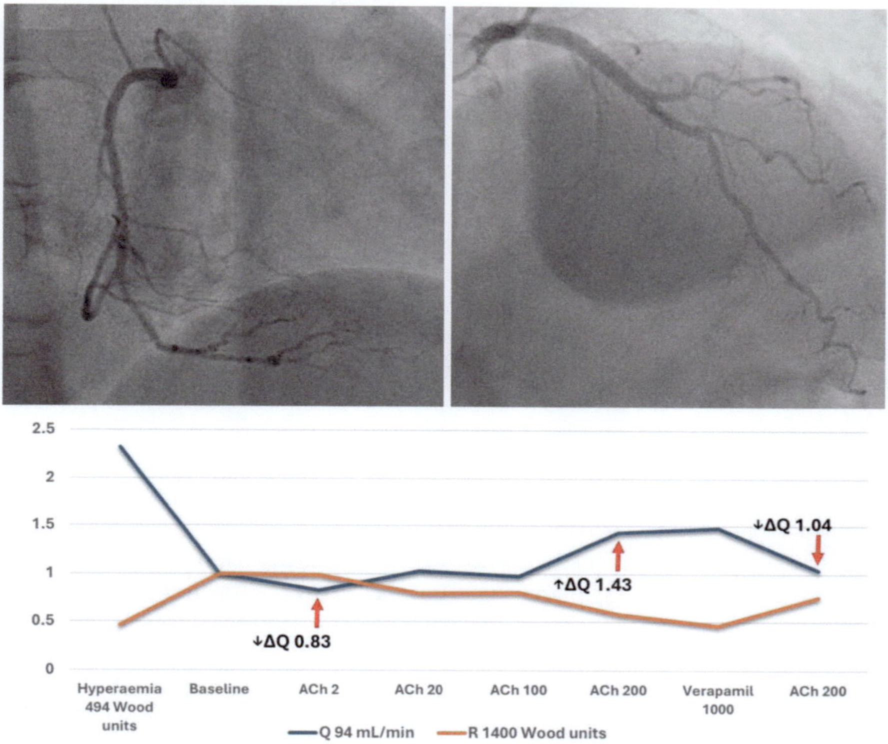

Fig. 11.2 (**Top, left and right panels**) Unobstructed co-dominant right coronary artery and a superselective left anterior descending (LAD) artery. (**Bottom panel**) Changes in flow and resistance in response to saline hyperaemia and to acetylcholine (ACh), verapamil and ACh rechallenge. There is intact vasodilatory reserve, fall in flow with low-dose ACh 2 µg which could be due to a reduction in LAD calibre, followed by either preserved or increased flow with microvascular endothelial function, albeit blunted (< 50%), which is abolished by verapamil pre-treatment, i.e. verapamil paradoxically worsens endothelial function

verapamil reduced microvascular response to ACh or negatively potentiated ACh, *despite preventing epicardial vasospasm theoretically microvascular vasospasm too,* thus the rechallenge with ACh-induced no epicardial vasospasm, yet the flow fell. The sequence was:

1. **ACh 200 µg Q↑43%**
2. **Verapamil 1 mg Q↑48%**
3. **ACh 200 µg Q↑4% (↓Δ39%)**

Verapamil usually at least doubles the flow (see Table 11.1 - 6), but in this case it was blunted, possibly suggesting that her endothelial vasodilatory pathway has shifted from NO to EDHF which technically is natural calcium channel blockade; her rest flow was within normal range or even slightly augmented at 92/94 mL/min. One potential mechanism was extravascular compression raising microvascular resistance. The sequence for biphasic ACh phenomenon:

1. **Low-dose ACh**
   Epicardial vasospasm in distal LAD → Q↓
2. **Medium-dose ACh**
   More epicardial vasospasm but autoregulation kicks in → Q↓↑
3. **High-dose ACh**
   More epicardial vasospasm but more non-NO pathways are recruited → Q↑↑
4. **Verapamil**
   Q↑ (blunted because of duplicated calcium channel blockade with baseline EDHF activation in the microvasculature)
5. **High-dose ACh rechallenge**
   Without "protective" epicardial vasospasm to impede pressure transmission, aortic pressure was transmitted to the microvasculature in full force that increased capillary hydrostatic pressure; this promoted ACh-induced postcapillary venular filtration, increased interstitial pressure which compressed the venules and in turn raised microvascular resistance → Q↓, if Q↑ this would mean flow diversion from the subendocardium to the epicardium, associated with coronary slow flow phenomenon (CSFP) (Chap. 8 case 3).

Dobutamine stress uncovered the LV contractile and diastolic reserve, without a rise in LVEDP and she was asymptomatic. Thus, her usual chest pain was not elicited during her comprehensive coronary physiology study. However, she has hypertensive heart disease; the raised NT-ProBNP reflected her day-to-day increased LVEDP, and at present she has reserve. Considering that she had a long trial period with high doses of diltiazem and continued to be symptomatic, it was switched to nebivolol, and the focus would be to treat her BP to target and a SGLT2i on reserve [38, 39].

11.4.2 Does a Contrast Agent with Twice the Blood's Viscosity Reflect Actual Flow?

A 68-year-old Chinese woman visiting from Beijing developed angina during a meal which was troponin I negative (< 12 ng/L). Her ECG showed non-specific flat ST/T changes with isolated R alternans in limb lead I (1.4 and 1.1 mV) and transition chest lead in V1 (R = S). Bedside echocardiogram showed mild LVH with septal bulge, dilated LA and mild to moderate aortic regurgitation with preserved LV systolic function. She had a coronary angiogram 18 years previously for chest pain and had been treated for hypertension for 20 years; she was taking amlodipine 5 mg od and olmesartan 20 mg od—her usual BP at home was ≤ 130 mmHg systolic, and she has mild reduction in estimated glomerular filtration rate (eGFR) 71 (≥ 90) mL/min/1.73m^2. Her NT-ProBNP was raised at 324 (< 125) ng/L. Her BMI was 23 kg/m^2.

Procedure Her LV is studied first; the LVEDP is elevated 15–20 mmHg with a central aortic systolic BP of 140 mmHg. LV angiogram reveals a normal EF of 65% with a hint of mid-LV hypokinesia (akin to Takotsubo syndrome, TTS) and an apical "nipple" sign suggesting a pressure-overloaded ventricle, which has been used as a distinguishing feature in separating TTS from anterior myocardial infarction; it is present in nearly a third of apical TTS cases (Fig. 11.3) [40, 41].

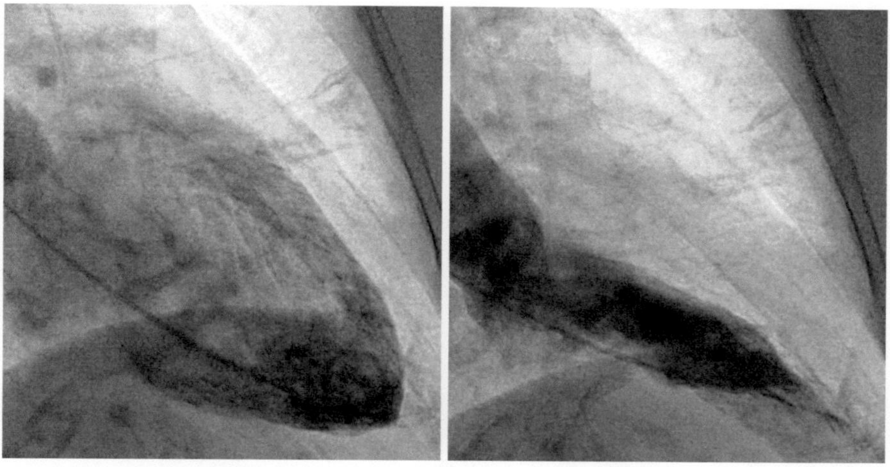

Fig. 11.3 (**Left and right panels**) Left ventricle at end diastole, and at end systole; note subtle mid-left ventricular hypokinesia and the "nipple" sign in the left ventricular apex, suggesting a pressure-loaded ventricle

Her coronary angiogram reveals unobstructed coronary arteries but with generalised CSFP (Fig. 11.4).

With Omnipaque 300 (iohexol, 465 mOsm/kg H_2O at 37 °Celsius) the flow from proximal LAD to apical LAD is 2.33 s, following GTN 200 μg—2.27 s, and with Visipaque 320, 3.27 s. The contrasts are injected with an 8 mL syringe into a 5 French EBU 3.5 guide catheter at a room temperature of 21.6 °Celsius. The corresponding corrected TIMI frame count, CTFC, are 41, 40 and 58 (> 27), respectively [42]. The relative viscosities at room temperature are 11.1 mPa·s and 24.1 mPa·s; thus Visipaque 320 (iodixanol, 290 mOsm/kg H_2O at 37 °Celsius) is 2.2 times more viscid than Omnipaque 300, which means 117% slower based on the Hagen-Poiseuille equation, where flow, $Q \propto 1/\text{viscosity}$:

Omnipaque 300 → 2.33 s
Visipaque 320 → 5.06 s (predicted), actual 3.27 s (1.79 s faster or 35.4% less time than predicted) likely due to rewarming with blood mixing. The discrepancy is corrected when the contrasts are rewarmed during injection from 21.6 → 32 °Celsius (normal blood stream temperature 37 °Celsius). At body temperature, Visipaque 320, which is a non-ionic dimeric (two benzene rings with six iodine atoms) iso-osmolar contrast is 1.89 times more viscid than Omnipaque 300, a non-ionic monomeric (one benzene ring with three iodine atoms) hyper-osmolar (x1.6 plasma osmolality) thus flow 53.5% slower. Omnipaque 300 being hyper-osmolar reduces capillary filtration, drawing interstitial fluid into the vascular compartment—osmotic stress that causes endothelial shrinkage and dysfunction with glycocalyx perturbation, hence more nephrotoxic. On the other hand, Visipaque 320, which is iso-osmolar, exerts shear stress on microvasculature. At a rewarmed temperature of 32 °Celsius it exerts twice the shear stress on the vascular endothelium, activating the vasodilatory mechanisms unless there is pre-existing endothelial dysfunction.

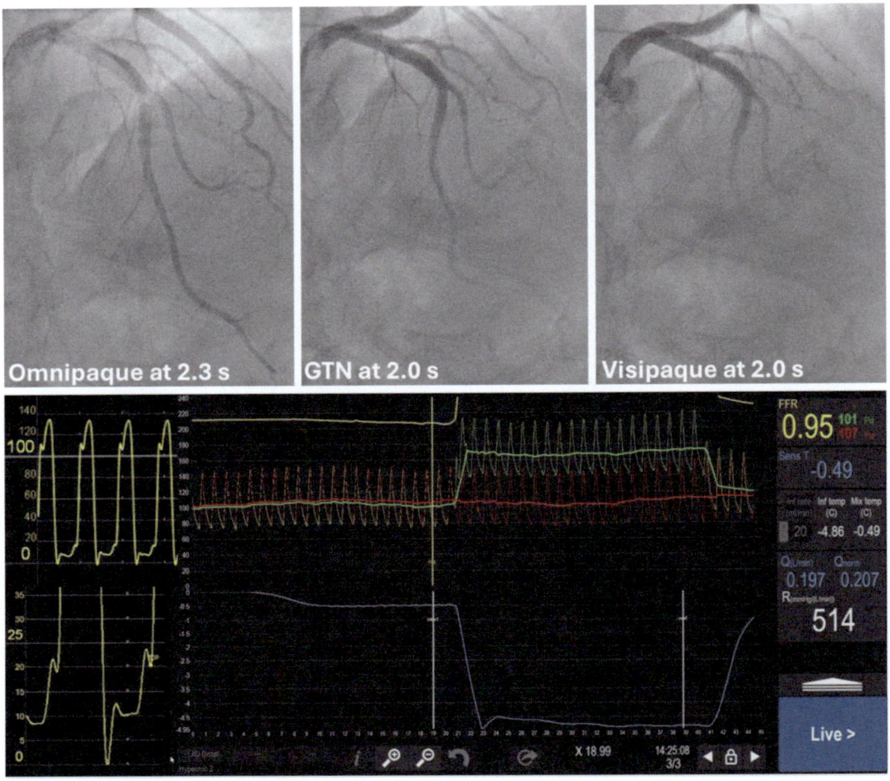

Fig. 11.4 (**Top, left and right panels**) Unobstructed left anterior descending (LAD) artery but coronary slow flow phenomenon (CSFP)—contrast in proximal LAD starts to clear by the time it reaches the LAD apex, with Omnipaque 300 corrected TIMI Frame Count, CTFC 41 (> 27), after GTN 200 μg—40, and with Visipaque 320, 58. (**Bottom, left and right panels**) Elevated LVEDP between 15 and 20 mmHg (*Bottom inset*), with an aortic systolic BP of 140 mmHg—overshoot with gradual rise after a small impulse gradient that opens the aortic valve, suggestive of a raised afterload from high systemic vascular resistance characteristic of chronic hypertension (*Top inset*), and hyperaemic flow of 197 mL/min (vs basal 64 mL/min, CFR 3.1) and raised hyperaemic resistance 514 Wood units

Continuous thermodilution is carried out in the LAD to understand if the CSFP is related to microvascular dysfunction. With the pressure wire in distal LAD, the Pd/Pa is 0.93 and RFR 0.91 (> 0.89). Hyperaemic flow is estimated with saline infusion rate of 20 mL/min in duplicates—197 and 197 mL/min with corresponded resistance of 490 and 514 Wood units. For basal flow, the saline infusion rate is reduced to 10 mL/min; first reading, 64 and second 48 mL/min with corresponding resistance of 1736 and 2269 Wood units. The second reading is obtained when she is restless with a full bladder and her aortic systolic BP rises to 150–160 mmHg. Her CFR is 3.1 and MRR is 3.4, if her hyperaemic minimal resistance is converted to IMR; this will be 26.

Interpretation This woman has unobstructed coronary artery with CSFP and preserved vasodilatory capacity, but raised LVEDP and increased coronary resistance, It is important to note that her Pd/Pa was > 0.9; when she had a BP rise, this rise was transmitted directly to her microvasculature. For example, when her BP rose by 20 mmHg due to stress of holding a full bladder, her coronary resistance rose by 24% and basal flow fell by 25%, illustrating the ever-changing basal state, as noted by Bernard de Bruyne which would significantly impact any threshold ratio such as the CFR. Similar to measuring the office BP, multiple readings are advisable.

The isometric strain of holding her full bladder increased her afterload, raising her end-systolic LV volume, coupled with preload provided the LV stretch to increase her BP (Anrep effect—Chap. 1). Her aortic mean BP was 116 mmHg, and her distal coronary BP was 110 mmHg, with resultant rise in coronary resistance and fall in flow. Her heart was operating at the upper limit of the Frank-Starling curve with her raised LVEDP. In hypertensives such as hers the autoregulatory curve shifts up and right; she was in the downward limb and was unable to mount a flow response at a relatively modest BP rise. Similarly noted in de Bruyne's case of a 78-year-old man with changing basal flow resulting in CFR ranging from 2.2 to 4.3 [43]. Bladder stress changed the CFR in this woman; if her stress basal flow of 48 mL/min was used as resting flow, it exaggerated her CFR to 4.1 (vs 3.1). This masked her underlying hypertensive myocardium but also illustrates the considerable reserve the heart has. Thus, the Gouldian CFR (< 2.0) threshold may not be strictly applicable to microvascular function which is dynamic and ever changing, compared to the fixed epicardial stenosis [44].

Fascinatingly, despite a demonstrably preserved microvascular vasodilatory function, she exhibited CSFP; this was associated with a high coronary resistance. There are enough studies to disprove the link between CSFP and CFR [45–48]. Research on CSFP has shifted focus to raised resting coronary resistance as in this case; yet CSFP is not consistently seen in such patients [49]. As proposed in Chap. 4, (pre-existing and non-acute) CSFP is a rheological artefact due to interaction between the contrast and the vessel wall. In this woman, changing contrast with twice the viscosity from Omnipaque 300 to Visipaque 320 was associated with significantly slower flow as predicted by the Hagen-Poiseuille equation; this suggests, in large part, that CSFP is due to flow rheology in the epicardial coronary artery, likely in the setting of endothelial dysfunction. Although very high LVEDP with extravascular compression potentially could cause a *phasic to-and-fro no reflow* (Chap. 5), and by extension, raised LVEDP would impact contrast flow.

Nevertheless, unprovoked CSFP is mostly due to the transit of contrast in the epicardial coronary artery. This has important implications in the use of contrast as a marker of microvascular function in both the cardiac catheter laboratory and CT angiogram-derived indices, i.e. contrast flow down the coronary artery may not reflect the true blood flow; after all, these are two very different mediums with disparate viscosities. At 32 °Celsius, after mixing at room temperature within the blood stream, Omnipaque 300 flows twice as slow as blood and Visipaque 320, four times as slow. Contrast viscosity is not systematically corrected for in non-invasive coronary imaging.

In summary, this lady has hypertensive HFpEF; the raised LVEDP coupled with elevated NT-ProBNP confirmed the diagnosis, and she was started on nebivolol and a SGLT2i [38, 39].

11.5 Closing Remarks

Isaac Newton's (1643–1727) gravitational laws, based on classical mechanics though put man on the moon in 1969, could not account for the anomalous orbit of Mercury when it comes close to the sun; this was later made predictable by Albert Einstein's (1879–1955) space-time-based general theory of relativity [50]. Similarly, cardiac ischaemia due to reduced flow from epicardial coronary disease fitted well within K. Lance Gould's hyperaemic flow reserve model which is the basis of non-invasive cardiac imaging stress testing techniques. This has been extrapolated to CMD. But there are noted inconsistencies by Attilio Maseri (1935–2021) and Gould himself as to how could angina occur with increased hyperaemic flow, and why would angina linger after any trigger has long passed. Maseri presciently proposed *flow diversion and islands of ischaemia*.

Use of continuous thermodilution has allowed actual flow to be measured, not the pressure-derived flow surrogates that have served fixed coronary artery disease well in guiding coronary revascularisation. The observation of cardiac ischaemia with increased absolute volumetric flow with ACh cannot be explained by the current framework. Looking through the literature, in 2001, Olaf Oldenburg had observed the same phenomenon but dismissed it as a washout effect of verapamil-induced vasodilatation (Table 11.1 - 6). For expediency, this is termed the Oldenburg Paradox, which is the question. The answer is in what exactly happens in the microvasculature; spasm would reduce flow. The *unmasking of microvascular spasm with nitrates* is debated [51–53]. The idea that nitrates, pre-treatment prevent epicardial coronary vasospasm, yet permit, or unmask microvascular spasm, is an implicit acknowledgment that non-nitric oxide (NO) pathways are augmented; yet endothelin antagonism has not transformed into clinical efficacy [54]. This would support the notion that other endothelial mechanisms are at play. Besides NO which is depleted in endothelial dysfunction, ACh endothelial M_3 receptor also activates more of the endothelium-dependent hyperpolarising factor (EDHF) system and to some extent, the prostanoids (Chap. 7). The interesting feature of the EDHF pathway is that it behaves like endogenous calcium channel blockade, which potentially explains the blunted flow response to verapamil in the woman in case 1, especially that adenosine-hyperaemia proves that there is vasodilatory capacity which is not recruited or matched by verapamil; thus NO has shunted to EDHF in the microvasculature.

11.6 Postscript

Nothing is truly new and there is no uncharted territory under the sun, paraphrasing King Solomon (Ecclesiastes 1:9–11). There is usually a precedent, examples from Chap. 1: Bayes' Theorem; Thomas Bayes (1702–1761) preceded Simon Pierre-Simon Laplace (1749–1827); Binary Theorem, which Gottfried W. Leibniz (1646–1716) saw in the Shào Yōng's (1012–1077) Yìjīng. The paradox of *cardiac ischaemia with increased flow* has been noted over thirty years ago with intracoronary papaverine, followed by verapamil (Table 11.1 - 6), but was then explained away as washout of pre-existing ischaemic metabolites or flow diversion via coronary steal with vasodilatation. However, adenosine increases flow yet without coronary sinus lactate overspill; this is because adenosine causes arteriolar and venular dilatation, while papaverine and verapamil preferentially increase arteriolar over venular dilatation, thus increasing capillary hydrostatic pressure and filtration. This is a well-recognised mechanism of calcium channel blockade in causing diuretic-resistant ankle oedema, which can be alleviated with angiotensin-converting enzyme inhibition (ACEi), that is proven efficacious in ANOCA [55, 56]; together with beta blockade and statin they are useful first-line triple therapy for ANOCA, which are also standard regimen for both stable coronary artery disease and acute coronary syndrome. Coincidentally, these therapies counteract the mechanisms by which the selfish heart perfuses itself at the expense of others, and perversely, vasospastic coronary arteries restrict overflow to the microvasculature, removing this with calcium channel blockade and nitrates paradoxical worsen interstitial fluid accumulation, and in the worst case scenario, hypothetically could precipitate Takotsubo syndrome (Chap. 8).

Progress is always about pulling together disparate and seemingly disconnected views with use of a new device. One prime example is recounted in Chap. 1: Rosalind Franklin's (1920–1958) **fine-focus X-ray tube crystallography**, and the formulation of the structure of deoxyribonucleic acid (DNA) by James Watson (1928–2025) and Francis H. C. Crick (1916–2004), which took them just 26 days to finalise in 1953. This was triggered by a key piece of Franklin's data, not photograph 51 of *rehydrated* DNA which clearly showed a helical structure as is popularly believed. DNA as a helical structure was well accepted by then, but molecular packing of *dehydrated* DNA that implied two strands of helices running in opposite directions. DNA's theoretical structure allowing replication was immortalised by Watson and Crick's throwaway remark, "It has not escaped our notice..." in their short Letter to the Editor of *Nature* on 25 April 1953, which was incidentally submitted a mere three weeks before. Their hypothesis was experimentally proven right five years later by Matthew S. Meselson and Franklin W. Stahl at California Institute of Technology, in double Laureate Linus Pauling's (1901–1994) laboratory, whose triple helix DNA hypothesis spurred Crick and Watson into action. Likewise, this book is about absolute volumetric coronary flow with the new technique of **continuous thermodilution**; for the first time quantitative analyses can be carried out in response to ACh with flow changes that track actual physiology. "*Chest pain with* *ischaemic ECG without epicardial spasm in response to ACh*" is the signature diagnosis of *microvascular spasm* restricting flow according to current guidelines [57, 58]. The *Oldenburg Paradox* emerges when such patients are rechallenged following verapamil; prior flow increase with ACh is attenuated.

The likely explanation is postcapillary venular compression from increased filtration with lagging lymphatic clearance of interstitial surge, without the "protective" epicardial vasospastic flow modulation. This potentially explains the efficacy of coronary sinus reducer (CSR) [59–61] in raising coronary venous pressure by about 5 mmHg over the right atrial pressure [62], and keeping the venules open by elevating Starling's "Pressure when Flow is 0" (PF_0), the minimal capillary pressure by which the venules collapse in diastole. Hence, redistributing flow from the subendocardium [59], which is also subject to extravascular compression from high LVEDP in ANOCA and HFpEF.

The writing of this book, the flow of which is inspired by Mark Forsyth's Etymologicon 2011; looking backward for a wider forward horizon, i.e. understanding how ideas evolve over time. Thus, *Oldenburg Paradox* is the question, and the answer is *microvascular transcapillary fluid dynamics*. The resulting series of propositions superficially are coherent, cohesive, congruent, consistent and credible, but will require wider validation. Oldenburg is etymologically "Old Fortress" in Germanic Saxon, perhaps "New Forest", after William the Conqueror's (c. 1028, r. 1066–1087) Nova Foresta enacted in 1079 in today's Hampshire, UK, where this book was first conceived, could be used to describe the black box physiology of coronary microvasculature, *New Forest Conjecture*, a rhetorical companion to *Old Fortress Paradox*.

References

1. O'Neill T, Kang P, Hagendorff A, Tayal B. The clinical applications of left atrial strain: a comprehensive review. Medicina (B Aires). 2024;60(5):693.
2. Lim PO, RJ MF, Clarkson PB, TM MD. Impaired exercise tolerance in hypertensive patients. Ann Intern Med. 1996;124(1 Pt 1):41–55. https://doi.org/10.7326/0003-4819-124-1_part_1-199601010-00008.
3. TA MD, Metra M, Adamo M, Gardner RS, Baumbach A, Böhm M, et al. ESC guidelines for the diagnosis and treatment of acute and chronic heart failure: developed by the task force for the diagnosis and treatment of acute and chronic heart failure of the European Society of Cardiology (ESC) with the special contribution of the heart failure association (HFA) of the ESC. Eur Heart J. 2021;42(36):3599–726. https://doi.org/10.1093/eurheartj/ehab368.
4. Heidenreich PA, Bozkurt B, Aguilar D, Allen LA, Byun JJ, Colvin MM, et al. 2022 AHA/ACC/HFSA guideline for the Management of Heart Failure: a report of the American College of Cardiology/American Heart Association joint committee on clinical practice guidelines. Circulation. 2022;145(18):e895–e1032. https://doi.org/10.1161/cir.0000000000001063.
5. Bruenn HG. Clinical notes on the illness and death of President Franklin D. Roosevelt. Ann Intern Med. 1970;72(4):579–91. https://doi.org/10.7326/0003-4819-72-4-579.
6. Andersson C, Johnson AD, Benjamin EJ, Levy D, Vasan RS. 70-year legacy of the Framingham heart study. Nat Rev Cardiol. 2019;16(11):687–98. https://doi.org/10.1038/s41569-019-0202-5.

7. Rossi R, Chiurlia E, Nuzzo A, Cioni E, Origliani G, Modena MG. Flow-mediated vasodilation and the risk of developing hypertension in healthy postmenopausal women. J Am Coll Cardiol. 2004;44(8):1636–40. https://doi.org/10.1016/j.jacc.2004.07.027.
8. Lim PO, Struthers AD, MacDonald TM. The neurohormonal natural history of essential hypertension: towards primary or tertiary aldosteronism? J Hypertens. 2002;20(1):11–5. https://doi.org/10.1097/00004872-200201000-00003.
9. Lim PO, Tzemos N, Farquharson CA, Anderson JE, Deegan P, MacWalter RS, et al. Reversible hypertension following coeliac disease treatment: the role of moderate hyperhomocysteinaemia and vascular endothelial dysfunction. J Hum Hypertens. 2002;16(6):411–5. https://doi.org/10.1038/sj.jhh.1001404.
10. Davies JE, Whinnett ZI, Francis DP, Manisty CH, Aguado-Sierra J, Willson K, et al. Evidence of a dominant backward-propagating "suction" wave responsible for diastolic coronary filling in humans, attenuated in left ventricular hypertrophy. Circulation. 2006;113(14):1768–78. https://doi.org/10.1161/CIRCULATIONAHA.105.603050.
11. Bellomo R. Noradrenaline: friend or foe? Heart Lung Circ. 2003;12(Suppl 2):S42–8. https://doi.org/10.1046/j.1443-9506.2003.t01-7-.x.
12. Feng XF, Hai JJ, Ma Y, Wang ZQ, Tse HF. Sudden cardiac death in mainland China: a systematic analysis. Circ Arrhythm Electrophysiol. 2018;11(11):e006684. https://doi.org/10.1161/CIRCEP.118.006684.
13. Taqueti VR, Di Carli MF. Coronary microvascular disease pathogenic mechanisms and therapeutic options: JACC state-of-the-art review. J Am Coll Cardiol. 2018;72(21):2625–41. https://doi.org/10.1016/j.jacc.2018.09.042.
14. Yang C, Alfadhel M, Saw J. Spontaneous coronary artery dissection: latest developments and new Frontiers. Curr Atheroscler Rep. 2020;22(9):49. https://doi.org/10.1007/s11883-020-00866-4.
15. Ghadri J-R, Wittstein IS, Prasad A, Sharkey S, Dote K, Akashi YJ, et al. International expert consensus document on Takotsubo syndrome (part I): clinical characteristics, diagnostic criteria, and pathophysiology. Eur Heart J. 2018;39(22):2032–46. https://doi.org/10.1093/eurheartj/ehy076.
16. Ghadri J-R, Wittstein IS, Prasad A, Sharkey S, Dote K, Akashi YJ, et al. International expert consensus document on Takotsubo syndrome (Part II): diagnostic workup, outcome, and management. Eur Heart J. 2018;39(22):2047–62. https://doi.org/10.1093/eurheartj/ehy077.
17. Kaur G, Lau E. Sex differences in heart failure with preserved ejection fraction: from traditional risk factors to sex-specific risk factors. Womens Health (Lond). 2022;18:17455057221140209. https://doi.org/10.1177/17455057221140209.
18. Taqueti VR, Solomon SD, Shah AM, Desai AS, Groarke JD, Osborne MT, et al. Coronary microvascular dysfunction and future risk of heart failure with preserved ejection fraction. Eur Heart J. 2018;39(10):840–9. https://doi.org/10.1093/eurheartj/ehx721.
19. Leening MJ, Ferket BS, Steyerberg EW, Kavousi M, Deckers JW, Nieboer D, et al. Sex differences in lifetime risk and first manifestation of cardiovascular disease: prospective population based cohort study. BMJ. 2014;349:g5992. https://doi.org/10.1136/bmj.g5992.
20. Torbati T, Shufelt C, Wei J, Noel Bairey Merz C. Premature menopause and cardiovascular disease: can we blame estrogen? Eur Heart J. 2022;43(40):4158–60. https://doi.org/10.1093/eurheartj/ehac321.
21. Naschitz JE. Flush hypertension during infusion of saline. QJM. 2015;108(1):63–5. https://doi.org/10.1093/qjmed/hcs097.
22. Cho L, Kaunitz AM, Faubion SS, Hayes SN, Lau ES, Pristera N, et al. Rethinking menopausal hormone therapy: for whom, what, when, and how long? Circulation. 2023;147(7):597–610. https://doi.org/10.1161/CIRCULATIONAHA.122.061559.
23. Zdravkovic M, Popadic V, Klasnja S, Klasnja A, Ivankovic T, Lasica R, et al. Coronary microvascular dysfunction and hypertension: a bond more important than we think. Medicina (B Aires). 2023;59(12):2149.

24. Radakrishnan A, Agrawal S, Singh N, Barbieri A, Shaw LJ, Gulati M, et al. Underpinnings of heart failure with preserved ejection fraction in women - from prevention to improving function. A co-publication with the American journal of preventive cardiology and the journal of cardiac failure. Amer J Prev Cardiol. 2025;23:100928. https://doi.org/10.1016/j.ajpc.2025.100928.
25. Johnson NP, Gould KL, De Bruyne B. Autoregulation of coronary blood supply in response to demand: JACC review topic of the week. J Am Coll Cardiol. 2021;77(18):2335–45. https://doi.org/10.1016/j.jacc.2021.03.293.
26. Desch S, Zeymer U, Akin I, Behnes M, Duerschmied D, Rassaf T, et al. Routine extracorporeal life support in infarct-related cardiogenic shock: 1-year results of the ECLS-SHOCK trial. Eur Heart J. 2024;45(39):4200–3. https://doi.org/10.1093/eurheartj/ehae610.
27. McGoldrick RB, Kingsbury M, Turner MA, Sheridan DJ, Hughes AD. Left ventricular hypertrophy induced by aortic banding impairs relaxation of isolated coronary arteries. Clin Sci. 2007;113(12):473–8. https://doi.org/10.1042/cs20070136.
28. González A, Ravassa S, López B, Moreno MU, Beaumont J, San José G, et al. Myocardial remodeling in hypertension. Hypertension. 2018;72(3):549–58. https://doi.org/10.1161/HYPERTENSIONAHA.118.11125.
29. Miyagi C, Miyamoto T, Kuroda T, Karimov JH, Starling RC, Fukamachi K. Large animal models of heart failure with preserved ejection fraction. Heart Fail Rev. 2022;27(2):595–608. https://doi.org/10.1007/s10741-021-10184-9.
30. Talle MA, Robbertse P-PS, Doubell AF, Lahri S, Herbst PG. Characterizing myocardial edema and fibrosis in hypertensive crisis with cardiovascular magnetic resonance imaging. Sci Rep. 2024;14(1):23509. https://doi.org/10.1038/s41598-024-74099-9.
31. Suradi H, Hijazi ZM. Current management of coarctation of the aorta. Glob Cardiol Sci Pract. 2015;2015(4):44. https://doi.org/10.5339/gcsp.2015.44.
32. Brown ML, Burkhart HM, Connolly HM, Dearani JA, Cetta F, Li Z, et al. Coarctation of the aorta: lifelong surveillance is mandatory following surgical repair. J Am Coll Cardiol. 2013;62(11):1020–5. https://doi.org/10.1016/j.jacc.2013.06.016.
33. National Institute, for H, Care E. Hyperparathyroidism (primary): diagnosis, assessment and initial management. London: NICE; 2019.
34. Grassi G. Reviewer critique of the sympathetic drive after acute myocardial infarction in hypertensive patients. Am J Hypertens. 2006;19(10):1077–8. https://doi.org/10.1016/j.amjhyper.2006.05.002.
35. Hogarth AJ, Mackintosh AF, DASG M. The sympathetic drive after acute myocardial infarction in hypertensive patients. Am J Hypertens. 2006;19(10):1070–6. https://doi.org/10.1016/j.amjhyper.2006.03.015.
36. Longhurst JC, ALSC T, Fu LW. Cardiac sympathetic afferent activation provoked by myocardial ischemia and reperfusion. Mechanisms and reflexes. Ann N Y Acad Sci. 2001;940:74–95. https://doi.org/10.1111/j.1749-6632.2001.tb03668.x.
37. Fryar CD, Ostchega Y, Hales CM, Zhang G, Kruszon-Moran D. Hypertension prevalence and control among adults: United States. NCHS Data Brief. Hyattsville: National Center for Health Statistics; 2015–2018. p. 2020.
38. Anker SD, Butler J, Filippatos G, Ferreira JP, Bocchi E, Böhm M, et al. Empagliflozin in heart failure with a preserved ejection fraction. N Engl J Med. 2021;385(16):1451–61. https://doi.org/10.1056/NEJMoa2107038.
39. Solomon SD, McMurray JJV, Claggett B, Boer RA, DeMets D, Hernandez AF, et al. Dapagliflozin in heart failure with mildly reduced or preserved ejection fraction. N Engl J Med. 2022;387(12):1089–98. https://doi.org/10.1056/NEJMoa2206286.
40. Desmet W, Bennett J, Ferdinande B, De Cock D, Adriaenssens T, Coosemans M, et al. The apical nipple sign: a useful tool for discriminating between anterior infarction and transient left ventricular ballooning syndrome. Eur Heart J Acute Cardiovasc Care. 2014;3(3):264–7.

41. Madias JE. "Nipple" and "hawk's beak" appearances on contrast left ventricular angiography in Takotsubo syndrome: what's in a sign? Int J Cardiol. 2014;173(2):326. https://doi.org/10.1016/j.ijcard.2014.03.053.
42. Gibson CM, Cannon CP, Daley WL, Dodge JT Jr, Alexander B Jr, Marble SJ, et al. TIMI frame count: a quantitative method of assessing coronary artery flow. Circulation. 1996;93(5):879–88. https://doi.org/10.1161/01.cir.93.5.879.
43. Mahendiran T, Wilgenhof A, De Bruyne B. The elusiveness of "rest": the challenges of assessing resting coronary physiology. Circulation. 2025;152(3):147–9. https://doi.org/10.1161/CIRCULATIONAHA.125.074343.
44. Gould KL, Johnson NP. Coronary physiology beyond coronary flow Reserve in Microvascular Angina. JACC. 2018;72(21):2642–62. https://doi.org/10.1016/j.jacc.2018.07.106.
45. Dutta U, Sinha A, Demir OM, Ellis H, Rahman H, Perera D. Coronary slow flow is not diagnostic of microvascular dysfunction in patients with angina and unobstructed coronary arteries. J Am Heart Assoc. 2023;12(1):e027664. https://doi.org/10.1161/JAHA.122.027664.
46. Harkin KL, Loftspring E, Beaty W, Joa A, Serrano-Gomez C, Farid A, et al. Visual estimates of coronary slow flow are not associated with invasive wire-based diagnoses of coronary microvascular dysfunction. Circ Cardiovasc Interv. 2024;17(6):e013902. https://doi.org/10.1161/CIRCINTERVENTIONS.123.013902.
47. Korjian S, Gibson CM. Flowing beyond conventions: rethinking coronary slow flow in the diagnosis of microvascular dysfunction∗. J Am Coll Cardiol Intv. 2024;17(7):930–2. https://doi.org/10.1016/j.jcin.2024.02.006.
48. Mayer M, Allan T, Harkin KL, Loftspring E, Saffari SE, Reynolds HR, et al. Angiographic coronary slow flow is not a valid surrogate for invasively diagnosed coronary microvascular dysfunction. J Am Coll Cardiol Intv. 2024;17(7):920–9. https://doi.org/10.1016/j.jcin.2024.02.025.
49. Zhu Q, Wang S, Huang X, Zhao C, Wang Y, Li X, et al. Understanding the pathogenesis of coronary slow flow: recent advances. Trends Cardiovasc Med. 2024;34(3):137–44. https://doi.org/10.1016/j.tcm.2022.12.001.
50. Janssen M, Rea EM. Einstein–Besso manuscript on the Perihelion motion of mercury sold for record amount. Ann Phys. 2022;534(2):2100563. https://doi.org/10.1002/andp.202100563.
51. Rahman H, Sinha A, Perera D. More is not always better: reassessing acetylcholine provocation in the diagnosis of coronary vasospasm. Circ Cardiovasc Interv. 2025;0(0):e015677. https://doi.org/10.1161/CIRCINTERVENTIONS.125.015677.
52. Rehan R, Wong CCY, Weaver J, Jain P, Adams M, Ng MKC, et al. Impact of nitroglycerin administration on acetylcholine provocation testing in angina with nonobstructive coronary arteries. J Soc Cardiovas Angiograp Interv. 2025:103668. https://doi.org/10.1016/j.jscai.2025.103668.
53. Seitz A, Feenstra R, Konst RE, Martínez Pereyra V, Beck S, Beijk M, et al. Acetylcholine Rechallenge: a first step toward tailored treatment in patients with coronary artery spasm. JACC Cardiovasc Interv. 2022;15(1):65–75. https://doi.org/10.1016/j.jcin.2021.10.003.
54. Morrow A, Young R, Abraham GR, Hoole S, Greenwood JP, Arnold JR, et al. Zibotentan in microvascular angina: a randomized, placebo-controlled, Crossover Trial. Circulation. 2024;150(21):1671–83. https://doi.org/10.1161/circulationaha.124.069901.
55. Turgeon RD, Pearson GJ, Graham MM. Pharmacologic treatment of patients with myocardial ischemia with no obstructive coronary artery disease. Am J Cardiol. 2018;121(7):888–95. https://doi.org/10.1016/j.amjcard.2017.12.025.
56. Vervaat FE, de Vos A, Schenk J, PAL T, Wijnbergen IF. Treatment modalities for angina with non-obstructive coronary arteries (ANOCA): a systematic review and meta-analysis. J Clin Med. 2025;14(12):4069.
57. Godo S, Takahashi J, Shiroto T, Yasuda S, Shimokawa H. Coronary microvascular spasm: clinical presentation and diagnosis. Eur Cardiol Rev. 2023;18:e07.2023. https://doi.org/10.15420/ecr.2022.50.

58. Vrints C, Andreotti F, Koskinas KC, Rossello X, Adamo M, Ainslie J, et al. ESC guidelines for the management of chronic coronary syndromes: developed by the task force for the management of chronic coronary syndromes of the European Society of Cardiology (ESC) endorsed by the European Association for Cardio-Thoracic Surgery (EACTS). Eur Heart J. 2024;45(36):3415–537. https://doi.org/10.1093/eurheartj/ehae177.
59. Cheng K, Alpendurada F, Bucciarelli-Ducci C, Almeida J, Kellman P, Hill JM, et al. Segmental redistribution of myocardial blood flow after coronary sinus reducer implantation demonstrated by quantitative perfusion cardiovascular magnetic resonance. J Cardiovasc Magn Reson. 2025;27(1):101868. https://doi.org/10.1016/j.jocmr.2025.101868.
60. Elshahat A, Husain MA, Elbataa A, Gadelmawla AF, Makhlouf HA, Ibrahim RA, et al. The efficacy and safety of coronary sinus reducer in refractory angina: a systematic review and meta-analysis. BMC Cardiovasc Disord. 2025;25(1):530. https://doi.org/10.1186/s12872-025-04617-8.
61. Foley MJ, Rajkumar CA, Ahmed-Jushuf F, Simader FA, Chotai S, Pathimagaraj RH, et al. Coronary sinus reducer for the treatment of refractory angina (ORBITA-COSMIC): a randomised, placebo-controlled trial. Lancet. 2024;403(10436):1543–53. https://doi.org/10.1016/S0140-6736(24)00256-3.
62. Benedetto D, Abawi M, Stella PR, Nijhoff F, Lakemeier MDM, Kortlandt F, et al. Percutaneous device to narrow the coronary sinus: shifting paradigm in the treatment of refractory angina? A review of the literature. Front Cardiovasc Med. 2016;3 https://doi.org/10.3389/fcvm.2016.00042.
63. Oldenburg O, Eggebrecht H, Gutersohn A, Schaar J, Brauck K, Haude M, et al. Myocardial lactate release after intracoronary verapamil application in humans: acute effects of intracoronary verapamil on systemic and coronary hemodynamics, myocardial metabolism, and norepinephrine levels. Cardiovasc Drugs Ther. 2001;15(1):55–61. https://doi.org/10.1023/A:1011162818809.
64. Takeuchi M, Nohtomi Y, Kuroiwa A. Intracoronary papaverine induced myocardial lactate production in patients with angiographically normal coronary arteries. Catheter Cardiovasc Diagn. 1996;39(2):126–30. https://doi.org/10.1002/(sici)1097-0304(199610)39:2<126::Aid-ccd4>3.0.Co;2-h.
65. Egashira K, Inou T, Hirooka Y, Yamada A, Urabe Y, Takeshita A. Evidence of impaired endothelium-dependent coronary vasodilatation in patients with angina pectoris and Normal coronary angiograms. N Engl J Med. 1993;328(23):1659–64. https://doi.org/10.1056/NEJM199306103282302.
66. Bates DO. Vascular endothelial growth factors and vascular permeability. Cardiovasc Res. 2010;87(2):262–71. https://doi.org/10.1093/cvr/cvq105.
67. Claesson-Welsh L, Dejana E, McDonald DM. Permeability of the endothelial barrier: identifying and reconciling controversies. Trends Mol Med. 2021;27(4):314–31. https://doi.org/10.1016/j.molmed.2020.11.006.
68. Cosson E, Pham I, Valensi P, Pariès J, Attali J-R, Nitenberg A. Impaired Coronary Endothelium–Dependent Vasodilation Is Associated With Microalbuminuria in Patients With Type 2 Diabetes and Angiographically Normal Coronary Arteries. Diabetes Care. 2006;29(1):107–12. https://doi.org/10.2337/diacare.29.01.06.dc05-1422.
69. Reitsma S, Slaaf DW, Vink H, van Zandvoort MA, oude Egbrink MG. The endothelial glycocalyx: composition, functions, and visualization. Pflugers Arch. 2007;454(3):345–59. https://doi.org/10.1007/s00424-007-0212-8.
70. Azhar SH, Lim HY, Tan B-K, Angeli V. The unresolved pathophysiology of lymphedema. Front Physiol. 2020; https://doi.org/10.3389/fphys.2020.00137.
71. Breslin JW. Edema and lymphatic clearance: molecular mechanisms and ongoing challenges. Clin Sci. 2023;137(18):1451–76. https://doi.org/10.1042/cs20220314.
72. Levick JR, Michel CC. Microvascular fluid exchange and the revised Starling principle. Cardiovasc Res. 2010;87(2):198–210. https://doi.org/10.1093/cvr/cvq062.

73. Woodcock TE, Michel CC. Advances in the Starling principle and microvascular fluid exchange; consequences and implications for fluid therapy. Front Vet Sci. 2021;8 https://doi.org/10.3389/fvets.2021.623671.
74. Borlaug BA, Jensen MD, Kitzman DW, Lam CSP, Obokata M, Rider OJ. Obesity and heart failure with preserved ejection fraction: new insights and pathophysiological targets. Cardiovasc Res. 2022;118(18):3434–50. https://doi.org/10.1093/cvr/cvac120.
75. Brakenhielm E, González A, Díez J. Role of cardiac lymphatics in myocardial edema and fibrosis: JACC review topic of the week. J Am Coll Cardiol. 2020;76(6):735–44. https://doi.org/10.1016/j.jacc.2020.05.076.
76. Crum Y, Hoendermis ES, van Veldhuisen DJ, van Woerden G, Lobeek M, Dickinson MG, et al. Epicardial adipose tissue and pericardial constraint in heart failure with preserved ejection fraction. ESC Heart Fail. 2024;11(3):1698–706. https://doi.org/10.1002/ehf2.14739.
77. Kataru RP, Park HJ, Baik JE, Li C, Shin J, Mehrara BJ. Regulation of lymphatic function in obesity. Front Physiol. 2020;11 https://doi.org/10.3389/fphys.2020.00459.
78. Timóteo AT, Barbas Albuquerque F, Lacerda Teixeira B. Pericardium, epicardial adipose tissue, and heart failure with preserved ejection fraction: Pathophysiology, quantification and treatment target1. Int J Cardiol. 2024;412 https://doi.org/10.1016/j.ijcard.2024.132303.
79. Chai K, Luo Y, Zhang M, Liu Y, Li Y, Cheng Y, et al. Effects of empagliflozin on cardiac structure, function and biomarkers in patients with heart failure with preserved ejection fraction: study protocol for a randomised, placebo-controlled prospective trial. BMJ Open. 2023;13(8):e070766. https://doi.org/10.1136/bmjopen-2022-070766.
80. Lam-Chung CE. Comprehensive review of SGLT2 inhibitors' efficacy through their diuretic mode of action in diabetic patients. Front Endocrinol. 2023;14 https://doi.org/10.3389/fendo.2023.1174692.
81. Baibhav B, Wang A. Hypertension and hypertrophic cardiomyopathy. In: Naidu SS, editor. Hypertrophic cardiomyopathy. Cham: Springer; 2025. p. 261–271. https://doi.org/10.1007/978-3-031-99282-7_19.

Abbreviations and Acronyms

AAOCA	Anomalous aortic origin of a coronary artery
ABPM	Ambulatory blood pressure monitoring
ACE	Angiotensin converting enzyme
ACh	Acetylcholine
ACT	Activated clotting time
ACTH	Adrenocorticotropic hormone
ADHD	Attention deficit hyperactivity disorder
AHI	Apnoea–hypopnoea index
AF	Atrial fibrillation
AI	Artificial intelligence
AICD	Automated implantable cardioverter defibrillator
AMH	Anti-Müllerian hormone
AMP	Adenosine diphosphate
ANOCA	Angina with non-obstructive coronaries
AP	Action potential
ARNi	Angiotensin receptor–neprilysin inhibitor
ARVC	Arrhythmogenic right ventricular cardiomyopathy
ATM	Artemether
ATP	Adenosine triphosphate
AUC	Area under the curve
AVN	Atrioventricular node
BAT	Brown adipose tissue
BER	Benign early repolarisation
BMI	Body mass index
BNP	B-type natriuretic peptide
BP	Blood pressure
BRCA	Breast cancer gene
BSA	Body surface area
BT	Bolus thermodilution

P. O. Lim, *Coronary Thermodilution*,
https://doi.org/10.1007/978-3-032-10734-3

CAA	Coronary artery anomalies
CABG	Coronary artery bypass grafting
CBD	Cannabidiol
CFC	Coronary flow capacity
CFI	Collateral flow index
CFR	Coronary flow reserve
CGRP	Calcitonin gene-related peptide
CMD	Coronary microvascular dysfunction
CMR	Cardiovascular magnetic resonance
CPAF	Coronary pulmonary artery fistula
CPAP	Continuous Positive Airway Pressure
CPP	Coronary pulse pressure
CLVA	Congenital LV aneurysm
CO	Cardiac output
COPD	Chronic obstructive pulmonary disease
COVID	Coronavirus disease
CRP	C-Reactive protein
CRT	Cardiac resynchronisation therapy
CRT-D	Cardiac resynchronisation therapy defibrillator
CRT-P	Cardiac resynchronisation therapy pacemaker
CSFP	Coronary slow flow phenomenon
CSR	Coronary sinus reducer
CT	Computer tomography
CTITU	Cardiothoracic intensive care unit
CTCA	CT coronary angiogram
CTFC	Corrected TIMI Frame Count
CTO	Chronic total occlusion
CVP	Central venous pressure
CYP11A1	Cytochrome P450 family 11 subfamily A member 1
Cx	Circumflex artery
DAPT	Dual antiplatelet therapy
DDDR	Dual chamber pacing mode with rate modulation
DES	Drug-eluting stent
dFFR	Diastolic fractional flow reserve
DHA	Dihydroartemisinin
DNA	Deoxyribonucleic acid
DPTI	Diastolic pressure time index
DCB	Drug-coated balloon
DCM	Dilated cardiomyopathy
DC shock	Direct current shock
DOAC	Direct oral anticoagulant
DSE	Dobutamine stress echocardiogram
DVI	Direct ventricular interaction
EAT	Epicardial adipose tissue
ECG	Electrocardiogram

EDHF	Endothelium-derived hyperpolarising factor
EDPVR	End-diastolic pressure-volume relationship
EDV	Left ventricular end-diastolic volume
EF	Ejection fraction
EFV	Epicardial fat volume
ESC	European Society of Cardiology
ESP	Left ventricular end-systolic pressure
ESPVR	End-systolic pressure-volume relationship
ESV(i)	Left ventricular end-systolic volume (index)
ET-1	Endothelin-1
ET-A/ET-B	Endothelin receptor subtypes
FEC	Fluorouracil–Epirubicin–Cyclophosphamide
FFA/NEFA	Free fatty acid/Non-esterified fatty acid
FFR	Fractional flow reserve
FMD	Flow-mediated dilation
FSH	Follicle stimulating hormone
5FU	5-Fluorouracil
GLP-1 RA	Glucagon-like peptide-1 receptor agonist
GMT	Greenwich Mean Time
GTN	Glyceryl trinitrate
HAC	Heart Attack Centre
HER2	Human epidermal growth factor receptor 2
HFpEF	Heart failure with preserved ejection fraction
HFrEF	Heart failure with reduced ejection fraction
HFsnEF	Heart failure with supranormal ejection fraction
HPO axis	Hypothalamic-pituitary-ovarian axis
HR	Heart rate
HRT	Hormone replacement therapy
HVMB	Helical ventricular myocardial band
IABP	Intra-aortic balloon pump
IASD	Interatrial shunt device
IC	Intracoronary
IgE	Immunoglobulin E
ILVAH	Isolated left ventricular apical hypoplasia
IMR	Index of microvascular (originally described as 'microcirculatory') resistance
IP_3	Inositol 1,4,5-trisphosphate
ISR	In-stent restenosis
ITU	Intensive care unit
IUD	Intrauterine device
IV	Intravenous
IVC	Inferior vena cava
IVCD	Intraventricular conduction defect
IVF	In vitro fertilisation
IVPG	Intraventricular pressure gradient

IVUS	Intravascular ultrasound
Kir	Inward-rectifier potassium channels
LA	Left atrium
LAD	Left anterior descending artery
LAS	London Ambulance Service
LBBB	Left bundle branch block
LBBP	Left bundle branch pacing
LER	Lactate extraction ratio
LGE	Late gadolinium enhancement
LH	Luteinising hormone
LIMA	Left internal mammary artery
LSD	Lysergic acid diethylamide
LM	Left main coronary artery
LV	Left ventricle
LVH	Left ventricular hypertrophy
LVEDP	Left ventricular filling pressure
LVMI	Left ventricular mass index
LVOTO	LV outflow tract obstruction
LVSD	Left ventricular systolic dysfunction
MASLD	Metabolic dysfunction–associated steatotic liver disease
MB	Myocardial bridge
MCO	Left ventricular midcavity obstructive
MELOS	Multicentre European Left bundle branch pacing Outcomes Study
MET	Metabolic equivalent of task
MFR	Myocardial flow reserve
MI	Myocardial infarction
MINOCA	Myocardial infarction with non-obstructive coronary arteries
MLA	Minimal luminal area
MPR	Myocardial perfusion reserve
MRC	Medical research council
MRR	Microvascular resistance reserve
MRSA	Methicillin-resistant *Staphylococcus aureus*
MVO	Microvascular obstruction
nAChR	Nicotinic acetylcholine receptor
NAFLD	Non-alcoholic fatty liver disease
NYHA	New York Heart Association
NO	Nitric oxide
NT-ProBNP	N-terminal pro B-type natriuretic peptide
OCT	Optical coherence tomography
ODI	Oxygen desaturation index
OSA	Obstructive sleep apnoea
PA	Pulmonary artery
PCAT	Pericoronary adipose tissue
PCI	Percutaneous coronary intervention

PCOS	Polycystic ovary syndrome
PCSK9	Proprotein convertase subtilisin/kexin type 9
PCWP	Pulmonary capillary wedge pressure
PDA	Posterior descending artery
Pd/Pa	Distal coronary to aortic pressure ratio
PEA	Pulseless electrical activity
PET	Positron emission tomography
PF_0	Pressure at which Flow is 0
PFO	Patent foramen ovale
PGI_2	Prostacyclin
PKA	Protein kinase A
PKP2	Plakophilin-2
PM	Permanent pacemaker
POS	Platypnea–orthodeoxia syndrome
PSI	Pressure per square inch
Pv	Venous pressure
PV loop	Pressure-volume loop
Pw	Wedge pressure
PWV	Pulse wave velocity
Q	Flow
RA(P)	Right atrial (pressure)
RCA	Right coronary artery
RCT	Randomised controlled trials
REM	Rapid eye movement
RFR	Rest full-cycle ratio
RH	Relative humidity
Rμ	Minimal coronary resistance
RNA	Ribonucleic acid
ROS	Reactive oxygen species
RPDA	Right posterior descending artery
RPP	Rate–pressure product
RV	Right ventricle
RVOT	Right ventricular outflow tract
RyR	Ryanodine receptors
S-AICD	Subcutaneous automated implantable cardioverter defibrillator
SCAD	Spontaneous coronary artery dissection
SEI	Subendocardial ischaemia
SGLT2i	Sodium–glucose cotransporter-2 inhibitor
SHBG	Sex hormone binding globulin
SNDRI	Serotonin–norepinephrine–dopamine reuptake inhibitor
SPTI	Systolic pressure time index
STEMI	ST-elevation myocardial infarction
SV(i)	Stroke volume (index)
SVR	Systemic vascular resistance
τ (Tau)	Time constant of LV relaxation (used in diastolic function analysis)

TCT	Transcatheter Cardiovascular Therapeutics. An annual scientific meeting organised by the Cardiovascular Research Foundation focusing on interventional cardiology in the US
TdP	Torsades de Pointes
TFC	TIMI frame count
TGF-β	Transforming growth factor beta
THC	Δ9-tetrahydrocannabinol
TIMI	Thrombolysis in Myocardial Infarction
Tmn	Mean transit time
TNF-α	Tumour necrosis factor alpha
TRPA-1	Transient receptor potential ankyrin 1
TRPV1	Transient receptor potential vanilloid 1
TSH	Thyroid stimulating hormone
TTS	Takotsubo syndrome
UCL	University College London
VAC	Ventriculo-arterial coupling
VF	Ventricular fibrillation
VO_2	Oxygen consumption
VSMC	Vascular smooth muscle cell
VTA	Ventral tegmental area
WHO	World Health Organization

Studies

CADILLAC
Controlled Abciximab and Device Investigation to Lower Late Angioplasty Complications Trial. Stone GW, Grines CL, Cox DA, Garcia E, Tcheng JE, Griffin JJ, et al. Comparison of Angioplasty with Stenting, with or without Abciximab, in Acute Myocardial Infarction. New England Journal of Medicine. 2002;346(13):957–66. https://doi.org/10.1056/NEJMoa013404.

CorMicA
Coronary Microvascular Angina Trial. Ford TJ, Stanley B, Good R, Rocchiccioli P, McEntegart M, Watkins S, et al. Stratified Medical Therapy Using Invasive Coronary Function Testing in Angina. JACC. 2018;72(23_Part_A):2841–55. https://doi.org/10.1016/j.jacc.2018.09.006.

EDIT-CMD
Efficacy of Diltiazem to Improve Coronary Vasomotor Dysfunction in ANOCA Trial. Jansen Tijn PJ, Konst Regina E, de Vos A, Paradies V, Teerenstra S, van den Oord Stijn CH, et al. Efficacy of Diltiazem to Improve Coronary Vasomotor Dysfunction in ANOCA. JACC: Cardiovascular Imaging. 2022;15(8):1473–84. https://doi.org/10.1016/j.jcmg.2022.03.012.

ENCORE
Evaluation of Nifedipine and Cerivastatin On Recovery of coronary Endothelial function Trial. Effect of nifedipine and cerivastatin on coronary endothelial function in patients with coronary artery disease: the ENCORE I Study (Evaluation of Nifedipine and Cerivastatin On Recovery of coronary Endothelial function). Circulation. 2003;107(3):422–8. https://doi.org/10.1161/01.cir.0000046488.52939.bf.

FAME 2
Fractional Flow Reserve versus Angiography for Multivessel Evaluation 2. Bruyne BD, Fearon WF, Pijls NHJ, Barbato E, Tonino P, Piroth Z, et al. Fractional Flow

P. O. Lim, *Coronary Thermodilution*,
https://doi.org/10.1007/978-3-032-10734-3

Reserve–Guided PCI for Stable Coronary Artery Disease. New England Journal of Medicine. 2014;371(13):1208–17. https://doi.org/10.1056/NEJMoa1408758.

IDEAL [Iberian-Dutch-English] Collaborators Study

Cook CM, Jeremias A, Petraco R, Sen S, Nijjer S, Shun-Shin MJ, et al. Fractional Flow Reserve/Instantaneous Wave-Free Ratio Discordance in Angiographically Intermediate Coronary Stenoses: An Analysis Using Doppler-Derived Coronary Flow Measurements. JACC: Cardiovascular Interventions. 2017;10(24):2514–24. https://doi.org/10.1016/j.jcin.2017.09.021.

ILIAS Registry

Inclusive Invasive Physiological Assessment in Angina Syndromes. van de Hoef TP, Lee JM, Boerhout CKM, de Waard GA, Jung J-H, Lee SH, et al. Combined Assessment of FFR and CFR for Decision Making in Coronary Revascularization: From the Multicenter International ILIAS Registry. JACC: Cardiovascular Interventions. 2022;15(10):1047–56. https://doi.org/10.1016/j.jcin.2022.03.016.

ORBITA 1

Objective Randomised Blinded Investigation With Optimal Medical Therapy of Angioplasty in Stable Angina trial. Al-Lamee R, Thompson D, Dehbi HM, Sen S, Tang K, Davies J, et al. Percutaneous coronary intervention in stable angina (ORBITA): a double-blind, randomised controlled trial. Lancet. 2018;391(10115):31–40. https://doi.org/10.1016/s0140-6736(17)32714-9.

Index

P. O. Lim, *Coronary Thermodilution*,
https://doi.org/10.1007/978-3-032-10734-3

MIX
Papier aus verantwortungsvollen Quellen
Paper from responsible sources
FSC® C105338

If you have any concerns about our products,
you can contact us on
ProductSafety@springernature.com

In case Publisher is established outside the EU,
the EU authorized representative is:
Springer Nature Customer Service Center GmbH
Europaplatz 3, 69115 Heidelberg, Germany

Printed by Libri Plureos GmbH
in Hamburg, Germany